Wellness

GUIDELINES FOR A HEALTHY LIFESTYLE

Wellness

FOURTH EDITION

GUIDELINES FOR A HEALTHY LIFESTYLE

Werner W.K. Hoeger
Boise State University

Lori W. Turner
University of Arkansas

Brent Q. Hafen
Brigham Young University

THOMSON

WADSWORTH

Australia • Brazil • Canada • Mexico • Singapore • Spain
United Kingdom • United States

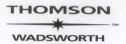

Wellness: Guidelines for a Healthy Lifestyle, Fourth Edition
Werner W.K. Hoeger | Lori W. Turner | Brent Q. Hafen

Executive Editor: Nedah Rose

Assistant Editor: Colin Blake

Editorial Assistant: Kate Franco

Technology Project Manager: Ericka Yeoman-Saler

Marketing Manager: Jennifer Somerville

Marketing Assistant: Catie Ronquillo

Marketing Communications Manager: Jessica Perry

Project Manager, Editorial Production: Sandra Craig

Creative Director: Rob Hugel

Art Director: Lee Friedman

Print Buyer: Doreen Suruki

Permissions Editor: Joohee Lee

Production, Illustration, Composition:
Ash Street Typecrafters, Inc.

Text and Cover Design: Ellen Pettengell Design

Photo Research: Norman Baugher

Copy Editor: Carolyn Acheson

Cover Image: John Terence Turner/Getty Images

Printer: Courier Corporation/Kendallville

ExamView® and ExamView Pro® are registered trademarks of FSCreations, Inc. Windows is a registered trademark of the Microsoft Corporation used herein under license. Macintosh and Power Macintosh are registered trademarks of Apple Computer, Inc. Used herein under license.

Library of Congress Control Number: 2006905206

ISBN 0-495-11112-0

Thomson Higher Education
10 Davis Drive
Belmont, CA 94002-3098
USA

For more information about our products, contact us at:
Thomson Learning Academic Resource Center
1-800-423-0563

For permission to use material from this text or product, submit a request online at **http://www.thomsonrights.com.**
Any additional questions about permissions can be submitted by e-mail to **thomsonrights@thomson.com.**

This book is dedicated to

Joanne Saliger for her

unconditional commitment

and dedication to my books

during the last 21 years.

WERNER

Brief Contents

Contents

© George Doyle/Stockbyte Platinum/Getty Images

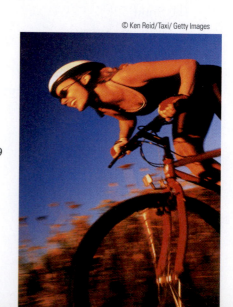

© Ken Reid/Taxi/ Getty Images

© Eric Glenn/DK Stock/Getty Images

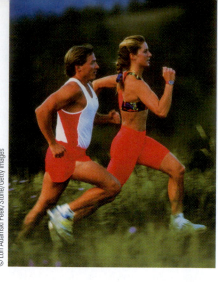

© Kate Powers/Taxi/Getty Images

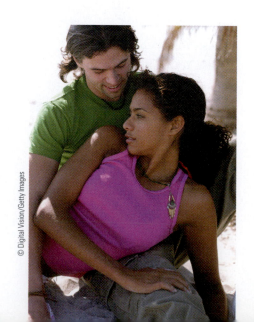

© Digital Vision/Getty Images

Preface

THE responsibility for enhancing health and wellness and developing a healthy lifestyle rests primarily with the individual. According to research literature, improving health, fitness, quality of life, longevity, happiness, and wellness is a matter of personal choice. The purpose of *Wellness: Guidelines for a Healthy Lifestyle* is not only to increase readers' understanding about health and wellness but also to help assess personal attitudes and behavior and, where necessary, to make appropriate changes. This book places a strong emphasis on fitness and nutrition, because the scientific evidence has shown clearly that one of the most effective ways to enhance wellness and longevity is to increase one's level of physical activity and fitness, and to adhere to a healthy diet. Self-responsibility is emphasized throughout the book, with the realization that enhancing wellness requires personal decision making and realistic goal setting, with positive and optimistic follow through.

Contemporary knowledge and ethical considerations suggest a broad approach to health behavior, involving the physical, social, emotional, mental, environmental, occupational, and spiritual natures and consequences. Our book explains, with support from the scientific literature, how each dimension contributes to wellness. In the pages that follow, you will learn what the research literature has to say about traditional wellness-related topics, as well as what we know about how emotions impact health and wellness. What is written here will help you appreciate what we know about the mind/body connection and the tremendous healing power of your mind.

Changes to the Fourth Edition

- **Chapter 1.** New contents in the opening chapter include an update about the underlying causes of death in the United States; current physical activity recommendations for health, weight gain prevention, and weight regain; the use of pedometers to monitor daily physical activity; and an expanded discussion on environmental influences on human behavior. All statistics related to this chapter have also been brought up to date.

- **Chapter 2.** The contents related to the mind-body connection and the implications for health and wellness have been updated according to recent advances in this field.

- **Chapter 3.** An expanded discussion on the impact of daily stressors and adequate coping strategies, as well as information on the post traumatic stress syndrome and hurricane Katrina, are provided in the chapter.

- **Chapter 4.** The section on the benefits of community involvement on health and wellness has been enhanced in this fourth edition.

- **Chapter 5.** The chapter has been reorganized to improve the flow of information and also contains a more inclusive approach regarding diverse religions.

- **Chapter 6.** Considerable changes were made to the Fitness Assessment for Wellness chapter, including a more extensive discussion on the definitions of physical fitness, health-related and skill-related fitness, and physiological fitness. The concept of responders and nonresponders, the benefits of pedometers to monitor daily physical activity, and the relevance of physical fitness assessments have been added to the chapter. A new Assessment to monitor daily physical activity was also added to the chapter.

- **Chapter 7.** The contents of the cardiorespiratory endurance, muscular strength, and muscular endurance guidelines for exercise prescription have been completely revised to conform with the newly released American College of Sports Medicine (ACSM) Guidelines for Exercise Testing and Prescription (2006). The importance of using a pedometer to quantify and increase daily physical activity to enhance health and quality of life is emphasized. Provided also are behavior modification techniques to pursue this goal.

- **Chapter 8.** The nutrition chapter includes updates on current dietary recommendations for healthy eating and a discussion and figure on MyPyramid guidelines. New to this chapter are tables on estimated caloric needs for adults and recommended amounts from each food group. A new figure with photos on the size of fast food portion today as compared to a few years ago is provided.

- **Chapter 9.** New to the Body Composition Assessment chapter are an introduction to the air displacement technique to assess body composition, updates on the role of body mass index (BMI) as the most widely used technique to determine overweight and obesity in the general population, the Waist Circumference (WC) technique to help identify individuals with high abdominal visceral fat, and the importance of BMI in combination with WC to identify individuals who are at increased risk for disease. The chapter Assessment was also revised to conform with updated standards for BMI and WC.

- **Chapter 10.** Changes to the Weight Management, Eating Disorders, and Wellness chapter include an update on the health consequences of being overweight or obese; information on low-carbohydrate/high protein diets; the binge-eating disorder; learning to make healthy food choices; the benefits of dietary calcium on weight management; the relationship between strength training, diet, and muscle mass; and the estimated energy requirement equations (EER) to determine daily caloric intake by the DRI committee of the Institute of Medicine of the National Academy of Sciences. Several behavior modification boxes to clarify misconceptions and help students make healthy-lifestyle decisions were also added throughout the chapter. A new Assessment: Healthy Dietary Plan for Weight Maintenance or Weight Gain, is also included.
- **Chapter 11.** Statistical updates on the prevalence of cardiovascular disease are provided in this chapter. Revisions were made to many of the coronary heart disease risk factors and the dietary guidelines to lower LDL-cholesterol. New information is provided on inflammation and C-reactive protein, the A1c test to screen for diabetes risk, and the metabolic syndrome condition.
- **Chapter 12.** Changes in this chapter include updates on the prevalence and number of deaths related to different cancer sites, risk factors for various cancer sites, and cancer prevention guidelines. A new Assessment: Cancer Prevention: Are You Taking Control? is also provided.
- **Chapter 13.** Information on addictive behavior and wellness has been revised and updated based on current data reported in this area.
- **Chapter 14 .** This chapter includes an enhanced discussion about communication regarding aspects of sexual involvement and sexually transmitted infections.

Ancillaries

- **Instructor's Manual with Test Bank.** The Instructor's Manual with Test Bank helps instructors plan and coordinate their lectures by offering detailed outlines of each chapter with specific transparency and Power-Point references. Instructor's Activities are included for each chapter. These activities offer instructors ideas for incorporating the material into classroom activities and discussions. A set of Key Point Transparencies is provided. A full test bank containing approximately 30 questions per chapter is also provided.

- **Transparencies.** Approximately 80 color transparency acetates of graphs, tables, and illustrations from the text can be used to enhance lectures. The transparencies will also be available on the Web and on a CD-ROM. Also provided is a set of Key Point Transparencies—text-only transparencies that list important terms from each chapter.

- **ThomsonNOW™.** Class-tested and student-praised, **ThomsonNOW™** for Health offers a variety of features that support course objectives and interactive learning. This online tutorial and self-assessment program for students offers a **Personalized Behavior Change Plan,** pre- and post-tests, a wellness journal, and a variety of activities all designed to get students involved in their learning progress and to be better prepared for class participation, class quizzes, and tests. Students log on to **ThomsonNOW™** by using the access code available with this text.

- **Diet Analysis+ 8.0 Online and Win/Mac CD-ROM.** This market-leading diet assessment program allows students to create their own personal profiles based on height, weight, age, sex, and activity level. Its dynamic interface makes it easy for students to track the types and serving sizes of the foods they consume, from one day to 365 days! Now including even more exciting features, the updated 8.0 version includes an 18,000+ food database, a 500+ activity database, ten reports for analysis (including MyPyramid), the ability to print single- and multiple-day reports, a food recipe feature, the latest Dietary References, and goals and actual percentages of essential nutrients, vitamins, and minerals. Students can use this information to adjust their diet and gain a better understanding of how nutrition relates to their personal health goals.

- **ExamView®—Computerized Testing.** Create, deliver, and customize tests and study guides (both print and online) in minutes with this easy-to-use assessment and tutorial system. ExamView offers both a Quick Test Wizard and an Online Test Wizard that guide you step-by-step through the process of creating tests, while its unique "WYSIWYG" capability allows you to see the test you are creating on the screen exactly as it will print or display online.

- **Multimedia Manager for** *Wellness: Guidelines for a Healthy Lifestyle.* This link tool includes a wide array of lecture-specific PowerPoint slides, images from the Hoeger texts, digitized ABC video clips, an electronic instructor's manual and an electronic test bank.

- **ABC Videos for Health and Wellness**. These videos allow you to integrate the news-gathering and programming power of the ABC News networks into the classroom to show students the relevance of course topics to their everyday lives. The videos include news clips correlated directly with the text and can help you launch a lecture, spark a discussion, or demonstrate an application. Students can see firsthand how the principles they learn in the course apply to the stories they hear in the news.

- **Relaxation Video.** Explores techniques to decrease vulnerability to stress, enhance sports performance, and manage time more effectively.
- **Wadsworth Video Library for Fitness, Wellness, and Personal Health.** A comprehensive library of videos is available to adopters of this textbook. Topics include weight control and fitness, AIDS, sexual communication, peer pressure, compulsive and addictive behaviors and the relationship between alcohol and violence. Contact your local Thomson representative for a detailed list of video options.
- **Wellness Worksheets.** Forty detachable self-assessments and a complete wellness inventory are included.
- **Trigger Video Series.** Exclusive to Thomson Wadsworth! This video is designed to promote classroom discussion on a variety of important topics related to physical fitness and stress. Each 60-minute video contains five 8–10 minute clips, followed by questions for answer or discussion and material appropriate to the chapters in this text.
- **InfoTrac® College Edition.** This extensive online library gives professors and students access to the latest news and research articles online—updated daily and spanning four years! Conveniently accessible from students' own computers or the campus library, InfoTrac® College Edition opens the door to the full text of articles from hundreds of scholarly and popular journals and publications.
- **The Wadsworth Health & Wellness Resource Center Web Site:**

  www.thomsonedu.com/health

  When you adopt *Wellness: Guidelines for a Healthy Lifestyle*, you and your students will have access to a rich array of teaching and learning resources you won't find anywhere else. This outstanding site features both student and instructor resources for this text, including self-quizzes, Web links, suggested online readings, and discussion forums for students— as well as downloadable supplementary resources, PowerPoint® presentations, and more for instructors.

Acknowledgments

We wish to thank the reviewers, whose valuable comments helped us improve this and previous editions:

Diana Avans, Sam Houston State University
Carol Biddington, California University of Pennsylvania
John Buckholtz, Rochester Institute of Technology
Lenda B. Dillard, Macon State College
Terri Edwards, Bacone College
Robert Emery, Plattsburgh State University
Tony Evans, Pacific Lutheran University
Carol Foust, Colorado State University, Pueblo
Jeanne Freeman, California State University, Chico
Steve Hartman, Citrus College
Jerolyn F. Hughes, Alabama A&M University
Connie R. Kunda, Muhlenberg College
Ann Neilson, St. Rose College
Christine Lottes, Kutztown University
Mark Lund, Grant MacEwan College
Chet Martin, Tarleton State University
Susan M. Moore, Western Illinois University
Linda Ramsey, University of Tennessee at Martin
Misti Reisman, Tarleton State University

1

Introduction to Wellness

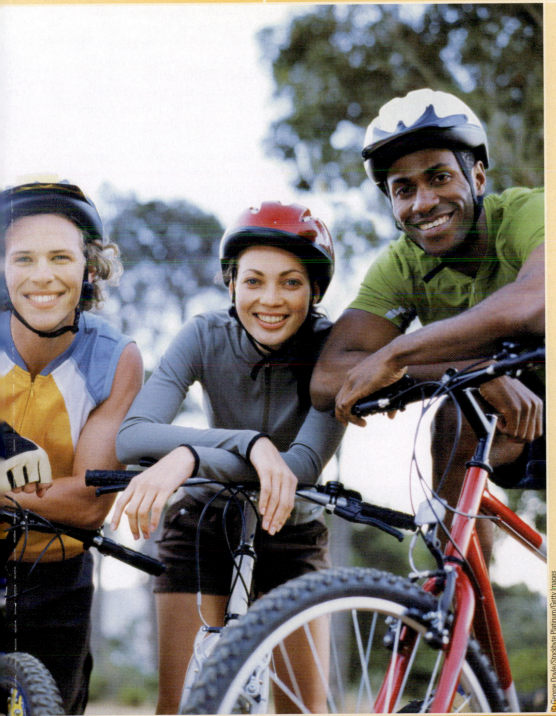

OBJECTIVES

Identify leading health problems in the United States.

Describe the characteristics of wellness.

Name the dimensions of wellness.

Recognize risk factors that compromise wellness.

List main goals of the Year 2010 National Health Objectives.

Discuss at least four things you can do as part of a personalized approach to health and wellness.

At the beginning of the 20th century, the most common health problems in the United States were infectious diseases such as influenza, diphtheria, polio, and tuberculosis. Scientific advances enabled us to wipe out many of those diseases or, at the least, to reduce dramatically the deaths they caused. Those same scientific advances, however, also heralded an age of convenience characterized by a sedentary lifestyle, more alcohol consumption, tobacco use, and a diet permeated by saturated and trans fats and sugars. The result was America's new health problem, **chronic diseases**, such as heart disease, cancer, obesity, diabetes, emphysema, and cirrhosis of the liver.

The focus at the turn of the 20th century was treatment. Researchers confronted with infectious diseases searched for a cure and often met with success. Our focus at the beginning of the 21st century, however, must be on prevention because the health problems that face the population are, in large measure, the result of lifestyle decisions. Emphatic statements released year after year by the U.S. Surgeon General's Office point out that the leading causes of premature death and illness in the United States could be prevented through positive lifestyle habits. The solution to those health problems, then, is largely within our control.

Until recently the American health-care system did not address prevention. It has been, instead, a sickness-care system. More than $1.7 trillion—about 13 percent of the gross national product—is spent on the nation's health care, encompassing hospitals, doctors, health maintenance organizations, pharmaceuticals, and other related companies.

According to World Health Organization figures, in terms of yearly health-care costs, the United States spends more per person than any other industrialized nation. In 2003, U.S. health-care costs were about $5,800 per capita and are expected to reach almost $9,000 per capita in 2010. Yet, in terms of overall health, the health care system ranks only 37th in the world. People in Japan, who spend half of what the United States does per person on health care, outlive us by an average of 5 years.

A fundamental reason for the low overall ranking of the United States is the overemphasis on state-of-the-art cures instead of prevention programs. The United States is the best place in the world to treat people once they are sick, but we do a poor job of keeping people healthy in the first place. The U.S. system also fails to provide good health care for all: 44 million residents do not have health insurance.

Further, Americans have a higher age-adjusted mortality rate than most industrialized nations. The current U.S. **life expectancy** averages 77.6 years (about 75 for men and 80 for women). The World Health Organization has calculated **healthy life expectancy (HLE)** estimates for 191 nations. HLE is obtained by subtracting the years of ill health from total life expectancy. The United States ranked 24th in this report with an HLE of 70 years; Japan was first with an HLE of 74.5 years (see Figure 1.1).

The U.S. ranking was a major surprise, given its status as a developed country with one of the best medical-care systems in the world. The rating indicates that Americans die earlier and spend more time disabled than people in most other advanced countries. The World Health Organization points to several factors that may account for this unexpected finding:

1. The extremely poor health of some groups such as Native Americans, rural African Americans, and the inner-city poor. Their health status is more characteristic of poor developing nations than a rich industrialized country.
2. The HIV epidemic, which causes more deaths and disability than in other developed nations.
3. The high incidence of tobacco use.
4. A high incidence of coronary heart disease.
5. Fairly high levels of violence, notably homicides, as compared to other developed countries.

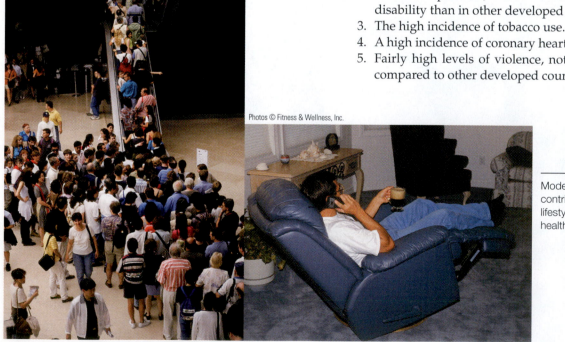

Photos © Fitness & Wellness, Inc.

Modern technology has contributed to a sedentary lifestyle and accompanying health problems.

FIGURE 1.1 Year 2000 Healthy Life Expectancy and Life Expectancy for Selected Countries

Country	Healthy life expectancy	Life expectancy
Ireland	69.6	75.8
USA	70.0	76.8
Germany	70.4	76.9
United Kingdom	71.7	77.2
Austria	71.6	77.4
Belgium	71.6	77.9
Greece	72.5	78.0
Netherlands	72.0	78.1
Norway	71.7	78.6
Spain	72.8	78.7
Italy	72.7	78.8
Canada	72.0	79.1
Switzerland	72.5	79.3
France	73.1	79.3
Sweden	73.0	79.5
Japan	74.5	81.0

Years: 60 65 70 75 80

■ Healthy life expectancy ■ Life expectancy

Source: World Health Organization, http://www.who.int/inf-pr-2000/en/pr2000-life.html. Retrieved June 4, 2000.

Further, of 20 countries that researchers at Northwestern University Medical School in Chicago studied, the typical American diet was highest of all in the percentage of fat. Only a few nations ranked higher in the amount of artery-clogging cholesterol consumed. The typical American diet also is the lowest in dietary fiber. As a result, the United States is one of the fattest nations in the world. Approximately two-thirds of middle-aged U.S. men are overweight, compared with only 3 percent of the middle-aged men in Japan. As if that isn't enough, the United States has the highest rate of heart disease of all developed nations, and some of the highest rates in the world of cancers of the colon, rectum, breast, and lung.

Considering how much the nation spends on medical care, it should outshine the world in health and wellness, but it doesn't, because it has failed to make prevention a top priority. Critical to a focus on prevention, say health care experts, is a change in attitude by patients and health care providers alike. Patients have to stop demanding medication for every ailment and hospitalization or surgery for every illness. In turn, physicians have to be more

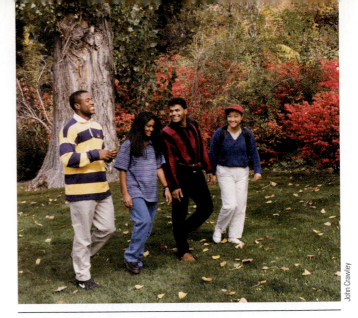

John Crawley

Health and wellness encompass physical, mental, emotional, social, environmental, occupational, and spiritual dimensions.

conservative in their approach to disease. According to Joseph A. Califano, former Secretary of Health, Education and Welfare, America's doctors need to be "more skeptical in resorting to surgery and less promiscuous in dispensing pills."

The problem, in essence, lies with us, not with the medical establishment. Of all the people who die in the United States every year, only about 10 percent die because of inadequate health care, and approximately 20 percent die because of environmental or biological factors. The rest die as the direct result of an unhealthy lifestyle.

Leading Health Problems in the United States

According to the U.S. Surgeon General, about 83 percent of all deaths before age 65 in the United States could have been prevented. Of all deaths in people of all ages, about 53 percent is attributable to lifestyle factors. More than half of all disease is what health experts call "self-controlled"; we can influence it through lifestyle changes and other preventive methods.

At the beginning of the 20th century, almost one-third of all deaths in the United States resulted from tuberculosis, influenza, and pneumonia. Millions died of influenza

Chronic diseases Illnesses that linger over time and may get progressively worse.

Life expectancy Number of years a person is expected to live based on the person's birth year.

Healthy life expectancy (HLE) Number of years a person is expected to live in good health; this number is obtained by subtracting ill-health years from overall life expectancy.

FIGURE 1.2 Leading Causes of Death in the United States, 1900 and 2003

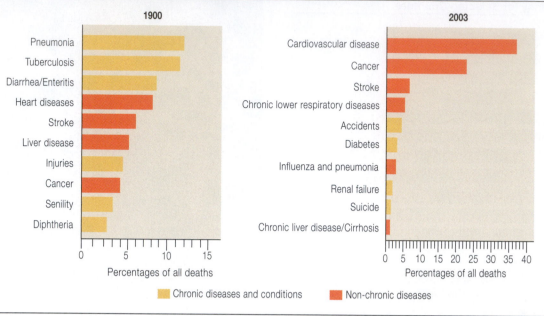

Source: Centers for Disease Control and Prevention. Atlanta, GA.

in a 1918 epidemic. Fewer than 5 percent died from cancer, and only about 10 percent died from cardiovascular disease. Today, death from tuberculosis is a rarity. Less than 5 percent die from influenza and pneumonia. More than half of all deaths in the United States are caused by cardiovascular disease and cancer[1] (see Figure 1.2). Close to 80 percent of those deaths can be prevented by making lifestyle changes—things as basic as eating a healthier diet, being more active and getting regular exercise, and quitting smoking.

The other top two causes of death—chronic lower respiratory diseases (diseases of the respiratory system including emphysema and chronic bronchitis) and accidents—also are largely preventable. Most chronic lower respiratory disease cases are caused by cigarette smoking. Many fatal accidents are the result of alcohol abuse, drug abuse, or failure to use seatbelts.

The underlying causes of death in the United States (see Figure 1.3) indicate that eight of the nine causes are related to lifestyle and lack of common sense. Of the approximately 2.4 million deaths in the United States each year, the "big three"—tobacco use, poor diet and inactivity, and alcohol abuse—are responsible for about 632,000 deaths each year.

Cigarette smoking is the single largest preventable cause of death in the United States, accounting for 435,000 deaths each year. According to the American Council on Science and Health, four of the five leading causes of death are related directly to cigarette smoking. Smoking is responsible for an estimated 30 percent of all cancer deaths, 30 percent of all heart disease fatalities, and 83 percent of all deaths from chronic bronchitis and emphysema. It also is an "unquantifiable risk factor" for cerebrovascular disease.

FIGURE 1.3 Underlying Causes of Death in United States.

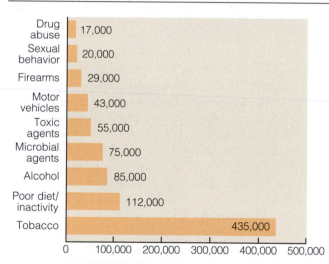

Source: Centers for Disease Control and Prevention, Atlanta, GA.

The Council also has stated that infant and fetal mortality can be reduced substantially by reducing cigarette smoking. Smoking is responsible for higher rates of spontaneous abortion and stillbirth and accounts for up to 14 percent of all premature births in the United States. Cigarette smoking is the most important health issue that we face in our time. The official position of the World Health Organization on smoking is clear:

> The control of cigarette smoking could do more to improve health and prolong life in developed countries than any other single action in the whole field of preventive medicine.[2]

What are Health and Wellness?

The World Health Organization defines health as "a state of complete physical, mental, and social well-being, and not merely the absence of disease or infirmity." The key word in that definition is possibly "well-being," and true health may actually be a condition in which we are able to avoid illness, even if we are predisposed to it.

More than five decades ago, health care education pioneer Jesse Williams proclaimed that health is a condition that allows one to do the most constructive work, render the best possible service to the world, and experience the highest possible enjoyment of life. "Health as freedom from disease is a standard of mediocrity," he said. "Health as a quality of life is a standard of inspiration and increasing achievements."

Williams was ahead of his time. Most Americans have taken decades to catch on to his vision. A series of Gallup polls finally hinted at his much broader scope of health and wellness. In increasing numbers, Americans now are defining health as the energy to do the things we care about.

HEALTH

The word **health** is derived from the Old English "hal," which means whole. Researchers on the cutting edge consider health to be a continuum, a perpetual but ever-changing balance of the various dimensions that make us whole.

Everything with which you interact—the place you live, the air you breathe, the food you eat, the job you have, the people you associate with—affects your position on the health continuum. The same series of Gallup polls shows that Americans are beginning to understand the influence of these interactive factors. When ranking their health priorities, their top concern was staying free of disease, but the third highest concern was living in an environment with clean air and water.

WELLNESS

Wellness combines seven dimensions of well-being (physical, mental, emotional, social, environmental, occupational, and spiritual) in a quality way of living. Wellness is the ability to live life to the fullest, to have a zest for life, to maximize personal potential in a variety of ways. Illness and health are opposite states, but you can be ill and still enjoy wellness if you have a purpose in life, a deep appreciation for living, a sense of joy.

People who are bound by the strictures of traditionally defined physical health wait until some disease has crept up on them, then consult a professional to evaluate their condition and prescribe treatment. Simply put, they turn over their physical health to someone else. Wellness, by contrast, places responsibility on the individual. Wellness

becomes a matter of self-evaluation and self-assessment, continually working on learning and on making changes that will enhance wellness. You take the reins. Rather than delegating your physical health to someone else, you make a deep personal commitment to wellness.

Whereas physical health is a fairly simple concept, wellness is multifaceted and involves much more than simple physical condition. Physical health is not available to everyone, but everyone can enjoy wellness—despite physical limitations, disease, and disability. Wellness fully integrates its seven dimensions (see the Dimensions of Wellness, page 6) in a complex interaction that leads to a quality life. It is not something that is "achieved" once and stays with you thereafter; it is a horizon that we move toward throughout life. We move along a continuum, and the important factor is the direction in which we are moving. Finally, wellness affects more than the individual. It also can encompass the family and society as a whole.

If we are to accept a definition of wellness that goes beyond mere freedom from disease, we also must accept a notion that calls for a dramatic change in the way we deal with health. For centuries the emphasis has been on identifying bacteria, classifying viruses, and waging a determined war on devastating diseases. We have

Health A state of complete well-being and not just the absence of disease or infirmity.

Wellness Full integration of physical, mental, emotional, social, environmental, occupational, and spiritual well-being into a quality life.

concentrated on treatment. If we are to redefine health to reflect a condition of wellness, though, we must redefine the ultimate goal of our health efforts: to prevent disease. Inherent in that challenge is the recognition that behavior plays a key role in the development of disease and also in our ability to resist disease and maintain optimum health.

Embodied in the definition of wellness is a philosophy calling for consideration of the whole person, not a fractionalization into separate parts. We must consider ourselves as we interact in our environment, not as separate complaints or body parts in a sterile laboratory or in the unnatural environs of a physician's examining room. Wellness emphasizes a conscious and active commitment by the individual who understands that optimum health is *not* something that just happens. Most significantly, it calls for concentrating on the factors that precede illness instead of being concerned solely with the anatomy of disease once it strikes.

THE DIMENSIONS OF WELLNESS

Writing in *The History and Future of Wellness*, author Donald Ardell points out that living by the principles of wellness is considered a richer way to be alive.[3] Optimum wellness balances seven dimensions: physical, mental, emotional, social, environmental, occupational, and spiritual. These are depicted in Figure 1.4.

Physical Wellness The dimension most commonly associated with being healthy is **physical wellness**. A person who is physically well eats a well-balanced diet, gets plenty of physical activity and exercise, maintains proper weight, gets enough sleep, avoids risky sexual behavior, tries to limit exposure to environmental contaminants, and restricts intake of harmful substances such as alcohol, tobacco, caffeine, and drugs. Physical wellness is characterized by good cardiorespiratory endurance, muscular strength and endurance, muscular flexibility, proper body composition, and the ability to carry out daily tasks.

To remain well requires that you take steps to protect your physical health. This begins with self-exams and thorough physical examinations, including appropriate screening tests, from a physician. It also involves taking effective measures if you do become sick, such as seeking medical care and using medications conservatively.

Physical wellness entails confidence and optimism about one's ability to take care of health problems. These conditions need not prevent one from enjoying life. Physical wellness brings with it a remarkable resistance to disease. The proper combination of nutrition, exercise, and sleep renders healthy people capable of resisting the common colds and influenza that wipe out others.

People who enjoy physical wellness are intelligent about their health. When they develop an unusual or irritating symptom, they do what is necessary to relieve it. If symptoms persist, they check with a doctor.

Irrespective of whether healthy individuals are muscular, they usually are physically powerful. Exercise tunes

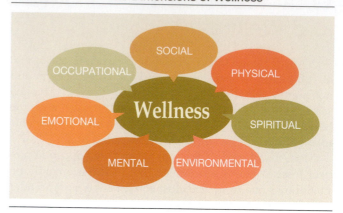

their muscles and endows them with a high level of physical coordination and self-confidence. Instead of shying away from physical challenge, they accept it with enthusiasm, confident they can make their body work for them. Their reaction time is good, strength is obvious, and endurance is high.

People characterized by physical wellness lead an active lifestyle. They like to be outdoors. They enjoy a fast-paced bicycle ride along a roadside cloaked

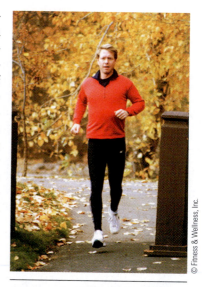

A person who is physically well exercises regularly.

with apple blossoms or a vigorous game of touch football on a crisp autumn afternoon. They have the energy they need to do the things they enjoy, as well as the energy they need to complete demanding tasks at work, breeze through final exams without feeling exhausted, or clear the debris from last year's vegetable garden.

People who are physically well respect and like their own body. They have a natural grace and ease. You can see their health in the way they move. Beauty in the traditional sense of the word has little to do with it. People with physical wellness make the most of their body, and they delight in it.

Mental Wellness Just as the physical dimension of wellness embodies much more than the mere absence of disease, so does **mental wellness**. Pioneers in the field of psychoneuroimmunology are proving scientifically what philosophers such as Homer, Plato, and Aristotle speculated more than 5,000 years ago: The mind has a striking influence on the body (and, therefore, on health and wellness).

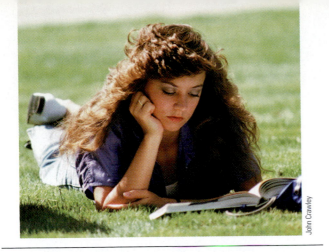

Mentally well people are curious and have an inquisitive mind.

Education shouldn't stop with commencement exercises. Mental wellness involves unbridled curiosity and ongoing learning. This dimension of wellness implies that you can apply the things you have learned (whether at home or on the job), that you create opportunities to learn more, and that you engage your mind in lively interaction with the world around you.

People who are mentally well think clearly, are quick to pick up new concepts, and catch on rapidly to new ideas. Instead of being intimidated by facts and figures with which they are unfamiliar, they embrace the chance to learn something new. Their confidence and enthusiasm enable them to approach learning situations with eagerness that leads to success.

Mental wellness breeds creativity. In contrast to people who seem burdened with getting a job done, mentally well people are able to approach the same task in a new way. They don't seem restricted by what they have always done before. They are willing to tackle the chore from a different angle, one that lets them exercise creativity and initiative.

Logic is a basic attribute of mental wellness. People who are confronted suddenly with an unfamiliar situation tend to experience mild panic. Mental wellness brings with it common sense and logic that enable those who are mentally well to reason their way through.

A genuine sense of curiosity leads mentally well people into a world that is constantly new and challenging. Whereas others accept what life has to offer with quiet resolve, mentally well people grasp each aspect of life with a desire to understand. They are the people who know why the surface of a lake is so blue, how a newspaper is printed, how a robin can tell that spring has arrived. They know the answers because they ask the questions. Some people pass a flowering hedge and notice that it is beautiful. Mentally healthier people want to know why the blooms are pink, what kind of hedge it is, how they can grow one like it.

Along with alertness and brightness, mental wellness brings capability with it. Mentally well people have a good memory and use it to their best advantage. They are skilled in their chosen area of expertise, and they are open to new ideas and suggestions. They relish the chance to improve themselves and to learn something new.

Mental wellness brings with it vision and promise. More than anything else, mentally well people are open-minded and accepting of others. Instead of being threatened by those who are different from themselves, they show respect and curiosity without feeling they have to conform. They are faithful to their own ideas and philosophies and allow others the same privilege. Their self-confidence guarantees that they can take their place in the world without giving up part of themselves and without requiring others to do the same.

Emotional Wellness Emotions involve both the mind and the body, and, as a result, they can bridge the gap between the two. Emotions are a contributing factor in a number of diseases, such as rheumatoid arthritis, bronchial asthma, peptic ulcer, ulcerative colitis, hypertension, and dermatitis.

What constitutes **emotional wellness**? Foremost is probably the ability to understand your own feelings, to accept your limitations, and to achieve emotional stability. It also involves being comfortable with your emotions. Understanding and accepting your own feelings helps you understand and accept the emotions of others, which leads to the ability to maintain intimate relationships with other people. Emotional wellness also implies the ability to express emotions appropriately, adjust to change, cope with stress in a healthy way, and enjoy life despite its occasional disappointments and frustrations.

The hallmark of emotional wellness is a deep and abiding happiness—not a happiness that depends on some frail set of circumstances but, rather, a happiness that stems from powerful inner contentment. Instead of being dependent on a certain income or status in life, the happiness that signals real wellness is an emotional anchor that gives meaning and joy to life.

In the Declaration of Independence, Thomas Jefferson promised three things to all Americans: the rights to life, liberty, and the pursuit of happiness. He did not promise happiness itself, because he knew that the government could not deliver it. Happiness is not a fleeting emotion tied to a single event but, rather, a long-term state of mind that permeates the various facets of life and influences our outlook. We can experience true happiness and temporary unhappiness at the same time. Happiness may seem to vanish temporarily, giving way to bursts of

Physical wellness Flexibility, endurance, strength, and optimism about your ability to take care of health problems.

Mental wellness A state in which your mind is engaged in lively interaction with the world around you.

Emotional wellness The ability to understand your own feelings, accept your limitations, and achieve emotional stability.

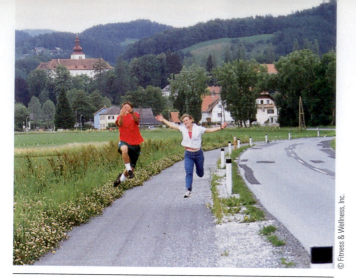

Emotionally well people enjoy friends, play, and leisure time, and they laugh often.

Ten Qualities of Wellness

1. Deeply committed to a cause outside oneself.
2. Physically able to do whatever one wants with intensity and great energy; seldom sick.
3. Caring and loving; a person others can lean on in a crisis.
4. In tune with the spiritual, having a clear sense of purpose and direction.
5. Intellectually sharp, able to handle information, possessing an ever-curious mind and a good sense of humor.
6. Well organized and able to accomplish plenty of work.
7. Able to live in and enjoy the present rather than focusing on the past or looking toward the future.
8. Comfortable with experiencing the full range of human emotions.
9. Accepting of one's limitations, handicaps, and mistakes.
10. Able and willing to take charge of one's life, to practice positive self-care, and to be assertive when necessary.

depression or disappointment, but it returns. As Harry Emerson Fosdick stated:

> One who expects to completely escape low moods is asking the impossible. Like the weather, life is essentially variable, and a healthy person believes in the validity of his high hours even when he is having a low one.[4]

No one has ever come up with a simple recipe for producing happiness, but researchers agree that certain ingredients seem universal among those who have the kind of true, abiding happiness that characterizes emotional wellness. Those who are happy usually are part of a family. They are partners, parents, or children. They love others, and they feel loved themselves. Healthy, happy people enjoy friends, work hard at something fulfilling, get plenty of exercise, and enjoy play and leisure time. They know how to laugh, and they laugh often. They give of themselves freely to others and seem to have found deep meaning to life.

An attitude of true happiness signals freedom from the tension and depression that many people endure. Emotional wellness obviously is subject to the same kinds of depression and unhappiness that plague all of us once in a while, but the difference lies in the ability to bounce back. Well people take minor setbacks in stride and have the notable ability to enjoy life despite it all. When something unhappy happens, they put it behind them. They don't waste energy or time recounting the situation, wondering how they could have changed it, or dwelling on the past.

The spirit of optimism basic to healthy, happy individuals enables them to focus their energy on the present. They recognize that the past can hold powerful lessons, but they do not let it control the here-and-now.

In addition to avoiding the pitfalls of the past, they avoid the temptation to pin all their hopes and dreams on the future. They are goal-oriented and ambitious and at the same time are able to enjoy themselves today. They aren't waiting until they graduate from college, until they marry, until they pay off their home, or until they are the president of a company. Instead, they are happy today in the circumstances they are in. Although they may aspire to graduate with honors, marry their sweetheart, pay off the mortgage, or gain the top spot at the firm, they are happy regardless. They know that happiness is not the product of a particular thing but instead is a condition.

Part and parcel of happiness is acceptance of self. Healthy people value themselves as having something to contribute and being worthwhile. Healthy people enjoy a sense of success—not as measured traditionally by the world but as measured against their own standards. They know what is important to them, and they are confident they can achieve it. They are in touch with self to the point that they have a clear definition of their own needs.

Emotional wellness brings with it a certain stability, an ability to look both success and failure squarely in the face and to keep moving along a predetermined course. When success is evident, the emotionally well person radiates the expected joy and confidence. When failure seems evident, the emotionally well person responds by making the best of circumstances and moving beyond the failure. Wellness enables us to learn from failure, identify ways to avoid it in the future, and then go on with the business at hand.

Emotional wellness also embodies the ability to get in touch with your own feelings. Because healthy people have a good self-image, they do not worry about showing their feelings or sharing them with others. They are not concerned with what others think of them. They do not feel the need to prove themselves to others, nor do they feel they have to force others to accept their point of view. They quietly, peacefully accept themselves and are able to move freely beyond that to accept others.

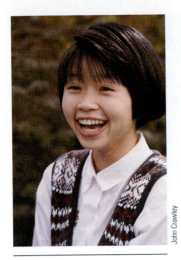

A good sense of humor is an important part of wellness.

John Crawley

Sensitive, yet independent, emotionally well people accept themselves to an extent that they are extremely insightful about themselves and others. Emotional wellness brings with it a necessary frame of mind that allows involvement with other people. A truly healthy person is one who enjoys others and who is not threatened by what other people might do or say.

Emotional wellness also brings with it a maturity that allows the individual to forgive others. Emotionally well people accept responsibility for their own happiness instead of blaming others when they are unhappy. They are free from anger and resentment because they recognize that anger is almost always destructive. By accepting responsibility for their own emotional well-being, they free themselves to achieve it.

More than dictating happiness and optimism, emotions play a profound part in physical health and avoiding disease. Biobehavioralist Norman Cousins maintained that what you think, what you believe, and how you react to experiences can impair or aid the workings of the body's immune system.

Studies of terminally ill cancer patients reveal that those who survive have one characteristic in common: their utter refusal to give up hope. Cousins said:

> Nothing is more wondrous about the fifteen billion neurons in the human brain than their ability to convert thoughts, hopes, ideas, and attitudes into chemical substances. Every emotion, negative or positive, makes its registrations on the body's systems. . . . The most important thing I have learned about the power of belief is that an individual patient's attitude toward serious illness can be as important as medical help. It would be a serious mistake to bypass or minimize the need for scientific treatment, but that treatment will be far more effective if people put their creative hopes, their faith, and their confidence fully to work in behalf of their recovery.[5]

Harvard-trained surgeon Bernie Siegel, who has spent his medical career working with cancer victims, remarked:

> I can say from my own experience that patients who have given up, who have come to me feeling defeated and desperate, feeling that nothing can possibly help them, have often made their own predictions come true. The fighter-type patients who are willing to try anything that has a chance to help them, who have real faith in their survival, always do better.[6]

Social Wellness Social wellness, with its accompanying self-image, endows us with the ease and confidence to be

outgoing, friendly, and affectionate toward others. Social wellness goes beyond a concern for the individual, to an interest in humanity and the environment as a whole.

One of the hallmarks of social wellness is the ability to relate to others, to reach out to other people, both within the family unit and outside it. Healthy people are honest and loyal. Their own balance and sense of self allow them to extend respect and tolerance to others. They are confident of themselves and don't feel threatened by opening up to others.

People who are socially healthy are able to develop and maintain intimacy but are not promiscuous. They organize themselves in family groups and are loyal and faithful to family members. They are trustworthy and loyal to those outside the family unit and have the ability to make and keep friends. They treat others with fairness and respect.

Social wellness goes hand-in-hand with social graces. Socially healthy people are affectionate, polite, and helpful toward others; can handle conflict without exploding; and are true to their ideals and beliefs while allowing others to be true to theirs. They do not interpret a difference of opinion as the basis for destruction. Instead, they are tolerant, respectful, and secure. They can say "no" when they should and are sensitive in responding to others' needs without sacrificing their own.

Socially well people love themselves. This is not a vain, self-centered kind of love that causes them to develop an overinflated image of themselves. Instead, it

Social wellness The ability to relate well to others, both within and outside the family unit.

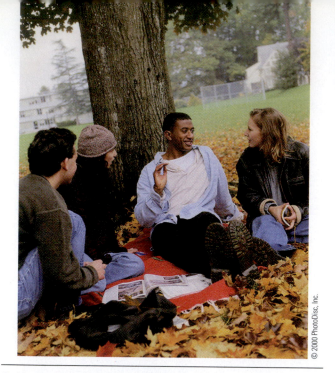

Group activities enhance social wellness.

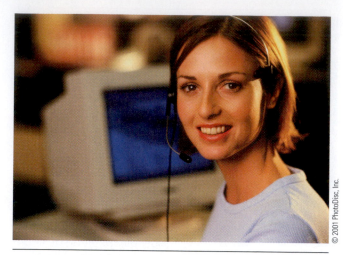

Occupational wellness provides important personal rewards.

is the kind of love that enables individuals to feel secure enough, confident enough, and good enough about themselves to reach out to others. Before you can love others, you must be able to love yourself.

The socially well person relishes touch, especially hugging, as a vital, irreplaceable means of communicating caring and concern for others. Long-term research by experts in a variety of disciplines has confirmed that touch is crucial to well-being. San Diego psychologist James Hardison wrote:

> It is through touching that we are able to fulfill a large share of our human needs and, in doing so, to attain happiness. By touching someone, we can affirm our friendship or approval, communicate important messages, promote health, and bring about love.[7]

Unfortunately, Hardison continues, too many people put up barriers to the language of touch, equating touching "with either sex or violence. Consequently many people avoid the simple acts of touching—pats on the back, heartfelt handshakes, cordial hugs—that affirm goodwill."

Socially well people—whether at home, in the classroom, or at work—develop a spirit of teamwork with those around them. They do not view others with suspicion, jealousy, or contempt. They find no satisfaction in the thought of outdoing, putting down, or getting ahead of others. They find great joy in cooperation, mutual support, and working together to accomplish something of lasting value for all.

Occupational Wellness Some models also include a sixth dimension of wellness: **occupational wellness**. Occupational wellness is not tied to high salary, prestigious

position, or extravagant working conditions. Any job can bring occupational wellness if it provides rewards that are important to the individual. Salary might be the most important factor to one person, whereas another might place a much greater value on creativity.

People with occupational wellness face demands on the job, and they also have some say over demands placed on them. Any job has routine demands, but occupational wellness means that they are mixed with new, unpredictable challenges that keep a job exciting. Occupationally well people are able to maximize their skills, and they have opportunities to broaden existing skills or gain new ones. They welcome opportunities for advancement and appreciate recognition of achievement.

Occupational wellness also brings some sense of control. People are given the chance to participate in long-term planning and are able to determine some corporate policies, including policies on discipline. People with occupational wellness control the machines they work with, not the other way around. Feedback from both customers and management is given freely. Occupational wellness encourages collaboration among co-workers, fostering a sense of teamwork and support, with frequent interaction. When problems arise, democratic procedures are used to solve them; those with a grievance have an accepted and effective way to solve problems.

A workplace free from physical stressors promotes occupational wellness. Among the many things in the workplace that can cause stress are noise, poor temperature control, crowding, poor arrangement of space, lack of privacy, and poor lighting (lights are too bright, too dim, too glaring, or flickering). Occupational wellness also implies freedom from safety hazards on the job, such as dangerous machinery, toxic chemicals, air pollution, or the threat of nuclear accidents.

People with occupational wellness work consistently toward a satisfying balance between the time and energy spent at work and the time and energy spent in family and leisure activities. At a healthy job, people share responsibilities so everyone has time (and energy) left for activities away from work.

Environmental Wellness The quality of today's environment has a direct effect on personal wellness. To enjoy health, we require clean air, pure water, quality food, adequate shelter, satisfactory work conditions, and personal safety. **Environmental wellness** is a broad dimension that also encompasses our human environment and relationships.

Health is affected negatively when we live in a polluted, toxic, unkind, and unsafe environment. To enjoy environmental wellness, we must take responsibility by educating ourselves about and protecting ourselves from environmental hazards. We also must do everything we can to protect the environment so we, our children, and future generations can enjoy a safe and clean environment.

Environmental wellness is tied closely to physical wellness and goes beyond the above-mentioned factors. Behavioral therapists have established that most of the behaviors we adopt are a product of our environment—the forces of social influences we encounter and our thought processes. This environment includes family, friends, peers, homes, schools, workplaces, television, radio, and movies, as well as our communities, country, and culture in general.

We are so habituated to the toxic factors in our environment that we miss the subtle ways it influences our behaviors, personal lifestyle, and health each day. From a young age, we observe, we learn, we emulate, and without realizing it, we incorporate into our own lifestyle the behaviors exhibited by people around us. We are transported by parents, relatives, and friends to nearly any place we need to go. We also watch them drive short distances to run errands. We see adults take escalators and elevators and ride moving sidewalks at malls and airports. We notice that they use remote controls, pagers, and cell phones. We observe as they stop at fast-food restaurants and pick up super-sized, calorie-dense, high-fat meals. We notice that they watch television and surf the Net for hours at a time. Some smoke, some drink heavily, and some have addictions to hard drugs. Others engage in risky behaviors by not wearing seatbelts, by drinking and driving, and by having unprotected sex. All of these unhealthy habits can be passed along, unquestioned, to the next generation.

Among the leading underlying causes of death in the United States are physical inactivity and poor diet. Yet, most activities of daily living—which a few decades ago required movement or physical activity—now require almost no effort and negatively impact health, fitness, and body weight. Small movements that have been streamlined out of daily life add up quickly, especially when we consider these over seven days a week and 52 weeks a year.

To be considered active, health experts recommend that a person accumulate the equivalent of 5 to 6 miles of

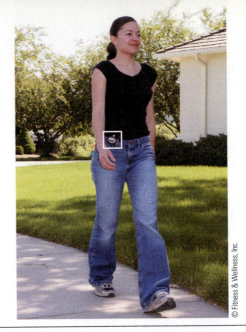

The pedometer is an excellent tool to determine daily physical activity by monitoring the total number of steps taken each day.

TABLE 1.1 Daily Physical Activity Recommendations

Total Time	Outcome
30 minutes	Health benefits
60 minutes	Weight gain prevention
60–90 minutes	Weight regain prevention

walking per day. This level of activity equates to about 10,000 to 12,000 daily steps (see Table 1.1). If you have never clipped on a **pedometer**, try to do so. A pedometer is a great motivational tool to help increase, maintain, and monitor daily physical activity that involves lower body motion (walking, jogging, running). When you look at the total number of steps displayed at the end of the day, you may be shocked by the low number of steps you have taken. Use of pedometers most likely will increase in the next few years to help promote and quantify daily physical activity (additional information on pedometer use is provided in Chapter 6, page 107).

Modern-day architecture also reinforces unhealthy behaviors. Elevators and escalators are often of the finest workmanship and located in convenient places. Many of our newest, showiest shopping centers and convention centers don't provide accessible stairwells, so people are

Occupational wellness The ability to perform your job skillfully and effectively under conditions that provide personal and team satisfaction and adequately reward each individual.

Environmental wellness The capability to live in a clean and safe environment that is not detrimental to health.

Pedometer An electronic device that senses body motion and counts footsteps. Some pedometers also record distance, calories burned, speeds, "aerobic steps," and time spent being physically active.

all but forced to ride escalators. If they want to walk up the escalator, they can't because the people in front of them obstruct the way. Entrances to buildings provide electric sensors and automatic door openers. Without a second thought, people walk through automatic doors instead of taking the time to push open a door.

With the advent of cell phones, people now move even less. Family members call each other on the phone even within the walls of their own home. Some individuals don't get out of the car anymore to ring doorbells, instead, they stop out front and use the cell phone to call and wait for the person to come out.

Leisure time is no better. When people arrive home after work, they surf the Net, play computer games, or watch television for hours at a time. Current data indicate that in the average household, television watching consumes close to 8 hours of programming each day.[8]

Our nutrition patterns are also shaped by the environment. According to the USDA's Center for Nutrition Policy and Promotion, the amount of daily food supply available in the United States is about 3,900 calories per person, before wastage. This figure represents a 700-calorie rise over the early 1980s,[9] which means that we have taken the amount of food available to us and tossed in a Cinnabon for every person in the country.

The overabundance of food increases pressure on food suppliers to advertise and try to convince consumers to buy their products. The food industry spends more than $33 billion each year on advertising and promotion, and most of this money goes toward highly processed foods. The few ads and campaigns promoting healthy foods and healthful eating simply cannot compete. Most of us would be hard-pressed to recall a jingle for brown rice or kale. The money spent advertising a single food product across the United States is often 10 to 50 times more than the money the federal government spends promoting MyPyramid or encouraging us to eat fruits and vegetables.[10]

Coupled with our sedentary lifestyle, many activities of daily living in today's culture are associated with eating. We eat during coffee breaks, when we socialize, when we play, when we watch sports, at the movies, during television viewing—in addition to when the clock tells us it's time for a meal. Our lives seem to revolve around food, a nonstop string of occasions to eat and overeat. As a nation, we now eat out more often than in the past, portion sizes are larger, and the variety of foods to choose from is endless. We also snack more than ever before. No wonder we are becoming a nation of overweight and obese people!

Unfortunately, all the modern conveniences of the 21st century lull us into overconsumption and sedentary living. By living in America, we adopt behaviors that put our health at risk. And though we understand that lifestyle choices affect our health and well-being, we still have an extremely difficult time making changes.

Spiritual Wellness Spiritual wellness—comprising the ethics, values, and morals that guide us—gives meaning

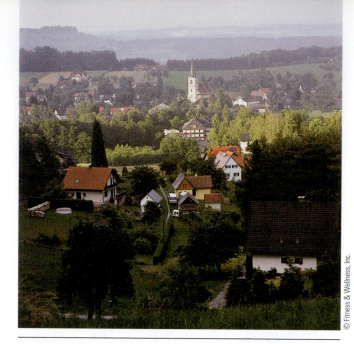

Spiritual wellness includes enjoying the wonder and beauty of nature.

and direction to life. Every human being needs the sense that life is meaningful, that life has purpose and direction, and that some power (nature, science, religion, or some higher power) brings all of humanity together. In essence, spiritual wellness entails a search for greater value in life.

Spiritual wellness embodies a worthwhile purpose, faith, and peace, an undaunted comfort with life and its outcome. It is characterized by faith and optimism, by a hope that sustains us through whatever life has to offer. It entails developing the inner self and identifying a purpose to life. Spiritual wellness is optimum when you are able to discover, articulate, and act on that purpose.

Spiritually well people have the unique ability to see beyond the isolated event, to envision the whole picture. The spiritually well person sets realistic goals and goes about reaching them with hope, enthusiasm, and determination. Those goals are never the end result. They are part of the whole, cogs in the larger machine of life. Spiritually healthy people are not merely content with what they have accomplished in the past. They are enthused about what lies ahead.

That's not to say that spiritually well people are immune from disappointment. Spiritually healthy people, however, are able to bridge the gap from one success to another, able to develop the fortitude necessary to keep going. Spiritually healthy individuals don't dwell on discouragement. They mobilize their inner resources to reach the next pinnacle. Instead of envisioning disappointments or setbacks as craggy stone walls, spiritually well people see them as smooth stepping stones, inviting

Critical Thinking

1. Now that you understand the seven dimensions of wellness, rank them in order of importance to you, and explain your rationale in doing so.

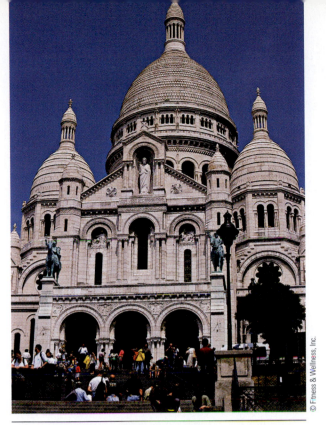

Spiritual wellness recognizes a power higher than oneself.

them to keep going, inviting them to make their way, carefully but securely, to the other side.

BEHAVIORAL HEALTH

Behavioral health brings with it solutions that seem simple in comparison to the array of scientific tests, the complex chemical formulas, the powerful lens of the microscope, and the elaborate assortment of available treatments. Researchers have found that the following simple lifestyle habits can add significantly to longevity.

1. Eat a well-balanced diet high in grains, fruits, and vegetables and low in saturated fat, trans fats, and cholesterol.
2. Eat a good breakfast every day.
3. Get at least 30 to 60 minutes of **moderate-intensity physical activity** most days of the week.
4. Maintain recommended body weight (through adequate nutrition and physical activity).
5. Get a good night's sleep.
6. Lower your stress levels and surround yourself with a supportive network of friends and family.
7. Implement personal safety measures—things as simple as wearing seatbelts, observing speed limits, and locking doors to your home.
8. Stay informed about the environment and avoid potential contaminants whenever you can.
9. Take any medication your doctor prescribes and follow the instructions precisely.
10. Limit your intake of alcohol.
11. If you smoke, quit.

12. Increase education to enhance healthy lifestyle choices and wellness.

Wellness Challenges of the 21st Century

With the landmark 1979 publication of *Healthy People*, the U.S. Surgeon General's report on health promotion and disease prevention, the government embarked on a plan to establish broad national goals intended to promote wellness among all Americans. Those goals were converted into specific health objectives a year later, with a precise list of measurable goals we had hoped to attain by the year 1990.

Americans were successful at some of these goals and we failed at others. After assessing what had been achieved and what still had to be done, the U.S. Public Health Service conducted hearings with health professionals from a variety of settings across the nation. The result was publication of the Year 2000 National Health Objectives, a set of goals aimed at taking Americans into the 21st century with a higher level of health and wellness. Again, we met a few of the goals but came up short in many others.

2010 HEALTH OBJECTIVES

A new set of more realistic goals have been set forth with the intent to improve the health of all Americans as we start the first decade of the new millennium. Two unique goals of the new 2010 objectives are that they emphasize increased quality and years of healthy life and they seek to eliminate health disparities among all groups of people (see Figure 1.5).

The objectives address three important points:

1. *Personal responsibility.* Individuals need to become ever more health-conscious, and responsible and informed behavior is the key to good health.
2. *Health benefits for all people.* Lower socioeconomic conditions and poor health are often interrelated. Extending the benefits of good health to all people is crucial to the health of the nation.
3. *Health promotion and disease prevention.* A shift from treatment to preventive techniques will drastically cut health-care costs and help all Americans achieve a better quality of life.

Spiritual wellness The sense that life is meaningful, that life has purpose, and that some power brings all humanity together; the ethics, values, and morals that guide us and give meaning and direction to life.

Behavioral health The effects of lifestyle behaviors on health.

Moderate-intensity physical activity Activity that uses 150 calories of energy per day, or 1,000 calories per week.

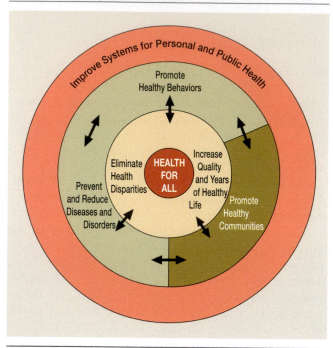

FIGURE 1.6 Selected Health Objectives for the Year 2010

1. Increase quality and years of healthy life.
2. Eliminate health disparities.
3. Improve the health, fitness, and quality of life of all Americans through the adoption and maintenance of regular, daily physical activity.
4. Promote health and reduce chronic disease risk, disease progression, debilitation, and premature death associated with dietary factors and nutritional status among all people in the United States.
5. Reduce disease, disability, and death related to tobacco use and exposure to secondhand smoke.
6. Increase the quality, availability, and effectiveness of educational and community-based programs designed to prevent disease and improve the health and quality of the American people.
7. Promote health for all people through a healthy environment.
8. Reduce the incidence and severity of injuries from unintentional causes, as well as violence and abuse.
9. Promote worker health and safety through prevention.
10. Improve access to comprehensive, high quality health care.
11. Ensure that every pregnancy in the United States is intended.
12. Improve maternal and pregnancy outcomes and reduce rates of disability in infants.
13. Improve the quality of health-related decisions through effective communication.
14. Decrease the incidence of functional limitations due to arthritis, osteoporosis, and chronic back conditions.
15. Decrease cancer incidence, morbidity, and mortality.
16. Promote health and prevent secondary conditions among persons with disabilities.
17. Enhance the cardiovascular health and quality of life of all Americans through prevention and control of risk factors, and promotion of healthy lifestyle behaviors.
18. Prevent HIV transmission and associated morbidity and mortality.
19. Improve the mental health of all Americans.
20. Raise the public's awareness of the signs and symptoms of lung disease.
21. Increase awareness of healthy sexual relationships and prevent all forms of sexually transmitted diseases.
22. Reduce the incidence of substance abuse by all people, especially children.

Development of the 2010 Health Objectives involved more than 10,000 people representing 300 national organizations, including the Institute of Medicine of the National Academy of Sciences, all 50 state health departments, and the federal Office of Disease Prevention and Health Promotion. Selected objectives are provided in Figure 1.6. By living the wellness guidelines provided in this book, you will be an active participant in achieving the Healthy People 2010 Objectives and you will enhance the quality of your life.

SURGEON GENERAL'S REPORT

A major report on the influence of regular physical activity on health was released by the U.S. Surgeon General in 1996. That report stated that regular moderate physical activity provides substantial benefits in health and well-being for the vast majority of Americans who are not physically active. The report became a call to nationwide action.

According to the Surgeon General, improving health through physical activity poses a serious public health challenge. Benefits of leading a moderately active lifestyle include a significant reduction in the risk of developing or dying from heart disease, diabetes, colon cancer, and high blood pressure. Regular physical activity also helps to maintain a high quality of life into old age. Additional information on the Surgeon General's report is given in Chapter 6.

Moderate physical activity has been defined as any activity that requires an energy expenditure of 150 calories per day, or 1,000 calories per week. The general health recommendation is that people strive to accumulate at least 30 minutes of physical activity per day most days of the week (see Table 1.2). Examples of moderate physical activity are walking, cycling, playing basketball or volleyball, swimming, water aerobics, dancing fast, pushing a stroller, raking leaves, shoveling snow, washing or waxing a car, washing windows or floors, and even gardening.

TABLE 1.2 Adult Activity Levels Based on Total Number of Steps Taken per Day

Steps per Day	Category
<5,000	Sedentary lifestyle
5,000–7,499	Low active
7,500–9,999	Somewhat active
10,000–12,499	Active
≥12,500	Highly active

Source: C. Tudor-Locke, and D. R. Basset. "How Many Steps/Day are Enough? Preliminary Pedometer Indices for Public Health," *Sports Medicine* 34:1–8, 2004.

Because of the ever growing epidemic of obesity in the United States, a 2002 guideline by American and Canadian scientists from the Institute of Medicine of the National Academy of Sciences increased the recommendation to 60 minutes of moderate-intensity physical activity every day.[11] This recommendation was based on evidence indicating that people who maintain healthy weight typically accumulate 1 hour of daily physical activity.

Subsequently, the 2005 Dietary Guidelines for Americans released by the USDA, recommend that up to 60 minutes of moderate- to vigorous-intensity physical activity per day may be necessary to prevent weight gain; and between 60 and 90 minutes of daily moderate-intensity physical activity is recommended to sustain weight loss for previously overweight people.[12] Although health benefits are derived with 30 minutes per day, people with a tendency to gain weight need to be physically active for 1 to 1½ hours daily to prevent weight gain. Further, a regimen of 60 to 90 minutes of activity per day provides additional health benefits, including lower risk for cardiovascular disease and diabetes.

A Personalized Approach to Health and Wellness

Experts who were instrumental in formulating the national objectives and the report on physical activity and health point to the commitment of the government toward achieving wellness goals. They also invite the commitment and involvement of each American in accepting responsibility for their own health and wellness.

Vital to achieving health and wellness is your willingness to take personal responsibility for your behaviors and choices. We know enough about disease and premature death to formulate a set of goals that applies to the nation as a whole. How you achieve those goals, however, requires a personal decision. It entails careful, intelligent planning. What will work for someone else won't necessarily work for you. How you apply the principles you'll learn in this book has to be highly personalized.

Moderate-Intensity Physical Activities

Here are some examples of moderate activity going from less to more vigorous:

- Washing and waxing a car for 45–60 minutes.
- Playing volleyball for 45 minutes.
- Playing touch football for 30–45 minutes.
- Gardening for 30–45 minutes.
- Wheeling self in wheelchair for 30–40 minutes.
- Walking 1¾ miles in 35 minutes (20-minute mile).
- Basketball (shooting baskets) for 30 minutes.
- Bicycling 5 miles in 30 minutes.
- Dancing fast for 30 minutes.
- Pushing a stroller 1½ miles in 30 minutes.
- Raking leaves for 30 minutes.
- Walking 2 miles in 30 minutes.
- Doing water aerobics for 30 minutes.
- Swimming laps for 20 minutes.
- Playing basketball for 15–20 minutes.
- Jumping rope for 15 minutes.
- Running 1½ miles in 15 minutes.
- Shoveling snow for 15 minutes.
- Stairwalking for 15 minutes.

Source: Physical Activity and Health: A Report of the Surgeon General, 1996.

As you study the information in this book on achieving wellness, the following personalized approach may be helpful:

- If you're smoking now, determine how you are going to stop. Find out what community resources are available to help you. If you need to, talk to your doctor. Outline a specific course of action that will work for you.
- If you have a drinking problem or a drug dependency, find out specifically where you can get help. Make an appointment. Follow through. Start by figuring out why you started using drugs or alcohol to begin with. Your personal motives have a lot to do with your ability to kick the habit.
- If you have a weight problem, start your lifetime weight management program using the contents of Chapter 10. With guidance from your instructor or another health care professional, determine specifically how you are going to change your eating and exercise habits so you can lose weight safely and permanently.
- Increase your level of physical activity—up to 90 minutes a day if necessary (see Chapter 10). Before you do, however, take a critical look at your situation and determine whether you need a doctor's okay. If you do, schedule an appointment for a thorough physical examination, discuss your objectives with your physician, and get the go-ahead for a safe, effective fitness

program. Then design a program that works for you, based on your situation and preferences.

- Pinpoint your individual sources of stress. You probably can eliminate some of them. You can respond to others differently. If you have a particularly difficult class, for example, get on top of things by scheduling an extra hour every day to study that subject or talk to the professor about getting individualized help from a teaching assistant. Stress has a major influence on disease. A wellness plan demands that you handle stress with determination and commitment.

At the end of this chapter you will find a Health Assessment and a Wellness and Longevity Potential Test (Assessments 1.1 and 1.2). These two assessments will help you determine how well you are living your life and can help you identify areas in which you can make improvements. Keep in mind that at the center of wellness is self-responsibility. No one else can make you eat better, exercise more regularly, stop smoking, use alcohol in moderation, or cope with stress. Accepting the challenge

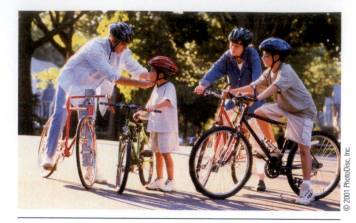

Objectives for enhancing health and wellness are aimed at protection, promotion, and prevention.

to achieve wellness implies that you are willing to make lifelong changes in your lifestyle. Wellness doesn't happen in a day. It involves an ongoing process of healthy choices throughout the rest of your life.

WEB Interactive

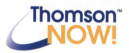

Don't forget to check out the wealth of resources on the ThomsonNOW website at **www.thomsonedu.com/ ThomsonNOW** that will:

- Coach you through identifying target goals for behavior change and monitoring your personal change plan throughout the semester
- Help you evaluate your knowledge of the material
- Allow you to take an exam-prep quiz
- Provide a Personalized Learning Plan targeting resources that address areas you should study.

WEB ACTIVITIES

Healthy People 2010 Healthy People is a national health promotion and disease prevention initiative that lists a series of goals for improving health of all Americans by the year 2010.

http://www.health.gov/healthypeople

Mayo Clinic Online This comprehensive consumer site, sponsored by the renowned Mayo Clinic, features the following: current health topics, diseases and conditions "A to Z," condition centers (comprehensive resources for cancer, heart disease, and other medical conditions), healthy living centers (practical advice about nutrition, fitness, women's health, men's health, family life, and other topics), "Take Charge of Your Health" (personal health scorecard, healthy lifestyle planners, disease self-management, and health decision guides), drug information, and first-aid and self-care guides.

http://www.mayohealth.org

Healthy Lifestyle Quiz All of us want good health, but many of us do not know how to be as healthy as possible. Health experts now describe lifestyle as one of the most important factors

affecting health. It is estimated that as many as 7 of the 10 leading causes of death could be reduced through commonsense changes in lifestyle. Take this quiz to determine which habits to change!

http://www.rochester.edu/uhs/healthtopics/GeneralHealth/ lifestylequiz.html

Self-Care Flow Charts This excellent, patient-friendly site, sponsored by the *American Family Physician* journal, features a comprehensive list of symptoms and flowcharts to help you seek out the most appropriate type of medical care at the most appropriate time (based on urgency). Some of the symptoms listed include abdominal pain (acute and chronic), chest pain, headaches, fever in adults and children, cold and flu, cough, diarrhea, sore throat, eye problems, foot problems, tooth problems, and lots more.

http://familydoctor.org/symptom.xml

InfoTrac®

You can find additional readings related to wellness via InfoTrac® College Edition, an online library of more than 900 journals and publications. Follow the instructions for accessing InfoTrac® that came packaged with your textbook, then search for articles using a key word search.

Suggested Reading Healthy doctors, healthy communities. (Healthy People 2010) by Donna Cameron: Ellen Katch; Patricia Anderson; Mary A. Furlong. *The Journal of Ambulatory Care Management*, Oct–Dec 2004 v27 i4 p328 (11).

1. What health behaviors typically characterize medical students?
2. Why did the American Medical Student Association (AMSA) initiate the Train the Trainer program designed to promote student wellness in medical schools nationwide?

3. Describe three evaluation and assessment techniques presented by the authors.
4. What are the Multidimensional Model of Wellness and the Stages of Change Model as described in the medical students' course experiences?

Web Activity

Live Well Personal Wellness Assessment

http://wellness.uwsp.edu/Other/livewell/index.htm

Sponsor University of Wisconsin—Stevens Point

Description This colorful and comprehensive site features 100 multiple-choice self-assessment questions encompassing 10 dimensions of wellness. The site analyzes your overall state of health based on your composite score using a percentage scale for excellent, good, average, fair, and poor.

Available Activity

1. Take the self-assessment, which contains 10 lifestyle questions in each of the following 10 wellness dimensions: physical fitness, nutrition, self-care, drugs and driving, social environment, intellectual, occupational, spiritual, emotional awareness, and emotional control.

Web Work

1. From the University of Wisconsin–Stevens Point home page, click the Services tab.
2. You will see a list of three interactive programs. Click on Live Well.
3. Honestly answer all of the 10 multiple-choice questions describing your lifestyle, beliefs, and behaviors in each of the ten categories of wellness.

Helpful Hint

After answering all questions, click on the "Evaluate" button to receive your personalized results.

For additional Web activities, links, and suggested readings, visit our Health, Fitness, and Wellness Resource Center at http://health.wadsworth.com.

Notes

1. U.S. Department of Health and Human Services, Centers for Disease Control and Prevention, National Center for Health Statistics, National Vital Statistics Reports: *Deaths, Preliminary Data for 2003* (February 28, 2005) 53:15.
2. World Health Organization, Ch-1211 Geneva 27, Switzerland; Donald Ardell, *The History and Future of Wellness* (Dubuque, IA: Kendall Hunt, 1985).
3. Robert Moats Miller, *Preacher, Pastor, Prophet* (New York: Oxford University Press, 1988).
4. Norman Cousins, *Head First: The Biology of Hope* (New York: E. P. Dutton, 1989).
5. Bernie Siegel, *The Complete Book of Cancer Prevention* (Emmaus, PA: Rodale Press, 1986).
6. James Hardison, *Let's Touch: How and Why To Do It* (Englewood Cliffs, NJ: Prentice Hall, 1980).
7. Television Bureau of Advertising website, "Time Spent Viewing Per TV Home: Per Day Annual Averages," available at http://www.tvb.org/nav/build_frameset.asp?url=/rcentral/index.asp, accessed March 26, 2005.
8. S. Gerrior, L. Bente, and H. Hiza, "Nutrient Content of the U.S. Food Supply, 1909–2000," *Home Economics Research Report No. 56* (Washington, DC: U.S. Department of Agriculture, Center for Nutrition Policy and Promotion, 2004): 74 (Available online at http://www.usda.gov/cnpp/nutrient_content.html, accessed April 18, 2005).
9. Marion Nestle, *Food Politics,* (Berkeley: University of California Press, 2002), 1, 8, 22.
10. National Academy of Sciences, Institute of Medicine, *Dietary Reference Intakes for Energy, Carbohydrates, Fiber, Fat, Protein and Amino Acids (Macronutrients)* (Washington, DC: National Academy Press, 2002).
11. U.S. Department of Health and Human Services, Department of Agriculture, *Dietary Guidelines for Americans 2005* (Washington, DC: Government Printing Office, 2005).

Assess Your Behavior

1. Are you aware of family health history and lifestyle factors that may negatively impact your health?
2. Do you accumulate at least 30 minutes of moderate-intensity physical activity on most days of the week?
3. Do you make a constant and deliberate effort to stay healthy and achieve the highest potential for well-being?

Evaluate how well you understand the concepts presented in this chapter by answering the following questions.

1. Scientific advances during the last century have led to
   a. an increased rate of chronic diseases.
   b. an increase in daily physical activity.
   c. a higher rate of infectious diseases.
   d. a reduction in health care costs.
   e. All of the choices are correct.

2. Healthy life expectancy
   a. in the U. S. exceeds that of all other countries in the world.
   b. is calculated by subtracting years of ill health from total life expectancy.
   c. is determined according to the health-related components of fitness.
   d. in the U. S. is so good because we do a good job keeping people healthy in the first place.
   e. All of the choices are correct.

3. The leading cause of death in the United States is
   a. cancer.
   b. accidents.
   c. COPD.
   d. diseases of the cardiovascular system.
   e. drug-related deaths.

4. Which of the following is not a dimension of wellness?
   a. physical
   b. emotional
   c. health
   d. environmental
   e. occupational

5. Wellness living requires
   a. responsibility on the individual.
   b. self evaluation.
   c. self assessment.
   d. continuous learning.
   e. all of the above.

6. Among the benefits of regular physical activity and exercise are significantly reduced risks for developing or dying from
   a. heart disease.
   b. diabetes.
   c. colon cancer.
   d. high blood pressure.
   e. All of the above are correct choices.

7. The state in which your mind is engaged in lively interaction with the world around you is known as
   a. physical wellness.
   b. social wellness.
   c. emotional wellness.
   d. occupational wellness.
   e. mental wellness.

8. Emotional wellness incorporates
   a. a genuine sense of curiosity.
   b. a state of happiness that stems from powerful inner contentment.
   c. a high level of physical coordination.
   d. tolerance and respect for others.
   e. faith and optimism to sustain us throughout life.

9. Moderate-intensity physical activity
   a. requires an energy expenditure of 150 calories per day.
   b. helps to maintain a high quality of life into old age.
   c. provides substantial health benefits to inactive individuals.
   d. should be conducted for at least 30 minutes on most days of the week.
   e. All of the above are correct choices.

10. The National Academy of Sciences recommends that people attain
    a. 30 minutes of moderate-intensity physical activity every day.
    b. 20 to 30 minutes of activity in the appropriate target zone 3 to 5 days per week.
    c. 60 minutes of moderate-intensity physical activity every day.
    d. 30 minutes of vigorous-intensity activity 3 days per week.
    e. 60 to 90 minutes of daily activity.

Correct answers can be found on page 369.

Health Assessment

Name: _____ **Date:** _____ **Grade:** _____

Instructor: _____ **Course:** _____ **Section:** _____

Assessing mental health and stress is a complex task and difficult to do in limited space. The following assessment instruments represent a sampling of stress and mental-health indicators.

Self-Esteem Assessment

Write *a* in front of each statement that describes you and *b* in front of each statement that does not describe you.

____ **1.** People generally like me.
____ **2.** I am comfortable talking in class.
____ **3.** I like to do new things.
____ **4.** I give in easily.
____ **5.** I'm a failure.
____ **6.** I'm shy.
____ **7.** I have trouble making up my mind.
____ **8.** I'm popular with people at school.
____ **9.** My life is all mixed up.
____ **10.** I often feel upset in my home, room, or apartment.
____ **11.** I often wish I were like someone else.
____ **12.** I often worry.
____ **13.** I can be depended on.
____ **14.** I often express my views.
____ **15.** I think I am doing okay with my life.
____ **16.** I feel good about what I have accomplished recently.

Scoring/Interpretation

Determine how many matches you have with the following key. Total that number.

1. a	4. b	7. b	10. b	13. a	16. a
2. a	5. b	8. a	11. b	14. a	
3. a	6. b	9. b	12. b	15. a	

From the total number of matched, interpret as follows:

12–16 high self-esteem
8–11 moderately high self-esteem
4–7 moderately low self-esteem
0–3 low self-esteem

Depression Assessment

Indicate which of the following reflect what you do or how you feel. Indicate by marking an *X* in the space provided if it is like you.

____ **1.** I use drugs to relax or have fun.
____ **2.** I need to see a professional about how sad I feel.
____ **3.** I have trouble making it to class.
____ **4.** I think I would be better off dead.
____ **5.** My life seems hopeless.
____ **6.** I have thought through how I would kill myself.
____ **7.** People around me would be better off if I were gone.
____ **8.** I change my moods often.
____ **9.** I'm not interested in much anymore.
____ **10.** I can't seem to concentrate.
____ **11.** I feel unloved and unwanted.
____ **12.** I have a quick temper.
____ **13.** I feel guilty.
____ **14.** I take things too hard.
____ **15.** I have been thinking a lot about death lately.

Scoring/Interpretation

If you have marked number 2, 4, 5, 6, 7, or 11, you should talk with someone right away about your feelings and needs. You may want to talk to your instructor about where to go for help.

If you have marked any of the other responses (number 1, 3, or 8–13) in conjunction with number 15, then you should also talk with someone about how you feel.

If you have marked three or more of the remaining statements (number 1, 3, or 8–13), you also may want to seek help.

Assertiveness Assessment

Indicate what you would do in the following situations by circling *a*, *b*, or *c*.

1. A professor gives you a grade that is lower than you had expected.
  a. Ask the professor to recalculate the grade because you feel he or she is in error.
  b. Complain to the professor but accept the grade.
  c. Say nothing.

2. In a cafeteria line after waiting some time to get something to eat, a group of people recognize the person in front of you and crowd in line.
  a. Ask them to please move to the back of the line and wait like everyone else.
  b. Make a comment but not ask them to move back.
  c. Say nothing.

3. Someone near you is smoking in a nonsmoking section.
  a. Ask him or her to notice the no smoking sign and please put out the cigarette.
  b. Make a comment like, "Can't you read?" but don't ask him or her to put it out.
  c. Say nothing.

4. You have waited for ten minutes at a department secretary's office to get course information, and she is obviously making a personal call.
  a. Get her attention and say, "Can you help me?"
  b. Sigh heavily and give frustrated looks.
  c. Wait patiently.

Scoring/Interpretation

Assign the following number of points to each of your answers. Total your points.

    a = 4   b = 2   c = 0

Interpret as follows:

12–16 assertive
6–11 moderately assertive
0–6 unassertive

Stress Index

To identify the types and degrees of stress you are experiencing, complete the following index. Circle the number that corresponds to your reaction to each statement. Total the numbers in each column and add them to arrive at a subtotal for each section.

	Always	Often	Sometimes	Rarely	Never
1. I get upset when I have to wait in lines.	5	4	3	2	1
2. I work by the clock to see how much I can get done in a short time.	5	4	3	2	1
3. I get upset if something takes too long.	5	4	3	2	1
4. I make almost every activity I do competitive with myself or others.	5	4	3	2	1
5. I feel guilty when I'm not working on something.	5	4	3	2	1
Section subtotal					
6. I get upset when I can't do something my way.	5	4	3	2	1
7. I get upset when my accomplishments depend on others' actions.	5	4	3	2	1
8. I get anxious when my plans become disrupted.	5	4	3	2	1
9. All good things are worth waiting for.	1	2	3	4	5
10. When I set a goal I can't reach, I simply alter it.	1	2	3	4	5
Section subtotal					
11. I have been given too much responsibility.	5	4	3	2	1
12. I get depressed when I think of everything I have to do.	5	4	3	2	1
13. People demand too much of me.	5	4	3	2	1
14. I often find myself without enough time to complete my work.	5	4	3	2	1
15. Sometimes I feel that my head is spinning, or I get confused because so much is happening.	5	4	3	2	1
Section subtotal					
16. I succeed in most things and try even when the task is difficult.	1	2	3	4	5
17. I am comfortable being with members of the opposite sex.	1	2	3	4	5
18. I am generally comfortable around teachers, bosses, and other superiors.	1	2	3	4	5
19. I prefer that others make decisions for me.	5	4	3	2	1
20. I don't think I have too much going for me.	5	4	3	2	1
21. I'm most relaxed when I'm busy.	5	4	3	2	1
22. I throw away old clothes, toys, and other mementos.	1	2	3	4	5
23. I enjoy being alone.	1	2	3	4	5
24. I feel the need to belong to a social group.	5	4	3	2	1
25. I get homesick easily.	5	4	3	2	1
Section subtotal					
26. I often feel my stomach knotting, my mouth getting dry, and my heart pounding when I get nervous.	5	4	3	2	1
27. When I get nervous, I can feel my muscles tense, my hands and fingers shake, and my voice become unsteady.	5	4	3	2	1
28. After a crisis I relive the experience over and over in my mind, even though it is resolved.	5	4	3	2	1
29. I know I must resolve a crisis or it will bother me for a long time.	5	4	3	2	1
30. When I'm nervous, I imagine the worst possible outcomes of the original crisis.	5	4	3	2	1
Section subtotal					
TOTAL =					

Scoring/Interpretation

By summing all the subtotals on the index, you estimate your overall susceptibility to stress based on social situation and personality. Interpret your score as follows:

100 or higher – High stress   **50–99** – Moderate stress   **49 or below** – You are doing well for now; keep it up.

The Wellness and Longevity Potential Test

Name: _____ Date: _____ Grade: _____

Instructor: _____ Course: _____ Section: _____

Changeable Lifestyle Factors

1. Tobacco

(1 pipe = 2 cigarettes, 1 cigar = 3 cigarettes)

Never smoked	+20	
Quit smoking	+10	
Smoke up to one pack per day		−10
Smoke one to two packs per day		−20
Smoke more than two packs per day		−30

Pack-years smoked (number of packs smoked per day, times number of years smoked):

7–15	−5
16–25	−10
Over 25	−20

2. Alcohol

(1 beer or 1 glass of wine = 1.25 oz. alcohol)

1.25 oz. per day or less	+10	
Between 1.25 and 2.5 oz. per day		−4
−1 more for each additional 1.25 oz. per day		−___

3. Exercise

(20 min. or more moderate aerobic exercise)

3 or more times per week	+20	
2 times per week	+10	
No regular aerobic activity		−10
Work requires regular physical exertion or at least 2 miles walking per day	+3	
+1 more for each additional mile walked per day	+ ___	

4. Weight

Maintain recommended weight for height	+5	
5–10 lbs. over recommended		−1
11–20 lbs. over recommended		−2
21–30 lbs. over recommended		−3
−1 more for each additional 10 lbs.		−___
Yo-yo dieting		−10

5. Nutrition

Eat a well-balanced diet	+3	
Do not eat a well-balanced diet		−3
Regularly eat meals at consistent times	+2	
Do not regularly eat meals at consistent times		−2
Snack or eat meals late at night		−2
Eat a balanced breakfast	+2	
Eat fish or poultry as primary protein source (totally replacing red meat)	+5	
Do not eat grains and fish as primary protein source		−2
Eat at least 5 servings of green leafy vegetables per week	+3	
Eat at least 5 servings of fresh fruit or juice per day	+3	
Try to avoid fats	+5	
Do not try to avoid fats		−5

For each of the following foods eaten 2 or more times per week:

Beef, veal, or pork	−1
Bacon or sausage	−1
Luncheon meat or hot dogs	−1
Fast food	−1
Fried food	−1
Processed food/TV dinners	−1
Eggs	−1
Cheese	−1
Butter	−1
Whole milk or cream	−1
Pastries, doughnuts, muffins	−1
Candy, chocolate	−1
Pretzels, potato chips	−1
Ice cream	−1

Eat some food every day that is high in fiber (whole-grain bread, fresh fruits and vegetables)	+3	
Do not eat some food every day that is high in fiber		−3
Take a daily multivitamin/mineral supplement	+10	
Women: Take a calcium supplement	+5	
Subscribe to health-related periodicals	+2	

	A	G
Subtotal:		

Fixed Factors

1. Gender

Male		−5
Female	+10	

2. Heredity

Any grandparent lived to be over 80	+5

This test was developed for the average healthy person. If you already have a serious health condition, such as heart disease, diabetes, cancer, or kidney disease, ask your physician for a health-risk assessment designed especially for you.

Reproduced by permission of *Longevity,* © 1990, Longevity International, Ltd.

Average age all four grandparents lived to:

60–70	+5
71–80	+10
Over 80	+20

3. Family history

Either parent had stroke or heart
attack before age 50 —10

–5 for each family member (grandparent,
parent, sibling) who prior to age 65
has had any of the following:

Hypertension	–___
Cancer	–___
Heart disease	–___
Stroke	–___
Diabetes	–___
Other genetic diseases	–___

Subtotal B: ___ + ___

Partially Fixed Factors

1. Family income

0–$5,000	–10
$5,001–$14,000	–5
$14,001–$20,000	+1

+1 for each additional $10,000,
up to $200,000 + ___

2. Education

Some high school (or less)	–7
High school graduate	+2
College graduate	+5
Postgraduate or professional degree	+7

3. Occupation

Professional	+5
Self-employed	+6
In the health-care field	+3
Over 65 and still working	+5
Clerical or support	–3
Shift work	–5
Unemployed	–7
Possibility for career advancement	+5
Regularly in direct contact with pollutants, toxic waste, chemicals, radiation	–10

4. Where you live

Large urban area	–5
Near an industrial center	–7
Rural or farm area	+5
Area with air-pollution alerts	–5
Area where air pollution has curtailed normal daily activities	–7
High crime area	–3
Little or no crime area	+3
Home has tested positive for radon	–7

Total commuting time to and from work:

0–1/2 hour	+3
1/2 hour–1 hour	+0
–1 for each 1/2 hour over 1 hour	–___
Within 30 miles of major medical/trauma center	+3
No major medical/trauma center in area	–3

Subtotal C: ___ + ___

Changeable Health Status and Maintenance Factors

1. Health status

- Present overall physical health:

Excellent	+15
Good	+12
Fair	+5
Poor	–10

Normal or low blood pressure	+5
High blood pressure	–10
Don't know	–5

Low cholesterol (under 200)	+10
Moderate cholesterol (200–240)	+5
High cholesterol (over 240)	–10
Don't know	–5

HDL cholesterol 29 or less	–25
30–36	–20
37–40	–5
41–45	+5
Over 45	+10
Don't know	–5

Have medical insurance coverage	+10
Able to use physicians of your choice	+5

2. Preventive and therapeutic measures

Physical exams (every 3 to 4 years
before age 50, every 1 to 2 years
over 50) +3

Women:

Yearly gynecological exam and Pap smear	+2
Monthly self breast exam	+2
Mammogram (35–50, every 3 years; over 50, every year)	+2
Smoke and use oral contraceptives	–5

Men:

Genital self-exam every 3 months	+2
Rectal or prostate exam (yearly after age 30)	+2

All:

Current on mumps, measles, rubella, diphtheria and tetanus immunizations	+2
Tested for hidden blood in stool (over 40, every 2 years; over 50, every year)	+2

If over age 50:

    Yearly sigmoidoscopy of the
        lower bowel   +2

All:

    Regularly use sunscreen and avoid
        excessive sun   +2

    Actively involved in a life-extension,
        prevention, or comprehensive
        wellness program   +10

3. Accident control

Always wear seatbelt as driver and
    passenger   +7

Do not always wear seatbelt as driver
    and passenger   −5

Never drink and drive or ride with a driver
    who has been drinking   +2

−10 for each arrest for drinking while
    under the influence of alcohol in the
    past 5 years   −___

−2 for every speeding ticket or accident in
    the past year   −___

For each 12,000 miles per year driven
    over 12,000 (national average)   −1

Primary car weighs more than 3,500 lbs.   +10

Subcompact   −5

Motorcycle   −10

−2 for every fight or attack you were
    involved in, or witness to, in the
    past year   −___

Smoke alarms in home   +1

    Subtotal D: ___ + ___

Changeable Psychosocial Factors

Married or in long-term committed
    relationship   +5

Satisfying sex life   +3

Children under 18 living at home   +3

For each 5-year period living alone   −1

No close friends   −10

+1 for each close friend (up to 5)   +___

+2 for each active membership in a
    religious community or volunteer
    organization (up to 4)   +___

Have a pet   +2

Regular daily routine   +10

No regular daily routine   −10

Hours of uninterrupted sleep per night:

    Less than 5 hours   −5

    5–8 hours   +5

    8–10 hours   −7

−1 for each additional hour over 10   −___

Not consistent   −7

Regular work routine   +5

No regular work routine   −5

−2 for every 5 hours worked over
    40 in a week   −___

Take a yearly vacation from work
    (at least 6 days)   +5

Regularly use a stress-management
    technique (yoga, meditation, music, etc.)   +3

    Subtotal E: ___ + ___

Changeable Emotional Stress Factors

N = Never   **R** = Rarely   **S** = Sometimes
A = Always (or as much as possible)

	N	R	S	A
Generally happy	−2	−1	+1	+2
Have and enjoy time with family and friends	−2	−1	+1	+2
Feel in control of personal life and career	−2	−1	+1	+2
Live within financial means	−2	−1	+1	+2
Set goals and look for new challenges	−2	−1	+1	+2
Participate in creative outlet or hobby	−2	−1	+1	+2
Have and enjoy leisure time	−2	−1	+1	+2
Express feelings easily	−2	−1	+1	+2
Laugh easily	−2	−1	+1	+2
Expect good things to happen	−2	−1	+1	+2

	A	S	R	N
Anger easily	−2	−1	+1	+2
Critical of self	−2	−1	+1	+2
Critical of others	−2	−1	+1	+2
Lonely, even with others	−2	−1	+1	+2
Worry about things out of your control	−2	−1	+1	+2
Regret sacrifices made in life	−2	−1	+1	+2

    Subtotal F: ___ + ___ + ___ + ___

    Scoring

    A + B + C + D + E + F = _____

    (Subtotal, up to 200*)

    Subtotal + G = Total

    Divide total by 2. This gives your chance
    (in %) of living to or beyond average life
    expectancy of a person your age.

        Total: _____ ÷ 2 =

        _____ %

---

* If this number is higher than 200, use 200 as your subtotal. Maintain those healthy habits that allowed you to score much higher than the average person (around 50%) and try to turn any of the negatives in section G (e.g., smoking) into positives. You have the very best chance of living a long and healthy life, because these factors are totally in your control.

— Linda Addlespurger

If you scored 100%, congratulations. But don't rest on your laurels. Keep looking for ways to improve your good health. And if you didn't score as well as you would have liked, it's never too late to begin improving your longevity potential.

Interpretation and Conclusions

Based on the results of Assessments 1.1 and 1.2, indicate what you have learned about how your lifestyle habits are affecting your health and wellness. Do you feel that these assessments provide an accurate analysis of your lifestyle habits?

_____
_____
_____
_____
_____
_____
_____
_____
_____
_____
_____

Please identify areas where you feel you can make improvements in your daily living habits that will be conducive to better health and wellness.

_____
_____
_____
_____
_____
_____
_____
_____
_____
_____
_____

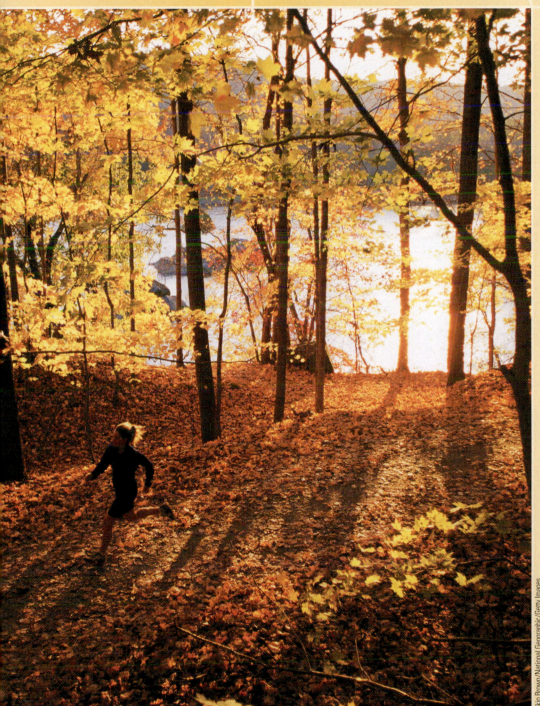

2

CHAPTER

The Mind-Body Connection

OBJECTIVES

Identify some physiological manifestations of emotions.

Define psychoneuroimmunology and explain the links among the mind, the brain, and the immune system.

Identify the connection between personality and disease.

Describe the characteristics of the coronary-prone personality.

Define the relaxed, cancer-prone, and distressed personalities.

Explain the differences between anger and hostility and the health effects of each.

Discuss the health effects of depression.

List the warning signs of suicide and know what to do to help someone who is considering suicide.

List the stages in the grief process.

Explain the "three C's of hardiness.

Virtually every illness known to modern humanity—from arthritis to migraine headaches, from the common cold to cancer—is influenced for good or bad by our emotions. Emotions affect our susceptibility to disease and our **immunity,** influencing our likelihood of recovering from illness, as well as whether we become ill in the first place. The feelings we have and the way we express them can either boost our immune system or weaken it.

Emotional health is a dimension of wellness with both indirect and direct ties to the physical health dimension. Indirectly, most emotionally healthy people take care of themselves physically—eating well, exercising, and getting enough rest. They strive to develop supportive personal relationships. By contrast, many people who are emotionally unhealthy are self-destructive. Typical self-destructive behaviors are abuse of alcohol and other drugs. Or people may overwork, reflecting an imbalance in their lives.

Emotional health affects what we do, who we meet, who we marry, how we look, how we feel, the course of our lives, and even how long we live. And emotions cause physiological responses that can influence health. Certain parts of the brain are associated with specific emotions and specific hormone patterns. The release of specific hormones is associated with various emotional responses. Those hormones affect health and may contribute to the development of disease.[1]

Negative physiological responses to emotion may weaken the immune system over time. The wide range of resulting conditions includes allergies, asthma, angina, heart disease, high blood pressure, arthritis, back pain, cancer, dental cavities, diabetes, gastric ulcers, insomnia, irritable bowel syndrome, and a variety of skin problems.

Emotions have to be expressed somewhere, somehow. If they are suppressed repeatedly, or if individuals don't express them appropriately, emotions can reveal themselves through physical symptoms. As an exercise to see if you cultivate emotional well-being, Assessment 2.1 is provided at the end of the chapter.

The Science of Psychoneuroimmunology

The scientific investigation of how the brain affects the body's immune cells and how behavior can affect the immune system is called **psychoneuroimmunology**. Psychoneuroimmunology focuses on the links among the mind, the brain, and the immune system. As a science, it has received the endorsement of the National Institutes of Health. Research indicates the following effects, among others, of the mind–body connection:[2]

- Positive emotions can help protect the heart.
- Among people with heart disease, pessimism can be deadly, but a healthy outlook promotes healing.
- Remaining calm during emotional conflict reduces the risk of heart attack.

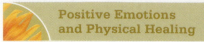

Positive Emotions and Physical Healing

The late Norman Cousins, former editor of the *Saturday Review* and member of the UCLA medical faculty, twice intrigued the medical community and the larger public by overcoming usually fatal conditions—once a massive heart attack and another time an advanced case of a degenerative spinal disease. Cousins followed his physicians' regimens each time and also infused himself with vast doses of positive emotions and laughter. According to Cousins himself, he was healed not only by the miracle of modern medicine but also by the healing emotions of love, hope, faith, confidence, and a tremendous will to live.

- Anxiety and suppressed anger increase the risk for premature death, as does depression.

Research in this field is booming, and a number of medical schools have integrated psychoneuroimmunology into their curricula. Almost every important conference on immunology includes seminars on the relationship between the brain and the immune system, and an increasing number of physicians acknowledge that the way a patient thinks and feels can be a powerful determinant of physical health.

THE BRAIN

The brain is a privileged organ. The heart supplies the brain with blood; the lungs supply it with oxygen; the intestines supply it with nutrients; and the kidneys remove poisons from its environment. The brain is the most important part of the nervous system. For the body to survive, the brain must be nurtured. When the entire body is under severe stress, all other organs sacrifice to keep the brain alive and functioning.

Major functions of the brain are as follows:

- The brain directs nerve impulses to be carried throughout the body.
- The brain controls *voluntary* processes, such as the direction, strength, and coordination of muscle movements and the processes involved in smelling, touching, and seeing.
- The brain controls *involuntary* or *automatic* functions over which you have no conscious control. Among these are breathing, heart rate, digestion, control of the bowels and bladder, blood pressure, and release of hormones. The voluntary and involuntary functions are illustrated in Figure 2.1.
- The brain is the cognitive center of the body, the place where ideas are generated, memory is stored, and emotions are experienced.
- The brain provides a powerful and complex link between the emotions and the immune system. The emotions generated in the brain produce physical responses, including effects on the immune system.

FIGURE 2.1 Voluntary and Involuntary Processes Controlled By the Brain

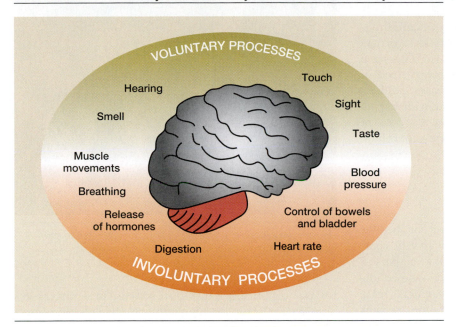

VOLUNTARY PROCESSES

Hearing

Touch

Smell

Sight

Taste

Muscle movements

Blood pressure

Breathing

Release of hormones

Control of bowels and bladder

Digestion

Heart rate

INVOLUNTARY PROCESSES

Critical Thinking

Now that you understand the concept of psychoneuroimmunology, describe the connections between the mind, the brain, your emotions and your immune system.

Personality and Health

Personality is the total physical, intellectual, and emotional structure of an individual, including abilities, interests, and attitudes. Personality is the manifestation of your habits, attitudes, and traits that combine to make the person that is uniquely you. In keeping with your personality, you act in a similar way from one day to the next, and when you are placed in various situations, you still tend to act in a generally consistent way. Your personality, in essence, is the pattern of behavior that distinguishes you from everybody else. Personality depends partly on biology and genetics (the unique set of genes you inherited from your parents) but also is greatly affected by the family you grow up in, the environment that surrounds you, and the culture and subcultures that influence you.

The theory that personality affects health is, as world-renowned psychologist Hans Eysenck put it, a theory based on centuries of observations made by keen-eyed physicians.[3] The notion that a certain personality type leads to heart disease dates back more than 2,000 years to Hippocrates, and the belief that a certain personality is associated with cancer goes back several centuries, and much current scientific research substantiates these notions.[4]

This is not to say that people always bring illness on themselves. This viewpoint may lead to inhumanity and a lack of compassion for people who need it the most.

THE IMMUNE SYSTEM

The brain's natural chemicals form literal communication links among the brain, its thought processes, and the cells of the body, including those of the immune system. The immune system patrols and guards the body against attackers. This system consists of about a trillion cells called **lymphocytes** and about a hundred million trillion molecules called **antibodies**. The brain and the immune system are closely linked in a connection that allows the mind to influence both susceptibility and resistance to disease.

A number of immune system cells—including those in the thymus gland, spleen, bone marrow, and lymph nodes—are laced with nerve cells. Cells of the immune system are equipped to respond to chemical signals from the central nervous system. For example, the surface of the lymphocytes contains receptors for a variety of central nervous system chemical messengers, such as catecholamines, prostaglandins, serotonin, endorphins, sex hormones, the thyroid hormone, and the growth hormone. Certain white blood cells have the ability to receive messages from the brain.

Receptors on lymphocytes allow physical and psychological stress to alter the immune system. (Chapter 3 addresses the topic of stress.) Stress causes the body to release several powerful neurohormones that bind with these receptors and suppress immune function. Corticosteroids, for example, have been found to be such powerful suppressors of the immune system that they are used widely to treat allergic conditions (such as asthma and hayfever) and **autoimmune disorders** (such as rheumatoid arthritis and rejection of transplanted organs). Other brain chemicals unleashed by the hypothalamus have equally profound effects on the immune system.

Immunity The function that guards the body from invaders, both internal and external.

Psychoneuroimmunology (PNI) The scientific investigation of how the brain affects the body's immune cells and how the immune system can be affected by behavior.

Lymphocytes Specialized immune system cells.

Antibodies Substances produced by the white blood cells in response to an invading agent.

Autoimmune disorder A condition in which the immune system attacks the body.

Personality The whole of a person's behavioral characteristics.

Instead we can use this information to protect and preserve our health status.

People associate certain personalities with certain illnesses: Workaholics tend to have heart attacks. Worriers tend to get ulcers. People who get too uptight often have asthma attacks. In reality, can people be categorized so neatly? No. Yet, researchers have made tremendous strides in proving that personality does have an impact on health. They have found that the way we look at things, as determined by our personality, may contribute to illness or help keep us well.

PERSONALITY TYPES

Personality traits may be health-harming or health-enhancing.[5] Some researchers believe that a specific combination of personality traits may make a person susceptible to a general classification of disease conditions, not just a specific disease. Researchers have categorized people into broad personality types to help determine if a person is more likely to become ill or stay well. People in general are not exclusively one type but, instead, fluctuate between the traits of each personality.

The Coronary-Prone Personality (Type A) The most prominent in research is what has been labeled the **Type A** or **coronary-prone personality**.[5] This person is characterized by a hard-driving and competitive person who is also hostile, angry, and suspicious—all of which leads to aggressive, time-urgent, impatient behaviors and a hostile style of living. Although the Type A personality can result from a number of influences, including genetic and environmental factors, most prominent is a hostile, angry, nonsupportive family environment.

Type A has been dubbed the "hurry sickness." Type A personalities never seem to slow down. They[6]

- try to do two or more things simultaneously;
- have a sense of time-urgency;
- are impatient when waiting in lines or in traffic;
- are involved in car accidents more frequently than other personality types;
- are extremely competitive and tend to keep score in even trivial situations;
- are aggressive;
- make forceful, rapid, or "staccato" gestures;
- speak loudly and interrupt people;
- eat and walk rapidly;
- are insecure about their status;
- are hard-driving and ambitious;
- have a high need for achievement;
- have a high level of job involvement; and
- sometimes harbor an unconscious drive to self-destruct.

These traits add up to joyless striving. The Type A personality is in a chronic state of vigilant observation.

In the physical manifestations of a Type A person, the hormones (particularly epinephrine and cortisol) are

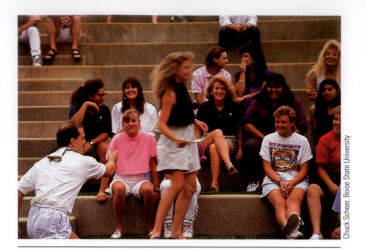

Research suggests that personality may play a role in health and wellness.

Chuck Scheer, Boise State University

released continually, causing an increase in serum cholesterol and fat levels, leaching of blood platelets, overworking of the heart and arteries, excessive insulin secretion, and suppression of the immune system. Type A behavior also is associated with calcification of the arteries,[7] resulting in a higher risk for heart disease. If a person with Type A personality also exhibits two other risk factors for heart disease (such as cigarette smoking and high blood pressure), that person's risk for developing coronary heart disease is even greater.

The traits that are most predictive of coronary disease are said to be anger, cynicism, suspiciousness, and excessive self-involvement.[8] Probably the most detrimental trait of the **toxic core** is continuous hostility, a continuous state of anger that hovers quietly until some trivial incident causes it to erupt.

Fortunately, Type A behavior can be modified to reduce the risk for disease. A group of Type A insurance representatives participated in behavior therapy targeted at reducing the negative effects of Type A actions. The therapy was shown to significantly reduce the intensity of Type A behavior and in particular the element of time-urgency.[9]

Apparently a person can have many of the characteristics typically associated with Type A personality—such as competitive drive, an ambitious personality, and time urgency—without running the risks of a heart attack as long as the person is not hostile. The hostility component, which includes anger directed outward, frequent angry outbursts, and explosive responses, is a more accurate predictor of coronary heart disease than the more general notion of Type A behavior.[10]

Fortunately, not all components of the Type A personality are harmful to health. Some people do not have to slow down—as long as they are not driven by hostility. Those who have many of the Type A traits without the toxic core that harms health and who are positive and enthusiastic possess characteristics that can be protective, not harmful.

- Make a contract with yourself to slow down and take it easy. Put it in writing and post it in a conspicuous spot, then stick to the terms you set up. Be specific. Abstracts such as "I'm going to be less uptight" don't work.
- Work on only one or two things at a time. Wait until you change one habit before you tackle the next one.
- Eat more slowly, and eat only when you are relaxed and sitting down.
- If you smoke, quit.
- Cut down on your caffeine intake, as it increases the tendency to become irritated and agitated.
- Take regular breaks throughout the day—even as brief as 5 or 10 minutes—when you totally change what you're doing. Get up, stretch, get a drink of cool water, and walk around for a few minutes.
- Fight impatience. If you're standing in line at the grocery store, study the interesting things people have in their carts instead of getting upset.
- Work on controlling hostility. Keep a written log. When do you flare up? What causes it? How do you feel at the time? What preceded it? Look for patterns and figure out what sets you off. Then do something about it. Either avoid the situations that cause you hostility or practice reacting to them in different ways.
- Plan some activities just for the fun of it. Load a picnic basket in the car and drive to the country with a friend. After a stressful physics class, stop at a theater and see a good comedy.
- Choose a role model, someone you know and admire who does not have a Type A personality. Observe the person carefully, then try some techniques the person demonstrates.

- Simplify your life so you can learn to relax a little bit. Figure out which activities or commitments you can eliminate right now, then get rid of them.
- If morning is a problem time for you and you get too hurried, set your alarm clock half an hour earlier to give you more time.
- Take time out during even the most hectic day to do something truly relaxing. Because you won't be used to it, you may have to work at it at first. Begin by listing things you'd really enjoy that would calm you. Include some things that take only a few minutes: Watch a sunset, lie out on the lawn at night and look at the stars, call an old friend and catch up on news, take a nap.
- If you're under a deadline, take short breaks. Stop and talk to someone for 5 minutes, take a short walk, or lie down with a cool cloth over your eyes for 10 minutes.
- Pay attention to what your own body clock is saying. You've probably noticed that every 90 minutes or so, you lose the ability to concentrate, get a little sleepy, and have a tendency to daydream. Instead of fighting the urge, put down your work and let your mind wander for a few minutes. Use the time to imagine and let your creativity run wild.
- Learn to treasure unplanned surprises: a friend dropping by unannounced, a hummingbird outside your window, a child's tightly clutched bouquet of wildflowers.
- Savor your relationships. Think about the people in your life. Relax with them and give yourself to them. Give up trying to control others, and resist the urge to end relationships that don't always go as you'd like them to.

The Relaxed Personality (Type B) The relaxed personality type called Type B is opposite from the Type A personality. The **Type B personality** is characterized as relaxed, easy-going, noncompetitive, and laid-back. Type B people have little hostility. They are not as driven as the Type A and do not strive as hard to reach goals. This personality type has been associated with low levels of heart disease. At the extreme, Type B individuals who lack goals and report boredom may be at risk for impaired health.

The Cancer-Prone Personality (Type C) Some research has suggested that a certain set of personality traits may dispose a person to cancer. Thus, this personality type has been called the **cancer-prone personality**. Also designated as the **Type C personality**, these people show little emotion and appear ambivalent toward self and others. They have been described as consistently serious, overly cooperative, overanxious, painfully sensitive, passive, and apologetic. Some cancer patients have been characterized as "too nice," displaying passivity about most things, including their cancers. In this area the findings are inconsistent.[11] Not every study has found a link between cancer and personality.[12]

Type A personality Sometimes referred to as "hurry sickness," a person who is hard-driving and competitive and also hostile, angry, and suspicious; also known as coronary-prone behavior.

Coronary-prone personality A hard-driving, competitive person who is also hostile, angry, suspicious, and at increased risk for heart attack; also known as Type A personality.

Toxic core Type A personality traits most detrimental to health: anger, cynicism, suspiciousness, and excessive self-involvement.

Type B personality Known as the relaxed personality; a person who is easy-going and generally free of hostility, anger, and suspicion.

Cancer-prone personality Also called the Type C personality; an emotionally unexpressive person who demonstrates ambivalence and is at increased risk for cancer; sometimes called Type C personality.

Type C personality Also called the cancer-prone personality; an emotionally unexpressive person who demonstrates ambivalence and is at increased risk for cancer.

Emotional States That Affect Health

Emotion has been defined as a felt tendency to move toward something assessed as favorable or away from something assessed as unfavorable. The terms "emotions" and "feelings" often are used interchangeably. These states are normal and healthy, but sometimes the way we handle our feelings is not healthy. Following is a discussion of some emotions, as well as some ways to handle them effectively.

ANGER

Anger usually is a temporary emotion that combines physiological and emotional arousal. It can range in severity all the way from intense rage to "cool" anger that doesn't really involve arousal at all (and might be defined more accurately as an "attitude," such as resentment). Although the terms "anger" and "hostility" (described next) are often used interchangeably, they are not the same. Among other differences, anger, unlike hostility, is a temporary emotion.

To be healthy, people have to express anger appropriately—that is, at the right time and in a nondestructive manner. We have to confront the things that are making us angry and to work through the anger. Problems arise when anger is misdirected, and when anger is expressed through miscommunication, emotional distancing, escalation of conflicts, rehearsing of grievances, assuming a hostile disposition, acquiring angry habits, making a bad situation worse, losing self-esteem, and losing the respect of others. Misdirected anger buries the real problem and creates more problems along the way.

Serious problems also result from suppressed anger. Bottling up anger can lead to many health consequences—among them, heart disease, cancer, rheumatoid arthritis, hives, acne, psoriasis, peptic ulcer, epilepsy, migraine, and high blood pressure. Expressing anger is healthy, but it must be done in a way that does not cause damage or harm.

Chronic repression of anger has physical effects similar to those of chronic stress (see Chapter 3). One of the major physiological effects is the release of chemicals and hormones, principally adrenaline and noradrenaline, which

The Distressed Personality (Type D) Another type of personality that may hasten mortality, the **Type D personality**, is also called the distressed personality because it is characterized by negative emotions and social inhibition. People who think negatively and isolate themselves from others have a greater risk for heart disease and are more prone to depression.[13]

The distressed personality has been associated with irritation of an existing disorder rather than a cause of disease.[14] This personality is characterized by excessive dependence on others, low levels of social support, excessive worry, annoyance, and fear of common situations or circumstances. Whereas other people are able to "bend" with stress, distressed people tend to "break."

People with this trait may experience the same number of stressful situations as others, but distressed people perceive the situations as being far more negative than do other people. Fortunately, people with Type D personalities can modify the unhealthy ways they deal with emotions and can learn to improve their social relations.[15]

- Recognize the anger for what it is. Don't be afraid of it or try to suppress it.
- Figure out what made you so angry, then decide whether it's worth being so upset. Chances are that it's really a minor irritation or hassle.
- Stop before you act. Calm down first. Count to 10, take a deep breath, mentally recite the words to a favorite verse, or initiate some other distracting and relaxing activity. Then get ready to deal with the anger.
- If you're ticked off at somebody else, use calm tact to say why, without ripping into the other person. Tell him or her how you're feeling, and try to negotiate a resolution.
- Be generous with the other person. Maybe he just failed an exam. Maybe she just heard bad news from home. Maybe he's having a rotten day. Listen carefully to her side of things and sincerely try to understand.
- When all else fails, forgive the other person. Everyone makes mistakes. Carrying a grudge will hurt you more than it hurts the other person.

Physiological Reactions Accompanying Anger

This list includes physiological reactions to momentary and chronic anger. Monitor yourself for these symptoms. If anger is not managed, you may experience the effects of chronic anger.

Momentary Anger

changes in muscle tension	lower skin temperature
scowling	excessive sweating
grinding teeth	skin redness
glaring	hives
clenching fists	itching
flushing	tension headache
goosebumps	migraine headache
chills/shudders	belching
prickly sensations	hiccupping
numbness	diarrhea
choking	intestinal cramping
twitching	
sweating	**Chronic Anger**
losing self-control	loss of appetite
feeling hot or cold	frequent colds
fatigue	acne
jaws clenching	peptic ulcers
neck or jaw pain	chronic indigestion
ringing in the ears	constipation

affect proper functioning of the heart and the amount of constriction or dilation of the arteries. This effect is a major contributor to arterial diseases.

Research also indicates a possible link between anger and cancer. The effect of anger on cancer may result from its effect on the immune system. Anger may lead to interactions among body systems that can lower immune functioning and resistance to disease.

HOSTILITY

Hostility comes from the Latin word *hostis*, which means "enemy." Simply stated, hostility is an ongoing accumulation of anger and irritation. It is a permanent kind of anger that shows itself in its response to trivial happenings. People experience real problems that warrant anger, but hostile people get equally angry about major injustices and trivia. Generally, a hostile person has an orientation toward hurting other people, either physically or verbally.

Hostility is characterized by anger, resentment, and suspicion. It is marked by explosive and vigorous vocal mannerisms, competitiveness, impatience, and irritability. Hostile people typically reveal the following characteristics:

- Even when they're smiling, they look uptight and tense; they appear ready to fight at a moment's notice.
- They have an intense need to win in sports and in games, even when other people are playing just for relaxation or fun.
- They are extremely sensitive to any perceived criticism against them and at the same time are loudly critical of others and of themselves.
- They argue incessantly, even over trivial issues. Every conversation becomes an angry debate, and they refuse to lose an argument.

Although almost everyone exhibits one or more of these traits occasionally, hostile people demonstrate them all the time. Life has become a sordid battle for them, and they charge into the fight armed with anger and irritation.

Type D personality A distressed personality characterized by negative emotions, social inhibition, and isolation.

Anger A feeling of extreme hostility, indignation, or exasperation; rage.

Hostility An ongoing accumulation of anger and irritation; a permanent, deep-seated type of anger that hovers quietly until some trivial incident causes it to erupt.

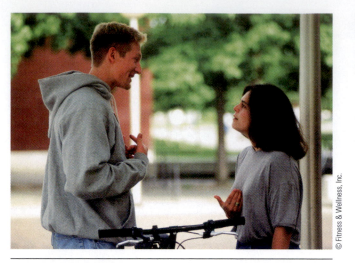

A person who is unable to manage anger is at particular risk for disease.

norepinephrine, cortisol, prolactin, and testosterone. These hormones cause blood pressure to increase, the heart to beat harder and faster, blood volume to increase, the blood to move from the skin and organs to the brain and muscles, the liver to release stored sugar, and breathing to speed up. Those reactions in themselves are not harmful if they happen only occasionally and if the body can use physical activity to dispel the hormones. With hostility, though, the body is not allowed to recover from the stress. Hostility disallows the body's built-in calming mechanism.

The autonomic nervous system has two main branches:

1. the "emergency branch," (the sympathetic branch), which pumps out hormones and prepares the body to respond in case of emergency, and
2. the "calming branch" (the parasympathetic branch), which switches off the hormones when the emergency is over. The calming branch soothes the body, preventing it from remaining in an aroused state too long, which can result in disease.

Because hostility weakens the parasympathetic (calming) branch of the nervous system, the body does not recover from the surge of stress hormones, does not calm down, and remains in a state of prolonged, harmful arousal.

Hostility is an independent risk factor for coronary heart disease. Hostility has been shown

• to cause coronary blockages, coronary heart disease, and coronary death;
• to contribute significantly to a second heart attack; and
• to lead to the premature death of people with existing heart disease.

Hostility also is a significant factor in determining which heart-attack patients will have a second heart attack. In addition, hostile people who seek revenge are much more likely to have another heart attack than hostile people

Harmful traits are associated with hostility. These include cynical beliefs that others are inherently bad, selfish, mean, and not to be trusted; frequent angry feelings when these negative expectations are fulfilled; and overt expression of the angry feelings in aggressive acts toward others. The effects of hostility are especially devastating to the body for two reasons:

1. Hostility causes a continuous release of hormones that destroy health in a variety of ways.
2. Hostility weakens the branch of the nervous system designed to calm the body after an emergency.

In essence, the hostile person goes throughout the entire day in a stressed condition. Many hostile people don't even get relief while sleeping because stress hormones are secreted 24 hours a day.

Hostility, like stress and fear, causes the body to release a sequence of stress hormones including epinephrine,

TIPS FOR ACTION Overcoming Hostility

Hostility can be overcome. Here are some ways to do it:

• This may sound too simple, but when you realize you're feeling hostile, tell yourself to stop. You might have to shout it aloud at first. Later, as you get better at it, you can change to a silent command.
• Talk to yourself about how you're feeling. Evaluate the situation. Figure out why you're so upset. Decide to respond to the situation in a healthy way.
• Don't let yourself get trampled. If your anger is justified, deal with it calmly and rationally. Stand up for yourself. Work to correct a wrong. If a classmate fails to recognize your contribution on an important project, for example, don't just blow up and seethe with hostility. Talk to the professor, set the record straight, and spell out how you contributed to the project. Then confront your classmate calmly and express your feelings.

• Learn to trust other people. This might be hard at first, and, strange as it sounds, you might have to practice. Start with a minor situation in which you usually take control. Then let someone else be in charge.
• Be tolerant and nonjudgmental of others. The source of anger and hostility is often our response to someone else. Put yourself in the other's shoes and consider the situation from the other's point of view. Gain empathy for that person.
• Cut down on things that speed up your system. These include sugar, caffeine, nicotine, and the hidden sources of caffeine such as soft drinks, chocolate, and many over-the-counter and prescription drugs.
• If all else fails, distract yourself. If you're caught in traffic, turn on the radio. Visualize the last concert you went to. Do something to take your thoughts off the situation.

who are less retributional. Assessment 2.2 addresses hostility related to heart health, and Assessment 2.3 asks you to respond with how you deal with resentment.

PERFECTIONISM

Upholding high standards and striving to reach challenging goals are healthy behaviors. But the compulsive pursuit of unrealistically high standards for yourself and those around you is unhealthy and has been labeled **perfectionism**. One example of perfectionism is the student who begins exercising to improve her health, then finds herself exercising and dieting excessively in the pursuit of the ideal body.

Perfectionism actually can hinder academic and other performance. For example, some people who are perfectionistic have an obsessive attention for detail and may spend hours straightening out their desk but miss project deadlines. Too, procrastination often stems from perfectionism, as people put off projects because they fear they will make a mistake.

Also, perfectionism can hinder relationships with others. The fear of making a mistake might lead students to take so much time proofreading a paper that they neglect the overall content. And if they rigidly hold others to unrealistic standards, they can project negative feelings when you fail to meet their expectations.

SELF-ESTEEM

People who are emotionally healthy have high self-esteem; they know and like themselves. These people accept that they are not perfect but they cherish their positive qualities and work to improve their negative traits. Table 2.1 lists characteristics of emotionally healthy and unhealthy people.

Self-esteem is so crucial for emotional health that some psychologists select attitudes toward the self as the criteria for evaluating mental health. Poor self-esteem is linked closely to alcoholism, drug abuse, crime and violence, child abuse, teenage pregnancy, prostitution, welfare dependency, and failure of children to learn. High self-esteem facilitates emotional growth and helps those around you. People who take care of themselves have more energy to offer their families, friends, and society.

WORRY AND ANXIETY

Worry is a state in which we dwell on something so much it causes us to become apprehensive. **Anxiety** is the psychological and physiological response to worry and causes physical changes, such as a racing pulse and rapid breathing. Worry is the thinking part of anxiety.

Anxiety often translates into negative physical symptoms and changes, which can impair the immune system and result in physical illness. Worry and anxiety have been shown to affect the heart and the circulatory system

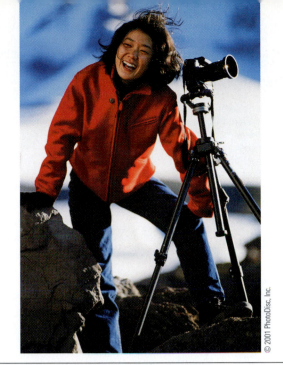

Positive self-esteem is associated with good health.

© 2001 PhotoDisc, Inc.

as a whole, causing irregular heartbeat, high blood pressure, and various abnormalities involving the arteries. Our thoughts and feelings are closely related to heart health. Further, worry and anxiety can cause the body to produce the chemical acetylcholine, which causes the airways to contract and can result in asthma.

One specific kind of worry, *uncertainty*, has been shown to cause a particularly devastating kind of stress. Uncertainty keeps a person in a constant state of semi-arousal, which puts an extreme burden on the body's adaptive resources and resistance. The result is often disease, particularly gastrointestinal disease.

When worry and anxiety escalate, the outcome is **fear**. Fear causes the heart to race, the head to spin, the palms to sweat, the knees to buckle, and breathing to become labored. Fear signals the body to secrete adrenaline, which has a powerful effect on the heart. Both the rate and strength of heart contractions increase, and blood pressure rises. The body is stimulated, in turn, to release other hormones. If the fear is intense enough, all systems can be overloaded fatally.

Perfectionism The compulsive pursuit of unrealistically high standards.

Worry A state in which we dwell on something so much that we become apprehensive.

Anxiety A state of intense worry that is not grounded in reality.

Fear A state of escalated worry and apprehension that causes distinct physical and emotional reactions.

TABLE 2.1   Characteristics of Emotionally Healthy People Versus Emotionally Unhealthy People

Emotionally Healthy People	Emotionally Unhealthy People
Have high self-esteem.	Have low self-esteem.
Are confident that their behavior is normal.	Guess at what normal behavior is.
Are honest.	Often lie when it would be just as easy to tell the truth.
Accept themselves.	Judge themselves without mercy.
Can have fun.	Have difficulty having fun.
Don't take themselves too seriously.	Take themselves very seriously.
Recognize that other people can enhance their lives but are not the sole source of their happiness.	Are certain that their happiness hinges on others.
Can have intimate relationships.	Have unusual difficulty with intimate relationships.
Don't try to control things beyond their control.	Try to control things they cannot control.
Are able to affirm themselves.	Constantly seek approval and affirmation from others.
Communicate openly and assertively about their needs and wants.	Communicate indirectly and try to meet their needs using aggressiveness or manipulation.
Usually think they are similar to other people.	Usually feel they are different from other people.
Take responsibility appropriately, but don't take too much responsibility for others.	Are either super-responsible or super-irresponsible.
Be loyal when it is appropriate and deserved.	Are extremely loyal, even when loyalty is undeserved.
Consider consequences before acting.	Act impulsively without considering consequences.
Deal with emotional pain by feeling it and expressing it.	Deal with emotional pain by resorting to addictions and compulsive behaviors.
Continue to mature mentally, emotionally, and spiritually throughout their lives.	Tend to remain immature; their mental, emotional, and spiritual growth is blocked.
Live with balance, not extremes.	Live life punctuated by extremes.
Validate and acknowledge their observations, feelings, and reactions.	Invalidate and repress their observations, feelings, and reactions.
Attend to their physical and psychological needs.	Neglect their needs.
Disclose family problems when appropriate.	Hide family or other secrets.
Refuse to tolerate inappropriate behavior.	Have a high tolerance for inappropriate behavior.
Feel emotional pain; are able to grieve when they suffer.	Are unable to grieve losses to completion.
Cope with stress in positive ways, and therefore are not prone to stress-related illnesses.	Are prone to stress-related illnesses.

Sources: Adapted from *Adult Children of Alcoholics*, J. G. Woititz, (Deerfield Beach, FL: Health Communications, 1983); *Love Is a Choice,* R. Hemfelt, F. Minirth, and P. Meier, (Nashville, TN: Thomas Nelson, 1989), pp. 9–16).

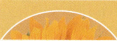

TIPS FOR ACTION Dealing with Fear

The following is a simple strategy for overcoming fear:

- First, admit you're afraid. List the things that cause you fear. As you mentally re-create those fears, try to imagine them without the emotion of fear. It takes some practice, but you can do it.
- Next, confront your fear. Do whatever it is you're so afraid of. Realize that your fear will intensify as you face it, but do it anyway. Go back to your mental pictures and try to imagine that the situation is not fearful.

- Do at least three times whatever it is that you're so afraid of. Chances are, you'll be less afraid each time. Chances are even better that you were afraid because you were unsure.
- As you confront your fear, call it something else—excitement or a challenge, for example.

DEPRESSION

Depression is much more than an occasional sad mood. Depression is characterized by apathy and a feeling of hopelessness. In a low-energy state, the person feels apathetic and withdraws from others. A depressed person does less and less, loses interest in people, abandons hobbies, and gives up in school or work. An estimated 10 to 14 million Americans suffer from depression at any given time.[16]

Sometimes depression follows the loss of something valued or someone important—the death of a loved one, divorce, aging, the diagnosis of serious illness, an automobile accident, termination of employment, retirement, or children leaving home. Under those circumstances, feeling sad or discouraged is a normal response.

In other cases depression is caused by biological factors—a chemical imbalance in the brain, a physical illness, a disturbance in the nervous system or neurotransmitters,

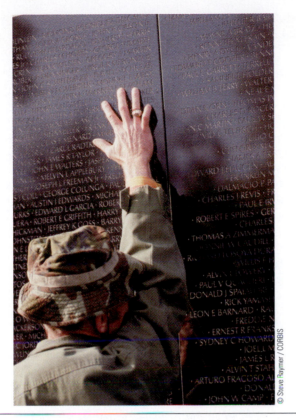

To become free of pain, one may have to go through it.

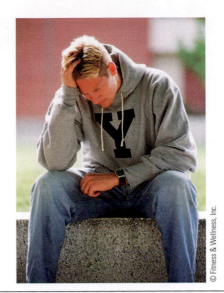

Worry may trigger or increase the stress response.

or an injury involving brain tissue. These cases require medical attention, and sometimes an antidepressant drug is prescribed.

In addition to the increased risk of suicide among depressed people, depression can shorten life in other ways. Depressed people have significantly higher mortality rates in general than people who are not depressed. Depression can become a potent risk factor in determining whether a person will die sooner than expected, either of natural causes or of underlying disease.

Depression consistently predicts poor health outcomes, and correlates with self-rated physical health. People who are depressed tend to believe their physical health is poor even when physical exams show no clinically-defined illness.

Also, depression impairs the immune system in a variety of ways, one of the most significant being its impact on the immune cells that assist the body in its surveillance against tumors and its resistance to viral disease. Natural killer cell activity is impaired in people who are depressed, and the more severe the depression, the greater this impairment. Other components of the immune system are crippled by depression as well. Depression causes a striking reduction in white blood cells, an upset in the ratio of helper and suppressor cells, and overall suppression of immune function.

The hormones triggered by depression—especially cortisol and norepinephrine—have significant damaging

Depression and Heart Disease

Each year in the United States, mild or major depression affects 50 percent of the people who survive a heart attack, and up to 40 percent of the nation's 350,000 heart-bypass patients.

Until recently, doctors treated their patients' mind only after they treated their heart. Now it's known that patients who aren't treated for depression are at far greater risk for a second heart attack and death.

At highest risk for post-cardiac depression are women (who often outlive their husbands and have to face illness alone), people with a history of depression, and those who are socially isolated or recently bereaved.

Memory loss—a common but temporary side effect of heart surgery—also can trigger depression. Symptoms to watch for include lethargy, sleeplessness, and weight changes.

Source: National Institutes of Health, Hope Heart Institute.

effects on the heart. Norepinephrine speeds up heart rate, encourages blood clotting (which can lead to heart attack), increases the level of harmful cholesterol in the blood, and impairs the heart's ability to adapt when demands increase. The cortisol that is produced during depression leads to a particularly dangerous kind of irregular heartbeat and encourages fat storage around the abdomen (another risk factor for heart disease). Thus, depression increases the risk of heart disease and worsens the outcomes for people who already have heart disease.

To combat depression, behavioral counseling, lifestyle modifications and sometimes medications have been helpful. The result may be reduced risk for heart disease, improved quality of life, and increased survival.

If your depression is caused by biological factors, you need medical help. If your depression is mild or your physician rules out biological factors, try these coping measures:

- Start by admitting you are depressed, then try to figure out why. Once you have identified a cause, you might be able to eliminate it.
- As much as you can, stick to your normal routine. Change, even positive change, is a source of stress and can intensify depression.
- If you can, plan some quiet times each day when you can relax, pamper yourself, do something you enjoy, or just get away from stresses you might feel. If you've been feeling depressed for a while, you might start by actually making a list of things you'd like to do: Read the newest book on the best-selling list, take a watercolor class, travel to a new area.

- Find a confidant, someone you can talk to about your feelings. If you're lucky, you'll find someone who will listen without judging. Whatever you do, don't choose another depressed person as your confidant. You'll only end up dragging each other down.
- Do something you're good at: Write an essay for a literary magazine, enter a local bicycle race, volunteer to play the piano at a local retirement center, ask your landlord if you can plant flowers around your apartment building. You'll get an immediate boost.
- Get regular exercise. Studies have shown that exercise is one of the best ways to conquer depression. Exercise in the outdoors may offer an extra mood-lifting benefit. Be sure the exercise is in a form you enjoy.
- Whatever you do, don't try to get rid of depression by using alcohol or drugs. They only make things worse.

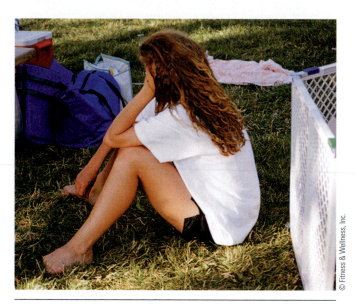

© Fitness & Wellness, Inc.

Depression can range from a mild case of the blues to severe clinical depression.

SUICIDE

Severe depression can lead to suicide. Most people who commit suicide suffer from deep despair, loneliness, and hopelessness. They feel that their lives are completely out of their control and that the only way they can regain control is to take their lives. Suicide among young people is an epidemic problem. Signs of depression that may warn of impending suicide include:

- Withdrawing from friends
- Losing interest in hobbies and activities
- Slackening of interest in schoolwork and decline in grades
- Not caring what happens, good or bad; passivity
- Feeling bad about oneself, pessimistic, and helpless

- Ceasing to groom oneself or care for one's room, possessions, or clothes
- Failing to meet responsibilities (pay bills, return phone calls or answer the phone)
- Changes in eating or sleeping habits, alcohol or drug use
- Abrupt changes in personality; aggressive, hostile behavior or impulsiveness; sudden mood swings
- Anxiety at times of separation
- Inability to concentrate
- Refusing to leave the room or the bed
- Obsession with death; a death wish.

If you suspect an imminent suicide attempt, take the person seriously and get involved. Don't wait to see what develops, because tomorrow may be too late. Do not be afraid to ask outright if the person is planning suicide. The two most important actions to take if a person seems on the verge of making a suicide attempt are

- Phone a suicide hotline or crisis intervention center immediately. They will be able to help. Dial 911, the operator, or the police.
- Stay with the person until help arrives.

These suggestions may help you to intervene when a friend or family member is considering suicide. However, it's important to know that, if someone you know does follow through with taking their own life, it is not your fault.

THE GRIEF PROCESS

Losses evoke what is called the grief process. To maintain emotional—and physical—health, it is beneficial to allow oneself to feel the pain and share the sadness with safe and supportive others. This permits grieving to move along through its stages until one is free of it. If people do not learn how to navigate this process, they accumulate a lifetime of unresolved grief, an unhealthy condition.

Stages of grief that people typically experience with loss are the following:[17]

- Denial: "No, it can't be!"
- Anger: "Why me? I don't deserve this!"
- Bargaining: "I'll do anything; just let this not happen."
- Depression (including withdrawal and loss of hope): "I'll never get over this."
- Acceptance: "I can make it."
- Hope for the future: "I can move on now."

Everyone does not necessarily go through these stages in the above sequence. The grief process is different for everyone. Nevertheless, anyone who represses the feelings associated with losses carries a heavy load of unresolved, lifelong grief in the form of chronic anxiety, tension, fear, anger, resentment, emptiness, confusion, or shame. Learning to go through the pain is a way to be free of it.

WHAT'S "NORMAL" GRIEF?

When you experience a loss significant enough to cause grief, you can expect the following:

- For the first few days, you'll be in a state of shock and denial. It will be difficult to accept the loss, and you're likely to feel numb. You'll probably cry a lot during this time, too.
- For the next 2 or 3 months, you'll go through a series of emotions. You'll feel anger and may "bargain" with God, offering all kinds of things in exchange for what was lost. You'll feel sad, tearful, and preoccupied. You may have vivid memories of the lost person and may even sense his or her presence. You may lose your appetite, as well as interest in things you used to enjoy. These feelings tend to peak about a month after the loss and usually last for 3 or 4 months but can last as long as a year.
- About a year after the loss, most people are able to resume ordinary activities and are able to generate happy memories about the lost person. You'll feel sad less often and finally will be able to resolve the loss within yourself.

PROTECTING YOUR IMMUNE SYSTEM WHILE YOU GRIEVE

To keep your immune system in shape:

- Get plenty of rest. Take naps if you need them, and try to maintain your normal sleep pattern at night.
- Eat a balanced diet—three solid meals a day with choices from all food groups. When you feel hungry in between meals, eat low-fat snacks high in complex carbohydrates.

- Get plenty of fluids, but avoid those that contain alcohol or caffeine.
- Exercise regularly. Choose an activity you enjoy, and do it for at least half an hour at least three times a week. Bicycling, walking, and swimming are good choices.

Above all, stay connected to other people! Social support, as you will learn in Chapter 4, is especially important to keep your immune system healthy.

Hardiness

Some people enjoy remarkably good health and longevity in what has been described as **hardiness**. The personality traits of hardiness are the "three Cs": commitment, control, and challenge.

1. *Commitment* entails a commitment to yourself, your work, your family, and the other important values in your life. This is not a fleeting involvement but, instead, a deep and enduring interest. People who are committed are involved with their work and their families, hold a belief that their life has meaning, and have a pervasive sense of direction in their lives.
2. *Control* is a belief that you can influence a negative event in a more positive way. It is a belief that you can cushion the hurtful impact of a situation by the way you look at it and react to it. The kind of control that keeps a person healthy is the opposite of helplessness. It is the firm belief that you can influence how you will react and the willingness to act on that basis. It is the refusal to be victimized.

   Control does not mean controlling your environment, your circumstances, or other people. That kind of an attitude leads to illness, not health. The control that keeps you healthy is a belief that you can control yourself and your reactions to what life hands you.

   Control is associated with hardiness. When faced with difficulties, hardy people use active strategies to either change the way they think about a problem or to attempt to resolve the issue by dealing directly with it. The healthiest students approach problem-solving with a sense of control instead of passivity. People who believe they have little or no control over their health and their lives are less likely to take positive actions and are more likely to be depressed and anxious. The healthiest and hardiest people are those who focus on what they can control and ignore the rest. They believe that every problem has a solution through skill, planning, and diligent attention to detail.
3. *Challenge* means the ability to see change as an opportunity for growth and excitement. Excitement is vital,

Hardiness A set of personality traits marked by commitment, control, and challenge.

because boredom puts people at a high risk for disease. People who are challenged constructively are healthier. One of the biggest foes of human happiness is boredom.

A person who is not hardy views change through a lens of helplessness and alienation. A hardy person, by contrast, faces change with confidence, self-determination, eagerness, and excitement. Change becomes an eagerly sought-after challenge, not a threat.

These three characteristics come into play when illness threatens. Illness often is preceded by a series of events. First a person perceives a distressing life situation. For whatever reason, he or she is not able to resolve the distressing situation effectively. As a result, the person feels helpless and anxious. Those feelings of helplessness weaken the immune system and resistance to disease, and the person becomes more vulnerable to disease-causing agents that are ever present in the environment.

The traits of a disease-resistant or hardy personality, which include the 3Cs, interrupt this cycle and thereby help to prevent illness. The personality trait of hardiness also has been termed *emotional intelligence*. Emotionally intelligent people remain positive, even under adverse circumstances.[18] Healthy people and ill people view things in entirely different ways. Healthy people tend to maintain reasonable personal control in their lives. If a problem crops up, they look for resources and try out solutions. If one solution doesn't work, they try another one.

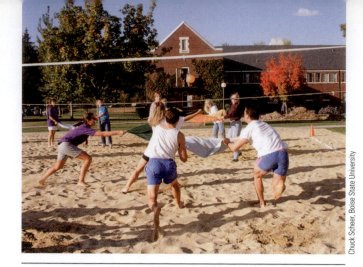

Chuck Scheer, Boise State University

Hardy people are characterized by the "three Cs": commitment, control, and challenge.

Critical Thinking

Now that you understand the concept of hardiness, describe the three Cs and how you can develop this trait.

Emotional health influences our physical health. Emotions cause physiological responses that affect disease and healing. Personality plays a role in our health outcomes. People can improve their emotional health through knowledge and positive attitudes and behaviors.

TIPS FOR ACTION Developing Hardiness

- Figure out what is causing you stress. Make a list, then divide it into two columns—things you can control and things you can't control. Map out a strategy to help you change the things you can control. Then map out a strategy to help you overcome— ignore or move away from—the things you can't control. Don't waste time struggling against things you can never change.
- Look back on ways you've handled your stress during the last month. It may help to write it down. Summarize the situation, then write down the way you handled it. Now evaluate. Did you respond appropriately? How could you have done it better? Finally, describe how you could have better dealt with the stress. Use that alternative as your blueprint for the future.
- Do self-examination a couple of times a day. Are you uptight? Is your stomach tied up in knots? Are you clenching your fists or grinding your teeth? Take a minute and ask yourself why. Then relax. Learn some meditation or relaxation techniques and use them to take control.
- Practice changing your attitude. When you're confronted with a problem, intentionally tell yourself that it's a challenge instead. Try to see some excitement in it. Try to find some pleasure.
- Do whatever you can to create some situations in your life when you are in control: Paint your room, direct a play, take charge of a simple class project. Keeping control over some things in your life reassures you that you can be in control and hones your skills for the times you're not so sure of yourself.

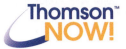

Don't forget to check out the wealth of resources on the ThomsonNOW website at **www.thomsonedu.com/ThomsonNOW** that will:

- Coach you through identifying target goals for behavior change and monitoring your personal change plan throughout the semester
- Help you evaluate your knowledge of the material
- Allow you to take an exam-prep quiz
- Provide a Personalized Learning Plan targeting resources that address areas you should study.

WEB ACTIVITIES

Dr. Koop—Mental Health Site This comprehensive site features reliable information on a variety of mental health topics, including depression, stress, attention deficit disorder, phobias, post-traumatic stress disorder, medications, as well as interactive self-assessment tools for depression and stress.

http://www.drkoop.com/channel/93/1329.html

World Health Organization: Mental Health This comprehensive site features a wealth of information on mental and neurological topics. The topics include global statistical information on depression, suicide, and women's mental health, among others.

http://www.who.int/mental_health

The Mind–Body Connection: Granny Was Right This interesting site, sponsored by the University of Rochester Medical Center, presents research findings involving the physiological link between the mind and the body.

http://www.rochester.edu/pr/Review/V59N3/feature2.html

Do You have a "Type A" Personality? This site features 17 questions designed to determine if you have characteristics of a "Type A" personality.

http://www.queendom.com/typea2.html

InfoTrac®

You can find additional readings related to wellness via InfoTrac® College Edition, an online library of more than 900 journals and publications. Follow the instructions for accessing InfoTrac® that came packaged with your textbook, then search for articles using a key word search.

Suggested Reading "Depressive Illness," by Alan Doris, Klaus Ebmeier, and Polash Shajahan, *The Lancet* 354, no. 9187 (Oct. 16, 1999): 1369.

1. What constitutes depressive symptoms that are pathological?
2. Describe the relative contributions of genetics and environment in relation to the cause and pathophysiology of major depressive illness.
3. In the treatment of depression, what are some of the pharmacologic and alternative forms of therapy?

Web Activity

Depression Screening Test

http://www.depression-screening.org/index.htm

Sponsor National Mental Health Association

Description This interactive site features a series of confidential multiple-choice questions designed to assess whether you are suffering from depression.

Available Activities Review the following site features:

1. A confidential depression screening test
2. Several links dealing with depression, including depression symptoms and treatments, "Depression can affect anyone" link, personal stories, education and advocacy opportunities, as well as sources of help

Web Work

1. From the home page, click on the violet box entitled "Confidential Screening Test."
2. Honestly answer the series of 10 multiple-choice questions.
3. Once the questionnaire is completed, the site automatically provides you with a personal analysis and recommendations if your answers suggest that you might be suffering from clinical depression.

Helpful Hints

1. This site's strong disclaimer informs the user that online screening tests are *not* intended to provide a diagnosis for clinical depression, but they *may* help identify any depressive symptoms and determine whether a further evaluation by a medical or mental health professional is indicated. As with any other illness, you should see your doctor if you think you might have symptoms of depression.
2. After completing the test and receiving your recommendations, also click on the "Follow-up Survey" link to answer a question regarding what you plan to do with these results. Choices include calling 911 or seeking professional help.

For additional Web activities, links, and suggested readings, visit our Health, Fitness, and Wellness Resource Center at http://health.wadsworth.com.

Notes

1. E. Reiche, S. Nunes, H. Morimoto, "Stress, Depression, the Immune System, and Cancer," *The Lancet*, 5 (October 2004): 617–625.

2. S. Bunker et al., "Stress and Coronary Heart Disease: Psychosocial Risk Factors," *Australian Medical Journal* 178 (2003): 272–279.

3. H. J. Eysenck, "Personality, Stress, and Cancer: Prediction and Prophylaxis," *British Journal of Medical Psychology* 61 (March 1988): 57–75.

4. See Note 3.

5. G. E Miller, K. E. Freedland, R. M. Carney, C. A. Stetler, and W. A. Banks, "Cynical Hostility, Depressive Symptoms, and the Expression of Inflammatory Risk Markers for Coronary Heart Disease," *Journal of Behavioral Medicine* 26 (2003): 501–515.

6. L. Karlberg et al., "Is There a Connection Between Car Accidents, Near Accidents, and Type A Drivers?" *Behavioral Medicine* 24 (Fall 1998): 99; N. Koivula et al., "Type A/B Behavior Pattern and Athletic Participation: Attitudes and Actual Behavior," *Journal of Sport Behavior* 21 (June 1998): 148–166.

7. B. Sparagon et al., "Type A Behavior and Coronary Atherosclerosis," *Atherosclerosis* 156 (2001): 145–149.

8. See Note 5.

9. A. Moller et al., "Effects of a Group Rational-Emotive Behavior Therapy Program on the Type A Behavior Pattern," *Psychological Reports* 78 (June 1996): 947–961.

10. B. C. Sirois, M. Burg, "Negative Emotion and Coronary Heart Disease," *Behavior Modification* 27 (2003): 83–102.

11. K. Lillberg et al., "Personality Characteristics and the Risk of Breast Cancer," *International Journal of Cancer* 100 (2002): 361–166.

12. M. Price et al., "The Role of Psychosocial Factors in the Development of Breast Carcinoma: Part 1. The Cancer Prone Personality," *Cancer* 91 (2001): 679–685.

13. M. E. Habra, W. Linden, J. C. Anderson, J. Weinberg, "Type D Personality is Related to Cardiovascular and Neuroendocrine Reactivity to Acute Stress, *Journal of Psychosomatic Research* 55 (2003): 235–245.

14. Centers of Disease Control and Prevention. Have a stressful job? You must have an ulcer, right? Retrieved October 30, 2004 from http://www.cdc.gov/ulcer/myth.htm.

15. J. Denollet, G. Van Heck, "Psychological Risk Factors in Heart Disease: What Type D Personality is (Not) About," *Journal of Psychosomatic Research* 51 (2001): 465–468.

16. K. Wells et al., "Impact of Disseminating Quality Improvement Programs for Depression in Managed Primary Care: A Randomized Controlled Trial," *Journal of the American Medical Association* 283 (January 12, 2000): 212–218.

17. E. Kübler-Ross, *On Death and Dying* (New York: Springer, 1969).

18. M. Soderstrom, C. Dolbier, J. M. Steinhartd, "The Relationship of Hardiness, Coping Strategies, and Perceived Stress to Symptoms of Illness," *Journal of Behavioral Medicine* 23 (2000): 311–328.

Assess Your Behavior

1. Do you have a health-promoting or health-hindering personality type?

2. What actions are you taking to improve the effect of your personality on your health?

3. Do you know the signs of depression and suicide?

4. What can you do to help yourself or a friend if you are facing one of these conditions?

Assess Your Knowledge

Evaluate how well you understand the concepts presented in this chapter by answering the following questions.

1. Psychoneuroimmunology involves the interrelationships between
   a. mind and body.
   b. emotions and immunity.
   c. biology and genetics.
   d. a and b.
   e. a and c.

2. The Type A personality is at risk for
   a. cancer.
   b. heart disease.
   c. passivity.
   d. apathy.
   e. all of the above.

3. Which of the following is likely to result from perfectionism?
   a. high academic achievement
   b. high self-esteem
   c. procrastination
   d. obesity
   e. cancer

4. People who are overly-sensitive to perceived criticism against them but are loudly critical of others are likely to possess this trait:
   a. Type B.
   b. perfectionism.
   c. hostility.
   d. euphoria.
   e. raised immunity.

5. Depression is associated with high levels of which chemical(s)?
   a. serotonin
   b. cortisol
   c. norepinephrine
   d. a and b
   e. b and c

6. To help someone who is talking about suicide, you should
   a. phone a suicide hotline or crisis intervention center immediately and stay with the person until help arrives.
   b. do not ask if the person is planning suicide.
   c. Ignore the talk because the person probably just wants attention.
   d. All of the above.
   e. None of the above.

Correct answers can be found on page 369.

Do You Cultivate Emotional Well-Being?

Name: _____   Date: _____   Grade: _____

Instructor: _____   Course: _____   Section: _____

Try answering these questions to get an idea. Don't take your score too seriously; this is just for fun.

1. I spend time doing work that I enjoy.

   a. almost always

   b. sometimes

   c. almost never

2. I find it easy to relax.

   a. almost always

   b. sometimes

   c. almost never

3. In my spare time, I participate in activities that I enjoy.

   a. almost always

   b. sometimes

   c. almost never

4. When I am about to be in a stressful situation, I realize it ahead of time and I prepare for it.

   a. almost always

   b. sometimes

   c. almost never

5. I handle anger:

   a. by expressing it in ways that hurt neither myself nor other people.

   b. by bottling it up so that no one knows I'm angry.

   c. I never am angry, or I express my anger aggressively.

6. I participate with group organizations such as school, sports, church, or community activities.

   a. quite often

   b. very seldom

   c. never

7. I find it easy to express my feelings.

   a. almost always

   b. sometimes

   c. almost never

8. I can talk to close friends, relatives, or others about personal matters.

   a. almost always

   b. sometimes

   c. almost never

9. When I need help with personal matters, I seek it out.

   a. almost always

   b. sometimes

   c. almost never

10. When I am under stress, I make extra sure to exercise regularly to work off my tension.

   a. almost always

   b. sometimes

   c. almost never

For each *a* answer, give yourself 2 points; for each *b* answer, give yourself 1 point; for each *c* answer, give yourself 0 points. A score of 18 to 20 is excellent; 16 or 17 is very good; 14 or 15 is good; and 13 or below means that you may benefit from making some small changes.

Source: Adapted from U. S. Department of Health and Human Services, *Health Style,* HHS publication no. (PHS) 81-50155, 1981 (a self-test distributed by National Health Information Clearinghouse).

Hostility Could Harm Your Heart

Name: _____   Date: _____   Grade: _____

Instructor: _____   Course: _____   Section: _____

Experts now conclude that feelings of hostility increase your risk of heart disease. Dr. Redford Williams, Duke University Medical Center, has designed a questionnaire to help you determine whether you have a hostile personality. Circle the answer that most closely fits how you would respond to the given situation:

1. **A person drives by my yard blasting the car stereo:**
   A. I begin to understand why some people can't hear.
   B. I can feel my blood pressure starting to rise.

2. **A boyfriend/girlfriend calls at the last minute "too tired to go out tonight." I'm stuck with two $15 tickets:**
   A. I find someone else to go with.
   B. I tell my friend how inconsiderate he/she is.

3. **Waiting in the express checkout line at the super-market where a sign says "No More Than 10 Items Please":**
   A. I pick up a magazine and pass the time.
   B. I glance to see if anyone has more than 10 items.

4. **Most homeless people in large cities:**
   A. Are down and out because they lack ambition.
   B. Are victims of illness or some other misfortune.

5. **At times when I've been very angry with someone:**
   A. I was able to stop short of hitting him/her.
   B. I have, on occasion, hit or shoved him/her.

6. **When I am stuck in traffic:**
   A. I am usually not particularly upset.
   B. I quickly start to feel irritated and annoyed.

7. **When there's a really important job to be done:**
   A. I prefer to do it myself.
   B. I am apt to call on my friends to help.

8. **The cars ahead of me start to slow and stop as they approach a curve:**
   A. I assume there is a construction site ahead.
   B. I assume someone ahead had a fender-bender.

9. **An elevator stops too long above where I'm waiting:**
   A. I soon start to feel irritated and annoyed.
   B. I start planning the rest of my day.

10. **When a friend or co-worker disagrees with me:**
    A. I try to explain my position more clearly.
    B. I am apt to get into an argument with him or her.

11. **When I was really angry in the past:**
    A. I have never thrown things or slammed a door.
    B. I've sometimes thrown things or slammed a door.

12. **Someone bumps into me in a store:**
    A. I pass it off as an accident.
    B. I feel irritated at their clumsiness.

13. **When my spouse/significant other is fixing a meal:**
    A. I keep an eye out to make sure nothing burns.
    B. I talk about my day or read the paper.

14. **When someone is hogging the conversation at a party:**
    A. I look for an opportunity to put him/her down.
    B. I soon move to another group.

15. **In most arguments:**
    A. I am the angrier one.
    B. The other person is angrier than I am.

Score one point for each of these answers: 1. B, 2. B, 3. B, 4. A, 5. B, 6. B, 7. A, 8. B, 9. A, 10. B, 11. B, 12. B, 13. A, 14. A, 15. A. If you scored 4 or more points you may be hostile. Questions 1, 6, 9, 12, and 15 reflect anger. Questions 2, 5, 10, 11, and 14 reflect aggression. Questions 3, 4, 7, 8, and 13 reflect cynicism. If you scored 2 points in any category, you may want to explore ways that you can make changes in response to situations.

Adapted from *Anger Kills: 17 Strategies*, by Redford B. Williams and Virginia Williams. Copyright © 1993 by Redford B. Williams, M.D., and Virginia Williams, Ph.D. Reprinted by permission of Times Books, a division of Random House, Inc.

How Well Do You Express Resentments?

Name: _____   **Date:** _____   **Grade:** _____

Instructor: _____   **Course:** _____   **Section:** _____

This is a measure of how likely you are to respond assertively, aggressively, or passively to various situations. (Some items may not apply to you. Try to imagine that they do.)

1. Your mother has emphasized that she wants you with the family at 6 o'clock today. At 5 o'clock, a friend invites you to a get-together you can't refuse. You:
   a. Go with your friend, stay through 6, and explain to your mother later.
   b. Call your mother and tell her that you will be going with your friend.
   c. Complain to your mother that she is too demanding, but stay home.
   d. Tell your friend you can't go, and say nothing to your mother.

2. Several of your friends and you studied together for a test. All of your friends got good grades. You wrote the same kinds of answers on the test but got a low grade. You think your work was just as good as theirs. You:
   a. Write an anonymous note to the instructor's supervisor saying that the test grades are obviously unfair.
   b. Take your test to the instructor and ask why your grade was low.
   c. Complain to all your friends, and say nothing to the instructor.
   d. Keep your mouth shut so the instructor won't be even more unfair to you the next time.

3. You have just cleaned up the kitchen area. The next person puts a greasy frying pan on the countertop and starts to leave. You:
   a. Wait until you are alone, and then put the greasy frying pan between the bedsheets, where the person will be sure to find it.
   b. Tell the person, "Please wash your frying pan before you leave."
   c. Make a general remark about inconsiderate people who leave dirty dishes for others to clean.
   d. Say nothing, and wash it yourself later.

4. You are on your first date with someone you have admired from a distance for a long time. At the end of the evening, the other person gets much more sexual than you want to be. You:
   a. Back off, and leave as quickly as you can without saying anything.
   b. Tell the other person that things are going too far for you.

   c. Keep pulling away, and let the other person guess the message.
   d. Say nothing and go along because you want to date the person again.

5. You get home with a newly bought bag of groceries, only to find that the chicken you bought is already spoiled in the package. You:
   a. Storm back into the store and make a scene so all the other customers will know you were sold some rotten chicken.
   b. Go back to the store, ask to see the manager, and explain that the chicken you just bought is spoiled.
   c. Never shop in that store again.
   d. Do nothing.

6. You are in your room studying for a big exam. Your neighbor is playing the stereo loudly. You:
   a. Knock on your neighbor's door, walk in, and switch off the stereo.
   b. Ask your neighbor to turn down the volume and explain why.
   c. Go someplace else to study and never speak to your neighbor again.
   d. Give up and stop trying to study.

7. Your friends like horror movies, but you don't enjoy them at all. Your friends are making plans to see the latest horror movie this Saturday night. You:
   a. Tell them you think horror movies are for mental midgets and you're not going.
   b. Tell them you don't enjoy horror movies and ask if they'd consider another movie.
   c. Go to the movie and afterward make some humorous negative remarks about it, hoping they will get the message.
   d. Stay home Saturday night.

8. You occasionally babysit for Mrs. Harper's three children. Lately she has been making excuses when it comes time to pay you. You:
   a. Tell her that you're fed up and that you won't babysit for her anymore.
   b. Tell her that it's inconvenient for you to be paid late.
   c. Decide you won't work for her again.
   d. Say nothing.

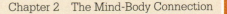

9. You and your friend are in a store together and you see your friend slip a CD into a coat pocket. You:
   a. Grab the CD, put it back on the shelf, and threaten to turn in your friend.
   b. Tell your friend how you feel about shoplifting and recommend replacing the CD.
   c. Say nothing, but resolve never to go shopping with your friend again.
   d. Act as if nothing has happened.

10. Your parents have given you some money to spend on clothes and they have told you exactly what they want you to buy. You need clothes, but you disagree with the style they are urging on you. You:
    a. Buy what you want, and tell them they are way out of touch with today's styles.
    b. Tell them how you'd rather spend the money and why it's important to you.
    c. Buy what they want you to have and try to trade it for something else latter.
    d. Buy what they want you to have, wear it, and thank them for it.

Scoring

Give yourself 10 points for each *a* answer, 8 for each *b*, 6 for each *c*, and 4 for each *d*. Add them up. If you scored:

85 to 100: You have no trouble asserting yourself, but your behavior borders on aggressiveness. You know what you want, but you may want to give more thought to how you go about getting it.

70 to 84: You have a good sense of what you want, and you speak your mind. You are assertive.

45 to 69: You may consider voicing your opinions and speaking up for your rights.

Below 45: You almost never voice an opinion. You may be building up some resentments. Start practicing assertiveness. Be honest with yourself and direct with others. This may improve your quality of life.

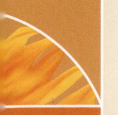

3

Stress and Health

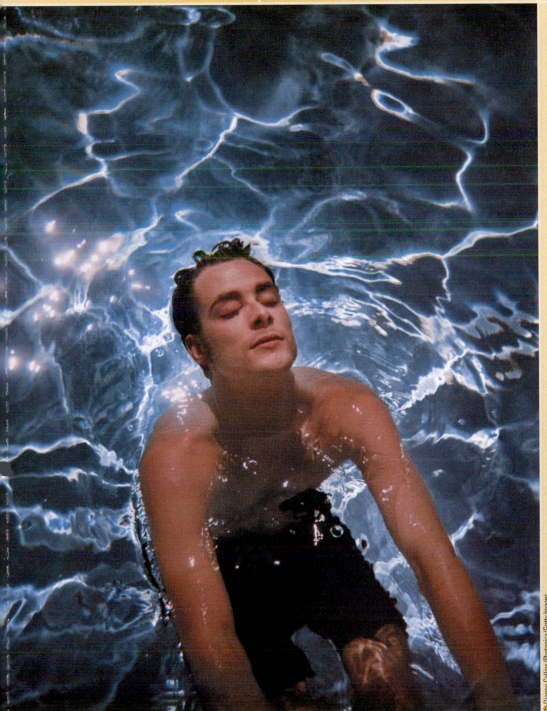

© Dianne Collins/Photonica/Getty Images

OBJECTIVES

Define stress, and identify common sources of stress.

Define the variants of eustress and distress.

Explain the relationship between stress and illness.

Recognize the signs and symptoms of stress.

Identify the body systems affected by stress.

Recognize the importance of diet, exercise, and sleep in relation to stress.

Describe some effective time-management strategies.

Define burnout and suggest how to help prevent it.

Identify stress reduction techniques, including meditation, progressive relaxation, autogenics, biofeedback, and yoga.

When you say, "I'm stressed!" what do you mean? Stress means different things to different people, and what causes stress for one person may not produce stress in someone else. Stress is not the same as frustration, anxiety, or conflict, though it can lead to all of those emotions.

Stress is a biological response to demands made upon an individual. It is the combination of a **stressor** (anything that makes us adapt) and our response to the stressor. Stressors can be physical (such as fatigue or a bacterial infection), emotional (such as pent-up anger or hostility), social (such as rejection or embarrassment), intellectual (such as confusion), and spiritual (such as guilt). Scientifically speaking, stress is any challenge to **homeostasis**, or the body's internal sense of balance. The biological and biochemical process of stress begins in the brain and spreads through the autonomic nervous system, causing the release of hormones.[1]

Good Stress or Bad Stress?

Dr. Hans Selye, the father of stress research,[2] was the first to explore the notion of "desirable" stress, the stress that keeps life interesting and provides opportunity for growth (such as marriage, birth, new job, new friends, or an exciting vacation). This kind of stress, which he termed **eustress**, is the physiological stress essential for maintaining life (such as the churning of the digestive tract and the rhythmic contractions of the heart). **Distress**, its opposite, is negative and results from stressors that are too intense or persist for a long time.

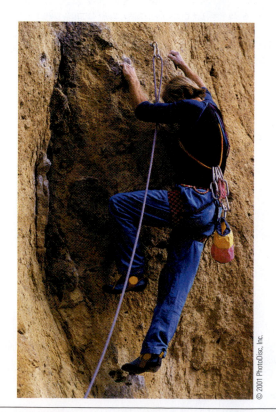

Challenges can be stressful—and beneficial.

Signs and Symptoms of Stress

- pounding, racing, or irregular heartbeat
- chest pain
- cold, sweaty hands
- inability to concentrate; loss of memory
- lack of creativity
- low self-esteem
- shortness of breath, rapid breathing, asthma attacks
- insomnia, fatigue, nightmares
- anxiety, nervousness, irritability
- unexplained fearfulness
- depression
- forgetfulness
- emotional instability, mood swings
- impulsive behavior
- tearfulness
- difficulty completing tasks
- urge to hide
- changes in eating/smoking/drinking behaviors
- increased dependence on drugs
- acne, rashes
- excessive dryness of skin or excessive perspiration
- dryness of the mouth and throat
- loss of appetite
- difficulty swallowing
- diarrhea or constipation
- grinding of the teeth
- increased cravings
- abdominal pain, nausea or queasiness, indigestion, vomiting
- frequent urination
- twitching or shakiness
- headache, including migraine
- neck or back pain; stiff muscles

The way we perceive stress drives how it affects us. Some stress promotes curiosity and exploration; it is challenging, stimulating, and rewarding. And stress can be altered by perceptions and attitude. For example, when confronted by the stress of an upcoming final exam in a difficult class, you may react either by becoming extremely anxious and unable to study (distress) or by welcoming the challenge by studying twice as long and enlisting the help of study companions (eustress).

Sources of Stress

Sources of stress vary throughout our lives. College students face a variety of stressors, and some researchers believe that the college years may be the most stressful in life. The following are some common kinds of pressures that students face.[3]

- *Pressures to achieve.* Students may create their own pressure if they have high internal standards. Or students may feel pressure from parents and teachers to perform according to their high expectations.

- *Financial burdens*. Many students have to work while earning their degrees. These students have to balance employers' expectations with academic goals. For those with families to support, the stress is even more intense.
- *Family stressors*. Students who have specific family stressors such as divorce of parents, health problems of a family member, or family conflict are burdened with stress.
- *Living adjustments*. Many students are living away from home, usually for the first time, and have not established a network of social support, which is crucial for coping.
- *Social pressure*. Students are confronted with choices regarding alcohol, drug use, and sexuality. The current epidemic of sexually transmitted diseases adds even more pressures.

Figure 3.1 illustrates these and other stressors. Assessment 3.1 may help you identify specific things that are causing stress in your life. Assessments 3.2 and 3.3 will provide you with more insights into how stress affects you personally.

Physical sources of stress include agents and conditions that challenge the body. Infection by bacteria, viruses, parasites, fungi, and protozoa can produce stress. So can fever, pain, trauma, injury, and deformity. Use of alcohol and other drugs can stress the body by interfering with the body's natural ability to recover.

The environment is another source of stress. Temperature, humidity, and weather extremes cause stress. So do pollutants in the air and water. Noise can be a significant source of environmental stress; the stress response is triggered by noise over 85 decibels (a loud television, garbage disposal, motorcycle, lawn mower, vacuum cleaner). Something as simple as being in a room that is too hot or too cold can cause stress. More dramatic examples of environmental stress include catastrophic events such as severe storms, long-term drought, famine, fires, earthquakes, tornadoes, hurricanes, floods, and war.

Other stressors are emotional and social. One of the most common sources of stress is **conflict**, which occurs when we are faced with incompatible needs, demands, motives, opportunities, or goals.[4] Some of the most pervasive stressors are daily **hassles**—the seemingly minor, irritating annoyances that happen every day, such as losing your car keys, getting stuck in a slow line at the supermarket, waking up to a miserable snowstorm, being kept waiting for an appointment, having unexpected company, or getting stuck in traffic.[5] These seemingly trivial problems actually may be more damaging to health and wellness than major stressors, partly because they occur frequently, and the net effect of an accumulation of daily hassles can lead to reduced ability to cope.

FIGURE 3.1   Some Stressors in the Lives of Students

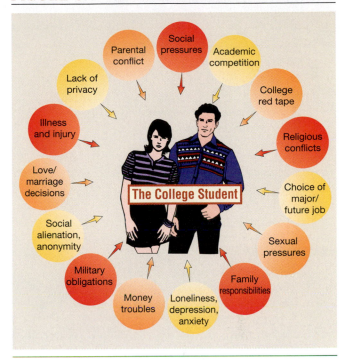

Occupational factors have been recognized as significant sources of stress,[6] including

- physical demands, such as uncomfortable seating, extremes in temperature, inadequate lighting;
- role demands, such as conflict or ambiguity in an employee's role;
- conflicts between work and family;
- interpersonal demands, such as an abrasive boss, passive leaders, or abusive co-workers; and
- task demands, such as repetition, too few or too many changes, job insecurity, or overload, the latter of which is a huge source of stress.

Unmanaged stressful demands such as these can arouse anxiety, which in turn can lead to mental and physical harm, as the next sections describe.

Stress An automatic biological response to stressors, or demands made on an individual; the result of any event or condition that requires adaptation.

Stressor Any situation or demand that requires adaptation.

Homeostasis A stable sense of physiological balance wherein all of the body's systems are functioning normally.

Eustress Positive, desirable stress.

Distress Negative stress, usually consisting of too much stress in a short time, chronic stress over a prolonged time, or a combination of stressors.

Conflict The stress that results from two opposing and incompatible goals, demands, or needs.

Hassles Seemingly minor, irritating, everyday annoyances that increase the level of stress.

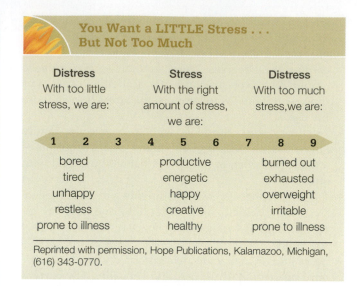
Critical Thinking

1. Describe common sources of stress.
2. Discuss why all stress is not negative.
3. Identify examples of eustress and discuss how these influence health.

Stress and Disease

Research has indicated that stress is a major factor in neuromuscular disorders, respiratory and allergic ailments, immunologic disorders, gastrointestinal disturbances, skin conditions, dental problems, and other disorders. Among other risk factors, stress influences a number of conditions, including:

- *cardiovascular diseases*.[7] Stress causes an increase in blood cholesterol, blood pressure, and stroke. Coronary artery disease and congestive heart failure both are partly caused or aggravated by stress.
- *gastrointestinal diseases*. Stress impairs the gastrointestinal tract, resulting in diarrhea, constipation, and ulcerative colitis (deterioration of the membranes lining the colon). Stress can alter eating patterns, causing severe loss of appetite in some people and eating disorders or obesity in others.
- *musculoskeletal disorders*. One of the most common results of stress is the tension headache, caused by chronic tension in the muscles of the scalp and neck. Another type of headache—the migraine, in which the blood vessels of the scalp become dilated and exert extreme pressure—also is worsened by stress. Other musculoskeletal disorders associated with stress include rheumatoid arthritis, chronic muscle tension, low back pain,[8] and temporomandibular joint (TMJ) syndrome, which interferes with chewing.
- *respiratory distress*. Stress may induce shortness of breath and rapid breathing. Also, asthma and hayfever, both allergic reactions, have been strongly linked to stress. Significant emotional stress can precipitate an attack even in the absence of the allergen.

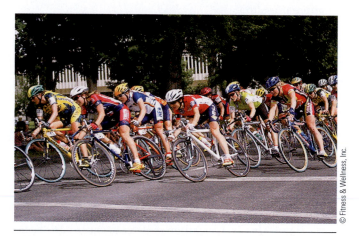

Some physical stress is positive.

Stress also is a factor in a number of skin conditions (such as hives, eczema, and psoriasis), metabolic disorders (such as thyroid malfunctions and diabetes), menstrual irregularity, and gout.

How the Body Reacts to Stress

In an ideal state, the body enjoys homeostasis, a physiological balance in which all systems function smoothly. When stress leads to a disruption of homeostasis, the body goes through an adaptive response in an effort to reestablish this balance. When faced with an intense stressor, the body undergoes the **fight-or-flight response**. This consists of a series of physiological changes that occur in succession to enable people, when confronted with physical harm, to face their enemies (fight) or run (flight) for their lives.

A student with communication anxiety giving an oral presentation in front of a class has a physiological

FIGURE 3.2   The Stress Response: Two Different Outcomes

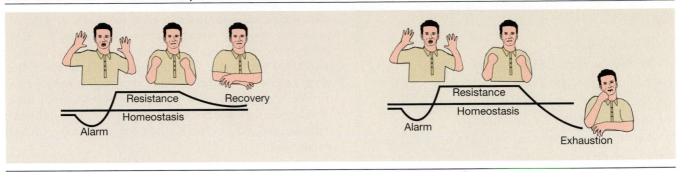

FIGURE 3.3   Physiological Manifestations of the Alarm Reaction

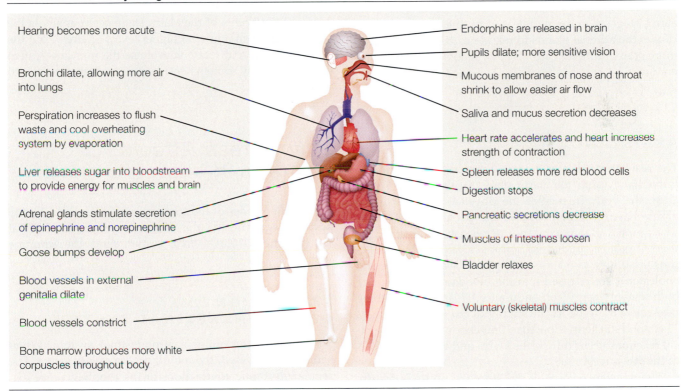

- Hearing becomes more acute
- Bronchi dilate, allowing more air into lungs
- Perspiration increases to flush waste and cool overheating system by evaporation
- Liver releases sugar into bloodstream to provide energy for muscles and brain
- Adrenal glands stimulate secretion of epinephrine and norepinephrine
- Goose bumps develop
- Blood vessels in external genitalia dilate
- Blood vessels constrict
- Bone marrow produces more white corpuscles throughout body

- Endorphins are released in brain
- Pupils dilate; more sensitive vision
- Mucous membranes of nose and throat shrink to allow easier air flow
- Saliva and mucus secretion decreases
- Heart rate accelerates and heart increases strength of contraction
- Spleen releases more red blood cells
- Digestion stops
- Pancreatic secretions decrease
- Muscles of intestines loosen
- Bladder relaxes
- Voluntary (skeletal) muscles contract

response similar to a person who faces physical danger. The stress response, termed the **general adaptation syndrome**, occurs in three general stages—alarm, resistance, and recovery or exhaustion—as depicted in Figure 3.2.

ALARM STAGE

The **alarm stage** of the stress response begins when a person is faced with a stressor. Rapid physical reactions follow the initial emotional reaction to a stressor: The brain triggers an immediate response from the autonomic nervous system (the branch of the nervous system that regulates body functions we cannot consciously control). All body systems mobilize and prepare for defense. Manifestations of the alarm reaction are depicted in Figure 3.3.

The mouth gets dry, and the palms get sweaty. Air sacs in the lungs dilate and breathing rate increases, infusing the blood with oxygen. Adrenaline and other hormones are pumped throughout the body, signaling the heart to deliver oxygen-rich blood to the muscles. Digestion is delayed so the much-needed blood is not diverted to the stomach. The liver releases glucose, which the muscles use as fuel. The muscles get tense, preparing for a workout. The senses—sight, hearing, smell, and taste—become acute, ready to identify any "danger."

Fight-or-flight response A series of rapid-fire physical reactions to stress that provides maximum physical readiness to face threats in the environment.

General adaptation syndrome A three-stage attempt of the body to react and adapt to stressors that disrupt its normal balance.

Alarm stage The first phase of the general adaptation syndrome, characterized by the release of stress hormones.

If stress is prolonged, further changes occur during the alarm stage. A hormone released by the pituitary gland causes the adrenal glands to release cortisol.[9] As a result, more stored nutrients are made available to the body for energy.

RESISTANCE

The **resistance stage** of the stress response begins almost immediately after the alarm stage begins. During resistance, the body intensifies the physical changes of the alarm stage in anticipation of the perceived challenge. The adrenal glands continue to release adrenaline, the thyroid pumps out thyroid hormones, and the hypothalamus continues to release endorphins. More glucose and cholesterol are released into the bloodstream, providing both instant energy and endurance. Heart and breathing rates increase to boost the supply of oxygen to the body. The blood thickens. More than 1,400 known physiochemical reactions occur during the alarm and resistance stages of the stress response.

The resistance stage of the stress response is ideally suited to meeting the challenges of short-term stress. Simply stated, the body tries to adapt or meet the challenge so it can later return to the balance (homeostasis) that existed before the stress occurred.

This reaction is designed to cope with physical threats. The body is prepared for energy to be expended physically. But our body experiences the same physical response when confronted with psychological stressors. Consider what happens if you experience alarm and resistance but you take no physical action in response. The body prepares for exercise, mobilizing its resources (blood sugar, fats, and hormones), but doesn't use them. Your muscles are tense, and your blood is rich with fuels that can accumulate and damage your heart.

If the stressful situation is short-term and subsides, the body is able to adapt and return to a state of balance or recovery. If the stress becomes chronic, however, the body eventually loses its ability to adapt and becomes exhausted. Thus, remaining in a state of chronic arousal and resistance can result in physical damage.

EXHAUSTION OR RECOVERY

Although most people experience the alarm and resistance stages of the stress response frequently, the final stage of the stress response varies. Preferably, the stressor will leave you before your resources run out. Thus, this stage can take the form of either **recovery** or **exhaustion**. If you recover, you relax and recuperate. Normal functioning resumes, needed repairs take place, fuel stores are refilled, and you become ready for the next round of excitement.

If you remain in a stressful state for too long, however, your resources may become depleted. People with chronic stress reach the exhaustion stage, in which the body's resources are depleted and its adaptive abilities are lost. Many of the events of the alarm stage occur again as the body attempts to adjust to higher levels of stress, but the resulting wear and tear compromise the immune system and injure body systems and organs—which can lead to illness.

How Stress Affects the Body Systems

Repeated episodes of the stress response can impair body systems—specifically, the digestive or gastrointestinal system, the cardiovascular system, and the immune system.

EFFECTS ON THE GASTROINTESTINAL SYSTEM

Stress affects the entire gastrointestinal system. When someone is stressed, the mouth produces less saliva. The regular rhythmic contractions of the esophagus are disrupted, making swallowing difficult. The stomach secretes more hydrochloric acid and thins the gastric mucus that normally protects the stomach lining, which can cause ulcers. The liver releases excess glucose, and the pancreas can become chronically inflamed. Increased hydrochloric acid and disruption of normal action in the intestinal tract can contribute to duodenal ulcers and chronic diarrhea or constipation.

EFFECTS ON THE CARDIOVASCULAR SYSTEM

Excessive stress affects the cardiovascular system, resulting in increased heart rate, damaged blood vessels, high blood pressure, and a boost in serum cholesterol levels, all of which increase the risk of cardiovascular disease. The heart itself beats more forcefully and pumps more blood during stress. Research has shown a strong link between stress and all kinds of cardiovascular disease. Stress can cause blood pressure to rise, resulting in

Conditions caused or aggravated by stress include the following, among others:

- heart disease
- arteriosclerosis
- atherosclerosis
- high blood pressure
- coronary thrombosis
- stroke
- angina
- respiratory ailments
- ulcers
- irritable bowel syndrome
- ulcerative colitis
- gastritis
- pancreatitis
- diabetes
- migraine headache
- myasthenia gravis
- epileptic attacks

- chronic backache
- kidney disease
- chronic tuberculosis
- allergies
- rheumatoid arthritis
- psoriasis
- eczema
- cold sores
- shingles
- hives
- asthma
- Raynaud's disease
- multiple sclerosis
- cancer
- endocrine and auto-immune problems

In 2005, Hurricane Katrina severely damaged areas and displaced people from their homes and jobs. Immediate problems included lack of water, food, shelter, and sanitation facilities. News reports clearly conveyed the physical devastation of this disaster, but the potential mental health consequences were not as well reported. As victims of this disaster struggled to rebuild their lives, some had deep mental health reactions that lingered for weeks or even months.

People often experience strong emotional and physical responses to disasters, including anxiety, depression, hopelessness, helplessness, sleeplessness, physical pain, confusion, fear, anger, grief, shock, guilt, and mistrust of others. Depending on the individual, these feelings vary in intensity and duration. If these reactions last for more than a month, a person may have Post Traumatic Stress Disorder (PTSD), a mental health disorder that most often develops in some people after being exposed to an event that invoked grave physical harm. People with PTSD may repeatedly re-experience a traumatic event through nightmares or frightening thoughts, especially when something reminds them of the trauma. They perceive that they are in danger even after it has passed.

For some people, the emotional recovery from Hurricane Katrina was the most difficult aspect. The good news is that effective treatments and services are available. Mental health resources are available to aid those affected by one of the biggest urban disasters the nation has ever seen.

For more information about coping with traumatic events, visit http://www.nimh.nih.gov/healthinformation/traumaticmenu.cfm

permanent hypertension if stress persists over time. Severe shock can even cause the heart to stop, and research has shown the link between cardiovascular disease and death.

For people with existing heart disease, mental stress may be just as hard on the heart as intense physical exertion. Stress causes blood vessels to constrict instead of expand, reducing the amount of blood that can be circulated. Stress causes the body to release cholesterol into the bloodstream. When the bloodstream carries too much cholesterol or other fats, fatty deposits build up on the walls of the coronary arteries, narrowing them and restricting blood flow to the heart. If the arteries eventually become clogged, blood flow to a certain part of the heart stops, that part of the heart muscle dies, and the victim has a heart attack.

In the alarm stage of the fight-or-flight reaction, the blood thickens. As a result, it coagulates more easily. Blood platelets build up along fatty deposits in the coronary arteries, worsening existing arteriosclerosis.

EFFECTS ON THE IMMUNE SYSTEM

Stress is potentially harmful to the immune system, making the body less capable of fighting disease and infection.[10] Stress suppresses the immune system's ability to produce and maintain lymphocytes (the white blood cells necessary for killing infection) and natural killer cells (the specialized cells that seek out and destroy foreign invaders), both of which are crucial in the fight against

infection and disease. Stress impairs the key players in immunity, from the body's levels of interferon (a protein that causes cells to produce infection-fighting enzymes) to the organs (such as the thymus) that are vital to immune system functioning.

Also, stress increases the risk for inciting allergic reactions, contracting infectious diseases, and developing autoimmune diseases such as rheumatoid arthritis. Stress suppresses the body's production of T lymphocytes, the immune cells that fight bacterial and viral infections, fungi, and cancer cells.

Resistance stage The second phase of the general adaptation syndrome, characterized by meeting the perceived challenge.

Recovery stage The return to homeostasis after a stressful event.

Exhaustion The final stage in the general adaptation syndrome, characterized by depletion of the body's resources and loss of adaptive abilities.

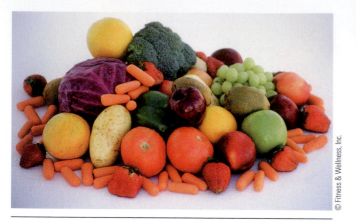
Proper nutrition is a key element in overall stress management.

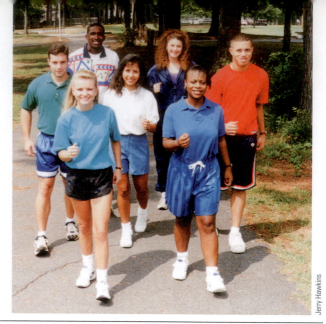
An active lifestyle buffers the effects of stress.

RESILIENCY

People who can withstand extreme stress without suffering the negative consequences have been said to be resilient or hardy. The hardiness concept (described in Chapter 2) incorporates the three Cs: commitment, control, and challenge. All three contribute to a healthier response to stress. People can work to build resiliency.[11] Developing close relationships and increasing connections with other people are among the positive ways to deal with stress.

Coping With Stress

Some people turn to unwise behaviors to cope with stress, such as using tobacco, alcohol, or other drugs. These behaviors are unhealthy in themselves, and they only mask the cause of the stress. Successful coping strategies provide long-term solutions to stressful problems without harming the body. Assessment 3.4 addresses your stress management skills.

Just as each individual reacts differently to stress, each individual has **adaptation energy stores**, the physical, mental, and emotional reserves that enable us to cope with stress. Professionals view these in two layers: a deep layer surrounded by a superficial layer. The energy stores in the superficial layer are used first and are easy for the body to access. These reserves can be replaced through positive health behaviors. The deep energy stores seem to be determined in part by heredity. They cannot be replaced, and when they are spent, the body dies.

Coping with stress successfully allows you to replenish adaptation energy stores. It prepares you to deal with stress. People who are educated about stress management strategies are better able to cope than those who are not, and people who maintain strong programs of personal wellness during ordinary life are best able to withstand crises when they arise. Eating well, sleeping well, being physically active, cultivating joy and laughter, and nurturing spiritual health can promote your ability to cope successfully with stress.

DIET AND PHYSICAL ACTIVITY

A balanced diet containing foods low in fat and high in fiber will help you physically cope with stress. A balanced diet follows the guidelines discussed in Chapter 8. Most of your calories should come from complex carbohydrates—grains, pastas (primarily whole grain), vegetables, and fruits.

Physical activity decreases the intensity of stress, lessens its effects, reduces the time needed to recover from stress, and even minimizes the physiological reactions of the stress response.[12] An active lifestyle reduces the risk of getting sick, even for those who are experiencing severe or chronic stress. Exercise reduces hostility, improves mental acuity, increases energy, eases muscle tension, and floods the system with endorphins.

As a word of caution: If you have not been exercising, start slowly. If you try too much at first, you are more likely to get injured or, at the least, stiff and sore. The resulting discouragement might keep you from exercising at all. If you are just starting out, take it easy. Try 10 to 15 minutes at a time, then extend the session as you get more conditioned. (Information on developing and implementing an active lifestyle and a regular exercise program is provided in Chapter 7.)

ADEQUATE SLEEP

Sleep is essential to coping with stress. If you've had your rest, it's easier to face almost anything. Sleep offers other, not-so-obvious benefits, too, including the relaxation that is so important to minimizing the effects of the stress response.

If you're feeling fatigued, try the following strategies to aid sleep:

• Try to establish a regular sleep pattern. Go to bed at about the same time every night and wake up at the

Sleep Stealers

- stress
- depression
- alcohol
- nicotine
- caffeine
- exercising too close to bedtime
- going to bed/getting up at differing times
- shift work
- jet lag
- bed partner with sleep problems
- bedroom that's too hot/too cold/too noisy/too bright
- arthritis, hormonal shifts (*e.g.*, menopause), asthma, sleep apnea, pain
- medications (side effect)

Source: National Sleep Foundation.

same time every morning instead of skimping on sleep during the week and sleeping until noon on weekends.

- If you really need to, take a short nap during the day, about 20 minutes. Shorter than that doesn't give you enough sleep, and more than that can make you sluggish.
- If you're having trouble falling asleep at night, don't nap during the afternoon, eat a light dinner, and avoid caffeine after 6 p.m.
- Use your bedroom only for sleeping. Don't watch television, study, or do work in bed. You need to associate your bed and your bedroom with sleep.
- Most people need 6 to 9 hours of sleep a night to function well and feel refreshed, but that requirement can vary from one person to another. To discover how much sleep you really need, go to sleep at the same time every night, then sleep until you wake up. It will take a couple of weeks to determine how much sleep you need.

Critical Thinking

Identify the body systems that are harmed by stress and connect the ways that diet, exercise, and sleep can benefit the body when in a state of stress.

A POSITIVE ATTITUDE

A positive attitude is a valuable component of stress management. For many, it involves reframing thoughts. **Reframing** means changing the way you look at things, learning to be an optimist instead of a pessimist. The way you think can reduce the negative effects of stress and increases your resilience.[13] To help reframe your thinking:

- Listen carefully to the words you use to describe yourself and your situation. Are they positive or negative?

Listen to yourself for a few weeks. Then, if you need to, use different phrases and descriptions.

- Role-play, either by yourself or with a friend. Start by relating a stressful situation you have experienced lately and tell how you reacted. Then come up with some different ways in which you could have reacted to the situation. If you're role-playing with a friend, ask for feedback or suggestions. Next, imagine some plausible stressful situations and outline how you'd handle them. Concentrate on positive responses.
- For one week, look for the good in every person and every situation you encounter. This can be tough, but you always can find something! This kind of exercise is like conditioning your attitudes. Before long, it can become a habit.
- Avoid words that signal defeat: always, never, should have, ought to. Replace them with more benign choices. Instead of saying, "I always fail quizzes in class," say, "I'm sometimes unprepared when the teacher springs a quiz on us."

EFFECTIVE TIME MANAGEMENT

One of the leading sources of stress is simply too much to do in too little time. We are living in a fast-paced society, and the mere speed at which we move can be a significant stressor. Learning to manage the time you have can alleviate stress and reduce anxiety.

To better manage your time:

- Figure out where your time goes. Keep a diary for 2 weeks. You may be surprised at the results!
- Determine your peak performance time. Are you a "morning person," or do you get your second wind when most people are quitting for the day? Plan and schedule your most demanding tasks—studying, working—for the time you are at your peak.
- Plan your breaks. Before writing anything else on your daily calendar, schedule a break or two to do what you want. Knowing you can look forward to a few breaks can help you face the day's stressful periods more effectively.
- Prioritize. Not every demand is a top priority. Decide which tasks are essential, important, and trivial, and spend your time and attention on the ones you've labeled as essential and important.
- Attack tasks one at a time. Don't try to accomplish everything at once. Make a list, and decide on a plan that lets you move through it calmly.
- Be realistic. Most people underestimate by about 50% how long a task will take, so get into the habit of adding 50% to the time you think you will need to complete a task.

Adaptation energy stores Reserves of physical, mental, and emotional energy that give us the ability to cope with stress.

Reframing Changing the way you look at things.

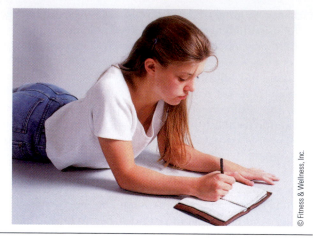

Planning and prioritizing your daily activities will simplify your life.

- Delegate when you can. If something doesn't require your personal attention, ask someone else to do it.
- Plan ahead. Before bedtime, write a schedule for the next day, including priorities and breaks.
- Set challenging, but realistic goals. Break them into manageable pieces; keep track of your progress and reward yourself for making that progress.
- Say "no" without guilt. You can do only so much in a day. If you start to feel overwhelmed, back off. Learning to say no also will help you by increasing your assertiveness (the ability to express yourself and satisfy your needs). Stress increases when people behave nonassertively (denying their own needs or wishes to make someone else happy) or aggressively (trying to get their own way at someone else's expense).

Critical Thinking

1. Discuss how time management helps with stress management.
2. What do you use for time management strategies?

PREVENTING BURNOUT

Stress—especially chronic stress—can lead to **burnout**, a state of physical and mental exhaustion with few remaining resources. Accompanying physical symptoms may include headache, indigestion, fatigue, and muscle soreness. Mental symptoms might be depression, resentment, apathy, inability to cope, or loss of enjoyment in life. Assessment 3.5 is a quiz on burnout.

To prevent burnout:

- Surround yourself with a strong social network. Have at least one friend in whom you can confide.
- Do something different to gain a fresh perspective. Distract yourself from your routine by trying something new and completely different.
- Take time for pure enjoyment. When you get bogged down, indulge in something fun or silly at least once a day. Laughter strengthens the immune system.

Laughter as Medicine

The physical benefits of laughter are many. It lowers blood pressure, increases muscle flexibility, and triggers a flood of beta endorphins, the brain's natural compounds that induce euphoria.

Laughter's most profound effects are on the immune system. Gamma-interferon, a disease-fighting protein, rises with laughter—as do B-cells, which produce disease-destroying antibodies, and T-cells, which orchestrate the immune response.

Laughter also shuts off the flow of stress hormones, the fight-or-flight compounds that come into play during times of stress, hostility, and rage.

Stress hormones suppress the immune system, raise blood pressure, and increase the number of platelets, which can cause fatal blockages in the arteries.

The average child laughs hundreds of times a day. The average adult laughs a dozen times. We need to find these lost laughs—and use them to our advantage.

Sources: Lee Berk, M.D. and Stanley Tan, M.D., American Association for Therapeutic Humor; Loma Linda University.

- Take a class for fun. Select something fun you have always wanted to try.

Relaxation Techniques

Any of a host of techniques can bring on the body's relaxation response—a process opposite from the response to stress, which counteracts the harmful effects of unmanaged stress. Invoking the relaxation response directly reduces the negative effects of stress and also gives you a more positive mental outlook, eases anxiety, and brings on a sense of control (essential to overcoming the negative aspects of stress). Regular relaxation exercises can reduce stress, increase resistance to stress-induced illness, minimize the symptoms of illness (such as headache), lower your blood pressure, and alleviate pain.

Some relaxation exercises are based on deep relaxation, with its myriad benefits. Others (such as deep breathing or a quick massage) reduce immediate stress and are a good way of leading into more extensive relaxation exercises. As with physical exercise, learning about various relaxation exercises takes some time. Before you decide which ones to try, you should consider your likes and dislikes, your personality, and your situation. You can learn some techniques on your own, and you will need some training for others. The techniques discussed here are meditation, prayer, progressive relaxation, deep breathing techniques, autogenics, biofeedback training, and yoga. With a little research, you will be able to find others.

A note of caution: If you are taking medication for high blood pressure, heart conditions, diabetes, epilepsy, or psychological conditions, consult with your health-care practitioner before you begin practicing relaxation techniques. These exercises can cause physiological changes.

MEDITATION

Simply stated, **meditation** is an exercise in which you become mindful. Mindfulness allows you to influence and monitor your thoughts and, thus, your body processes and responses to stressors.[14] Meditation helps many people lower their stress levels. It improves concentration, reduces mental distraction, drifting attention, and unfocused thoughts.

During meditation, a person focuses exclusively on a specific positive thought or object. Heartbeat and breathing slow down, blood pressure drops (often for as long as 12 to 24 hours after the meditative period), and the body's metabolism slows, decreasing its need for oxygen and other nutrients. As the person becomes relaxed, blood flow to the arms and legs increases, which eases muscle tension. Laboratory studies have shown that people who meditate have fewer blood lactates, the enzymes associated with stress and anxiety.[15]

To be effective, meditation has to be done in a comfortable position in a quiet place, free of distractions. No specific posture is required for meditation, but because the physiological processes of meditation are different from those of sleep, some people often sit so they will not fall asleep during meditation.

For maximum effect, experts recommend meditating 20 minutes at a time, twice during the day. The procedure is as follows:

1. Find a quiet room as free from distraction as possible. Lighting and temperature are a matter of individual preference. Just make sure you're comfortable. Turn off your phone and other distractors. Alert others that you don't want to be disturbed. (At first, it's important to have quiet surroundings; later, after you've practiced for a while, you will be able to meditate in almost any situation.)
2. Loosen your clothing if it is tight, especially at the wrists, neck, and waist. Get in the most comfortable position you can, in a chair or on a couch. Some recommend a straight-backed chair to prevent you from falling asleep. Place your feet flat on the floor and rest your hands in your lap.
3. Inhale slowly and deeply through your nose, hold your breath briefly, then exhale slowly. As you begin to breathe deeply, let the tension flow out of your body. Do not force it or concentrate on it. Just let it happen.
4. If you are concentrating on an unchanging object, close your eyes partially so the object appears blurred. Focus on it softly without bringing in any of the sharp details. Gradually focus all your attention on that object. Do not let any other thoughts invade your meditation.

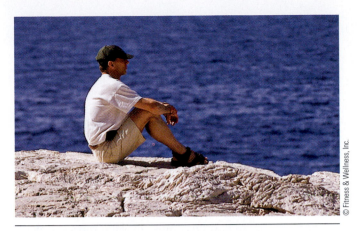
Meditation is an effective stress-reduction technique.

5. Continue meditating for approximately 20 minutes. Do not worry about the exact time. You will probably have to work up to it at first. Learning to sit still for 20 minutes at a time takes a lot of practice, especially when you are concentrating so intensely on a single object or phrase.
6. When you have finished meditating, give yourself time—at least several minutes—to readjust. Open your eyes, focus on various objects around the room, and return gradually to your normal rate and pattern of breathing. While still seated, stretch your arms, legs, back, shoulders, and neck. Finally, stand up slowly.

After meditating, it is important to let your body readjust. If you stand up too soon or too quickly, you may get dizzy, because your heart rate and blood pressure drop during meditation.

PRAYER

Some people combine prayer and meditation, claiming that either prayer alone or the combination of prayer and meditation enhances the effectiveness of stress management. Prayer involves communicating spiritually. When people pray, they seek help for problems and situations. By obtaining spiritual assistance, they reduce their perceptions of stress. (Prayer is discussed in more detail in Chapter 5.)

PROGRESSIVE RELAXATION

Progressive relaxation is a technique for physically relaxing the nerves and muscles. Practitioners learn to

---

Burnout A state of physical and mental exhaustion in which few resources remain.

Meditation A mental exercise to help gain control over thoughts.

Progressive relaxation A method of reducing stress that consists of tensing, then relaxing, small muscle groups.

recognize muscle tension and how to distinguish tense muscles from relaxed muscles. This technique is simple, with only three basic steps, but it takes practice:

1. Contract (tense) a small muscle group such as those in your fingers, toes, or forehead.
2. Relax the muscle group.
3. Concentrate on how different the two sensations feel.

You then proceed to other muscle groups until you have contracted and relaxed all the muscles of the body.

Progressive relaxation helps relieve tension headache, migraine headache, back pain, and other conditions related to muscle tension. It even has been shown to relax the smooth, or involuntary, muscles (like those in blood vessels of the digestive tract). It also has been shown to reduce anxiety, relieve depression, and improve sleep patterns.

You can design your own routine—working from your head to your toes, for example, or from your feet to your head—as long as all major groups in the body are involved eventually. When you start doing progressive relaxation, you should first tense the muscles as hard as you can, then relax them.

Unlike meditation, in which you work to detach your thoughts and awareness from your body, progressive relaxation requires you to concentrate on what is happening to your muscles. For the best results, you have to be acutely aware of the relaxed condition of your body.

Regardless of your individual routine, follow this procedure:

1. Take off your shoes and loosen any restrictive clothing. Stretch out on the floor on your back in the most comfortable position possible. Support your neck with a small pillow. If you need it, put a pillow under your knees. Close your eyes and rotate your ankles outward. Depending on which is most comfortable, either put your arms at your sides or rest your hands on your abdomen.
2. First tense, then relax, each muscle group. (Make sure you move to all major muscle groups in the body. Don't forget your face—including your forehead, eyes, nose, mouth, cheeks, and tongue).
3. As you move to each muscle group, contract the muscles as tightly as you can and hold the contraction for 20 or 30 seconds. If you experience pain or cramping, release the contraction immediately.
4. Concentrate on the dramatic difference in feeling between a tensed muscle and a relaxed one.

BREATHING TECHNIQUES

Breathing exercises also can be an antidote to stress. These can be learned in only a few minutes and require less time than other relaxation methods.

In breathing exercises, the person concentrates on "breathing away" the tension and inhaling fresh oxygen to the entire body. To be effective, the breathing must be so deep that the belly is expanded with each breath—a sign that the diaphragm is being expanded. Following is an example of a breathing exercise:

1. Lie in a comfortable position on your back and place your hands lightly over your lower abdomen.
2. Keeping your eyes open, imagine a balloon lying beneath your hands.
3. Begin to inhale slowly through your nose, concentrating on the warm air entering your nose and slowly filling the balloon. As you breathe in, you should be able to feel your lower abdomen rise. When the "balloon" is full (this should take 3 to 4 seconds initially), pause for a second, then slowly exhale to empty the balloon, feeling your chest and abdomen relaxing.
4. Repeat the entire process two or three times.
5. When finished, sit quietly for a few minutes before getting up. If you feel dizzy at any point, stop the procedure.

AUTOGENICS

Similar to progressive relaxation, **autogenics** is self-induced relaxation that causes all major muscle groups in the body to feel relaxed, heavy, and warm. It begins with a routine that relaxes all the major muscles (much like that of progressive relaxation), followed by **imagery** (vivid mental visualization) that extends the relaxed state.

Although autogenics and meditation both result in relaxation, they do it in different ways. In meditation, you first relax the mind, which causes the body to relax. In autogenics, you first relax the body, which causes the mind to relax.

The general sensations resulting from autogenics are feelings of warmth and heaviness, especially in the arms and legs, caused by dilation of blood vessels and relaxation of muscles. Autogenics and the associated imagery reduce heartbeat and breathing rates, ease muscle tension, and increase the brainwaves associated with deep relaxation.

Autogenics requires time, motivation, commitment, and practice. Commercial tapes are available to guide you through the relaxation exercises. You also may make your own tape or simply repeat the phrases aloud as you move through the exercises. As with progressive relaxation, you may want to design your own routine.

1. In a quiet room with mild temperatures, free of distractions, sit in the most comfortable position you can. Experts recommend sitting in a straight-backed but comfortable chair with your feet flat on the floor, your head hanging loosely forward, your eyes closed, and your hands in your lap with your palms turned upward. Loosen any restrictive clothing.
2. Imagine that you have just had a strenuous workout. You might begin with your legs. As you inhale and exhale deeply and slowly, repeat, "My legs are so tired. My legs are so heavy. My legs are very heavy and warm." As you repeat these phrases, feel the

heaviness and warmth in your legs. With practice, your legs should become so heavy and relaxed that you can lift them only with considerable struggle.

3. Move to other muscle groups—buttocks, abdomen, chest, arms, shoulders, and so on. You even might imagine your internal organs, such as your stomach and your heart, relaxed and warm.

4. Concentrate on how cool your forehead feels. For you to feel refreshed and alert, your forehead must feel cool.

5. Once your entire body is relaxed, visualize an image that you find relaxing. It might be waves lapping against a sandy beach, a cloud drifting lazily across the afternoon sky, an eagle soaring silently across a mountain. The image is different for everyone, but it should lead you to total relaxation.

For the greatest benefit, experts recommend that you practice twice a day for 10 minutes at a time. As with other kinds of relaxation exercises, autogenics requires practice, starting out slowly, then working up to a 10-minute period of visualization and relaxation.

BIOFEEDBACK TRAINING

Essentially, **biofeedback** is a method of measuring physiological functions you normally are not aware of (such as skin temperature and blood pressure) and then training yourself to control those functions. It has three basic stages:

1. Measuring the physiological function,
2. Converting the measurement into something meaningful, and
3. Feeding back the information.

Unlike some other forms of relaxation exercises, you can't learn biofeedback training on your own. It requires that you be monitored by equipment, then taught to regulate your own physiological responses. Biofeedback training is valuable as a stress management technique because it allows you to control your body's responses to stress. Most people can learn effective biofeedback techniques in a few sessions from a trained therapist.

YOGA

Yoga is known to induce calm, invigorate the mind, and reduce the biological effects of stress. This is an excellent exercise for improving muscular strength, flexibility, and endurance. **Yoga** consists of precise postures done in a specific sequence combined with an exact breathing rhythm designed to reduce tension and inflexibility. Yoga means union and involves stretching exercises to induce relaxation.

Some yoga postures are difficult and complex, requiring training and practice. Some simpler ones will help you get started, and many of the more difficult ones may be modified until you can perform the original pose.

One goal of yoga is relaxation, so you should not force positions that make you tense or could cause injury.

A number of good yoga instruction books and videotapes are available in the marketplace, and yoga classes are taught throughout the United States. Most experts recommend practicing yoga for 15 to 45 minutes a day in a place free of distraction. Many people sign up for classes, where they actually perform yoga daily.

Critical Thinking

1. What stress management techniques have you tried?
2. What was the result?

Checkmate for Stress

Like improving your game of chess, you can develop strategies to put stress in check. You don't want to eliminate stress completely because minimal or moderate stress enhances immunity. Too little stress leaves you feeling restless, bored, unhappy, and tired. Conversely, with too much stress, you feel exhausted, irritable, and burned out. Just the right amount of stress can help you feel energetic, creative, happy, and productive. The key is to achieve the middle ground.

Three more techniques for coping are the following:

1. *Situational reconstruction*: When a stressful event occurs, replay it in your mind to gain understanding and pinpoint where the anxiety is coming from. If you have had an argument, what contribution did you make? What did the other person do? Next, get some perspective by imagining both how the situation could get worse and how it could get better. Finally, ask yourself what you could do to increase the likelihood of it getting better, and put your answer into action.

2. *Compensatory self-improvement*: When you can't think of anything you could do to make the situation better, you may be confronting something you cannot change. If this is the case, accept the reality gracefully without succumbing to bitterness and self-pity. One way to do this is by choosing another problem related to the first one and work on that problem instead. Rather than feeling victimized or overwhelmed,

Autogenics A relaxation technique in which the person is trained, with the aid of specialized equipment, to relax all major muscle groups through a form of self-hypnosis, followed by imagery.

Imagery Vivid mental visualization.

Biofeedback A relaxation technique that involves measuring and controlling physiological functions.

Yoga An exercise technique involving stretching, used to relieve stress and induce calm.

The following strategies are designed to reduce the amount and extent of stress in your life, not to cause you more stress. To reach that goal:

- Don't overload yourself with too many strategies at once.
- Know your own strengths and skills, as well as what you enjoy, and what social support you have for beneficial changes.
- With stress management, one size doesn't fit all; be flexible, know when you need to change, and be willing to do so.

- Don't expect one new strategy to make you stress-free; you may need to add several new habits over time.
- Know your limits. You can't control everything and will have to accept some things and move on.
- See the positive side of negative stress. Meeting stressors as challenges and opportunities for learning and growth will help you counter that stress.

---

say to yourself, "I may not be able to fix everything, but I can improve some things."

3. Find humor in yourself and situations.[16] Allow yourself to relax and laugh, as laughter is health-enhancing.

In short, start with yourself. There are few situations that cannot be improved by working on your own personal changes. Stress management offers techniques that you can master to enhance your overall quality of life.

WEB Interactive

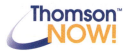

Don't forget to check out the wealth of resources on the ThomsonNOW website at **www.thomsonedu.com/ ThomsonNOW** that will:

- Coach you through identifying target goals for behavior change and monitoring your personal change plan throughout the semester
- Help you evaluate your knowledge of the material
- Allow you to take an exam-prep quiz
- Provide a Personalized Learning Plan targeting resources that address areas you should study.

WEB ACTIVITIES

Stress Management: A Review of Principles This online series of lectures is presented by Wesley E. Sime, Ph.D., M.P.H., professor of Health and Human Performance at the University of Nebraska, Lincoln. It features stress-management information on the psychobiology of stress and relaxation, as well as pathophysiology of stress.

http://www.unl.edu/stress/mgmt

Exercise Can Help Control Stress This site, sponsored by the American Council on Exercise, lists several ways to help manage stress through regular exercise.

http://www.acefitness.org/fitfacts/fitfacts_list.aspx

InfoTrac®

You can find additional readings related to wellness via InfoTrac® College Edition, an online library of more than 900 journals and publications. Follow the instructions for accessing InfoTrac® that came packaged with your textbook, then search for articles using a key word search.

Suggested Reading Dusselier, Laurie et al. "Personal, health, academic, and environmental predictors of stress for residence hall students," *Journal of American College Health*, July–August 2005 v54 i1 p15 (10).

1. Which students reported greater levels of stress? Why do you think this is so?
2. What were the most frequent predictors of chronic stress?
3. What is the relationship between depression and stress?

Web Activity

Stress Assess

http://wellness.uwsp.edu/Other/stress/

Sponsor National Wellness Institute, University of Wisconsin— Stevens Point

Description This three-part on-line educational tool, developed by the National Wellness Institute, is in the form of a questionnaire designed to increase your knowledge about stress. It features separate evaluations for stress sources, distress symptoms, and stress-balancing strategies. Based on these results, you will learn healthy strategies to better manage your specific stressors.

Available Activities Select from the following three evaluations:

1. *Stress Sources* Helps you evaluate the sources of stress in your life. Each stage of life is accompanied by its own unique stress sources: family, social, individual, environment, work, and college. This assessment measures the various sources of stress in your life at the current time.
2. *Distress Symptoms* Helps you identify your symptoms of stress. In answering the questions, you select your symptoms and signs of distress (feelings, behaviors, body reactions).
3. *Stress-Balancing Strategies* Provides you with information to help you handle stress.

Web Work

1. From the home page, click on the "Stress Sources" link first. Answer these questions honestly to determine your major stressors.

2. Upon completing the "Stress Sources" evaluation, click on the "Distress Symptoms" link from the home page to help you identify your symptoms of stress. In the "Distress Symptoms" section, answer the demographic information and then the questions, using the pull-down menu.
3. Complete the questions for the "Signs of Distress" section for all three areas (feelings, behaviors, and body reactions). When you're finished, click on the "Perform Your Stress Assessment" button to obtain your results for this section.
4. Repeat these directions for the other two evaluations available at this site.

Helpful Hint

"Stress Assess" is an educational tool designed to enhance your knowledge about stress. It is not a clinical instrument or diagnostic tool.

For additional Web activities, links, and suggested readings, visit our Health, Fitness, and Wellness Resource Center at http://health.wadsworth.com.

Notes

1. E. R. DeKloet, "Hormones, Brain and Stress," *Endocrine Regulations* 37 (2003): 51–68.
2. R. R. Ross and E. M. Altmaier, *Intervention in Occupational Stress* (London: Sage Publications, 1994).
3. P. A. Bovier, E. Chamot, T. V. Perneger, "Perceived Stress, Internal Resources, and Social Support as Determinants of Mental Health Among Young Adults," *Quality of Life Research* 13 (2004): 161–170.
4. R. M. D'Souza, L. Strazdins, L. Lim, D. H. Broom, B. Rodger, "Work and Health in a Contemporary Society: Demands, Control, and Insecurity," *Journal of Epidemiology and Community Health* 57 (2003): 849–854.
5. M. Pohanka, S. Fitzgerald, "Urban Sprawl and You: How Sprawl Adversely Affects Worker Health," *American Association of Occupational Health Nurses* 52 (2004): 242–246.
6. V. A. Lambert, C. E. Lambert, H. Yamase, "Psychological Hardiness, Workplace Stress and Related Stress Reduction Strategies," *Nursing and Health Sciences* 5 (2003): 181–184.
7. D. S. Krantz et al., "Effects of Mental Stress in Patients with Coronary Artery Disease: Evidence and Clinical Implications," *Journal of the American Medical Association* 283 (2000): 1800–1802.
8. A. Feyer et al., "The Role of Physical and Psychological Factors in Occupational Low Back Pain: A Prospective Cohort Study," *Occupational and Environmental Medicine* 57 (2000): 116–120.
9. M. C. Rosal, J. King, Y. Ma, G. W. Reed, "Stress, Social Support, and Cortisol: Inverse Associations?" *Behavioral Medicine* 30 (2004): 11–21.
10. G. B. Stefano, G. L. Fricchione, B. T. Slingsby, H. Benson, "The Placebo Effect and Relaxation Response: Neural Processes and Their Coupling to Constitutive Nitric Oxide," *Brain Research Reviews* 35 (2001): 1–19.
11. C. C. Bell, "Cultivating Resiliency in Youth," *Journal of Adolescent Health*, 29 (2001): 375–381.
12. S. Stear, "Health and Fitness: The Importance of Physical Activity for Health," Journal of Family Care 13 (2003): 10–13.
13. K. Tusaie, J. Dyer, "Resilence: A Historical Review of the Construct," *Holistic Nursing Practice* 18 (2004): 3–8.
14. A. M. Tacon, J. McComb, Y. Caldera, P. Randolph, "Mindfulness Meditation, Anxiety Reduction, and Heart Disease: A Pilot Study, *Community Health* 26 (2003): 25–33.
15. J. H. Gruzelier, "A Review of the Impact of Hypnosis, Relaxation, Guided Imagery, and Individual Differences on Aspects of Immunity and Health," *Stress: The International Journal on the Biology of Stress* 5 (2002): 147–163.
16. A. Szabo, "The Acute Effects of Humor and Exercise on Mood and Anxiety," *Journal of Leisure Research* 35 (2003): 152–162.

Assess Your Behavior

1. List and describe the common sources of stress that are most likely to affect you. Can you identify the signs and symptoms of stress that you experience?

2. Are you obtaining adequate nutrients, exercise, and sleep to protect you from the negative effects of stress?

3. Have you experienced burnout recently and what strategies can you utilize to prevent it in the future?

Evaluate how well you understand the concepts presented in this chapter by answering the following questions.

1. A stressor is
   a. a virus.
   b. anything that requires adaptation.
   c. homeostasis.
   d. boredom.
   e. All of the above.

2. Positive challenges are called
   a. eustress.
   b. distress.
   c. anxiety.
   d. depression.
   e. burdens.

3. Excessive stress can worsen the following condition
   a. cardiovascular disease.
   b. gastrointestinal disease.
   c. musculoskeletal disorders.
   d. respiratory problems.
   e. All of the above.

4. The stress response always includes these stages:
   a. alarm.
   b. resistance.
   c. exhaustion.
   d. a and b.
   e. b and c.

5. Being able to withstand extreme stress without suffering the negative consequences is called
   a. coping.
   b. recovery.
   c. immunity.
   d. exhaustion.
   e. resiliency.

6. To prevent burnout
   a. surround yourself with a strong support network.
   b. take time for enjoyment.
   c. engage in laughter.
   d. engage in relaxation techniques.
   e. All of the above.

Correct answers can be found on page 369.

Scoring Your Stress: A Test to Pinpoint What's Eating You

Name: _____   Date: _____   Grade: _____

Instructor: _____   Course: _____   Section: _____

How Stressed Are You?

The answer depends in part on what's going on in your life, but it also depends on some other factors—such as what your attitudes are about those events and how much control you feel over what happens.

The first step in managing stress, of course, is to identify it. This assessment will help you do just that. It's simple: Read each question, then circle the number that most closely describes your situation or attitude. If you're completely neutral, circle 5; if a question doesn't apply to you at all, skip it.

Ready?

1. How often do you suffer stress-related physical symptoms, such as headaches, jaw pain, neck pain, back pain, indigestion, abdominal pain, diarrhea, loss of appetite, excessive perspiration, fatigue, or a pounding in your chest?

   Rarely or never   **Every day**
   1   2   3   4   5   6   7   8   9   10

2. Do you wash your hands before you eat?

   Always   **Rarely or never**
   1   2   3   4   5   6   7   8   9   10

3. Do you take measures to keep your food safe, such as cooking it adequately, storing it properly, and avoiding obvious contaminants?

   Almost always   **Rarely or never**
   1   2   3   4   5   6   7   8   9   10

4. How often do you eat fresh fruits, fresh vegetables, whole grains, and foods high in fiber?

   Every day   **Rarely or never**
   1   2   3   4   5   6   7   8   9   10

5. How often do you eat high fat or high-sugar foods—including candy, pastry, soft drinks, and food from fast-food restaurants?

   Occasionally   **Every day**
   1   2   3   4   5   6   7   8   9   10

6. How often do you exercise?

   Every day   **Rarely or never**
   1   2   3   4   5   6   7   8   9   10

7. How many hours of sleep do you get each day?

   8 or more hours   **Less than 4 hours**
   1   2   3   4   5   6   7   8   9   10

8. How many cups of coffee or caffeinated soft drinks do you drink each day?

   None   **Five or more**
   1   2   3   4   5   6   7   8   9   10

9. How often do you use alcohol, tobacco, over-the-counter drugs, or prescription drugs to relieve stress?

   Never   **Every day**
   1   2   3   4   5   6   7   8   9   10

10. If you have a relationship with a significant other, how would you describe that relationship?

   Mutually satisfying in many ways   **Marked by jealousy or insecurity**
   1   2   3   4   5   6   7   8   9   10

11. How do you feel when you have to say "no" to a request for your time, energy, talents, or money?

Confident and at ease   **Anxious and guilt-ridden**

1   2   3   4   5   6   7   8   9   10

12. How would you characterize your support system?

Broad-based, many sources   **Limited or no sources**

1   2   3   4   5   6   7   8   9   10

13. What kinds of friendships do you have?

At least several close friends/confidants   **No close friends**

1   2   3   4   5   6   7   8   9   10

14. What do you do if you have a problem you can't solve on your own?

Seek help immediately   **Suffer on my own**

1   2   3   4   5   6   7   8   9   10

15. How many major changes (such as entering or ending an intimate relationship, death of a family member, a change in your financial status, moving, starting a new job, a change in sleeping habits, a change in living conditions, or a change in the number of arguments you have with roommates) have occurred in your life during the last year?

None   **Many**

1   2   3   4   5   6   7   8   9   10

16. How do you react when you are confronted with a problem or stressful situation?

Put it aside to gain perspective then focus on solutions   **Feel overwhelmed or panic-stricken**

1   2   3   4   5   6   7   8   9   10

17. How often do you "retreat" temporarily when you start to feel overwhelmed by stress?

Most of the time   **Never**

1   2   3   4   5   6   7   8   9   10

18. How do you normally feel at the end of the day?

I got the important things done   **I didn't accomplish anything**

1   2   3   4   5   6   7   8   9   10

19. How many hassles do you have in a typical day?

A few   **A lot**

1   2   3   4   5   6   7   8   9   10

20. How much noise are you exposed to every day?

Not very much   **Most of the day is noisy**

1   2   3   4   5   6   7   8   9   10

21. How comfortable is your environment? (Consider temperature extremes, humidity, crowding, and environmental pollutants.)

Very comfortable   **Very uncomfortable**

1   2   3   4   5   6   7   8   9   10

22. Overall, how satisfying is your life?

Very satisfying   **Very disappointing**

1   2   3   4   5   6   7   8   9   10

Scoring

It's time to take a look at your stress level. This exercise will tell you two things: It will indicate your general stress level. Then it will help pinpoint the specific things that are causing you stress.

First, total your score by adding every number you circled. Now divide it by the number of questions you answered. This is one test on which you don't want a high score: The closer your average creeps toward 10, the higher your stress level is likely to be. (By the way, it's important to average your stress score this way; a high level of stress in a few areas won't cause your general stress level to skyrocket.)

Next, go back and isolate what's causing you problems. Look back through your responses. Find those in which you circled a number higher than 5. You've found your problem areas.

Now determine some stress-busting strategies.

How Stressed Are You?

Name: _____   Date: _____   Grade: _____

Instructor: _____   Course: _____   Section: _____

To find out your stress level, take the "stress scale"—a test developed by University of Washington researchers Thomas Holmes and Richard Rahe. The test rates life events known to produce stress. Check off the events that have happened to you in the past year. Add them up. If you score 300 or more, you are at highest risk of developing stress-induced disease.

Stress	Points		Stress	Points
1. Death of spouse	100		23. Son or daughter leaving home	29
2. Divorce	73		24. Trouble with in-laws	29
3. Marital separation	65		25. Outstanding personal achievement	28
4. Jail term	63		26. Spouse beginning or stopping work	26
5. Death of close family member	63		27. Beginning or ending school	26
6. Personal injury or illness	53		28. Change in living conditions	25
7. Marriage	50		29. Revision of personal habits	24
8. Fired from job	47		30. Trouble with boss	23
9. Marital reconciliation	45		31. Change in work hours or conditions	20
10. Retirement	45		32. Change in residence	20
11. Change in health of family member	44		33. Change in schools	20
12. Pregnancy	40		34. Change in recreation	19
13. Sexual difficulties	39		35. Change in worship activities at church or temple	19
14. Gain of new family member	39		36. Change in social activities	18
15. Business readjustment	39		37. Mortgage or loan less than $10,000	17
16. Change in financial state	38		38. Change in sleeping habits	16
17. Death of close friend	37		39. Change in number of family get-togethers	15
18. Change to different line of work	36		40. Change in eating habits	15
19. Change in number of arguments with spouse	35		41. Vacation	13
20. Mortgage over $10,000	31		42. Christmas	12
21. Foreclosure of mortgage or loan	30		43. Minor violation of the law	11
22. Change in responsibilities at work	29			

Total Points _____

Take Your Stress Temperature

Name: _____   Date: _____   Grade: _____

Instructor: _____   Course: _____   Section: _____

How Stressed Are You?

Let's play 20 questions. Check "yes" or "no" for the following:

		YES	NO
1.	Do you prefer to do everything yourself rather than let people help you?	☐	☐
2.	For you, is there only one right way to do things?	☐	☐
3.	Do you find it hard to make decisions?	☐	☐
4.	Do you forget to laugh?	☐	☐
5.	Do you never have time to daydream?	☐	☐
6.	Is it important to you that everyone likes you?	☐	☐
7.	When little things go wrong, does it ruin your whole day?	☐	☐
8.	Do you constantly feel exhausted?	☐	☐
9.	Have you had problems with insomnia?	☐	☐
10.	Do you grind your teeth?	☐	☐
11.	In the last year, have you had three or more illnesses that could have been triggered by stress—headaches, diarrhea, colds, flu?	☐	☐
12.	Do you hate it when the plan changes?	☐	☐
13.	Do you get upset when you have to wait in line?	☐	☐
14.	Are you easily bored?	☐	☐
15.	Do you find it hard to say no?	☐	☐
16.	Do you hate the shape your body is in but can't seem to do anything about changing it?	☐	☐
17.	Does your life feel out of control?	☐	☐
18.	Are you resentful that so many people make demands on your time?	☐	☐
19.	Have you moved, broken up with a boyfriend/girlfriend, lost a parent, or gone through any other big changes in the last year?	☐	☐
20.	Was the last time you had a vacation over a year ago?	☐	☐

Count one point for each "yes." The closer your total is to 20, the higher your stress level. If you rate 10 or above, be sure you do *something* because, with this level of stress in your life, you have a high risk of getting sick unless you learn to manage it.

Reprinted with permission from Elizabeth Somer, M.A.R.D., *Food & Mood,* 1999.

Stress Management Skills: What Do You Do?

Name: _____ **Date:** _____ **Grade:** _____

Instructor: _____ **Course:** _____ **Section:** _____

For each skill, circle the number that corresponds to your typical skill use.

I use the following skills . . .	Never	Rarely	Occasionally	Regularly
Personal Management Skills: Organizing Yourself				
Valuing: Investing self appropriately	1	2	3	4
Planning: Moving toward goals	1	2	3	4
Commitment: Saying yes and sticking to it	1	2	3	4
Time Use: Setting priorities	1	2	3	4
Pacing: Controlling the tempo	1	2	3	4
Relationship Skills: Changing the Scene				
Contact: Reaching out	1	2	3	4
Listening: Tuning in to others	1	2	3	4
Assertiveness: Saying no	1	2	3	4
Fight: Standing your ground	1	2	3	4
Flight: Leaving the scene	1	2	3	4
Nest-Building: Creating a home	1	2	3	4
Outlook Skills: Changing Your Mind				
Relabeling: Turning a spade into a diamond	1	2	3	4
Surrendering: Saying goodbye	1	2	3	4
Faith: Accepting your limits	1	2	3	4
Imagination: Laughing, creativity	1	2	3	4
Whispering: Talking nicely to oneself	1	2	3	4
Physical Stamina: Building Your Strength				
Exercise: Fine-tuning your body	1	2	3	4
Nourishment: Feeding your body	1	2	3	4
Gentleness: Wearing kid gloves	1	2	3	4
Relaxation: Cruising in neutral	1	2	3	4

Look down the column of 1s. These are your underdeveloped skills. Underline the ones you would like to use more often. **Look at the column of 4s.** These are probably your skills of habit. Mark those you tend to overuse. Which three individual coping skills do you use most often? For what kinds of stressors? As you identify your pattern of skill use, what insights and observations strike you?

Reprinted with permission from Donald A. Tubesing, *Kicking Your Stress Habits,* copyright 1981, 1989. Published by Whole Person Associates Inc., 210 West Michigan, Duluth, MN 55802, (218) 727-0500.

Burnout Quiz

Name: _____   **Date:** _____   **Grade:** _____

Instructor: _____   **Course:** _____   **Section:** _____

Take a look at all three aspects of your life—career/school, personal, and relationships—and ask yourself the following questions. If the answer is an emphatic yes, score 5 points. If it's definitely no, give yourself 0 points. If you're in between, score 1 to 4 points, depending on your level of discomfort.

Score

1. I feel more negative than positive lately.

2. I feel more fatigued than energetic.

3. I work harder and harder and accomplish less and less.

4. Joy is elusive, and I'm often invaded by a sadness I can't explain.

5. I'm increasingly irritable and choosing not to be with people.

6. I suffer from physical complaints (legs feel heavy, backache, headache, lingering colds).

7. I'm unable to laugh at a joke about myself.

8. I feel a loss of self-esteem, confidence, and can-do attitude.

9. Sex seems like more trouble than it's worth.

10. I'm increasingly judgmental, short-tempered, and disappointed in the people around me.

Total Points

Scoring

0–15:	You're doing fine.
16–25:	Oops! There are things you should be watching.
26–35:	You're a candidate for burnout.
36–45:	You're burning out.
46 and over:	Take special note. There are distinct threats to your health and well-being.

Reprinted with permission from Elizabeth Somer, M.A.R.D., *Food & Mood,* 1999.

4

CHAPTER

Social Support and Health

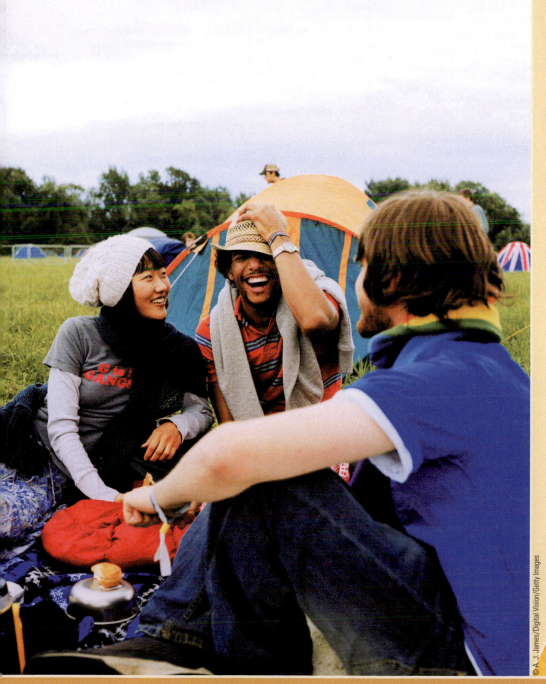

© A. J. James/Digital Vision/Getty Images

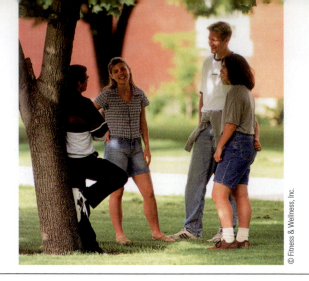

A network of social support can enhance and protect health.

The claim that our social connections are important to health is not new. What is new is the collection of hard evidence that supports the idea that social support is related to positive health practices and can protect people from a wide variety of diseases.[1]

People with positive social ties—regardless of their source—live longer than people who are isolated. People who are isolated are at greater risk of dying early from a number of causes. Being isolated contributes to higher rates of alcoholism, arthritis, depression, heart disease, suicide, and other problems. People who have close-knit networks of positive personal ties with other people seem to be better equipped for avoiding disease. They maintain higher levels of health and in general deal more successfully with life's difficulties.

Social Support and Social Networks

Social support consists of the human resources that people provide to each other. It tells a person that he or she can rely on other people for help with problems and in times of crises. It means giving and receiving help from others. A related term, **social network**, refers more specifically to the size, density, durability, intensity, and frequency of social contacts.

Four types of social support are:

1. *Instrumental support*: tangible aid such as a financial loan when needed, help running errands, or a ride to class when your car is being repaired.
2. *Emotional support*: affection, understanding, acceptance, and respect.
3. *Informational support*: information such as which classes to take, where to go to sign up for a club, and so on.
4. *Appraisal support*: feedback, advice, direction. People who provide this type of support can help when you are trying to make a decision or when you need to know how you are doing.

Benefits of Social Support

Social support protects health and reduces mortality. The number and strength of a person's close relationships are related closely to an individual's well-being and longevity. People who have frequent interactions with others and a variety of relationships generally have better health outcomes and are less likely to experience stress and its negative effects.[2]

People who have social support report having feelings of connectedness and feeling part of a community.[3] The most significant predictor against violence, stress, suicide, and substance abuse is a feeling of connectedness at home and in school. Individuals who lack the comfort of another human being may well lack one of nature's most powerful antidotes to stress. Dr. James Lynch, a social support researcher remarked:

> The mandate to love your neighbor as you love yourself is not just a moral mandate. It's a physiological mandate. Caring is biological. One thing you get from caring for others is you're not lonely; and the more connected you are to life, the healthier you are.[4]

Nearly 3,000 adults in Tecumseh, Michigan, were the subjects of one long-term study.[5] At the beginning of the study, each adult was given a thorough physical examination to rule out any existing illness that would force a person to become isolated. Researchers then watched these people closely for the next 10 years, making special note of their social relationships and group activities. Those who were involved socially were found to have optimal positive health status. When social ties were interrupted or broken, the incidence of disease increased significantly. The researchers concluded that interrupted social ties seemed to actually suppress the body's immune system. Those who conducted the study concluded that close personal relationships comprise a safety net and that people in the study without this safety net were most vulnerable to a wide variety of diseases.

Strong social support enables us to take better care of ourselves. In a national study, positive health behaviors such as engaging in physical activity, obtaining cholesterol and blood pressure screenings, and eating fruits and vegetables were all related to the extent of social contact in people's lives.[6]

If we want to live longer, happier lives, we need to surround ourselves with at least a few good people as friends and confidants. To provide benefit, these people must be positive and encouraging.

Critical Thinking

1. Define and describe social support and social networks.
2. List the number of people in your support network and rate the quality of support you give and receive from each person. Are your support relationships balanced?

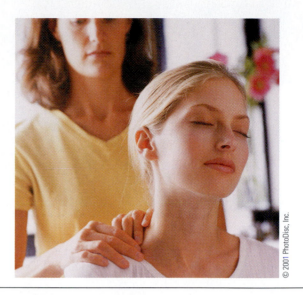

© 2001 PhotoDisc, Inc.

A therapeutic touch can hasten healing.

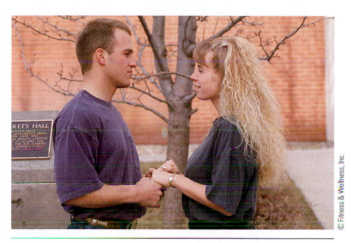

© Fitness & Wellness, Inc.

Appropriate touch is an important form of social support.

Landmark Study on Social Support

Dr. David Spiegel conducted a landmark study with women whose breast cancer had metastasized. One group received counseling and social support in addition to the proper medical care. The comparison group of women received only the appropriate medical care without the counseling or peer support. The latter group reported more pain and did not live as long as the group that had received social support from friends and family.

Source: *Healing and the Mind*, by Bill Moyers (New York: Doubleday, 1993), p. 157.

Touch: A Crucial Aspect of Social Support

Perhaps one of the most powerful components of social support is touch. People who appropriately touch others and welcome touch seem to reap positive health benefits. People who enjoy regular, satisfying touch—a pat on the back, a hug—receive both psychological and physical benefits.

To achieve benefits of stress reduction and physical and emotional healing, some people obtain therapeutic massage. The physical touch provided during massage can hasten healing and provide other emotional and physical health benefits.[7] It helps to reduce stress and fatigue and enhances relaxation.

Loneliness and Health

Loneliness is an unpleasant state of mind that results when a person's network of social relationships is significantly deficient in either quality or quantity.

Loneliness is not necessarily a consequence of being alone. Many people who live alone do not feel lonely. What for one person may be acceptable solitude is anguish for another. And people can feel lonely even when people surround them. Further, loneliness is related less to the number of people in our lives than to the satisfaction we have with those relationships. Loneliness sets in when our relationships do not meet our needs or when a positive relationship becomes negative.

Feelings of loneliness are worse when relationships lack true attachment. Also, people with low self-esteem seem to feel loneliness more keenly. Also, loneliness can

Social support The human resources that people provide to each other.

Social network The size, density, durability, intensity, and frequency of social contacts.

Loneliness A state of mind that occurs when a person's network of social relationships is significantly deficient in either quality or quantity.

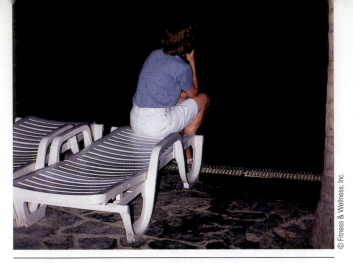

Loneliness may increase the risk for disease.

Loneliness and the Immune System

Bill Moyers interviewed David Felten, Professor of Neurobiology and Anatomy at the University of Rochester, about loneliness and health. He responded that loneliness consistently emerges as a predictor of diminished immune response in patients, leaving them vulnerable to a number of diseases. For example, in one study involving medical students, those who said they were lonely and had poor social support also had chronically diminished immune responses.

Source: *Healing and the Mind*, by Bill Moyers (New York: Doubleday, 1993), pp. 220–221.

stem from a person's sense of not belonging to an accepting community.

Loneliness carries with it a risk for health problems.[8] Loneliness, and the stress that accompanies it, have been connected to a host of physical and mental disorders and premature death. Loneliness is a significant risk factor for the range of conditions from colds to serious illnesses such as heart disease.[9] People who are not lonely have a better chance of staying healthy or recovering from disease than people who are lonely.

The Importance of Friendships

Close friendships clearly buffer stress and help overcome the unwanted effects of loneliness. Friendship involves certain attitudes that may in themselves help boost health. Friends enjoy trust, respect, and acceptance. A good friend accepts you as you are, without trying to make you change or become a different person. Friends support and help each other, act in the other's best interests, and respect what is important to the other. Friends share feelings and experiences with each other that they don't share with other people. And, despite occasional annoyances, friends enjoy each other most of the time.

Confiding in another person—having a confidant with whom you can share personal information—forges a powerful and lasting bond and can provide many health benefits. In some cases, friends are closer confidants than family members. Still, some risks are involved in sharing sensitive information with a friend. Before you confide in someone:

- Realize that sharing information about sensitive issues may strain the friendship. In most cases, confiding in someone helps the two of you grow closer, but if your friend feels threatened or hurt by what you say, it could change the nature of the relationship.
- Recognize that disclosing a past trauma may be difficult or uncomfortable for the listener to hear. If the information you divulge is upsetting, the listener may be so burdened by what you say that he or she, in turn, may have the urge to tell someone else.
- Explore your motive for sharing potentially hurtful information. Some people confide out of revenge (you hurt me, so I'm going to hurt you back). Revenge, anger, and the desire to inflict hurt are not constructive reasons for disclosing certain information.
- Recognize that there might be a better way to solve a problem than by discussing it with a friend. You might be able to take direct action, for example. If so, don't burden a friend.
- Before disclosing specific information, ask yourself three questions: Is it true? Will it be unhurtful? Is it necessary? If you can answer these questions in ways that reflect sincere motives for sharing information, go ahead and speak to a friend about it.

Enriching Your Support Network

Having a strong social network is stress-reducing and health-enhancing. If your social connections are weak, invest as much time and energy as you can toward building your support network. One way to enhance your social support is to enrich your existing friendships. Even though we are tempted to communicate by cell phone and e-mail in this fast-paced, high-tech society, it is vital to spend time with people in person. Face-to-face interactions provide benefits that cannot be obtained by talking on the phone or communicating on the Internet. Nonverbal communication and physical touch enhance relationships.

Another way to expand your social network is to increase diversity in your social interactions. Cultivate different types of friends. With some you will enjoy deep conversations. Others will be good companions to movies and social events. Seek friendships with people who have similar interests. You will find them readily in classes and clubs focusing on computers, poetry, sports activities, or other areas of common interest.

Establishing rituals for connecting is another good way to widen your support network. Getting together regularly to play golf, see the latest movies, or celebrate birthdays and holidays are possible friendship-building rituals.

Not all relationships are beneficial. Therefore, you should consciously become more involved in positive relationships and less involved in negative relationships. Some relationships are energizing and validating, and others are exhausting and unpleasant. Although people tend to gravitate toward relationships that enhance their self-esteem, some stay in touch with at least one person who is not good for them, often out of habit or obligation or because they cannot think of a way to end the relationship.

Having people around to talk with and relate to is health-enhancing only if the quality of those relationships is positive. One way to tell if a relationship is good for you is to reflect on how you feel after being with a friend —better or worse. If a person repeatedly leaves you feeling worse than before the visit, this relationship may not be helpful. Reducing the time involved with negative people and increasing your involvement with positive people will have a beneficial effect on your social network and, consequently, your health.

Becoming more involved in your community also can have significant health benefits. Trust in each other, willingness to help, and productive activities are indications of healthy community support systems whose residents perceive their own health as better.[10]

Another way to enrich a social network during a crisis or when coping with a difficult situation is to join a support group composed of members who are facing the same or similar problems. In support groups, participants share their experiences and feelings and offer coping strategies and informational help. Some support groups enlist experts to talk about related topics. Involvement in a support group can lower psychological stress, and reduce depression.

Critical Thinking

1. Thinking about your support network, how satisfied are you with the quality and quantity of this system?
2. What activities can you do to enrich your support network?
3. How can you minimize the effects of people in your network who are negative, and maximize the impact of people in your network who are positive?

The Importance of Pets

People aren't the only source of support. Pets can fulfill a variety of needs for their human companions. They meet our need to care for another being and our desire to feel loved. Pets return our affection.

As a form of social support, having a pet can have a positive effect on our physical health. If you have a dog that requires daily walks, for example, you will receive healthful exercise. Pet ownership has been associated with improved cardiovascular functioning, improved emotional stability, and better general health.[11]

Even though the health benefits of pets are positive, the decision to bring a pet into your home should not be taken lightly. Before making this type of commitment, you need to fully consider your life circumstances, including finances, type of housing, and time and energy available.

In consideration of the responsibilities involved, owning a pet has great advantages. In addition to physical health benefits:

- Pets bring cheerfulness, play, and laughter to your life. Watching a puppy or kitten play is entertaining and enjoyable.
- Pets help boost your self-esteem. After a hard day in class or at work, an enthusiastic greeting from your

---

TIPS FOR ACTION Choosing the Right Pet

Pets provide rewards—but they also require attention! Before you choose a pet, carefully consider your schedule and the demands on your time. You can expect the following from these pets:

- *Dogs*. Dogs offer the most intense interaction and also require the most care. They must be fed at the same time each day, usually must be exercised twice a day, and must be groomed several times a month. Larger dogs need plenty of space for exercise, and you must clean up after dogs.
- *Cats*. Cats require less care than dogs but more care than the pets listed below. You can leave sufficient water and dry food if you have to be gone for some time, and a cat will do just fine.

You also can train cats to use an indoor litter box, so cats can adapt to staying indoors. Cats preen themselves, so they usually do not need grooming and do not require you to provide exercise. Cats can adjust to even a small apartment. Even though they provide interaction, they also can be independent.

- *Birds, fish, hamsters, guinea pigs*. These and other less interactive pets require much less time and direct care than dogs and cats. You have to make sure they have food, and you have to clean their cages or bowls. Although they require less care, they also provide less social support.

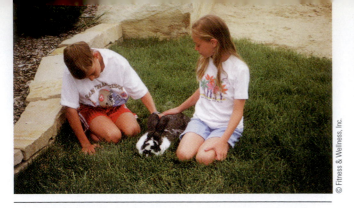

Pets can help meet our need and desire to be loved.

dog bounding to the door to meet you can make you feel appreciated.

- Pets can help satisfy physical touch needs. Caressing a purring cat, for example, can be soothing and comforting.
- Some pets, such as watchdogs, can contribute to your safety.

Critical Thinking

1. Do you have a pet?
2. If so, what benefits do you experience?
3. What responsibilities do you take on when you acquire a pet?

Marriage and Health

The greatest health benefits in our society are experienced by happily married people.[12] Marriage can protect people from illness and disease, help them recover more quickly if they do get sick, and even help people live longer. The health benefits of marriage result from a number of factors including good integration into the community, better social support, the tendency to eat more regular and nutritionally balanced meals, and higher economic status. At the same time, it must be said that marriage is not necessary for positive health. Single people are also able to achieve the health benefits that result from optimum social support.

What does happily married mean? Here are some characteristics of happy marriages.

- The partners find their prime source of joy in each other, while also maintaining separate identities. They are independent, and they have outside interests and hobbies that don't involve the partner.
- They are generous and giving out of love, not because they expect repayment or are keeping score.
- The partners enjoy a healthy and satisfying sexual relationship.
- The partners address conflict in a constructive way. For people in a healthy marriage, verbalizing issues of conflict offers a chance to air feelings and frustrations without implying that the other person is wrong or at

Factors Leading to a Happy Marriage

Your attitudes about marriage and the person you choose to marry play a large part in determining how happily married you'll be. Your marriage is more likely to be happy if you both want the marriage to succeed and you share the following attitudes about marriage with your partner:

- Marriage is a long-term commitment: "We're in this for good."
- Marriage is a spiritual, sanctified institution between two people.

Your chances for marital happiness are highest if you marry

- your best friend.
- someone you genuinely like as a person.
- someone who grows more interesting to you as time goes on.
- someone who shares your basic dreams, goals, and aspirations.

fault. They resolve issues without psychologically harming each other.

- The partners communicate with each other openly and honestly. This entails risk, but experts claim that the benefits are worth the risk if the communication is constructive.
- The two partners in the marriage trust each other. Even after a disagreement, they can reestablish a trusting relationship by working on it.
- The partners talk about their future together—a future they plan to share because they want to. They may dream about a house on the beach, a vacation to Europe, or a having a child. This kind of planning and talking indicates that both people intend to share their lives.

It must be pointed out, of course, that not all marriages are happy, and unhappily married people suffer in terms of health status and longevity.[13] Unhappily married people have poorer health outcomes than single people, as well as people who are divorced. Not surprisingly, marital dissatisfaction has a bearing on both physical health and mental health.

Over the long term, repeated issues of conflict can result in a much higher risk for all kinds of illness and

Critical Thinking

1. Are you married or are you considering marriage at some time in your life?
2. What are your expectations?
3. Are they realistic?
4. What traits do you need to develop before taking on the responsibilities associated with marriage?

reduced functioning of the immune system. Interactions characterized by hostility, sarcasm, and blame (refusing to take responsibility and demeaning the other partner) seem to be the most damaging. Physically, marital conflict in the extreme can be identified as spousal abuse and is potentially dangerous. For their safety, those involved in this sort of relationship would be wise to sever it.

Divorce and Its Consequences

In the United States, more than half of all marriages end in divorce. The parents of more than 1 million children divorce in the United States each year. Among the factors that lead to divorce are the following.

- Divorces are easier to obtain today than ever before.
- The former negative social stigma attached to divorce and divorced people no longer exists.
- Many people enter marriage without the proper preparation and with unrealistic expectations. Some couples think they should never argue, for example, when in reality "constructive fighting" is a characteristic of a healthy relationship. As a result, people too readily abandon the marriage when they have a fight.
- A large percentage of married women work outside the home, making them less financially dependent on their husbands, and thus making divorce a less devastating option.

When considering the circumstances of divorce, it is not surprising that it may pose health hazards. Men and women who are separated or divorced have poorer physiological and physical health than do widowed, happily married, or single adults.

Psychologically, divorced people are more likely to experience depression, alcoholism, traffic accidents and accidental death, psychiatric problems, and suicide and homicide. Physically, divorced people have higher rates of cancer, heart disease, diabetes, pneumonia, and high blood pressure than do married, single, or widowed persons. Both psychological and physiological conditions compromise the immune system, which helps explain why illness and death rates are higher among divorced people.

One reason that divorce compromises health is related to social support. Being married provides built-in social networks, economic ties, and instrumental support. People who are divorced often lose much of their social support and have to work harder to build new social networks.

In sum, divorced people and those who are unhappily married don't fare nearly as well as happily married people in terms of health and longevity. Cardiovascular function, endocrine function, and immunity are all influenced by the positive or negative behavior patterns exhibited in marriages.[14]

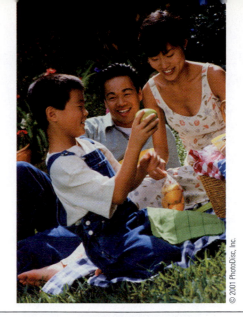

© 2001 PhotoDisc, Inc.

A strong family contributes to a long and healthy life.

Families and Health

A **family** is a group that shares common goals and values and works together to achieve those goals. A family may be a dual-career family, a single-parent family, or a "binuclear family" (in which the father and mother no longer live together but both provide a place for the children). What goes on in a family—the relationships between its members—can have a profound effect on the health and longevity of each member.

How children are perceived in the family can have great impact, even on their physical growth. An emotionally healthy family supports emotionally healthy development of each of its members. Conversely, a weak or unhealthy family is one with abnormal, impaired, or incomplete functioning that impairs the emotional health and self-esteem of family members.[15]

In all families, problems arise at times. No family is totally healthy nor totally unhealthy. Unhealthy or dysfunctional family dynamics both cause and result from several conditions. Among the most extreme are a result of:

- alcoholism and other chemical addictions, chronic mental illnesses, or disabling physical illnesses;
- dependence on, or obsession with, people who have such conditions;
- physical or sexual child abuse.

When these conditions persist, parents are not able to meet their children's emotional needs consistently. The more severe the dysfunction, the more the children are emotionally damaged. Table 4.1 compares characteristics of functional versus dysfunctional families.

Family A unique cluster of people who enjoy a special relationship by reason of love, marriage, procreation, and mutual dependence.

TABLE 4.1   Characteristics of a Functional Family Versus a Dysfunctional Family

Functional Family	Dysfunctional Family
Establishes rules for the sake of functioning cooperatively that are appropriate, consistent, and reasonably flexible.	Establishes rules for control's sake that are rigid and arbitrary.
Encourages its members to develop well-rounded personalities with many facets.	Establishes rigid roles for each member: For example, one is always the scapegoat, one is unnoticed, one is overly responsible, and one is the family clown.
Accepts its problems and treats them as factual.	Has deep, dark secrets that no one may ever disclose (alcoholism, infidelity, or other).
Welcomes outsiders into the system.	Resists allowing outsiders to enter the system.
Typically has members who are relaxed and have a sense of humor.	Has members who are usually serious and tense.
Permits members the right to personal privacy, so that they can develop a sense of self.	Permits members no personal privacy, so that they have difficulty defining themselves as individuals.
Fosters a spontaneous "sense of family," so that members feel free to leave and reenter the system.	Enforces loyalty to the family; members must always act as part of the system.
Allows and resolves conflict between members.	Denies and ignores conflict between members.
Continually changes.	Resists change.
Has spontaneous loyalty and a sense of wholeness.	Has no real unity; is fragmented.

People from dysfunctional families bear a painful legacy of confusion, fear, anger, and hurt. Then, because they instinctively seek what is familiar even if it is unpleasant, they tend to repeat the patterns they have learned. When developing relationships, they choose people who will interact with them in the same unhealthy ways that their families of origin did. Each person from a dysfunctional family is at high risk of marrying someone with alcoholism (or another such condition), repeating a life of addictions, or both.

In general, people from dysfunctional or weak families tend to have poor health outcomes. Families that are weak in structure and support have children with more disease symptoms, impaired physical health, and weakened emotional health.

Just as weak or stressed families can contribute to illness, strong families can contribute to good health and long lives. Individuals in healthy families have lower stress levels, fewer illnesses, and ability to recover from illness and disease much more rapidly than those in unhealthy families. A strong family helps an individual cope with stress, reducing the risk of illness and disease.

Evidence of the buffering effect of healthy families abounds. People in strong families recover more quickly from surgery, more often follow medical instructions and take medications as prescribed, maintain treatment recommendations, and recover more

12 Ways to Build Strong Family Values

1. Eat together as a family as often as possible, certainly several full family dinners a week. Involve everyone in meal preparation (for example, younger children can set the table and older ones can clean up after the meal).
2. Hold weekly gatherings to plan family activities, trips, and vacations, and discuss immediate and persistent problems.
3. Schedule daily stress-reduction periods when the entire household is quiet—no TV, CDs, DVDs, or computers. According to your family values, read, meditate, pray, exercise, or whatever works for your family.
4. Volunteer time and talent to worthy causes in the church or community.
5. Participate in your children's school. Become involved with teachers and administrators. Help with after-school and summer programs.
6. Do recreational activities as a family. Take walks or bike rides together.
7. Make or build things together. Share creative activities, and let children take the lead in some of these. Aim for accomplishment, not perfection.
8. As a family, plan organized trips to sporting events, concerts, and local fairs.
9. Bring children to work on occasion to let them see their parents' life away from home.
10. At least once a year travel away from home. Include the children in your vacation planning.
11. Limit TV watching and computer game playing. Monitor your children's activities closely.
12. Stay involved. Keep informed about community and national issues that concern you and your children. Let children know your concerns and opinions, and listen to theirs.

Excerpted and adapted from *A Better World for Children* (New York: National Press Books, 1994); as printed in the *Denver Post.* © Copyright by Benjamin Spock.

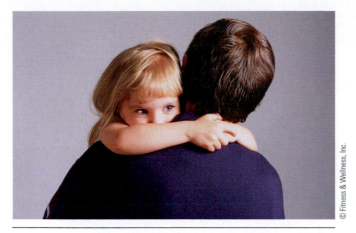

The decision to have a child should be made with deliberate thought and care.

How to Develop Parenting Skills

If you're thinking about becoming a parent, parent education is available—and well worth the time effort. You'll find out ahead of time what to expect, how to react, and how you can best build a healthy relationship between you and your child. To find a parent-education course, check the following:

- local public schools
- local churches or synagogues
- local community centers
- local institutions offering adult education courses, including school districts and local colleges
- YMCA
- your physician or health-care provider

quickly with fewer complications. People in strong families also tend to manage chronic illness better. As a result, they tend to live longer than people in weak families.

Should the family include children? The answer depends on you, your partner, your lifestyle, and your goals. Before you decide whether to have children:

- Talk openly and honestly with your partner. Is your relationship healthy? Do you both want a child? If one partner wants a child and the other does not, problems could result.
- Discuss your parenting philosophies. You should share similar views about discipline and techniques for correcting and guiding children. What about religion? Do you share the same religious views? If not, in which church will the child be reared?
- Consider why you want to have a child. A positive reason is to share your life and love. Having a child to realize an unfulfilled goal or dream is not healthy. Other unhealthy reasons for having a child include being pressured by your spouse or other people or hoping the child will make you happy or take care of you.
- Examine your lifestyle carefully. If you're both working, do you both want to keep working after you have a child? Are you ready to give up some of your freedom and independence that is necessary for making a commitment to a child?
- Assess your personal characteristics. Are you a person who gives love easily? Do you find it easy to share? Do you enjoy teaching others? Do you get along with your parents and your brothers and sisters? Most important, do you like children? If you don't enjoy children, you

Coping With Loss

- Try to keep things in your life as status quo as possible. Avoid things that could cause you stress right now, such as a new job, a vacation, or moving to a new house or apartment.
- Postpone decisions that can wait until later. You'll be thinking more clearly and won't be reacting under duress.
- Keep in touch with other people. Social support is especially important now. Let other people express their concern and help you out.
- Avoid the temptation to use drugs or alcohol to ease your feelings of grief; they only make things worse.
- Believe in yourself and your ability to recover. You have the right to go through the stages of grief, so don't be too hard on yourself.

need to take a hard look at your decision to become a parent.

Social Support in Times of Loss

Social support is vital to help people cope with loss and deal with grief. Losses range from minor disappointments to major losses. The loss of loved ones through death, separation, or divorce is particularly devastating and can result in both physical and psychological illness.

Grieving is necessary for healing. For grief to progress "normally," a person passes through the stages described in Chapter 2. People who don't go through the stages of grieving can get stuck in a stage and experience what professionals call "abnormal grief." The result can be serious illness and premature death.

Critical Thinking

1. What benefits do you receive from your family and friends?
2. How does this affect your health status?

Grieving a loss requires a tremendous amount of emotional and physical energy. Positive support systems can provide understanding, love, and comfort during these times. When a grieving person is ready, friends can assist in the transition back into enjoyable activities. A support network can be invaluable throughout the grief process and helping the person move on.

The best protection for grieving individuals is good social support, strong religious beliefs, rituals, and a conviction that one can control the bereavement.[15] These factors all increase the odds of good health and a long and fulfilling life.[16]

WEB Interactive

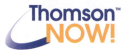

Don't forget to check out the wealth of resources on the ThomsonNOW website at **www.thomsonedu.com/ThomsonNOW** that will:

- Coach you through identifying target goals for behavior change and monitoring your personal change plan throughout the semester
- Help you evaluate your knowledge of the material
- Allow you to take an exam-prep quiz
- Provide a Personalized Learning Plan targeting resources that address areas you should study.

WEB ACTIVITIES

Friends' Health Connection This site is sponsored by the Friends' Health Connection—a nonprofit organization that connects people who have or have overcome the same disease, illness, disability, or injury—to provide a medium for mutual support. Participants are matched based upon a number of criteria including age, health problems, symptoms, lifestyle effects, tests and surgeries, attitude, occupation, hobbies, and interests. People of all ages participate, and their health problems range from the most common to very rare disorders. There is also an opportunity for networking friends and family members.

http://www.48friend.org/index.php

Relationship Skills and Heart Disease: A New Frontier This site is based on a lecture presented by Martin Sullivan, M.D., a cardiologist at Duke University. He describes the following "relationship risk factors" for cardiac disease: social isolation, sleep disorder and depression, hostility, repression of emotion, work stress, loss of meaning, and low affiliation/high power.

http://www.smartmarriages.com/healthyheart.html

InfoTrac®

You can find additional readings related to wellness via InfoTrac® College Edition, an online library of more than 900 journals and publications. Follow the instructions for accessing InfoTrac® that came packaged with your textbook, then search for articles using a key word search.

Suggested Reading Kathleen P. Pittman, Judith L. Wold, Astrid H. Wilson, Carolyn Huff, and Sharon Williams, "Community Connections: Promoting Family Health," *Family and Community Health* 23, no. 2 (July 2000): 72.

1. Who do most adolescents consider their most reliable source of critical health information?

2. Describe the multidimensional model, PCAP, that provided the framework for the development of the partnership between the College of Health and Human Sciences at Georgia State University, a major urban university, and M. L. King Middle School, an inner-city middle school.
3. What was the mission of the partnership?

Web Activity

"Go Ask Alice!"

http://www.goaskalice.columbia.edu

Sponsor Columbia University Health Education Department, a division of the University Health Service.

Description This site, sponsored by Columbia University Health Education Department, features a large interactive question-and-answer site. It contains its own search engine. The mission of "Go Ask Alice!" is to provide factual and nonjudgmental information written by health educators and health practitioners to assist readers' decision-making about their physical, emotional, sexual, and spiritual health.

Available Activity

1. Search the archives of more than 1,800 previously answered questions in the following six health disciplines: general health, fitness and nutrition, sexuality, relationships, sexual health, and alcohol and other drugs.

Web Work

1. From the home page, click on "Relationships."
2. Scroll down to read the different categories of questions, including general relationship "stuff"; gay, lesbian, bisexual, and nonconsensual relationships; talking with parents; friendship; roommate rumblings; miscellaneous.
3. Read the description of each question found on the links. When you see a question that interests you, simply click on that link.
4. Repeat this procedure for each question whose answer you would like to view.

Helpful Hints

1. "Go Ask Alice!" provides health information only and should not be viewed as providing personalized medical advice or diagnoses. You should consult with a qualified health care provider if you have specific symptoms or concerns. "Go Ask Alice!" does not respond immediately to your questions. Not all questions are answered.

2. Return to this site regularly to view new questions and answers on a variety of health topics of special interest to college students and young adults. Questions and answers on this site are updated weekly.

For additional Web activities, links, and suggested readings, visit our Health, Fitness and Wellness Resource Center at http://health.wadsworth.com.

Notes

1. P. A. Bovier, E. Chamot, and T. V. Perneger, "Perceived Stress, Internal Resources, and Social Support as Determinants of Mental Health Among Young Adults," *Quality of Life Research* 13 (2004): 161–170.
2. M. R. Janevic, N. K. Janz, J. A. Dodge et al., "Longitudinal Effects of Social Support of the Health and Functioning of Older Women with Heart Disease," *International Journal of Aging and Human Development* 59 (2004): 153–175.
3. S. S. Bunkers, "The Lived Experience of Feeling Cared For: A Human Becoming Perspective," *Journal of Clinical Nursing* 8 (2004): 63–71.
4. B. Q. Hafen and K. J. Frandsen, *In People Who Need People Are the Healthiest People: The Importance of Relationships* (Provo, UT: Behavioral Health Associates, 2000).
5. See Note 4.
6. E. S. Ford, I. B. Ahluwalia, and D. A. Galuska, "Social Relationships and Cardiovascular Disease Risk Factors: Findings from the Third National Health and Nutrition Survey," *Preventive Medicine* 30 (2000): 83–92.
7. A. G. Taylor, D. I. Galper, P. Taylor, et al., "Effects of Adjunctive Swedish Massage and Vibration Therapy on Short-term Postoperative Outcomes," *Journal of Alternative and Complementary Medicine* 9 (2003): 77–89.
8. J. T. Cacioppo, J. T. Hawkley, L. E. Crawford, J. M Ernst et al., "Loneliness and Health: Potential Mechanisms," *Psychosomatic Medicine* 64 (2002): 407–417.
9. A. Steptoe, N. Owen, S. R. Kunz-Ebrecht, and L. Brydon, "Loneliness and Neuroendocrine, Cardiovascular, and Inflammatory Stress Responses in Middle-aged Men and Women" *Psychoneuroendocrinology* 29 (2004): 593–611.
10. G. Kritsotakis and E. Gamarnikow, "What is Social Capital and How Does It Relate to Health?" *International Journal of Nursing Studies* 41 (2003): 43–50.
11. P. Raina et al., "Influence of Companion Animals on the Physical and Psychological Health of Older People: An Analysis of a One-Year Longitudinal Study," *Journal of the American Geriatrics Society*, 47 (1999), 323–329.
12. J. Bookwala, "The Role of Marital Quality in Physical Health During the Mature Years," *Journal of Aging and Health* 17 (2005): 85–104.
13. T. F. Robles and J. K. Kiecolt-Glaser, "The Physiology of Marriage: Pathways to Health," *Physiology and Behavior* 79 (2003): 409–416.
14. B. S. McEwen, "Early Life Influences on Life-long Patterns of Behavior and Health," *Mental Retardation and Developmental Disabilities Research Reviews* 9 (2003): 149–154.
15. E. Hallowell, "Strong Relationships Really Do Help Ensure Good Health," *Health* (2000), 3–4.
16. L. Ungar and V. Florian, "What Helps Middle-Aged Widows With Their Psychological and Social Adaptation Several Years After Their Loss?" *Death Studies* 28 (2004): 621–642.

Assess Your Behavior

1. Think about the people close to you. Do you have a positive support network?
2. Consider the four types of social support described in the chapter. Do you give and receive all types of social support? What areas are rich, and which areas are lacking?
3. What can you do to enrich your support network?

Evaluate how well you understand the concepts presented in this chapter by answering the following questions.

1. The types of social support are
   a. instrumental, emotional, information, appraisal.
   b. emotional, informational, network, appraisal.
   c. instrumental, intellectual, psychological, informational.
   d. emotional, physical, psycho-social, sexual.
   e. None of the above.

2. If a person gives you a ride to class when your car is being repaired, this type of support is
   a. instrumental.
   b. emotional.
   c. intellectual.
   d. informational.
   e. physical.

3. Before sharing sensitive information with a friend, you should consider
   a. that some issues may make your friend uncomfortable.
   b. your motive for sharing.
   c. that this may strain the friendship.
   d. that your friend may repeat the information to others.
   e. All of the above.

4. When thinking about sharing specific information that may be hurtful to a third party, ask yourself these questions:
   a. Is it true?
   b. Will sharing this be hurtful?
   c. Is it necessary?
   d. All of the above.

5. Benefits of pet ownership include
   a. positive effects on physical health.
   b. improved cardiovascular functioning.
   c. enhanced emotional stability.
   d. play and laughter.
   e. all of the above.

6. Situations that pose health risks include
   a. marriage.
   b. divorce.
   c. dysfunctional families.
   d. a and b.
   c. b and c.

Correct answers can be found on page 369.

Do You Have the Qualities of Friendship?

Name: _____   Date: _____   Grade: _____

Instructor: _____   Course: _____   Section: _____

Friendship is a two-way business. To make friends, you have to be a friend. The better friend you are, the more friends you are likely to have. This questionnaire lists some of the qualities of friendship.

Check "yes" or "no" to the questions. Then look at the scoring key at the end.

YES NO

1. Are people able to depend on you to keep your word?

2. Can they rely on you to respect their confidences?

3. Do you keep the friends you make?

4. Do you often put yourself to trouble and inconvenience to oblige other people?

5. Suppose they want to do something you are not particularly keen on. Would you go along with them and do what they want to do?

6. Are you quick to pay your share of the expenses?

7. Are you generous with your praise and appreciation?

8. Do you show affection when you feel it?

9. Is it easy for you to forgive and forget?

10. Do you readily give people the benefit of the doubt and make allowances?

11. In a sharp difference of opinion, would you speak first?

12. Do you own up when you are wrong, and say you are sorry?

13. You may like somebody very much, but would you feel the same if he or she were to become unpopular?

14. Are you quick off the mark to give sympathy and practical help when people need it?

15. Do you like to see others praised and fussed over?

16. Can you agree to differ and stay on the best of terms?

17. Are you an attentive and sympathetic listener?

18. Are you always the same, not full of welcome today and too busy to bother tomorrow?

19. Do you mind people having other friends and interests that you do not share?

20. Can you say you are much more interested in other people than in yourself?

Scoring

Count 5 points for every "yes." A score of 70 or over is good, and 60–70 is satisfactory. Under 60 is not satisfactory. You are not likely to be a good friend. Usually, when we are like this, we're wrapped up in ourselves. We like only the individuals who notice us and make a fuss over us and dislike anybody who is not interested in us or who will not do what we want. If you desire to be a good friend, you will have to be more interested in other people than in yourself and put them first.

Adapted from Singer Communications, Inc., Anaheim, California. Used by permission.

5

CHAPTER

Spirituality and Health

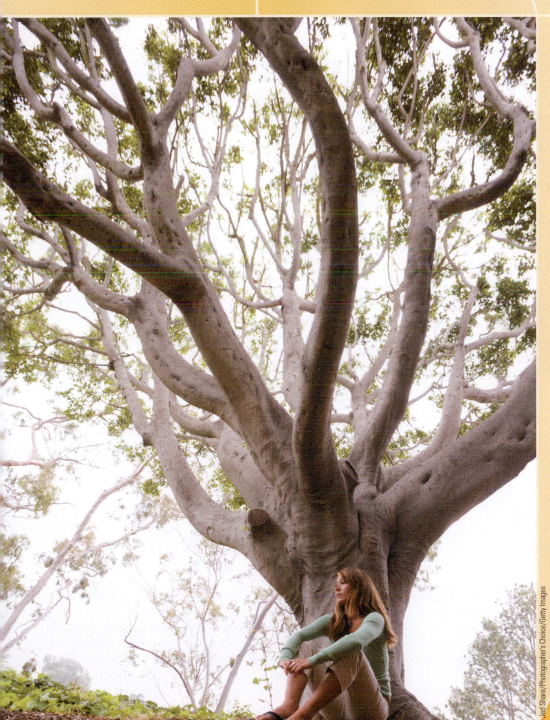

© Jed Share/Photographer's Choice/Getty Images

When people think about health and how to be healthy, they usually think first about nutrition, exercise, and how to reduce stress, and overlook the other important contribution of spirituality to health. This chapter covers spiritual concepts and their influence on total well-being.

Explanatory Style

We've all known people who seem perpetually upbeat, sometimes even in the face of great difficulties, and we've also known people who seem to see impending disaster in everything, even the smallest setback. The habitual manner in which people explain the things that happen to them is their **explanatory style**, a way of thinking when all other factors are equal and when there are no clear-cut right and wrong answers. The contrasting explanatory styles are **pessimism** and **optimism**. People with a pessimistic explanatory style interpret events negatively, and people with an optimistic explanatory style interpret events in the positive light that "every cloud has a silver lining."

The pessimistic explanatory style can be characterized as:

1. assuming a problem is never-ending, being convinced it will never go away.
2. believing a problem is global, that it applies in every situation instead of being an isolated incident.
3. internalizing most negative events ("It's my fault"), destructively assigning blame to self.

Explanatory style can be a potent predictor of physical health, affecting both emotional and physical well-being. In the emotional arena, a pessimistic explanatory style can lead to anxiety, depression, guilt, anger, or hostility. In the physical realm, a negative explanatory style can interfere with health in many ways. For example, it can delay healing, and worsen the course of a disease. In a study conducted at the Harvard School of Public Health, explanatory style was linked to decline in pulmonary function; more pessimistic men had greater declines in lung function than optimistic men.[1]

By contrast, an optimistic style tends to increase the quality and length of life.[2] Believing in a positive future and having positive coping styles tend to enhance health. An optimistic explanatory style and the positive emotions it embraces—such as love, acceptance, and forgiveness—promote health through psychological factors that in turn induce physiologic responses, which improve immunity and other processes.[3]

A positive explanatory style also may affect health through psychosocial aspects that promote a sense of control, positive social interactions, and other health-protective behaviors.[4] Positive-minded people are less likely to be socially isolated and more likely to be involved in health-enhancing behaviors including physical activity, good nutrition, satisfying interpersonal relationships, stress management, and spiritual connections. One

study showed that optimism was even linked to good dental habits and thereby lessened the risk for cardiovascular disease.[5]

Fortunately, people can cultivate optimism. Assessment 5.1 gives you the opportunity to assess your own optimism. To boost your optimism:

- Surround yourself with optimistic people who care about you and can encourage you. When you surround yourself with optimists, you begin to "catch" their attitude. Solicit their suggestions.
- Make an effort to genuinely like other people. Look for their good qualities, and respect their differences.
- Realize that changing your explanatory style requires a big commitment. In essence, you will have to change how you look at life. You didn't develop your explanatory style overnight, and you won't be able to change it overnight either. Be patient with yourself, and expect some hard work ahead of you. Get past the inevitable setbacks and disappointments. Look at these as challenges and don't let them deter you.
- Set small, attainable goals, and reward yourself in some way when you meet those goals. Celebrate your accomplishments.
- Look beyond yourself, realizing that the world doesn't revolve around you. Expand your horizons by getting involved in helping others, such as volunteer activities.
- Don't blow things out of proportion.
- An argument with a friend doesn't mean the friendship is collapsing. One poor exam score doesn't mean your college career is doomed.
- Avoid generalizing. One disappointment doesn't mean that nothing ever turns out right.
- Recount and embrace your past successes and the good things that have happened to you.
- Face your problems head-on. Develop strategies for solving them instead of trying to escape them.
- Above all, have fun. Learn to laugh at yourself, relax, and enjoy life.

Critical Thinking

Think about the two types of explanatory styles. If you had to assess your own style and that of selected friends, how would they rate?

Health Locus of Control

Our **health locus of control** is determined by the extent to which we believe that our behavior affects our health status. Control does not mean that we have to (or can) control everything around us. Control refers to how much we believe our actions can influence a situation. We can choose how to react and respond.

Each person's health locus of control lies somewhere along a continuum. At one end of the continuum shown in Figure 5.1 is the **external locus of control**. At the

FIGURE 5.1 Continuum of Locus of Control

LOCUS OF CONTROL

External

Internal

CONTINUUM ⟶

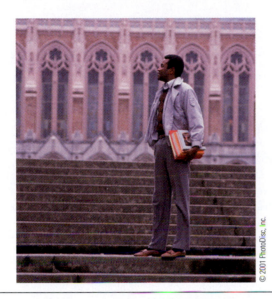

© 2001 PhotoDisc, Inc.

Attaining a goal affirms an internal locus of control.

People in stressful situations who believe they have some control over their situations experience less physiological damage normally associated with stress.[7] Internal locus of control functions as a buffer against stress.

Critical Thinking

1. Do you have an internal or external locus of control?
2. Think about others that you know. Where would you rate them in this area?

Self-Esteem

We have referred to **self-esteem** in earlier chapters. It is a way of viewing and assessing oneself. Positive self-esteem is a sense of feeling good about one's capabilities, goals, accomplishments, place in the world, and relationship to others. People with high self-esteem respect themselves.

Further, self-esteem is a powerful determinant of behaviors that lead to good health. A positive sense of self can boost the immune system, protect against disease, and aid in healing. Whether people get sick—and how long they stay that way—depends in part on the strength of their self-esteem. Low self-esteem has been shown to have detrimental health effects, including intensified chronic pain. Also, the higher the self-esteem, the more rapid is the recovery from illness. For those with high self-esteem, the outlook is good. For those with low

opposite end is the **internal locus of control**. People with an external locus of control believe the things that happen to them are unrelated to their own behavior and, therefore, are beyond their control. People with an internal locus of control, in contrast, believe that events are a consequence of their personal actions and, thus, potentially can be controlled.

As a whole, people with a strong sense of internal control have fewer illnesses because they practice healthier behaviors.[6] An internal locus of control has a significant influence over the body's release of hormones, which has been found to be a powerful determinant of health. Three of the hormones influenced by a lack of control are

1. *serotonin*, which regulates moods, relieves pain, and helps control the release of the pain-killing endorphins;
2. *dopamine*, largely responsible for a sense of reward and pleasure; and
3. *norepinephrine*, which, when depleted, causes depression.

When people perceive that they have little control, the level of corticosteroids in their bloodstream rises. The corticosteroids, released by the body during stress, have a variety of negative physical effects if they do not dissipate. They lower the body's resistance to disease and suppress the body's manufacture of the three hormones above.

Explanatory style The way people perceive the events in their lives, from an optimistic or a pessimistic perspective.

Pessimism A tendency to view life situations with negativity and gloom.

Optimism A tendency to expect the best possible outcome.

Health locus of control The extent to which people believe their behavior affects their health status.

External locus of control One's prevailing belief that the things that happen are unrelated to one's own behavior and are determined by outside forces.

Internal locus of control One's prevailing belief that events are a consequence of one's own actions and, thus, potentially can be controlled.

Self-esteem A sense of positive self-regard and self-respect.

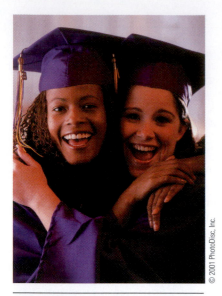

Self-esteem can enhance emotional and physical health.

© 2001 PhotoDisc, Inc.

FIGURE 5.2 Continuum Showing Attitudes Toward Serious Illness

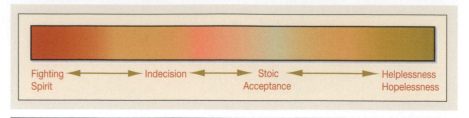

Fighting Spirit ←→ Indecision ←→ Stoic Acceptance ←→ Helplessness Hopelessness

self-esteem, their health can decline in direct proportion to their worsening attitude and negativity.

Belief in oneself is one of the most powerful weapons people have to protect their health and live longer, more satisfying lives. It has a dramatic impact on quality of life and overall wellness, and we can harness it to our advantage. Accomplishing worthwhile endeavors such as educational attainment enhances self-competence and contributes to positive self-esteem.[8] Assessment 5.2 is provided so you can assess your views about yourself.

Developing healthy self-esteem is one of the best things a person can do for overall health, both mental and physical.[9] To boost your self-esteem:

- Use **affirmations**. Prepare a list of your positive traits. Say positive things about you to yourself, such as, "I'm honest and open in expressing my feelings."
- Set positive goals, and develop a plan for accomplishing these goals. Focus on worthwhile achievements.
- When your "internal critic"—the negative inner voice in each of us—starts putting you down, tune it out. Redirect your thoughts to a situation that you handled well or something about yourself of which you're especially proud. Use Assessment 5.3 to gain insight into your thought patterns.

A Fighting Spirit

A **fighting spirit** involves the healthy expression of emotion and a willingness to face problems head-on and look for solutions. At the other extreme is hopelessness, a surrender to despair. In between these are attitudes of indecision and stoic acceptance.

A fighting spirit can play a major role in recovery from disease. People with a fighting spirit accept their disease diagnosis, adopt an optimistic attitude, seek information about how to help themselves, and are determined to

Case Study of a Fighting Spirit

In discussing the power of a fighting spirit, psychoneuro-immunology pioneer Dr. George Solomon told the story of a Harvard professor who had been stricken with cancer and had lesions in his head, lungs, and liver. Nonetheless, the professor continued teaching his classes, reassuring his friends and students.

Solomon says of the professor, "It was thrilling to see how powerful the fighting spirit can be. For most of a year, he battled that cancer. And he won. The most important thing he had to teach us came not out of his medical lectures but out of his own experience and example. He won against all the odds—against the predictions of the specialists and against the reports based on sophisticated technology."

What the professor taught all around him was, in essence, that if we are willing to fight, we can win.

fight the disease. Figure 5.2 depicts a continuum of attitudes toward serious illness.

A fighting spirit may be the underlying factor in what is called **spontaneous remission** from incurable illness. The fighting spirit appears to play a large role in the extent of psychological distress[10] and facilitates victory over disease. People with a fighting spirit are confident of being cured and use proactive strategies.[11] "Fighters" are not stronger or more capable than others. They simply do not give up. Thus, they enjoy better health and live longer, even when physicians and laboratory tests say they should not.

The Spiritual Link

Spirituality is an integral part of being human. The word **spirituality** itself is derived from the Latin word for "breath," or that which gives life to or animates a person. It denotes what is at the center of one's life. Spirituality is a belief in, and a person's relationship with, a Higher Being. Members of the Jewish and Christian faiths call this higher power God. People who practice Hinduism refer to it as Prana. Native Americans call it the Great Spirit. Muslims refer to Allah. The Chinese call the higher being Chi.

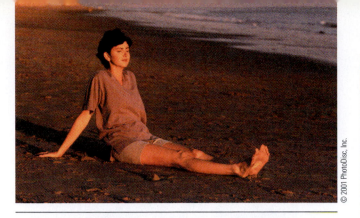

© 2001 PhotoDisc, Inc.

Spirituality entails a belief in a power higher than oneself.

Critical Thinking

1. Think about spirituality and health. Describe the connections considering the concepts of church attendance, prayer, forgiveness, and contentment.
2. Do you think most people in your support network are content?

Spirituality enhances meaning and purpose in life. It is a personal value system regarding the way people approach life, a dimension of a person that encompasses one's relationship with self, others, and the higher power. Spirituality involves finding meaning in life and in death.

All people have spiritual needs. They need to make sense of their particular circumstances, to find meaning and purpose in their days, relationships, and life. People need to feel connected. They need approval, and they need to know that their lives are of worth to themselves, their families, friends, and communities. People need hope, meaning in life, and forgiveness. They need to know that they are loved and that others care for them and find them worthwhile.

Spiritual health is the ability to discover and articulate our own purpose in life and to learn how to experience love, joy, peace, and fulfillment through that lens. It is the experience of helping ourselves and others achieve full potential. Through the spiritual dimension, we emphasize our connectedness to others.

The cultivation of spiritual health—which is a process or journey, not an endpoint—can enhance physical, mental, and emotional health, sometimes in dramatic ways. One study indicated that many professionally successful men and women have strong spiritual values and beliefs in spite of having suffered major psychological or physical traumas.[12] The researchers concluded that the subjects' spirituality enabled them to handle crises and develop effective styles of coping with life crises.

Spirituality seems to buffer stress. People with a deep sense of spirituality are not defeated by crises; they have traits of hardiness (see Chapter 2) that protect them from the negative effects of stress.[13] Spirituality helps people interpret crises in a growth-producing way and, as a result, they are able to use hardships, including illness, as a means of spiritual growth. One study indicated that spirituality was a valuable means of coping with chronic illnesses.[14] Behaviors associated with spirituality often promote a healthful lifestyle. In a targeted study of youth, those who had traits of spirituality were less likely to engage in early sexual behavior than those who lacked spirituality.[15] Even when disease claims a life, spirituality can make the experience one of positive growth for the bereaved.

RELIGION AND RELIGIOUS PRACTICE

Although **religion** is related to spirituality, the two concepts are different. Religion refers to the spiritual experience as part of an organized system of beliefs, practices, and knowledge. It is an expression of spirituality that involves the traditions, rituals, and practices that people utilize to express their relationship with God.

For some people, religion is an important part of spirituality. For others, spirituality means a quest for understanding life's ultimate questions and meaning and

Affirmations Positive statements that reinforce the positive aspects of personality and experience.

Fighting spirit Determination; the open expression of emotions, whether negative or positive.

Spontaneous remission Inexplicable recovery from incurable illness.

Spirituality A belief in and a person's relationship with a Higher Being.

Spiritual health Dimension of health related to a person's moral or religious nature; a relationship with a higher being.

Religion The system of how to know God, accompanied by rituals and places of worship.

purpose of living that doesn't incorporate religion. Thus, some people are not formally affiliated with a religious tradition but are still on a spiritual journey. People tend to define what spirituality means to them in an individual way.[16] One study found positive results of religious faith and spirituality in substance abuse recovery; most of the participants described themselves as spiritual rather than religious.[17] The authors of the study suggested that this may be a result of their associating the term *religious* with being judgmental.

People who are strongly affiliated with a place of worship generally enjoy better health. In a 6-year study of almost 4,000 older people, conducted at Duke University, participants who attended religious services once a week or more lived longer than the participants who did not attend religious services.[18] Another study showed that people who attended church at least once a week lived 7 years longer than people who never attended.[19] Those who frequently attended their places of worship reported more social support, less depression, and better health practices. They also had less anxiety, less substance abuse, fewer strokes, lower blood pressure, and overall enhanced well-being.

In a systematic review of research studies, one study reported the impact of religion on health.[20] Religious activities appeared to result in improved blood pressure, enhanced immunity, reduced depression, and lower risk of death.

Another study revealed that the participants who attended their place of worship weekly and prayed or studied the Bible at least daily had consistently lower blood pressure and recovered from bouts of depression more quickly than others.[21] Attending religious services improved social support, self-esteem, and coping skills. Lack of religious involvement was considered a risk factor for poorer health.

People who considered themselves religious, according to other researchers, experienced better health than those lacking religiosity or spirituality.[22] Probable ways by which religious participation protects health include the following:

- Many religious services prescribe behaviors that prevent illness, assist in treating illness, and discourage behavior that is harmful to health.
- Places of worship provide social support that can reduce loneliness and offer support groups for people in times of need.
- Most religions strongly emphasize marriage and the family, both of which have health benefits, as discussed in Chapter 4.
- People who attend religious services are more likely to pray and be prayed for, and prayer has been shown to benefit health.
- Religious people tend to have higher self-esteem and a stronger sense of control, as well as spiritual well-being.
- Places of worship promote positive approaches toward illness, pain, and disability, which can influence the

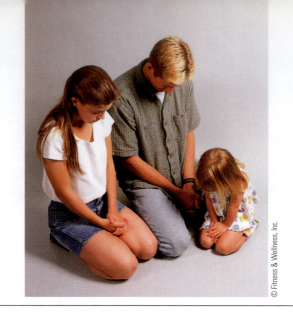

Prayer can enhance health and buffer stress.

outcome of disease. People with chronic disabling conditions, such as heart disease and diabetes, are less likely to become depressed if they call upon religion to adapt to stress.
- Religious faith and activity improve coping skills and instill in people a value system that helps them prioritize in times of indecision.

PRAYER

Prayer in Western cultures means communication with a higher power. Prayer is a manifestation of a commitment to a set of moral and ethical values and might include asking for guidance, wisdom, and strength. It is a signpost of our spirituality, at the core of most personal and spiritual experiences. In some Eastern cultures, this process is called **meditation** and involves sitting quietly while focusing on breathing. Eastern cultures have used meditation in a variety of ways for healing purposes. Some Native Americans believe that prayer and meditation are greatly enhanced outdoors where they can experience a greater connection with nature.

Prayer has powerful beneficial physiological effects on the body. A study of 100 cancer patients illustrated the positive impact of prayer on overall quality of life and reduced cancer symptoms.[23] In addition to its healing qualities, prayer prepares the mind to be receptive to treatment. It effectively induces the **relaxation response**, which is important in medical treatment and health status.

Prayer can exert a powerful benefit on people even when they do not know prayers are being offered in their behalf. In one interesting study, a group of people around the country prayed daily for 192 coronary-care patients at a hospital without telling the patients that anyone was praying for them. A separate group of 201 patients there were not prayed for. The praying continued for 10 months. The patients who were prayed for had significantly fewer complications while they were in the coronary-care unit.[24] The researchers advised that prayer be considered an effective adjunct to standard medical care. A critical review of this study stated that the remote effects of prayer should not be discounted, even if the mechanism involved is not completely understood.[25]

Non-Western cultures describe similar spiritual interventions. To promote physical healing, traditional Chinese medicine involves spirituality in a variety of schools of healing, utilizing life force or subtle bioenergy. These practices have some commonalities with the Western culture's practice of prayer.[26]

CONTENTMENT

Contentment means feeling satisfied, pleased, and happy. On the flip side, many people in today's society feel chronically dissatisfied with life. They suffer from emptiness and unhappiness. In response, some people look to external sources for fulfillment—a better job, more money, more things. Others seek wealth, popularity, and sometimes superficial highs. Often this pursuit leads to fleeting happiness. Most people, though, inwardly long for enduring contentment—a deep-down, soul-satisfying peace.

People who truly reach this level of contentment develop inner harmony through spirituality, and they learn to cultivate contentment by understanding that they are unconditionally loved and accepted by their higher power.

An important aspect of contentment is gratitude, which means appreciating what you have and not longing for what you do not have. The focus is on the positive aspects of life.

FORGIVENESS

Essential to a spiritual nature is **forgiveness**. Forgiving means releasing resentment, not holding wrongs against people, and not seeking revenge for their hurtful actions. To forgive is to give up the desire to punish or to pardon for wrongdoing. If you forgive someone, you do not hold hard feelings toward that person. You accept the core of every human being and do not judge them.

A negative, bitter attitude is harmful emotionally and physically. To understand the health benefits of forgiveness, we can examine what happens when people do not forgive. When we choose to hold hard feelings toward someone and feed anger and resentment, the body releases hormones that cause the heart to pound, blood pressure to rise, muscles to contract, and abdominal pain to develop. If the situation continues unchecked, the consequences can be gastric ulcers, gastritis, or irritable bowel syndrome.

Researchers have observed that people who think forgiving thoughts have an increased sense of control and reduced biological symptoms of stress.[27] They emphasize that forgiveness does not mean denying, ignoring, or tolerating the offense; rather forgivers release all negative thoughts and feelings they otherwise might hold toward someone.

Learning to Forgive

For day-to-day mishaps—a roommate offended you, you were served cold food in a restaurant—you can learn to forgive, and it may be easier than you think. Here's how you can do it:

- Start practicing forgiveness of minor infractions, things that are easy to forgive. Once you've learned this, it's easier to transfer forgiveness to more difficult problems.
- Set aside a "forgiveness hour." During that hour, forgive everything that happens, even the things you do. Then expand it to a "forgiveness day." Realize how great you feel to forgive someone instead of lugging around a burden of grudges and hard feelings.
- Take a hard look at the way you judge others. Your own judgment, not the action of someone else, is often what makes forgiveness difficult. Make it a policy to reserve judgment until you have all the facts. Better yet, have a hard-and-fast rule to postpone all judgments for one year. (Chances are that you will have forgotten the whole thing by then!)
- Don't say you've "forgiven" someone, then tell your roommates what happened. Forgiving entails forgetting.
- Learn to forgive yourself. If you have to, say it aloud ("I forgive myself for cutting class and not being upfront with the professor"). Learn from your mistakes, and turn them into positives instead of using them as ammunition against yourself forever.

Spiritual people are often more willing to forgive others because they have experienced forgiveness themselves. When people experience forgiveness, anger and resentment dissolve.

ALTRUISM

Another aspect of spirituality is **altruism**, a selfless giving to other people out of genuine concern without expecting something in return. It is an unselfish devotion to the interests and welfare of others. People who are altruistic are self-sacrificing for the benefit of others. During a selfless career, physician and philosopher Albert Schweitzer proclaimed that true happiness is to be found only by serving others.

Meditation To sit quietly while focusing on breathing.

Relaxation response The body's ability to enter a scientifically defined state of relaxation.

Forgiveness The ability to release from the mind all past hurts and failures, all sense of guilt and loss.

Altruism The act of giving of oneself out of a genuine concern for other people; unselfish devotion to the interests and welfare of others.

In the early 1960s, Bruce Randolph was almost 60 years old and nearly broke when he headed to Denver to be near his son. He began a little barbecue restaurant out of a house, using his mother's "secret sauce" recipe. Four years later he started a holiday meal tradition, feeding a few hundred people out of the back of a truck.

By the time he died in 1994, he was a household name in Denver. "Daddy Bruce" was the only name he needed. Annually for 30 years, he organized giant Thanksgiving dinners for thousands of needy people who had nowhere else to go for the holiday. And his philanthropy didn't end there. He often served free meals on Christmas and on his birthday. He collected and distributed clothing for the poor, and he organized Easter egg hunts in the park for children.

After his death at age 93, a street was named in his honor. A handpainted sign on the closed restaurant reads, "It is more blessed to give than to receive." No one would argue that one of Daddy Bruce's secrets to a long life was altruism, a giving spirit.

The ability to put another's needs above one's own also seems to contribute to a longer and healthier life. Physically, doing good for others benefits the nervous system and helps stabilize the immune system against the normal immunosuppressing effects of stress.

What makes a person altruistic? Some believe in an intrinsic "altruistic personality" that enables those who have it to automatically reach out to others. Others believe altruism is learned from the value systems and behaviors of surrounding people. In any case, most altruistic people grow up in families that are warm and nurturing. The emotional self-acceptance and compassion for others that is developed in such an environment encourages people to be generous, with the added bonuses of being creative, playful, and relaxed. It is generally agreed that altruism can be learned.

Altruistic people

- do not regard others as inferior to others;
- have a positive view of people in general;
- value human relationships more than money or material possessions;
- are concerned about others' welfare;
- believe that ethical values should be applied universally;
- believe in the right of innocent people to be free from persecution;
- have a healthy perspective about themselves;
- take personal responsibility for how other people are doing;
- are "connected" to others;
- have a profound sense of caring; and
- are willing to risk failure to control events and shape their own destiny.

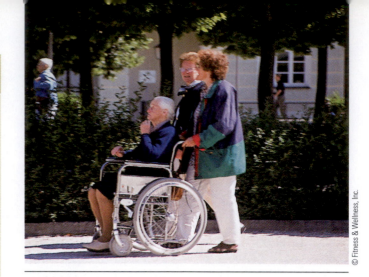

Altruism enhances health and well-being.

Characteristics of Volunteers

A true volunteer has the following characteristics:

- The helper actually connects with people—makes one-on-one contact. Writing out a check to a charity doesn't provide the same health benefits as working for a few hours at the local food bank.
- The helper has a desire to help.
- The helper likes what he or she is doing.
- The helper is consistent (the greatest health benefits have been reaped by those who do regular volunteer work at least once a week).
- The helper gives freely, not out of a sense of obligation. A person who swings a hammer on low-income housing because of her desire to see better housing for the poor will achieve more health benefits than a person who cleans up litter along the interstate highway as part of court-enforced community service requirements.

Volunteerism Altruistic people often engage in volunteer work, with the side benefit of better health, fewer visits to the doctor, and fewer medical complaints than others.[28] Places and groups that need volunteers include schools, churches, synagogues, homeless shelters, food pantries, thrift shops, libraries, zoos, animal shelters, museums, hospitals, and nursing homes. The best volunteer opportunities

- provide a regular schedule and a specific description of what the volunteers are expected to do;
- provide personal contact with the people the volunteers are going to help;
- utilize skills the volunteers have already or train them for something they'd like to be able to do;
- fall within volunteers' area of interest (it's easier to stick with the volunteer work if it's something they really enjoy doing); and
- expect a reasonable commitment (an initial commitment of 2 hours a week is suggested).

To guard against burnout, volunteers should adhere to the following guidelines:

- Don't try to do too much. A sensible goal is about 2 hours of volunteer work a week. If you have a tight schedule, just an hour a week may be advisable.
- Do something you enjoy and something you feel comfortable doing. A suicide hotline may be begging for volunteers, but if that kind of work makes you uncomfortable, another volunteer option would be better for you.
- Realize that any line of work, volunteer or paid, has occasional setbacks or bad experiences, but that plenty of good happens in the meantime.

- Realize that you aren't responsible for anyone else. You can't keep a person from committing suicide or an addict from returning to cocaine. You can provide help and support, but the responsibility is up to the person being helped.
- Get out of any situation that isn't right for you and look for something else. Just because the other volunteers seem to be doing well and enjoying themselves doesn't mean this specific situation is the best one for everybody.

Before making a commitment, the prospective volunteer should explore what is available in the area, visit the facility, watch what goes on, then narrow the choices. Before signing up for volunteer work, the volunteer should obtain as much information as possible and not be afraid to ask questions. This will enable the prospective volunteer to find the most satisfying outlet for altruism.

Volunteering can bring tremendous health benefits. As a note of caution, though: If volunteers overextend themselves or get involved in an activity that is not compatible, they may get burned out and run the risk of getting sick instead of protecting their health.

Random Acts of Kindness Another form of altruism consists of **random acts of kindness**—doing something anonymously for someone that will make his or her day easier or better in some way. This might mean paying a bridge toll for the driver behind you. Or you might see that an unknown person's parking meter has expired and deposit a quarter. Random acts of kindness are richly rewarding to the giver.

Critical Thinking

Think about some people you know or know of who are altruistic. What behaviors do they exhibit?

FAITH

Faith is a belief in something that is unseen, trusting without proof. History is replete with examples of people who have benefited from the healing power of faith. It is associated with an optimistic life orientation, social support, high resilience to stress, and low levels of anxiety.

Faith is an ingredient in Western medicine and every traditional system of healing. An example of the power of faith over physiological processes is the research showing that devoutly faithful groups of people have lower blood pressure than those who lack this quality.

HOPE

Hope is a belief that what one desires will happen—positive expectation or anticipation. Interpersonal connectedness and purpose in life, along with religious practice, are related aspects.

Hope is a way of coping with threatening situations by focusing on the positive. Hope often is challenged during crises and life transitions. No matter how dark or grim a situation may seem, optimistic people are able to extract the positive aspects and concentrate on them. They rely on support from family and friends and derive a sense of hope from their spiritual beliefs.[29]

An attitude of hope is not just a mental state. Hope promotes health and healing. It causes specific electrochemical changes in the body that benefit the strength of the immune system and even the workings of individual organs. Hope is so powerful that it can even influence the outcome of supposedly irreversible diseases such as cancer.

Medical history is replete with examples of "terminal" patients who, awash with hope, defied all medical odds. Some lived months or years longer than predicted. Others were healed. More and more, physicians are recognizing hope as a powerful tool in their work with patients.

Dr. Elisabeth Kübler-Ross, whose work with dying patients revolutionized the medical profession, stressed the importance of hope. Even if patients cannot hope for a

---

Random acts of kindness To engage in behavior that helps another person.

Faith Belief and trust in God or something that can't be proved.

Hope Positive anticipation and expectation, characterized by optimism.

cure, she said, they can hope for enriched relationships, freedom from pain, dignity, and peace.

If hope can influence health profoundly for the better, its opposite—**hopelessness**—can have the opposite effect. People who feel hopeless are desperate and despairing. Hopelessness is marked by negative expectations, the belief that the future holds nothing good or positive. It is accompanied by the inability to plan for and reach desired goals and a lack of motivation to take constructive action and gain control of life.

Spiritual Wellness

Spirituality has become a widely accepted dimension of wellness. Physicians are paying attention to patients' spiritual beliefs and addressing these as a part of health care support. Manifestations of spirituality—self-esteem, a fighting spirit, contentment, forgiveness, altruism, faith, hope—cannot only extend length of life but also can enhance quality of life, or wellness. How long we live is less important than how we embrace each day and experience an abundant and meaningful life.

> **Hopelessness** A mental state marked by negative expectations about the future; despairing.

WEB Interactive

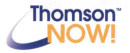

Don't forget to check out the wealth of resources on the ThomsonNOW website at **www.thomsonedu.com/ ThomsonNOW** that will:

- Coach you through identifying target goals for behavior change and monitoring your personal change plan throughout the semester
- Help you evaluate your knowledge of the material
- Allow you to take an exam-prep quiz
- Provide a Personalized Learning Plan targeting resources that address areas you should study.

WEB ACTIVITIES

Resources for Improving Self-Esteem, Self-Confidence, Self-Acceptance This site features links to a variety of resources, including online articles and books. The site also links to several self-assessment tests to provide you an opportunity to measure your self-esteem.

http://www.webheights.net/lovethyself/home.htm

ABC's of Personal Growth This is a self-help improvement site featuring psychology tests/quizzes on self-esteem and spiritual health, as well as educational articles about love, sex, violence, parenting, E-IQ test/quiz, self-esteem, dieting/weight loss, happiness, wellness, and mental health.

http://www.helpself.com

Optimism/Pessimism Test This site, sponsored by the award-winning QueenDom.com mental health Internet site, features an 18-question multiple-choice inventory designed to determine whether you have an optimistic or pessimistic viewpoint.

http://www.queendom.com/tests/index.html

Exploring Practical Spirituality Inspired by Mary Baker Eddy's *Science and Health with Key to the Scriptures*, this site features several links dealing with spirituality, including wellness, self-identity, relationships, career, and current events from a Christian Scientist perspective.

http://www.spirituality.com

InfoTrac®

You can find additional readings related to wellness via InfoTrac® College Edition, an online library of more than 900 journals and publications. Follow the instructions for accessing InfoTrac® that came packaged with your textbook, then search for articles using a key word search.

Suggested Reading Linda L. Barnes, Gregory A. Plotnikoff, Kenneth Fox, and Sarah Pendleton, "Spirituality, Religion, and Pediatrics: Intersecting Worlds of Healing," *Pediatrics* 16, no. 4 (Oct. 2000): 899.

1. Describe the different stages of James Fowler's faith-development theory.
2. How do spirituality and religion affect child development and improve self-esteem?
3. Give several examples of how religious engagement can contribute to children's pursuit of health-promoting and preventive health behaviors.

Web Activity

The Soul-Body Connection: Spirituality and Well-being Check-up

http://www.spiritualityhealth.com/newsh/items/selftest/item_234.html

Sponsor Jared Kass, Ph.D., professor of Counseling and Psychology and director of the Study Project on Well-Being, Graduate School of Arts and Social Sciences, Lesley College, Cambridge, Massachusetts.

Description This site features an easy-to-complete self-assessment questionnaire to determine your level of spirituality and how you can achieve greater personal fulfillment in the midst of a stressful life.

Available Activities This site features a three-part questionnaire to determine your level of spirituality and stress management, including

1. Questions in Part I determine your spiritual experience.
2. Part II questions determine your sense of wellness and include assessment of your energy level, goals, sources of stress, hopefulness, love, and life satisfaction.

3. Part III questions assess your stress load and how you respond to stress from the following areas: health, work, relationships, finances, daily hassles, and lifestyle choices.

Web Work

1. From the home page, click on the "Start the Tests" link. Answer all questions by clicking on the appropriate radio button.
2. Answer the questions in Part I, "Your Spiritual Experience."
3. Complete the 13 questions in the spiritual experiences table.
4. Answer the 32 questions in Part II, "Your Sense of Well-being," which immediately follows the Part I table.
5. Answer the questions in Part III, which immediately follows the Part II questions.
6. Once you have answered all questions, click on the "I'm finished" button to obtain your evaluation. You also have the opportunity to go back and change your answers if you choose.

For additional Web activities, links, and suggested readings, visit our Health, Fitness, and Wellness Resource Center at http://health.wadsworth.com.

Notes

1. L. D. Kubzansky, R. J. Wright, S. Cohen, S. Weiss, D. Sparrow, "Breathing Easy: A Prospective Study of Optimism and Pulmonary Function in the Normative Aging Study," *Annals of Behavioral Medicine* 24 (2002): 345–353.
2. T. Maruta, R. C. Colligan, M. Malinchoc, and K. P. Offord, "Optimists vs. Pessimists: Survival Rate Among Medical Patients over a 30-year period," *Mayo Clinic Proceedings*, 75 (2000): 140–143.
3. See Note 2.
4. C. Peterson and L. M. Bossio, "Optimism and Physical Well Being" in E. C. Chang (Ed), *Optimism and Pessimism: Implications for Theory, Research, and Practice.* Washington DC: American Psychological Association, 2000), pp. 127–146.
5. S. Mulkana and B. Hailey, "The Role of Optimism in Health-Enhancing Behavior," *American Journal of Health Behavior* 25 (2001): 388–395; P. V. Ylostalo, E. Ek, J. Laitinen, and M. L. Knuuttila, "Optimism and Life Satisfaction as Determinants for Dental and General Health Behavior— Oral Health Habits Linked to Cardiovascular Risk Factors," *Journal of Dental Research* 82 (2003): 194–199.
6. A. Steptoe and J. Wardle "Locus of Control and Health Behaviour Revisited: A Multivariate Analysis of Young Adults From 18 Countries," *British Journal of Psychology* 92 (2001): 659–672.
7. S. Schieman and S. C. Meersman, "Neighborhood Problems and Health Among Older Adults: Received and Donated Social Support and the Sense of Mastery as Effect Modifiers," *Journal of Gerontology* 59 (2004): S89–S97.
8. S. A. Murrell, N. L. Salsman, and S. Meeks "Education Attainment, Positive Psychological Mediators, and Resources for Health and Vitality in Older Adults," *Journal of Aging and Health* 15 (2003): 591–615.
9. M. Johnson, "Approaching the Salutogenesis of Sense of Coherence: The Role of 'Active' Self-esteem and Coping," *British Journal of Health Psychology* 9 (2004): 419–432.
10. C. Montgomery, M. Pocock, K. Titley, and K. Lloyd, "Predicting Psychological Distress in Patients with Leukaemia and Lymphoma," *Journal of Psychosomatic Research* 54 (2003): 289–292.
11. L. B. Link, L. Robbins, C. A. Mancuso, and M. E. Charlson, "How Do Cancer Patients Who Try to Take Control of Their Disease Differ From Those Who Do Not?" *European Journal of Cancer Care* 13 (2004): 219–226.
12. S. E. Kirby, P. G. Coleman, and D. Daley, "Spirituality and Well-Being in Frail and Nonfrail Older Adults," *Journal of Gerontology* 59 (2004): 123–129.
13. H. G. Koenig, L. K. George, and P. Titus, "Religion, Spirituality, and Health in Medically Ill Hospitalized Older Patients," *Journal of the American Geriatrics Society* 52 (2004): 554–562.
14. D. A. Pardini, T. G. Plante, A. Sherman, J. E. Stump, "Religious Faith and Spirituality in Substance Abuse Recovery: Determining the Mental Health Benefits," *Journal of Substance Abuse Treatment* 19 (2000): 347–354.
15. W. M. Doswell, M. Kouyate, and J. Taylor, "The Role of Spirituality in Preventing Early Sexual Behavior," *American Journal of Health Studies* 18 (2003): 195–202.
16. H. G. Koenig, "Taking a Spiritual History," *Journal of the American Medical Association* 291 (2004): 2881.
17. M. M. Rowe, R. G. Allen, "Spirituality as a Means of Coping With Chronic Illness," *American Journal of Health Studies* 19 (2004): 62–67.
18. H. Koenig et al., "Does Religious Attendance Prolong Survival? A Six-Year Follow-Up Study of 3,968 Older Adults," *Journal of Gerontology* 54A (1999): M370–M376.
19. R. A. Hummer et al., "Religious Involvement and U.S. Adult Mortality," *Demography* 36 (1999): 273–285.
20. M. Townsend, V. Kladder, H. Ayele, and T. Mulligan, "Systematic Review of Clinical Trials Examining the Effects of Religion on Health," *Southern Medical Journal* 95 (2002): 1429–1434.
21. "Therapeutic Efficacy of Prayer," *Archives of Internal Medicine* 160 (2000).
22. See Note 16.
23. E. S. T. Samano, P. T. Goldenstein, L. M. Ribero, F. Lewin, E. S. V. Filho, H. P. Soares, and A. Giglio, "Praying Correlates with Higher Quality of Life: Results From a Survey on Complementary/Alternative Medicine Use Among a Group of Brazilian Cancer Patients," *Sao Paulo Medical Journal* 122 (2004): 60–63.
24. W. Harris et al., "A Randomized, Controlled Trial of the Effects of Remote, Intercessory Prayer on Outcomes in Patients Admitted to the Coronary Care Unit," *Archives of Internal Medicine* 159 (1999): 2273–2278.
25. L. Dossey, "Prayer and Medical Science: A Commentary on the Prayer Study by Harris et al. and a Response to Critics," *Archives of Internal Medicine* 160 (2000).
26. J. Levin, "Spiritual Determinants of Health and Healing: An Epidemiologic Perspective on Salutogenic Mechanisms," *Alternative Therapies in Health and Medicine*, 9 (2003): 48–57.
27. C. V. Witvliet, T. E. Ludwig, and K. L. VanderLaan, "Granting Forgiveness or Harboring Grudges: Implications for Emotion, Physiology, and Health," *Psychological Science* 12 (2001): 117–123.
28. A. Luks with P. Payne, *The Healing Power of Doing Good: The Health and Spiritual Benefits of Helping Others* (New York: Ballantine Books, 1991).
29. J. Post-White "How Hope Affects Healing," *Creative Nursing* 1 (2003): 10–11.

Assess Your Behavior

1. Do you tend to be more of an optimist or a pessimist? What can you do to increase your level of optimism?

2. When thinking about health locus of control, do you tend to be more internal or more external? Do you take responsibility for your health status?

3. Do you possess a healthy sense of self-esteem? What behaviors do you engage in that reflect a high self-esteem that also nurture your health status?

4. Think about your spiritual health. Do you pray? Do you practice forgiveness of others?

5. Where do you derive your happiness? Are you able to be content in most circumstances?

6. Do you have traits of an altruistic personality? Think about how volunteering could help you personally.

Assess Your Knowledge

Evaluate how well you understand the concepts presented in this chapter by answering the following questions.

1. The habitual manner in which people describe the things that happen to them is called
   a. prayers.
   b. pessimism.
   c. explanatory style.
   d. self-esteem.
   e. health locus of control.

2. Pessimism can lead to
   a. anxiety.
   b. depression.
   c. guilt.
   d. anger.
   e. all of the above.

3. A positive explanatory style can lead to
   a. hostility.
   b. isolation.
   c. stress.
   d. lower quality of life.
   e. greater length of life.

4. The extent to which we believe that our behavior affects our health status is called
   a. health behavior.
   b. health cognition.
   c. health locus of control.
   d. health attitudes.
   e. healthy self-esteem.

5. People who believe that things that happen to them are unrelated to their own behavior are
   a. anxious.
   b. external in their locus of control.
   c. low in self-esteem.
   d. most likely to engage in positive health behaviors.
   e. internal in their locus of control.

6. People who have an internal locus of control
   a. are most likely to have fewer illnesses.
   b. are less likely to produce sufficient serotonin.
   c. are most likely to have high levels of corticosteroids.
   d. have more damage when exposed to stress.
   e. All of the above.

7. People with positive levels of self-esteem
   a. practice behaviors that lead to good health.
   b. have high levels of chronic pain.
   c. have reduced levels of quality of life.
   d. are less likely to take on worthwhile challenges.
   e. All of the above.

Correct answers can be found on page 369.

The Life Orientation Test:
Are You An Optimist?

Name: _____   Date: _____   Grade: _____

Instructor: _____   Course: _____   Section: _____

In the following spaces, write how much you agree with each of the items, using the following scale:

4 = strongly agree   3 = agree   2 = neutral   1 = disagree   0 = strongly disagree

1. In uncertain times, I usually expect the best.

2. If something can go wrong for me, it will.

3. I always look on the bright side of things.

4. I'm always optimistic about my future.

5. I hardly ever expect things to go my way.

6. Things never work out the way I want them to.

7. I'm a believer in the idea that "every cloud has a silver lining."

8. I rarely count on good things happening to me.

How to Score

For items 2, 5, 6, and 8, you will have to reverse the numbers. For example, if you strongly agree with statement 8, "I rarely count on good things happening to me," change your score from 4 to 0. Now total up your score.

Interpreting Your Results

This test has been used to demonstrate a relationship between an optimistic or a pessimistic outlook and physical well-being. When college students completed this test 4 weeks before final exams, the optimists (with 20 points and over) reported far fewer health problems. The pessimists complained of more dizziness, fatigue, sore muscles, and coughs.

How Do You Feel About Yourself?

Name: _____ Date: _____ Grade: _____

Instructor: _____ Course: _____ Section: _____

This scale is designed to help you understand your self-image. Positive attitudes toward oneself are important components of maturation and emotional well-being.

Self-Image Aspect	Strongly Agree	Agree	Disagree	Strongly Disagree
1. I'm a person of worth, at least on an equal plane with others.	A	B	C	D
2. I have a number of good qualities.	A	B	C	D
3. All in all, I am inclined to feel that I'm a failure.	A	B	C	D
4. I'm able to do things as well as most other people.	A	B	C	D
5. I don't have as much to be proud of as others.	A	B	C	D
6. I take a positive attitude toward myself.	A	B	C	D
7. On the whole, I'm satisfied with myself.	A	B	C	D
8. I wish I could have more respect for myself.	A	B	C	D
9. I certainly feel useless at times.	A	B	C	D
10. At times I think I'm no good at all.	A	B	C	D

How to Score

Use the following table to determine the number of points to assign to each of your answers. To determine your total score, add up all the numbers that match the letter (A, B, C, or D) you circled for each statement.

Statement	A	B	C	D
1.	4	3	2	1
2.	4	3	2	1
3.	1	2	3	4
4.	4	3	2	1
5.	1	2	3	4
6.	4	3	2	1
7.	4	3	2	1
8.	1	2	3	4
9.	1	2	3	4
10.	1	2	3	4

Total: [   ] This is your self-esteem score.

From *Society and the Adolescent Self-Image* by M. Rosenberg (Hanover, NH: Wesleyan University Press, 1986). Used by permission.

Interpreting Your Score

Classify your score in the appropriate score range.

Score Range	Current Self-Esteem Level
Less than 20	Low self-esteem
20–29	Below-average self-esteem
30–34	Above-average self-esteem
35–39	High self-esteem
40	Highest self-esteem

The higher your score, the more positive your self-esteem.

High self-esteem means that individuals respect themselves, consider themselves worthy, but do not necessarily consider themselves better than others. They do not feel themselves to be the ultimate in perfection; on the contrary, they recognize their limitations and expect to grow and improve.

Self-esteem is the most important variable in regard to human development and maturation. It is the master key that can open the door to the actualization of an individual's human potential.

Are Your Thoughts Helping or Hurting Your Longevity?

Name: _____   Date: _____   Grade: _____

Instructor: _____   Course: _____   Section: _____

Does an extraordinary challenge make you freeze up with fear? Do you let yourself dwell on minor slights? If so, you're prone to destructive thinking patterns that can prevent you from doing your best, fostering successful relationships, and, in general, coping well and living long. Pessimists are less likely to survive major surgery, for example. And anyone who's easily offended will have trouble enjoying the camaraderie that is a key to living a long life.

   The antidote for destructive thoughts is cultivating constructive ones. To help you do that, Seymour Epstein, Ph.D., professor of psychology at the University of Massachusetts and author of *You're Smarter Than You Think*, adapted the following quiz from a psychological test he uses to help patients strengthen their coping skills. This exercise will tell how constructive a thinker you are overall and identify the areas that could stand some pumping up.

Rate each statement from 1 to 5 according to this scale:

   1 = completely false   2 = mainly false   3 = undecided   4 = mainly true   5 = completely true

Be honest. Don't answer according to how you think you should be but how you naturally are.

1. I don't worry about things I can do nothing about.

2. I am the kind of person who takes action, not just complains about things.

3. I don't let little things bother me.

4. If I have an unpleasant chore to do, I try to make the best of it by thinking in positive terms.

5. I don't have to perform exceptionally well in order to consider myself a worthwhile person.

6. I look at challenges not as something to fear, but as opportunities to test myself and learn.

7. I tend to dwell more on pleasant than unpleasant incidents from the past.

8. When I have a difficult task, I think encouraging thoughts that help me do my best.

9. I tend not to take things personally.

10. When faced with upcoming unpleasant events, I usually think carefully how I will deal with them.

Total A

11. I believe that if people treat you badly, you should treat them in kind.

12. Talking about something I want to succeed usually ensures failure.

13. I believe in astrology.

14. There are two kinds of people: good and bad.

15. When something good happens to me, I believe it will be balanced by something bad.

16. I have at least one good-luck charm.

17. There are many wrong ways to do something, but only one right way.

18. I believe in good and bad omens.

19. I believe in ghosts.

20. I tend to classify people as being either for or against me.

21. I sometimes think that if I want something to happen too much, it probably won't.

22. I believe some people are able to read other people's thoughts.

23. I tend to be very judgmental.

24. I've learned not to hope for something too much—that usually means it won't happen.

Total B (90 minus total for 11–25)

Grand Total (A + B)

25. I believe there are people who can literally see into the future.

Scoring

Above 99 = VERY HIGH. You are a very constructive thinker. Keep up the good work.

89–99 = HIGH. You are a better-than-average constructive thinker. You usually expect good things to happen and they often do. But there's room for improvement.

74–88 = AVERAGE. Like most people, you're prone to some destructive thoughts. Go back through the exercise and try to identify a pattern. For example, statements 11, 14, 17, 20, and 23 represent categorical thinking—seeing situations and people as either good or bad; statements 12, 15, 18, 21, and 24 are examples of superstitious thinking; and 13, 16, 19, 22, and 25 show thinking that relies on belief in the paranormal. If you gave more than a 3 to these questions, try to catch yourself before lapsing into your usual assumptions. In addition, shore up your constructive thinking by reviewing the positive statements, 1 through 10, paying particular attention to those to which you gave less than a 3.

63–73 = LOW. Your habitual thinking is somewhat more destructive than most people's, and it interferes with your happiness and efficiency. Follow the advice given for average scorers. You have much to gain from working hard to improve your constructive thinking.

Below 63 = VERY LOW. Your destructive thinking is likely to be the source of serious problems. Work at identifying and correcting it. If you have trouble doing so, consider seeing a therapist. But regardless, don't expect your destructive thoughts to go away overnight.

6

Fitness Assessment for Wellness

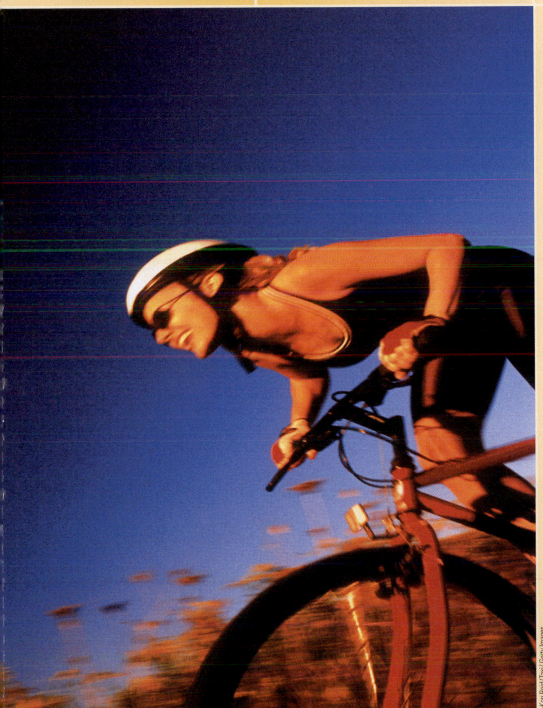

OBJECTIVES

Explain the differences between physical activity and exercise.

Understand the significance of the U. S. Surgeon General's Report on Physical Activity and Health.

Describe the role of the pedometer in monitoring physical activity.

Explain the relationship between physical fitness and health.

Describe the benefits and significance of lifetime physical activity.

Identify the impact of physical fitness on health-care costs and workplace productivity.

Identify the risk factors that may interfere with safe participation in exercise.

Define health-related fitness, skill-related fitness, and physiologic fitness and state the components of each.

Explain the relevance of assessing physical fitness.

Learn to assess cardiorespiratory endurance, muscular strength endurance, and muscular flexibility.

Be able to interpret the results of health-related fitness tests.

Modern technology has almost completely eliminated the need for physical activity in the daily life of most people. Physical activity is no longer a natural part of our existence. We live in an automated society in which most of the activities that used to require strenuous physical exertion can be accomplished by machines with the simple pull of a handle or push of a button.

Unfortunately, physical inactivity and a sedentary lifestyle pose a serious threat to our health and accelerate the deterioration rate of the human body. Physically active people live longer than their inactive counterparts, even if the latter become active later in life. According to the U.S. Centers for Disease Control and Prevention, more than 112,000 deaths each year are attributed to the lack of regular physical activity and improper dietary habits. A similar trend is found in most industrialized nations throughout the world.

During the late 1960s and in the 1970s, scientists began to realize that good fitness is important in the fight against chronic diseases, which had replaced infectious diseases as the leading causes of death.

We now recognize that health is largely self-controllable and that the leading causes of premature death and illness in the United States can be prevented by adhering to a healthy lifestyle. Physical activity is a crucial component.

Physical Activity Versus Exercise

The abundance of scientific research on physical activity and exercise over the last three decades, has established a clear distinction between physical activity and exercise. **Physical activity** is bodily movement produced by skeletal muscles that requires energy expenditure and produces progressive health benefits.[1] Examples of physical activity are walking to and from class, taking stairs instead of elevators and escalators, gardening, dancing, and washing the car by hand. The counterpart, physical inactivity, implies a level of activity that is lower than that required to maintain good health.

Exercise is a type of physical activity that requires "planned, structured, and repetitive bodily movement done to improve or maintain one or more components of physical fitness."[2] Examples of exercise are regular, continuous brisk walking, jogging, cycling, aerobics, swimming, strength training, and stretching exercises.

SURGEON GENERAL'S REPORT ON PHYSICAL ACTIVITY AND HEALTH

According to a 1996 landmark report by the U.S. Surgeon General, poor health resulting from lack of physical activity is a serious public health problem that we must meet

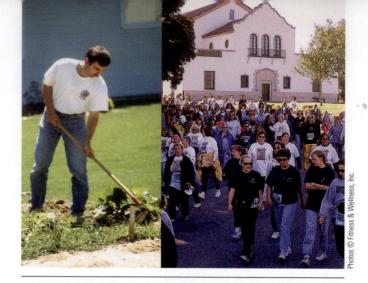

The U.S. Surgeon General has determined that moderate-intensity physical activity is beneficial to health and well-being.

head-on.[3] The general recommendation for health benefits issued by the Surgeon General is that people strive to accumulate at least 30 minutes of **moderate-intensity physical activity** per day most days of the week. The report also stated that physical inactivity is more prevalent in

1. women than men
2. African Americans and Hispanic Americans than Caucasians
3. older than younger adults
4. less affluent than more affluent people
5. less educated than more educated adults.

The report states that regular moderate-intensity physical activity can prevent premature death, unnecessary illness, disability, and provide substantial benefits in health and well-being for the vast majority of people who are not physically active. Individuals who are moderately active already can achieve even greater health benefits by increasing their physical activity.

Among the benefits of regular physical activity and exercise listed in the report and subsequent studies are significantly reduced risks for developing or dying from heart disease, stroke, Type 2 diabetes, colon and breast cancers, high blood pressure, and osteoporotic fractures.[4] Regular physical activity also is important for the health of muscles, bones, and joints, and it seems to reduce symptoms of depression and anxiety, improve mood, and enhance one's ability to perform daily tasks throughout life. It also can help control health-care costs and maintain a high quality of life into old age.

Critical Thinking

1. Do you consciously incorporate physical activity into your daily lifestyle?
2. Can you provide examples?
3. Do you think that you get sufficient daily physical activity to maintain good health?

FIGURE 6.1 Prevalence of Recommended Physical Activity in United States, 2003

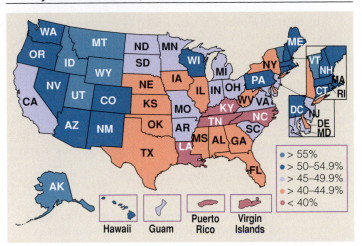

> 55%
> 50–54.9%
> 45–49.9%
> 40–44.9%
< 40%

Hawaii   Guam   Puerto Rico   Virgin Islands

Note: Recommended physical activity is moderate-intensity physical activity at least 5 days a week for 30 minutes a day, or vigorous-intensity physical activity 3 days a week for 20 minutes a day.

Source: Centers for Disease Control and Prevention, Atlanta, 2005.

MONITORING DAILY PHYSICAL ACTIVITY

According to the Centers for Disease Control and Prevention, the majority of U.S. adults are not sufficiently physically active to promote good health. The data indicate that only 46 percent of adults meet the minimal recommendation of 30 minutes of moderate physical activity at least 5 days per week; 25 percent report no leisure physical activity at all; and 16 percent are completely inactive (less than 10 minutes per week of moderate or vigorous-intensity physical activity). The prevalence of physical activity by state in the United States is displayed in Figure 6.1.

PEDOMETER USE

Other than carefully monitoring actual time engaged in an activity, an excellent tool to monitor daily physical activity is the **pedometer**. Pedometers are small mechanical devices that are used to count footsteps. Wearing a pedometer throughout the day allows you to determine the total steps taken in a day.

The pedometer is a motivational tool to help increase, maintain, and monitor daily physical activity that involves lower body motion (walking, jogging, running). Use of a pedometer most likely will continue to increase as a means of promoting and quantifying physical activity.

Before purchasing a pedometer, be sure to verify its accuracy. Many of the free and low-end cost pedometers provided by corporations for promotion and advertisement purposes are inaccurate, so they should be discouraged. A good pedometer costs about $25, and ratings are available online.

The typical male American takes about 6,000 steps per day, and women typically take about 5,300 steps per day.

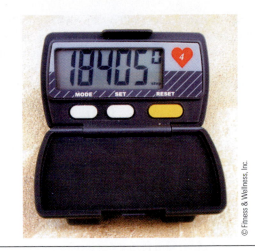

Pedometers frequently are used to help motivate and monitor daily physical activity.

A general recommendation for adults is 10,000 steps per day, and Table 1.2 in Chapter 1 (page 15) provides specific activity ratings based on the number of steps taken daily. For more accurate results, use an average of four days for your number of daily steps. You may then record this information in Assessment 6.2.

Fitness and Health

Several significant research studies linking physical activity habits and mortality rates have shown a decrease in premature mortality rates among physically active people. A study conducted by Dr. Ralph Paffenbarger and his colleagues involving 16,936 Harvard alumni showed that, as the amount of weekly physical activity increased, the risk of cardiovascular deaths decreased.[5] The greatest decrease in cardiovascular deaths was observed among alumni who used in excess of 2,000 calories per week through physical activity (see Figure 6.2).

Another major study, conducted by Dr. Steve Blair and his associates, upheld the findings of the Harvard alumni study.[6] Based on data from 13,344 people who were

Physical activity Bodily movement produced by skeletal muscles that requires energy expenditure and produces progressive health benefits.

Exercise Physical activity that requires planned, structured, and repetitive bodily movement done to improve or maintain one or more components of physical fitness.

Moderate-intensity physical activity Physical activity that uses 150 calories of energy per day or 1,000 calories per week.

Pedometer An electronic device that senses body motion and counts footsteps; some pedometers also record distance, calories burned, speeds, "aerobic steps," and time spent being physically active.

followed over an average of 8 years, the results confirmed that the level of cardiorespiratory fitness is related to mortality from all causes. In essence, the higher the level of cardiorespiratory fitness, the longer the life (see Figure 6.3). Death rates from all causes for the least-fit (group 1) men was 3.4 times higher than it was for the most-fit men. For the least-fit women, the death rate was 4.6 times higher than it was for the most-fit women.

The same study reported a much lower rate of premature deaths even at the moderate-fitness levels most adults can achieve. Even greater protection was attained when a higher fitness level was combined with eliminating other risk factors such as hypertension, high cholesterol, cigarette smoking, and excessive body fat.

Additional research that looked at changes in fitness and mortality found a substantial (44 percent) reduction in mortality risk when people abandoned a sedentary lifestyle and became moderately fit.[7] The lowest death rate was found in people who were fit and remained fit, and the highest rate was found in men who remained unfit (see Figure 6.4).

Subsequent research substantiated the previous findings and also indicated that primarily vigorous activities are associated with greater longevity.[8] **Vigorous activity**

FIGURE 6.2 Death Rates According to Physical Activity Index

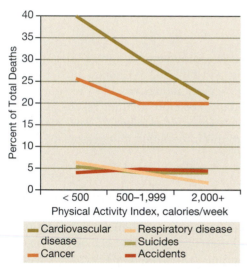

Based on 10,000 man-years of observation. One person-year indicates one person followed up 1 year later.

From "A Natural History of Athleticism on Cardiovascular Health," by R. S. Paffenbarger, R. T. Hyde, A. L. Wing, and C. H. Steinmetz. *Journal of the American Medical Association* 252 (1984): 491–495.

FIGURE 6.4 Five-year Follow-up in Mortality Rates Associated with Maintenance of and Improvements in Fitness

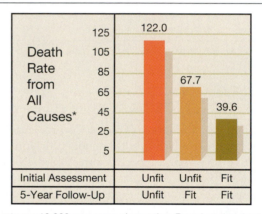

* Death rate per 10,000 man-years observation. Based on data from "Changes in Physical Fitness and All-Cause Mortality: A Prospective Study of Healthy Men," *Journal of the American Medical Association* 273 (1995): 1193–1198.

Source: "Changes in Physical Fitness and All-Cause Mortality: A Prospective Study of Healthy and Unhealthy Men" by S. N. Blair, H. W. Kohl III, C. E. Barlow, R. S. Paffenbarger, Jr., L. W. Gibbons, and C. A. Macera. *Journal of the American Medical Association* 273 (1995): 1193–1198.

FIGURE 6.3 Death Rates by Physical Fitness Groups

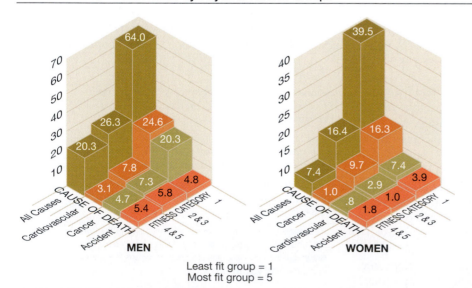

Least fit group = 1
Most fit group = 5

Note: Study included 13,344 people, followed for 10,000 person-years 1970–1985. One person-year indicates one person followed up 1 year later.

Based on data from "Physical Fitness and All-Cause Mortality: A Prospective Study of Healthy Men and Women," by S. N. Blair, H. W. Kohl III, R. S. Paffenbarger, Jr., D. G. Clark, K. H. Cooper, and L. W. Gibbons. *Journal of the American Medical Association* 262 (1989), 2395–2401.

was defined as any activity that requires a MET* level equal to or greater than 6 METs (21 ml/kg/min—see Health Fitness Standards, page 110). Examples of vigorous activities in the later study include brisk walking, jogging, swimming laps, squash, racquetball, tennis, and shoveling snow. The results also indicated that vigorous exercise is as important as maintaining recommended weight and not smoking.

The results of all these studies indicate clearly that fitness improves health, wellness, and longevity. If people are able to do vigorous exercise, it is preferable because it is most clearly associated with longer life.

Impact of Physical Fitness

Most people exercise because it improves their personal appearance and makes them feel good about themselves. The greatest benefit of all, however, is that physically fit individuals enjoy a better quality of life. These people live life to its fullest potential, with fewer health problems than inactive individuals (who may also indulge in other negative lifestyle patterns).

Health-Care Costs

Sedentary living can have a strong impact on a nation's economy. As the need for physical exertion in Western countries decreased steadily during the last century, health-care expenditures increased dramatically. Health-care costs in the United States rose from $12 billion in 1950 to $1.7 trillion in 2003, or about 13 percent of the gross national product (GNP). In 1980, health-care costs represented 8.8 percent of the GNP and they are projected to reach about 16 percent by the year 2010.

The United States is currently the best place in the world to treat people once they are sick, but the system

---

*One MET is the energy expenditure at rest, or approximately 3.5 ml/kg/min; 6 or more METs represents exercising at an oxygen uptake (VO$_2$) equal to or greater than 6 times the resting energy requirement.

does a poor job at keeping people healthy in the first place. The United States also fails to provide good health care for all: More than 44 million residents do not have health insurance.

Unhealthy behaviors are contributing to the staggering U.S. health care costs. Risk factors for disease such as obesity and smoking, for example, carry a heavy price tag. Estimates indicate that 1 percent of the people account for 30 percent of health care costs.[9] Half of the people use up about 97 percent of health-care dollars. Furthermore, the average health-care cost per person in the United States is almost twice as high as that in most other industrialized nations.

PROGRAMS IN THE WORKPLACE

In addition to better health, participation in fitness and wellness programs leads to lower medical costs and higher job productivity. As a result of the staggering rise in medical costs, many organizations offer health-promotion programs because keeping employees healthy costs less than treating them once they are sick.

Another reason that some organizations are offering health-promotion programs to their employees—overlooked by many because it does not seem to affect the bottom line directly—is top management's concern for employees' well-being. Whether the program lowers medical costs is not the main issue. More important, wellness helps individuals feel better about themselves and improve their quality of life.

Pre-Exercise Screening and Goals

Even though exercise testing and participation are relatively safe for most apparently healthy individuals under age 45, the reaction of the cardiovascular system to more intense levels of physical activity cannot always be predicted. Consequently, people face a small but real risk of some bodily changes during exercise testing or participation. These changes may include abnormal blood pressure, irregular heart rhythm, fainting, and, rarely, a heart attack or cardiac arrest.

Before you start an exercise program or participate in any exercise testing, you should fill out the Physical Activity Readiness Questionnaire (PAR-Q) in Assessment 6.1. This questionnaire, developed by the Ministry of Health in British Columbia, Canada, is used widely in the United States and Canada as a screening instrument prior to fitness testing.

If your answer to any of the PAR-Q questions is positive, you should consult a physician before participating

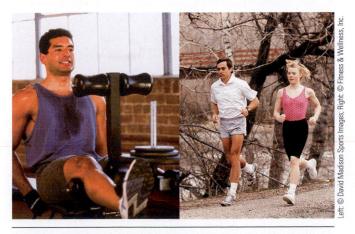

Regular participation in a lifetime exercise program increases quality of life and longevity.

Vigorous activity Any activity that requires a MET level equal to or greater than 6 METs (21 ml/kg/min).

in fitness testing or a fitness program. Exercise testing or participation is not advised under some of the conditions listed in the questionnaire and may require a stress electrocardiogram (ECG) test (see Chapter 11). If you have any questions regarding your current health status, you should consult your doctor before initiating, continuing, or increasing your level of physical activity.

As you work through this chapter and assess the various components of fitness, you will be able to develop a fitness profile. When you obtain the information pertaining to each component of fitness, you can enter your results on the profile in Assessment 6.2.

Once the results for each component have been established, either with your instructor's help or using your own judgment, you can set your own target goals to achieve over the next few weeks. You then may proceed with an exercise program as outlined in Chapter 7. Following 8 to 12 weeks of exercise training, you should retest each component to assess your improvements in physical fitness.

Physical Fitness

As the fitness concept has taken hold, it has become clear that several specific components contribute to an individual's overall level of fitness. **Physical fitness** is classified into health-related, skill-related, and physiologic fitness.

Health-related fitness is related to the ability to perform activities of daily living without undue fatigue and is conducive to a low risk of premature **hypokinetic diseases**.[10] The health-related fitness components are cardiorespiratory (aerobic) endurance, muscular strength and endurance, muscular flexibility, and body composition (Figure 6.5).

Skill-related fitness is more important in sports performance and may not be as critical to better health. The components are: agility, balance, coordination, power, reaction time, and speed.

FIGURE 6.5 Health-related Components of Physical Fitness

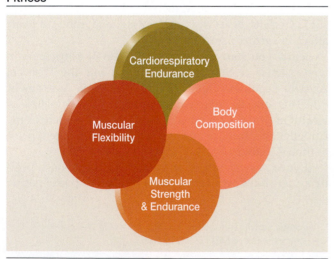

Critical Thinking

1. What role do the four health-related components of physical fitness play in your life?
2. Can you rank them in order of importance to you and explain the rationale you used?

Physiologic fitness is a term used primarily in the field of medicine with reference to biological systems affected by physical activity and the role the latter plays in preventing disease. Components of physiologic fitness are **metabolic fitness**, **morphologic fitness**, and **bone integrity**.[11]

Relevance of Physical Fitness Assessment

In terms of health and wellness, the main emphasis of fitness programs should be on the health-related components. The assessments of cardiorespiratory endurance, muscular strength and endurance, and muscular flexibility are discussed in this chapter. Assessment of body composition is covered in Chapter 9. Through these assessment techniques, you will be able to determine your level of physical fitness regularly as you engage in an exercise program. In comprehensive fitness testing, you will

- educate yourself regarding the various fitness components;
- assess your fitness level for each health-related fitness component and compare the results to health fitness and physical fitness standards;
- identify your areas of weakness for training emphasis;
- be motivated to participate in exercise;
- use your personalized exercise prescriptions as a starting point;
- evaluate the progress and effectiveness of your program;
- make adjustments in your exercise prescription, if necessary;
- reward yourself for complying with your exercise program (a change to a higher fitness level is a reward in and of itself).

Fitness Standards

Over time, two standards have emerged in physical fitness assessment: a health fitness standard and a physical fitness standard.

HEALTH FITNESS STANDARDS

As illustrated in Figure 6.6, although fitness (see VO_{2max} discussed on page 112) improvements with a moderate

FIGURE 6.6 Health and Fitness Benefits Based on Type of Lifestyle and Physical Activity Program

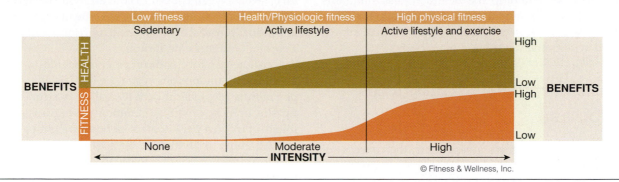

© Fitness & Wellness, Inc.

aerobic activity program are not as notable, significant health benefits are reaped with such a program. Only slightly better health benefits are obtained with a more intense exercise program. Benefits of health fitness include a reduction in blood lipids, lower blood pressure, less risk for diabetes, weight loss, stress release, lower risk for disease including cardiovascular diseases and cancer, and a lesser risk for premature mortality.

The health fitness standards proposed here are based on epidemiological data linking minimum fitness values to disease prevention and health. Attaining the health fitness standards requires only moderate physical activity. For example, a 2-mile walk in less than half an hour, five or six times per week, seems to be sufficient to achieve the health fitness standard for cardiorespiratory endurance.

PHYSICAL FITNESS STANDARDS

Physical fitness standards are set higher than the health fitness standards and require a more rigorous exercise program. Many experts believe that people who meet the criteria of "good" physical fitness should be able to do moderate to vigorous physical activity without undue fatigue and to maintain this capability throughout life. In this context, physically fit people of all ages will have the freedom to enjoy most of life's daily and recreational activities to their fullest potential. Current health fitness standards may not be enough to achieve these objectives.

Sound physical fitness gives the individual a degree of independence throughout life that many people no longer enjoy. Most older people should be able to carry out activities similar to those conducted in their youth, though not with the same intensity. A person does not have to be a championship athlete, but activities such as changing a tire, chopping wood, climbing several flights of stairs, playing a game of basketball or soccer, mountain biking, walking several miles around a lake, and hiking through a national park do require more than the current "average fitness" level of the American people.

In this book, fitness standards for cardiorespiratory endurance, strength, flexibility, and body composition include both a health fitness standard and a physical fitness standard. You will have to decide your own objectives. If

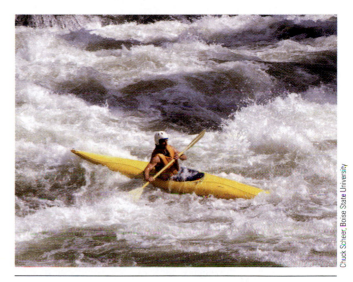

Chuck Scheer, Boise State University

A high level of fitness is needed to enjoy many of life's recreational and leisure activities.

Physical fitness The ability to meet the ordinary as well as the unusual demands of daily life safely and effectively without being overly fatigued and still have energy left for leisure and recreational activities.

Health-related fitness Fitness programs prescribed to improve the overall health of the individual.

Hypokinetic diseases Illnesses caused by lack of physical activity.

Skill-related fitness Fitness components important for success in skillful activities and athletic events.

Physiologic fitness A form of skill-related fitness used with reference to biological systems that are affected by physical activity and the role of activity in preventing disease.

Metabolic fitness A component of physiologic fitness that denotes reduction in the risk for diabetes and cardiovascular disease through a moderate-intensity exercise program in spite of little or no improvement in cardiorespiratory fitness.

Morphologic fitness A component of physiologic fitness used in reference to body composition (fat) factors such as percent body fat, body fat distribution, and body circumference.

Bone integrity A component of physiologic fitness used to determine risk for osteoporosis based on bone mineral density.

the main objective of a fitness program is to lower your risk for disease, attaining the health fitness standards may be enough. If you want to participate in more vigorous fitness activities, achieving a high physical fitness standard is recommended.

Variation in Physiological Response

Prior to introducing fitness assessments, the concepts of **responders** and **nonresponders** should be introduced. Individuals who follow similar training programs show a wide variation in physiological responses. Heredity plays a crucial role in how each person responds to and improves after beginning an exercise program. Several studies have documented that following exercise training, most individuals, the responders, readily show improvements, but a few, nonresponders, exhibit small or no improvements at all. This concept is referred to as the **principle of individuality**.

After several months of aerobic training, VO_{2max} increases are between 15 and 20 percent, on average, although individual responses can range from 0 percent (in a few selected cases) to more than 50 percent improvement, even when all participants follow exactly the same training program. Non-fitness and low-fitness participants, however, should not label themselves as nonresponders based on this discussion. Nonresponders constitute less than 5 percent of exercise participants. Although additional research is necessary, lack of improvement in cardiorespiratory endurance among nonresponders might be related to low levels of leg strength. A lower body strength-training program has been shown to help these individuals improve VO_{2max} through aerobic exercise.[12]

Following the assessment of cardiorespiratory fitness, if your fitness level is less than adequate, do not let that discourage you, but make it a priority to be physically active every day. In addition to regular exercise, lifestyle behaviors such as walking, taking stairs, cycling to work, parking farther from the office, doing household tasks, gardening, and doing yardwork provide substantial benefits. Nonresponders should monitor their daily physical activity and exercise habits in conjunction with fitness testing to evaluate compliance.

Assessment of Cardiorespiratory Endurance

Cardiorespiratory endurance has been defined as the ability of the lungs, heart, and blood vessels to deliver adequate amounts of oxygen to the cells to meet the demands of prolonged physical activity. As you breathe, part of the oxygen in the air is taken up in your lungs and transported in the blood to your heart. The heart then pumps the oxygenated blood through your circulatory system to all organs and tissues of your body. At the cellular level, oxygen is used to convert food substrates, primarily carbohydrates and fats, into the energy necessary to conduct physical activity, body functions, and maintain a constant internal equilibrium.

Cardiorespiratory endurance is measured in terms of the maximal amount of oxygen the body is able to utilize per minute of physical activity, called **maximal oxygen uptake**, or VO_{2max}. VO_{2max} commonly is expressed in milliliters of oxygen per kilogram of body weight per minute (ml/kg/min). Individual values can range from about 10 ml/kg/min in cardiac patients to 80 ml/kg/min or higher in male world-class runners and cross-country skiers (women values are about 10 to 15 percent lower).

Data from the research study presented in Figure 6.3 indicate that VO_{2max} values of 35 and 32.5 ml/kg/min for men and women, respectively, may be sufficient to significantly lower the risk for all causes of mortality. Although greater improvements in fitness yield a slightly lower risk for premature death, the largest drop is seen between the least fit (group 1) and the moderately fit (groups 2 and 3). Therefore, the 35 and 32.5 ml/kg/min values could be selected as the health fitness standards.

During physical exertion, more energy is needed. As a result, the heart, lungs, and blood vessels have to deliver more oxygen to the cells. During prolonged exercise, an individual with a high level of cardiorespiratory endurance is able to deliver the required amount of oxygen to the tissues quite easily. The cardiorespiratory system of a person with a low level of endurance has to work much harder, because the heart has to pump more often to supply the same amount of oxygen to the tissues and, consequently, fatigues faster. A higher capacity to deliver and utilize oxygen (oxygen uptake), then, indicates a more efficient cardiorespiratory system.

A sound cardiorespiratory endurance program greatly enhances health. With the exception of older adults, cardiorespiratory endurance is the single most important component of health-related physical fitness. Certain levels of muscular strength and flexibility are necessary in daily activities to lead a normal life. Even so, a person can get by without a lot of strength and flexibility but cannot do without a good cardiorespiratory system.

The most precise way to determine VO_{2max} is through **open-circuit indirect calorimetry** (also called direct gas analysis). This is done using a metabolic cart through which the amount of oxygen the body consumes can be measured directly. Because this type of equipment is not available in most health/fitness centers, several alternative methods of estimating VO_{2max} have been developed.

Even though most cardiorespiratory endurance tests probably are safe to administer to apparently healthy individuals (those with no major coronary risk factors or symptoms), the American College of Sports Medicine recommends that a physician be present for any **maximal exercise test** on apparently healthy men over age 45 and women over age 55.[13] A maximal test is any test that

TABLE 6.1 Estimated Maximal Oxygen Uptake (VO_{2max}) for the 1.5-Mile Run Test

Time	VO_{2max} (ml/kg/min)	Time	VO_{2max} (ml/kg/min)	Time	VO_{2max} (ml/kg/min)	Time	VO_{2max} (ml/kg/min)
6:10	80.0	9:30	54.7	12:50	39.2	16:10	30.5
6:20	79.0	9:40	53.5	13:00	38.6	16:20	30.2
6:30	77.9	9:50	52.3	13:10	38.1	16:30	29.8
6:40	76.7	10:00	51.1	13:20	37.8	16:40	29.5
6:50	75.5	10:10	50.4	13:30	37.2	16:50	29.1
7:00	74.0	10:20	49.5	13:40	36.8	17:00	28.9
7:10	72.6	10:30	48.6	13:50	36.3	17:10	28.5
7:20	71.3	10:40	48.0	14:00	35.9	17:20	28.3
7:30	69.9	10:50	47.4	14:10	35.5	17:30	28.0
7:40	68.3	11:00	46.6	14:20	35.1	17:40	27.7
7:50	66.8	11:10	45.8	14:30	34.7	17:50	27.4
8:00	65.2	11:20	45.1	14:40	34.3	18:00	27.1
8:10	63.9	11:30	44.4	14:50	34.0	18:10	26.8
8:20	62.5	11:40	43.7	15:00	33.6	18:20	26.6
8:30	61.2	11:50	43.2	15:10	33.1	18:30	26.3
8:40	60.2	12:00	42.3	15:20	32.7	18:40	26.0
8:50	59.1	12:10	41.7	15:30	32.2	18:50	25.7
9:00	58.1	12:20	41.0	15:40	31.8	19:00	25.4
9:10	56.9	12:30	40.4	15:50	31.4		
9:20	55.9	12:40	39.8	16:00	30.9		

Adapted from K. H. Cooper, "A Means of Assessing Maximal Oxygen Intake" *Journal of the American Medical Association* 203 (1968): 201–204; M. L. Pollock et al., *Health and Fitness Through Physical Activity*, (New York: John Wiley and Sons, 1978), and J. H. Wilmore, *Training for Sport and Activity* (Boston: Allyn and Bacon, 1982).

requires the participant's all-out or nearly all-out effort. For submaximal exercise tests, a physician should be present when testing higher risk/symptomatic individuals or diseased people, regardless of the participant's current age.

Two exercise tests frequently used to assess cardiorespiratory fitness are the 1.5-Mile Run test and the 1.0-Mile Walk test. Depending on fitness level and personal preference, you may choose either or both of these. The running test is recommended for individuals who exercise regularly, whereas the walking test is preferred for those who have not yet initiated an exercise program. Because these are field tests to estimate VO_{2max}, each test will not necessarily yield exactly the same results. To make valid comparisons, the same test should be used for pre- and post-assessments.

1.5-MILE RUN TEST

The 1.5-Mile Run test is the test used most frequently to predict cardiorespiratory fitness. VO_{2max} is estimated based on the time required to run (or walk) a 1.5-mile course (see Table 6.1).

The only equipment necessary to conduct this test is a stopwatch and a 440-yard track (six laps to complete the 1.5 miles) or a premeasured 1.5-mile course. A person should be cautious prior to doing the 1.5-mile run. Because the objective of this test is to cover the distance in the shortest time, it is considered a maximal exercise test. Therefore, its use should be limited to conditioned individuals who have been cleared for exercise. The 1.5-Mile Run test is not recommended for unconditioned beginners, men over

age 40, and women over age 50 without proper medical clearance, symptomatic individuals, and those with known disease or risk factors for coronary heart disease. Before taking this test, unconditioned individuals should participate in at least 6 weeks of aerobic training.

Before the actual run, you should warm up properly by doing some stretching exercises, walking, and slow jogging. Equally important, at the end of the 1.5-mile run,

Responders Individuals who exhibit improvements in fitness as a result of exercise training.

Nonresponders Individuals who exhibit small or no improvements in fitness as compared to others who undergo the same training program.

Principle of individuality Training concept stating that genetics plays a major role in individual responses to exercise training and that these differences must be considered when designing exercise programs for different people.

Cardiorespiratory endurance The ability of the lungs, heart, and blood vessels to deliver adequate amounts of oxygen to the cells to meet the demands of prolonged physical activity.

Maximal oxygen uptake (VO_{2max}) The maximum amount of oxygen the body is able to utilize per minute of physical activity, commonly expressed in ml/kg/min; the best indicator of cardiorespiratory or aerobic fitness.

Open-circuit indirect calorimetry (direct gas analysis) The most precise way to determine VO_{2max}, using a metabolic cart to measure the amount of oxygen consumed by the body.

Maximal exercise test Any test that requires the participant's all-out or nearly all-out effort.

Gender	Age	Fitness Category (in ml/kg/min)				
		Poor	**Fair**	**Average**	**Good**	**Excellent**
Men	<29	<24.9	25–33.9	34–43.9	44–52.9	>53
	30–39	<22.9	23–30.9	31–41.9	42–49.9	>50
	40–49	<19.9	20–26.9	27–38.9	39–44.9	>45
	50–59	<17.9	18–24.9	25–37.9	38–42.9	>43
	60–69	<15.9	16–22.9	23–35.9	36–40.9	>41
Women	<29	<23.9	24–30.9	31–38.9	39–48.9	>49
	30–39	<19.9	20–27.9	28–36.9	37–44.9	>45
	40–49	<16.9	17–24.9	25–34.9	35–41.9	>42
	50–59	<14.9	15–21.9	22–33.9	34–39.9	>40
	60–69	<12.9	13–20.9	21–32.9	33–36.9	>37

☐ Health fitness standard   ☐ High physical fitness standard

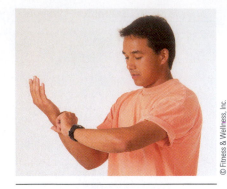

Pulse taken at radial artery.

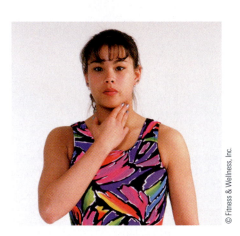

Pulse taken at carotid artery.

you should cool down by walking slowly or jogging another 3 to 5 minutes. You should not sit or lie down after the test. If any unusual symptoms arise during the run, the test should be terminated immediately, and you should cool down through slow jogging or walking. You may retake the test following 6 weeks of aerobic training.

Table 6.1 can be consulted to find the estimated VO_{2max}. The corresponding fitness categories based on VO_{2max} are found in Table 6.2. You can record the results of your 1.5-Mile Run test in the fitness profile in Assessment 6.2.

1.0-MILE WALK TEST[14]

For the walking test, either a 440-yard track (four laps to a mile) or a premeasured 1.0-mile course can be used. A stopwatch is required to determine total walking time and exercise heart rate. Prior to the walk, you will have to know your body weight in pounds.

You should walk the 1.0-mile course at a brisk pace in such a way that your exercise heart rate at the end of the test is above 120 beats per minute. At the end of the 1.0-Mile Walk, walking time is checked and the pulse is counted immediately for 10 seconds.

You can take your pulse on the wrist by placing two fingers over the radial artery (inside of the wrist near the base of the thumb) or over the carotid artery (in the neck just below the jaw next to the voice box). Next, the 10-second pulse count is multiplied by 6 to obtain the exercise heart rate in beats per minute (bpm).

Now the walking time is converted from minutes and seconds to whole-minute units. Because each minute has 60 seconds, the seconds are divided by 60 to obtain the fraction of a minute. For instance, a walking time of 12 minutes and 15 seconds equals 12 + (15 ÷ 60), or 12.25 minutes.

To obtain the estimated VO_{2max} in ml/kg/min for the 1.0-Mile Walk test, plug your values into the following equation:

$$VO_{2max} = 88.768 - (0.0957 \times W) + (8.892 \times G) - (1.4537 \times T) - (0.1194 \times HR)$$

Where:

W	=	weight in pounds
G	=	gender (use 0 for women and 1 for men)
T	=	total time for the mile walk (in minutes)
HR	=	exercise heart rate in beats per minute at the end of the mile walk

For example, a woman who weighs 140 pounds completed the mile walk in 14 minutes and 39 seconds with an exercise heart rate of 148 beats per minute. The estimated VO_{2max} is:

W	=	140 lbs
G	=	0 (female gender = 0)
T	=	14:39 = 14 + (39 ÷ 60) = 14.65 min
HR	=	148 bpm
VO_{2max}	=	88.768 − (0.0957 × 140) + (8.892 × 0) − (1.4537 × 14.65) − (0.1194 × 148)
VO_{2max}	=	36.4 ml/kg/min

As with the 1.5-Mile Run test, the fitness categories based on VO_{2max} are found in Table 6.2. The cardiorespiratory fitness test results can be recorded in Assessment 6.2.

Assessment of Muscular Strength and Endurance

Strength, a basic component of fitness and wellness, is crucial for optimal performance in activities of daily living, such as walking, running, lifting and carrying objects, doing housework, and even enjoying recreational activities. Strength also is of great value in improving posture, personal appearance, and self-image; in developing sports skills; and in meeting certain emergencies in life.

From a health standpoint, strength helps to maintain muscle tissue and a higher resting metabolism (see Chapter 10), facilitates weight loss and weight control, decreases the risk for injury, helps to prevent and correct chronic low-back pain, and is thought to help with child-bearing and delivery.

An important adaptation to strength training is that, with time, the heart rate and blood pressure response to lifting a heavy resistance decreases. This adaptation reduces demands on the cardiovascular system when performing activities such as carrying a child, the groceries, or a suitcase.

Adequate strength is especially important in advanced age, to maintain functional independent living. Many older adults lack sufficient strength to move about and perform simple tasks of daily living, such as being able to stand up or get out of bed without help, walk up a flight of stairs, or lift and carry small objects. Additional information on strength training and older adults is presented in Chapter 7.

STRENGTH VERSUS ENDURANCE

Although muscular strength and muscular endurance are interrelated, these components are different. Strength tests and training programs have been designed to measure and develop absolute muscular strength, muscular endurance, or a combination of both.

Muscular endurance (also referred to as localized muscular endurance) is the ability of a muscle to exert submaximal force repeatedly over a period of time. It depends to a large extent on muscular strength. Weak muscles cannot repeat an action several times or sustain it for a long time.

Muscular strength is the ability to exert maximum force against resistance. It usually is determined by the maximal amount of resistance—**one repetition maximum**, or **1 RM**, that an individual is able to lift in a single effort. This assessment gives a good measure of absolute strength, but it does require a considerable amount of time, because the 1 RM is determined through trial and error.

For example, the strength of the chest muscles is frequently measured with the bench press exercise. If the individual has not trained with weights, he or she may try 100 pounds and lift this resistance quite easily. Then 50 pounds are added, but the person fails to lift the resistance. The resistance then is decreased by 10 or 20 pounds, and finally, after several trials, the 1 RM is established. Fatigue also becomes a factor, because by the time the 1 RM is established, several maximal, or near-maximal attempts have been performed already.

Muscular endurance is commonly determined by the number of repetitions an individual can perform against a submaximal resistance, such as lifting 80 pounds 20 times. It also can be determined by the length of time a given contraction is sustained—for example, how long a chin-up can be maintained.

MUSCULAR ENDURANCE TEST

Muscular strength and endurance both are required to enjoy a good quality of life. Because muscular endurance depends to a large extent on muscular strength, a muscular endurance test has been selected to determine strength.

Three exercises, assessing the endurance of the upper body, lower body, and abdominal muscle groups, have been selected for the muscular endurance test. A stopwatch, a metronome, a bench or gymnasium bleacher 16¼ inches high, and a partner are needed to administer the following tests: Bench-Jump, Modified-Dip (men) or Modified Push-Up (women), and Bent-Leg Curl-Up (or abdominal crunch for individuals prone to low-back pain).

Bench-Jump The Bench-Jump requires a bench or gymnasium bleacher 16¼ inches high. Attempt to jump onto and off the bench as many times as possible in 1 minute. If you cannot jump the full minute, step up and down. A repetition is counted each time both feet return to the floor.

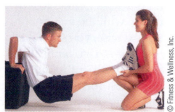

Bench-Jump.

Modified Dip The Modified Dip is an upper-body exercise performed by men only. Using the same bench or gymnasium bleacher 16¼ inches high, place your hands on the bench with fingers pointing forward. Have a partner hold your feet in front of you. Your hips should be bent at approximately 90°. Lower your body by flexing your elbows until the elbows are bent at a 90° angle, and then return to the starting position. A repetition does not count if your elbows do not reach 90°. Perform the repetitions to a two-step cadence (down–up),

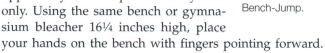

Modified Dip.

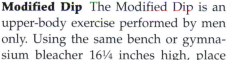

Muscular endurance The ability of a muscle to exert sub-maximal force repeatedly over a period of time.

Muscular strength The ability to exert maximum force against resistance.

One repetition maximum (1 RM) The maximal amount of resistance (weight) that an individual is able to lift in a single effort.

regulated with a metronome set at 56 beats per minute. Perform as many continuous repetitions as possible. The test is terminated if you fail to follow the metronome cadence.

Modified Push-Up Women are to perform the Modified Push-Up instead of the Modified Dip test. Lie face-down on the floor, bend your knees (raise feet up in the air), and place your hands on the floor by your shoulders with your fingers pointing forward. The lower body will be supported at the knees (rather than the feet) throughout the test. The objective is to raise and lower the upper body by fully extending and flexing the elbows. The chest must touch the floor on each repetition.

As with the Modified Dip test, the repetitions are performed to a two-step cadence (up–down) regulated with a metronome set at 56 beats per minute. Perform as many continuous repetitions as possible. The test is stopped when you cannot do any more repetitions or you no longer can follow the metronome cadence.

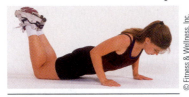
Modified Push-Up.

Bent-Leg Curl-Up In the Bent-Let Curl-Up, lie face-up on the floor and bend both legs at the knees at about 100° (see photo). Your feet should be on the floor, and you must hold them in place yourself throughout the test. Cross your arms in front of your chest, each hand on the opposite shoulder. Now raise your head off the floor, placing the chin against your chest. This is the starting and finishing position for each curl-up. The back of the head may not come in contact with the floor, the hands cannot be removed from the shoulders, nor may the feet or hips be raised off the floor at any time during the test. The test is terminated if any of these four conditions occur.

When you curl up, you must bring your upper body to an upright position before going back down. The repetitions are performed to a two-step cadence (up–down) regulated with the metronome set at 40 beats per minute. For this exercise, you should allow a brief practice period of 10 to 15 seconds to familiarize yourself with the cadence. The "up" movement is initiated with the first beat, then you must wait for the next beat to initiate the "down" movement; one repetition is accomplished every two beats of the metronome.

Count as many repetitions as you are able to perform following the proper cadence. This test also is terminated if you fail to maintain the appropriate cadence or if you accomplish 100 repetitions. Have your partner check the angle at the knees throughout the test to make sure the 100° angle is maintained as closely as possible.

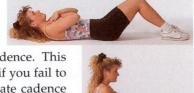
Bent-Leg Curl-Up.

Abdominal Crunch The Abdominal Crunch is difficult to perform correctly. Individuals often gain an unfair advantage by bending the elbows, shrugging the shoulders, or sliding the body during the test.[15] Test results are not valid unless the test procedure and the exercise form are monitored carefully.[16] Further, a large upper body mass and lack of spinal flexibility make it impossible or difficult for some individuals to reach the full range of motion required during the abdominal crunch.[17] This test, therefore, should be used only by individuals who, because of back pain or risk for low-back injury, cannot perform the Bent-Leg Curl-Up test.

To administer the test, tape a 3½ × 30-inch strip of cardboard onto the floor (for this test you may also use a Crunch-Ster Curl-Up Tester*). Lie face-up on the floor with your knees bent at approximately 100° and legs slightly apart (photo). Both feet should be on the floor, and you must hold them in place yourself throughout the test. Straighten your arms and place them on the floor alongside the trunk with the palms down and the fingers fully extended. The fingertips of both hands should barely touch the closest edge of the cardboard. Bring your head off the floor until the chin is 1 to 2 inches away from your chest. Your head should remain in this position during the entire test (do not move the head by flexing or extending the neck). You are now ready to begin the test.

The repetitions are performed to a two-step cadence (up–down) regulated with a metronome set at 60 beats per minute. As you curl up, slide the fingers over the cardboard until the fingertips reach the far edge (3½ inches) of the board, then return to the starting position.

Allow a brief practice period of 5 to 10 seconds to familiarize yourself with the cadence. The "up" movement is initiated with

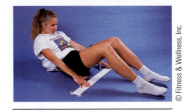
Abdominal Crunch: The fingertips of both hands should barely touch the closest edge of the cardboard.

Abdominal Crunch: As you curl up, slide the fingers over the cardboard until the fingertips reach the far edge of the board.

the first beat, and the "down" movement with the next beat. One repetition is accomplished every two beats of the metronome. Count as many repetitions as you are able to perform following the proper cadence. You may not count a repetition if the fingertips fail to reach the distant edge of the cardboard.

The test is terminated if (a) you fail to maintain the appropriate cadence, (b) your heels come off the floor, (c) your chin is not kept close to the chest, (d) you accomplish 100 repetitions, or (e) you can no longer perform the

* Available from Novel Products Figure Finder Collection, P.O. Box 408, Rockton, IL 61072-0408, (800) 624-4888.

TABLE 6.3 Percentile Ranks and Fitness Categories for Muscular Endurance Tests

Percentile Rank	MEN				WOMEN				Fitness Category
	Bench Jump	Modified Dip	Bent-Leg Curl-Up	Abdominal Crunch*	Bench Jump	Modified Push-Up	Bent-Leg Curl-Up	Abdominal Crunch*	
99	66	54	100	100	58	95	100	100	
95	63	50	81	100	54	70	100	100	Excellent
90	62	38	65	100	52	50	97	69	
80	58	32	51	66	48	41	77	49	
70	57	30	44	45	44	38	57	37	Good
60	56	27	31	38	42	33	45	34	
50	54	26	28	33	39	30	37	31	Average
40	51	23	25	29	38	28	28	27	
30	48	20	22	26	36	25	22	24	Fair
20	47	17	17	22	32	21	17	21	
10	40	11	10	18	28	18	9	15	Poor
5	34	7	3	16	26	15	4	0	

☐ High physical fitness standard   ☐ Health fitness standard

* Use this exercise only if you are unable to perform a Bent-Leg Curl-Up because of back pain or risk of lower back injury.

Abdominal crunches using Crunch-Ster Curl-Up Tester.

Photos © Fitness & Wellness, Inc.

Assessment of Muscular Flexibility

Flexibility is defined as the ability of a joint to move freely through its full range of motion. Sports medicine specialists believe that many muscular/skeletal problems and injuries, especially in adults, are related to a lack of flexibility. Improving and maintaining good range of motion in the joints throughout life enhances the quality of life.

Because flexibility is joint-specific—good flexibility in one joint does not necessarily indicate the same is true in other joints—two tests are used to obtain an indication of current flexibility levels: the Modified Sit-and-Reach and the Total Body Rotation tests. Before doing any flexibility testing, participants should warm up properly with a few stretching exercises. Assistance from another person is necessary to administer both tests.

test. Have your partner check the angle at the knees throughout the test to make sure that the 100° angle is maintained as closely as possible.

Look up the percentile rank based on the number of repetitions performed on each test and the respective strength fitness categories in Table 6.3. Record this information in Assessment 6.2.

MODIFIED SIT-AND-REACH TEST

To administer the Modified Sit-and-Reach test, you'll need an Acuflex I* flexibility tester or you may design your own equipment by placing a yardstick on top of a box 12 inches high. To perform the test, remove your shoes and sit on the floor with your hips, back, and head against a wall. Fully extend your legs with the bottom of your feet placed against the box (see photo).

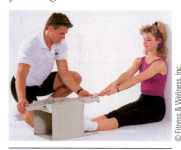

Determining starting position for Modified Sit-and-Reach test.

Position one hand on top of the other and reach forward as far as possible without letting your head or back come off the wall. The person assisting with the test then should slide the reach indicator (or yardstick) until the zero (end) point of the scale touches your fingers. He or she then must hold the indicator firmly in place throughout the rest of the test.

Your head and back now can come off the wall, and you should

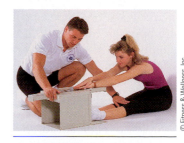

Modified Sit-and-Reach test.

© Fitness & Wellness, Inc.

* Available from Novel Products Figure Finder Collection, P.O. Box 408, Rockton, IL 61072-0408, (800) 624-4888.

Flexibility The achievable range of motion at a joint or group of joints without causing injury.

TABLE 6.4 Percentile Ranks and Fitness Categories for Modified Sit-and-Reach Test

	MEN						WOMEN				
	Age Category						Age Category				
Percentile Rank	<18	19–35	36–49	>50	Fitness Category	Percentile Rank	<18	19–35	36–49	>50	Fitness Category
99	20.8	20.1	18.9	16.2		99	22.6	21.0	19.8	17.2	
95	19.6	18.9	18.2	15.8	Excellent	95	19.5	19.3	19.2	15.7	Excellent
90	18.2	17.2	16.1	15.0		90	18.7	17.9	17.4	15.0	
80	17.8	17.0	14.6	13.3	Good	80	17.8	16.7	16.2	14.2	Good
70	16.0	15.8	13.9	12.3		70	16.5	16.2	15.2	13.6	
60	15.2	15.0	13.4	11.5	Average	60	16.0	15.8	14.5	12.3	Average
50	14.5	14.4	12.6	10.2		50	15.2	14.8	13.5	11.1	
40	14.0	13.5	11.6	9.7	Fair	40	14.5	14.5	12.8	10.1	Fair
30	13.4	13.0	10.8	9.3		30	13.7	13.7	12.2	9.2	
20	11.8	11.6	9.9	8.8	Poor	20	12.6	12.6	11.0	8.3	Poor
10	9.5	9.2	8.3	7.8		10	11.4	10.1	9.7	7.5	
05	8.4	7.9	7.0	7.2		05	9.4	8.1	8.5	3.7	
01	7.2	7.0	5.1	4.0		01	6.5	2.6	2.0	1.5	

□ High physical fitness standard   □ Health fitness standard

gradually reach forward as far as possible on the indicator, holding the final position at least 2 seconds. During the test, be sure that you keep the back of your knees flat against the floor.

Two trials are necessary, and the average of the two scores, each recorded to the nearest half inch, is used as the final test score. Flexibility fitness categories for this test are provided in Table 6.4.

TOTAL BODY ROTATION TEST

An Acuflex II* flexibility tester or a measuring scale with a sliding panel is needed to administer this test. The Acuflex II or scale is placed on the wall at shoulder height and should be adjustable to accommodate individual differences in height.

If you have to build your own scale, use two measuring tapes, each at least 30 inches long, and glue them above and below the sliding panel, centered at the 15-inch mark. Place one tape upside down so the 1-inch ends are opposite each other. If no sliding panel is available, simply tape the measuring tapes onto a wall so the panel is at your shoulder height. Also, draw a line centered on the 15-inch marks on the floor. The photos illustrate the measuring scales.

Stand sideways, an arm's length away from the wall, your feet straight ahead, slightly separated, and your toes right up to the corresponding line drawn on the floor. Hold out the arm opposite to the wall horizontally from your body, making a

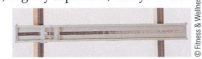
Acuflex II measuring device for the Total Body Rotation test.

fist with your hand. The Acuflex II, measuring scale, or tapes should be shoulder height at this time. Rotate your trunk, moving the extended arm backward and so it makes contact with the panel (as shown in the photo). Gradually slide the panel forward as far as possible. If no panel is available, slide your fist alongside the tapes as far as possible. Hold the final position for at least 2 seconds.

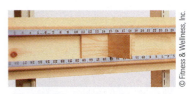
Homemade measuring device for Total Body Rotation test.

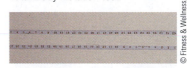
Measuring tapes for Total Body Rotation test.

Your hand should be positioned with the little finger side forward during the entire sliding movement. It is crucial to have the proper hand position. Many people attempt to open the hand or push with extended fingers or slide the panel with the knuckles, none of which is an acceptable test procedure. During the test, the knees can be slightly bent, but the feet cannot be moved; they always must point straight forward. The body must be kept as straight (vertical) as possible.

Conduct the test on either the right or the left side of the body. You are allowed two trials on the selected side. The farthest point reached,

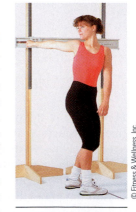
Total Body Rotation test.

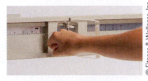
Proper hand position for the Total Body Rotation test.

* Available from Novel Products Figure Finder Collection, P.O. Box 408, Rockton, IL 61072-0408, (800) 624-4888.

TABLE 6.5 Percentile Ranks and Fitness Categories for Total Body Rotation Test

	Percentile Rank	Left Rotation				Right Rotation				Fitness Category
		<18	19–35	36–49	>50	<18	19–35	36–49	>50	
Men	99	29.1	28.0	26.6	21.0	28.2	27.8	25.2	22.2	Excellent
	95	26.6	24.8	24.5	20.0	25.5	25.6	23.8	20.7	
	90	25.0	23.6	23.0	17.7	24.3	24.1	22.5	19.3	
	80	22.0	22.0	21.2	15.5	22.7	22.3	21.0	16.3	Good
	70	20.9	20.3	20.4	14.7	21.3	20.7	18.7	15.7	
	60	19.9	19.3	18.7	13.9	19.8	19.0	17.3	14.7	Average
	50	18.6	18.0	16.7	12.7	19.0	17.2	16.3	12.3	
	40	17.0	16.8	15.3	11.7	17.3	16.3	14.7	11.5	Fair
	30	14.9	15.0	14.8	10.3	15.1	15.0	13.3	10.7	
	20	13.8	13.3	13.7	9.5	12.9	13.3	11.2	8.7	
	10	10.8	10.5	10.8	4.3	10.8	11.3	8.0	2.7	Poor
	05	8.5	8.9	8.8	0.3	8.1	8.3	5.5	0.3	
	01	3.4	1.7	5.1	0.0	6.6	2.9	2.0	0.0	
Women	99	29.3	28.6	27.1	23.0	29.6	29.4	27.1	21.7	Excellent
	95	26.8	24.8	25.3	21.4	27.6	25.3	25.9	19.7	
	90	25.5	23.0	23.4	20.5	25.8	23.0	21.3	19.0	
	80	23.8	21.5	20.2	19.1	23.7	20.8	19.6	17.9	Good
	70	21.8	20.5	18.6	17.3	22.0	19.3	17.3	16.8	
	60	20.5	19.3	17.7	16.0	20.8	18.0	16.5	15.6	Average
	50	19.5	18.0	16.4	14.8	19.5	17.3	14.6	14.0	
	40	18.5	17.2	14.8	13.7	18.3	16.0	13.1	12.8	Fair
	30	17.1	15.7	13.6	10.0	16.3	15.2	11.7	8.5	
	20	16.0	15.2	11.6	6.3	14.5	14.0	9.8	3.9	
	10	12.8	13.6	8.5	3.0	12.4	11.1	6.1	2.2	Poor
	05	11.1	7.3	6.8	0.7	10.2	8.8	4.0	1.1	
	01	8.9	5.3	4.3	0.0	8.9	3.2	2.8	0.0	

☐ High physical fitness standard   ☐ Health fitness standard

measured to the nearest half inch and held for at least 2 seconds, is recorded. The average of the two trials becomes the final test score. Flexibility fitness categories for the test are provided in Table 6.5.

After obtaining your flexibility scores, record your percentile ranks and flexibility fitness categories in the fitness profile provided in Assessment 6.2.

Exercise Prescription

Upon completing the health-related fitness assessment, Chapter 7 will help you learn how to develop and implement your own exercise programs for cardiorespiratory endurance, muscular strength, and muscular flexibility. In Chapter 9 you also will learn how to assess your body composition (the fourth component of health-related fitness) and compute your recommended body weight based on your current percent body fat. Guidelines for a weight management program are provided in Chapter 10.

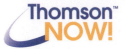

Don't forget to check out the wealth of resources on the ThomsonNOW website at **www.thomsonedu.com/ ThomsonNOW** that will:

- Coach you through identifying target goals for behavior change and monitoring your personal change plan throughout the semester
- Help you evaluate your knowledge of the material
- Allow you to take an exam-prep quiz
- Provide a Personalized Learning Plan targeting resources that address areas you should study.

WEB ACTIVITIES

American Council of Exercise Cardiovascular Fitness Facts This site features information about a variety of cardiovascular forms of exercise, including walking, running, jumping rope, swimming, spinning, cross-training, interval training, and others.

http://www.acefitness.org/fitfacts

Flexibility Exercises and Training Articles Use this archive of flexibility exercises and flexibility training pages and articles to improve your speed, strength, and stamina!

http://www.pponline.co.uk/encyc/flexibility-exercises.htm

Aerobics and Fitness Association of America This interactive site features "Exercise Gets Personal,™" in which you can create a customized exercise program that compiles activities you select, geared to your current level of fitness activity. Exercises include aerobics, muscular conditioning, and flexibility with descriptions and precautions for each activity.

http://www.afaa.com

InfoTrac®

You can find additional readings related to wellness via InfoTrac® College Edition, an online library of more than 900 journals and publications. Follow the instructions for accessing InfoTrac® that came packaged with your textbook, then search for articles using a key word search.

Suggested Reading Check "Health benefits of exercise," *JAAPA —Journal of the American Academy of Physicians Assistants,* Feb 2005 v18 i2 p30.

1. List five proven benefits of exercise.
2. What are some examples of moderate intensity activities?
3. Describe ways to get started exercising.

Web Activity

Shape Up America

http://www.shapeup.org

Sponsor Former U.S. Surgeon General Dr. C. Everett Koop in partnership with industry and non-profit organizations.

Description This interactive site will provide you with an excellent assessment of your level of physical fitness. It offers a battery of physical fitness assessments, including activity level, strength, flexibility, and an aerobic fitness test. You get started by entering your weight, height, age, and gender, and then taking a quick screen test to assess your physical readiness for physical activity. Your final results in each of these areas will be based on your personal data.

Available Activities This site contains five different self-assessments, each designed to provide you with reliable fitness and nutrition information. The interactive activities include:

1. PAR-Q test
2. Activity Level Assessment to determine whether your daily level of activity is Sedentary, Light, Moderate, Heavy, or Very Heavy
3. Flexibility Test to assess your range of movement
4. Muscular Strength and Endurance Test to assess the strength of the muscles in your upper body
5. Two tests for aerobic fitness

Web Work

1. From the home page, click on "Fitness Center" link.
2. Then click on the "Assessment" link.
3. Click on the "Take the PAR-Q Test" link to begin the self-assessment questionnaire to measure your readiness for physical activity.
4. Click on the radio button "Yes" or "No" that corresponds to the answers to each of the seven questions. Once completed, click on the "Continue" button.
5. The assessment will provide you with results concerning your ability to participate in physical activity. Then click on the "Return to the Assessment Main Page" link to continue with the other four assessments listed in the "Available Activities" above.

Helpful Hints

The information gathered from the results on these assessment tests will be used in other parts of the Fitness Center on this Web site. Therefore, you must complete the PAR-Q Test first.

For additional Web activities, links, and suggested readings, visit our Health, Fitness, and Wellness Resource Center at http://health.wadsworth.com.

1. National Institutes of Health, Consensus Development Conference Statement, "Physical Activity and Cardiovascular Health," Washington, DC, December 18–20, 1995.

2. See Note 1.

3. U.S. Department of Health and Human Services, *Physical Activity and Health: A Report of the Surgeon General* (Atlanta: Centers for Disease Control and Prevention, National Center for Chronic Disease Prevention and Health Promotion, 1996).

4. American College of Sports Medicine, *ACSM's Guidelines for Exercise Testing and Prescription* (Baltimore: Williams & Wilkins, 2006).

5. R. S. Paffenbarger, Jr., R. T. Hyde, A. L. Wing, and C. H. Steinmetz, "A Natural History of Athleticism and Cardiovascular Health," *Journal of the American Medical Association* 252 (1984): 491–495.

6. S. N. Blair, H. W. Kohl III, R. S. Paffenbarger, Jr., D. G. Clark, K. H. Cooper, and L. W. Gibbons, "Physical Fitness and All-Cause Mortality: A Prospective Study of Healthy Men and Women," *Journal of the American Medical Association* 262 (1989): 2395–2401.

7. S. N. Blair, H. W. Kohl III, C. E. Barlow, R. S. Paffenbarger, Jr., L. W. Gibbons, and C. A. Macera, "Changes in Physical Fitness and All-Cause Mortality: A Prospective Study of Healthy and Unhealthy Men," *Journal of the American Medical Association* 273 (1995): 1193–1198.

8. I. Lee, C. Hsieh, and R. S. Paffenbarger, Jr., "Exercise Intensity and Longevity in Men: The Harvard Alumni Health Study," *Journal of the American Medical Association* 273 (1995): 1179–1184.

9. "Wellness Facts," *University of California at Berkeley Wellness Letter* (Palm Coast, FL: The Editors, April 1995).

10. See Note 4.

11. See Note 4.

12. R. B. O'Hara et al., "Increased Volume Resistance Training: Effects upon Predicted Aerobic Fitness in a Select Group of Air Force Men," *ACSM's Health and Fitness Journal* 8, no. 4 (2004): 16–25.

13. See Note 4.

14. F. A. Dolgener, L. D. Hensley, J. J. Marsh, and J. K. Fjelstul, "Validation of the Rockport Fitness Walking Test in College Males and Females," *Research Quarterly for Exercise and Sport* 65 (1994): 152–158.

15. R. A. Faulkner, E. J. Sprigings, A. McQuarrie, and R. D. Bell, "A Partial Curl-Up Protocol for Adults Based on Analysis of Two Procedures," *Canadian Journal of Sports Science* 14 (1989): 135–141; P. A. Macfarlane, "Out with the Sit-Up, in with the Curl-Up!" *Journal of Physical Education, Recreation, and Dance* 64 (1993): 62–66; D. Knudson and D. Johnston, "Validity and Reliability of a Bench Trunk-Curl-Up Test of Abdominal Endurance," *Journal of Strength and Conditioning Research* 9 (1995): 165–169.

16. R. Kjorstad. "Validity of Two Field Tests of Abdominal Strength and Muscular Endurance," unpublished master's thesis, Boise State University, 1997; G. L. Hall, R. K. Hetzler, D. Perrin, and A. Weltman, "Relationship of Timed Sit-Up Tests to Isokinetic Abdominal Strength," *Research Quarterly for Exercise and Sport* 63 (1992): 80–84.

17. L. D. Robertson and H. Magnusdottir, "Evaluation of Criteria Associated with Abdominal Fitness Testing," *Research Quarterly for Exercise and Sport* 58 (1987): 355—359; see also Macfarlane, Note 15.

Assess Your Behavior

1. Do you make a conscious effort to incorporate as much physical activity as possible as you go though routine activities of daily living?

2. Are you aware of your current cardiorespiratory endurance, muscular strength, and muscular flexibility goals?

3. Are your fitness goals based on health-related or physical fitness standards?

Evaluate how well you understand the concepts presented in this chapter by answering the following questions.

1. Bodily movement produced by skeletal muscles is called
   a. physical activity.
   b. kinesiology.
   c. exercise.
   d. aerobic exercise.
   e. muscle strength.

2. Among the benefits of regular physical activity and exercise are significantly reduced risks for developing or dying from
   a. heart disease.
   b. type 2 diabetes.
   c. colon and breast cancers.
   d. osteoporotic fractures.
   e. All are correct choices.

3. Research on the effects of fitness on mortality indicates that the largest drop in premature mortality is seen between
   a. the average and excellent fitness groups.
   b. the least fit and moderately fit groups.
   c. the good and high fitness groups.
   d. the moderately fit and good fitness groups.
   e. the drop is similar between all fitness groups.

4. Individuals who show little or no improvement following a regular exercise training program are referred to as
   a. sedentary.
   b. unfit.
   c. nonresponders.
   d. untrainable.
   e. None of the above.

5. Cardiorespiratory endurance is determined by
   a. the amount of oxygen the body is able to utilize per minute of physical activity.
   b. the length of time it takes the heart rate to return to 120 bpm following the 1.5-Mile Run test.
   c. the difference between the maximal heart rate and the resting heart rate.
   d. the product of the heart rate and blood pressure at rest versus exercise.
   e. the time it takes a person to reach a heart rate between 120 and 170 bpm during the 1.0-Mile Walk test.

6. An "excellent" cardiorespiratory fitness rating in ml/kg/min for young male adults is about
   a. 10.
   b. 20.
   c. 30.
   d. 40
   e. 50.

7. The ability of a muscle to exert submaximal force repeatedly over time is known as
   a. muscular strength.
   b. plyometric training.
   c. muscular endurance.
   d. isokinetic training.
   e. isometric training.

8. A 70 percentile rank places an individual in the _____ fitness category.
   a. excellent
   b. good
   c. average
   d. fair
   e. poor

9. Muscular flexibility is defined as
   a. the capacity of joints and muscles to work in a synchronized manner.
   b. the achievable range of motion at a joint or group of joints without causing injury.
   c. the capability of muscles to stretch beyond their normal resting length without injury to the muscles.
   d. the capacity of muscles to return to their proper length following the application of a stretching force.
   e. the limitations placed on muscles as the joints move through their normal planes.

10. During the starting position of the Modified Sit-and-Reach test
    a. the hips, back, and head are placed against a wall.
    b. you measure the distance from the hips to the feet.
    c. you make a fist with the hands.
    d. you stretch forward as far as possible over the reach indicator.
    e. All of the above are correct choices.

Correct answers can be found on page 369.

Physical Activity Readiness Questionnaire (PAR-Q)
(A Questionnaire for People Age 15 to 69)

Name: _____   Date: _____   Grade: _____

Instructor: _____   Course: _____   Section: _____

Regular physical activity is fun and healthy, and increasingly more people are starting to become more active every day. Being more active is very safe for most people. However, some people should check with their doctor before they start becoming much more physically active.

If you are planning to become much more physically active than you are now, start by answering the seven questions in the box below. If you are between the ages of 15 and 69, the PAR-Q will tell you if you should check with your doctor before you start. If you are over 69 years of age, and you are not used to being very active, check with your doctor.

Common sense is your best guide when you answer these questions. Please read the questions carefully and answer each one honestly: check YES or NO.

YES	NO	
☐	☐	1. Has your doctor ever said that you have a heart condition <u>and</u> that you should only do physical activity recommended by a doctor?
☐	☐	2. Do you feel pain in your chest when you do physical activity?
☐	☐	3. In the past month, have you had chest pain when you were not doing physical activity?
☐	☐	4. Do you lose your balance because of dizziness or do you ever lose consciousness?
☐	☐	5. Do you have a bone or joint problem (for example, back, knee or hip) that could be made worse by a change in your physical activity?
☐	☐	6. Is your doctor currently prescribing drugs (for example, water pills) for your blood pressure or heart condition?
☐	☐	7. Do you know of <u>any other reason</u> why you should not do physical activity?

If you answered

YES to one or more questions

Talk with your doctor by phone or in person BEFORE you start becoming much more physically active or BEFORE you have a fitness appraisal. Tell your doctor about the PAR-Q and which questions you answered YES.

- You may be able to do any activity you want—as long as you start slowly and build up gradually. Or, you may need to restrict your activities to those which are safe for you. Talk with your doctor about the kinds of activities you wish to participate in and follow his/her advice.
- Find out which community programs are safe and helpful for you.

NO to all questions

If you answered NO honestly to <u>all</u> PAR-Q questions, you can be reasonably sure that you can:

- start becoming much more physically active—begin slowly and build up gradually. This is the safest and easiest way to go.
- take part in a fitness appraisal—this is an excellent way to determine your basic fitness so that you can plan the best way for you to live actively. It is also highly recommended that you have your blood pressure evaluated. If your reading is over 144/94, talk with your doctor before you start becoming much more physically active.

DELAY BECOMING MUCH MORE ACTIVE:

- if you are not feeling well because of a temporary illness such as a cold or a fever—wait until you feel better; or
- if you are or may be pregnant—talk to your doctor before you start becoming more active.

PLEASE NOTE: If your health changes so that you then answer YES to any of the above questions, tell your fitness or health professional. Ask whether you should change your physical activity plan.

<u>Informed Use of the PAR-Q</u>: The Canadian Society for Exercise Physiology, Health Canada, and their agents assume no liability for persons who undertake physical activity, and if in doubt after completing this questionnaire, consult your doctor prior to physical activity.

No changes permitted. You are encouraged to copy the PAR-Q but only if you use the entire form.

NOTE: If the PAR-Q is being given to a person before he or she participates in a physical activity program or a fitness appraisal, this section may be used for legal or administrative purposes.

"I have read, understood and completed this questionnaire. Any questions I had were answered to my full satisfaction."

Name _____

Signature _____   Date _____

Signature of Parent _____   Witness _____
or Guardian (for participants under the age of majority)

© Canadian Society for Exercise Physiology

Supported by: [🍁] Health Santé
Canada Canada

Note: This physical activity clearance is valid for a maximum of 12 months from the date it is completed and becomes invalid if your condition changes so that you would answer YES to any of the seven questions.

Source: Physical Activity Readiness Questionnaire (PAR-Q) © 2002. Reprinted with permission from the Canadian Society for Exercise Physiology. http://www.csep.ca/forms.asp.

Exercise Participation

Do you feel that it is safe for you to proceed with an exercise program? Explain any concerns or limitations that you may have regarding your safe participation in a comprehensive exercise program (which will include exercises to improve cardiorespiratory endurance, muscular strength and endurance, and muscular flexibility).

_____
_____
_____
_____
_____
_____
_____
_____
_____

In a few words, describe your previous experiences with sports participation, whether you have taken part in a structured exercise program, and express your own feelings about exercise participation.

_____
_____
_____
_____
_____
_____
_____
_____
_____
_____
_____
_____
_____
_____
_____
_____
_____

Physical Fitness Profile

Name: _____ **Date:** _____ **Grade:** _____

Instructor: _____ **Course:** _____ **Section:** _____

Necessary Lab Equipment:

Pre-measured 1.5-mile or 1.0-mile course, 16¼ inch bench, stopwatch, metronome, equipment for abdominal crunches, modified sit-and-reach box (Acuflex I), and total body rotation scale (Acuflex II).

Objective:

To assess your current level of cardiorespiratory endurance, muscular strength endurance, and muscular flexibility fitness.

Lab Preparation:

Wear appropriate exercise clothing, including a good pair of athletic (jogging/walking) shoes. Avoid strenuous physical activity for 36 hours prior to this lab.

PRE-TEST

Fitness Component	Test Data	Test Results	Fitness Category
Cardiorespiratory Endurance	Time	VO_{2max}	
1.5-Mile Run	_____ : _____	_____ . _____	
	Time		
1.0-Mile Walk	_____ : _____		
	Heart Rate	VO_{2max}	
	_____	_____ . _____	
Muscular Strength / Endurance	Reps	Percentile	
Bench Jumps			
Chair Dips or Modified Push-Ups			
Bent-Leg Curl-Ups or Abdominal Crunches			
Muscular Flexibility	Inches	Percentile	
Modified Sit-and-Reach			
Body Rotation (R/L)			

Number of Daily Steps
(Use an average of four days)

POST-TEST

Fitness Component	Test Data		Test Results		Fitness Category
Cardiovascular Endurance	Time		VO$_{2max}$		
1.5-Mile Run	☐	: ☐	☐	. ☐	☐
	Time				
1.0-Mile Walk	☐	: ☐			
	Heart Rate		VO$_{2max}$		
	☐		☐	. ☐	☐
Muscular Strength / Endurance	Reps		Percentile		
Bench Jumps	☐		☐		☐
Chair Dips / Modified Push-Ups	☐		☐		☐
Bent-Leg Curl-Ups or Abdominal Crunches	☐		☐		☐
Muscular Flexibility	Inches		Percentile		
Modified Sit-and-Reach	☐		☐		☐
Body Rotation (R/L)	☐		☐		☐
Number of Daily Steps (Use an average of four days)			☐ 🚶		☐

What I Learned and Where Do I Go From Here

Based on the results of your cardiorespiratory endurance test(s), muscular strength endurance, and muscular flexibility tests, interpret how these results relate to your present level of daily physical activity or exercise habits.

_____
_____
_____
_____

Please indicate the fitness components that you would like to improve, the fitness category that you wish to achieve by the end of the term, and what you intend to do to achieve your goal(s).

_____
_____
_____
_____

Wellness: Guidelines for a Healthy Lifestyle

7

CHAPTER

Exercise Prescription for Wellness

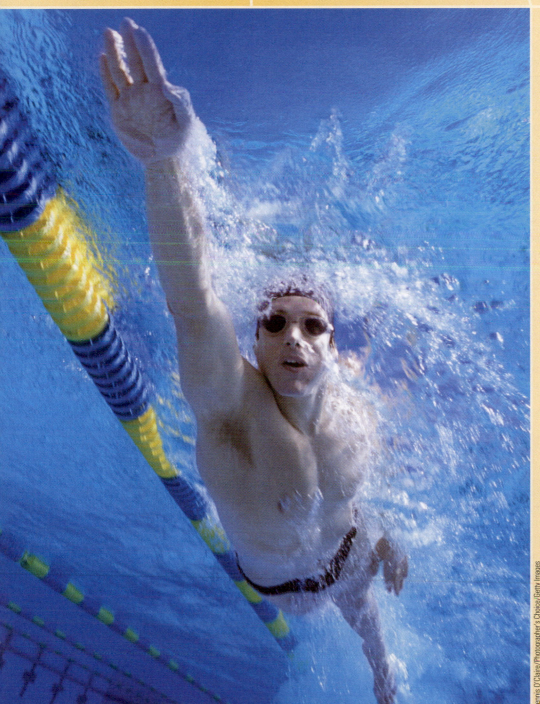

© Dennis O'Claire/Photographer's Choice/Getty Images

OBJECTIVES

Explain the benefits of an active lifestyle.

Describe how to use a pedometer to monitor daily activity.

Differentiate aerobic and anaerobic exercise.

Learn the guidelines for cardio-respiratory, strength, and flexibility exercise prescription.

Explain the association between physical activity and diabetes.

Describe the relationship between strength and metabolism.

Define and explain progressive resistance training.

Describe some causes, preventive measures, and treatment for low-back pain.

Become familiar with concepts for preventing and treating common exercise injuries.

Define and explain exercise intolerance.

Explain the transtheoretical model for behavior change.

Explain how to use behavior modification principles to promote adherence to exercise and change behavior.

The role of fitness in health is illustrated by George Snell from Sandy, Utah. At age 45, Snell weighed approximately 400 pounds, his blood pressure was 220/180, he was blind because of undiagnosed diabetes, and his blood glucose level was 487. Determined to do something about his physical and medical condition, Snell started a weight management program along with a walking/jogging program.

After about 8 months on this program, Snell had lost almost 200 pounds, his eyesight had returned, his glucose level was down to 67, and he was taken off medication. Two months later—less than 10 months after initiating his personal exercise program—he completed his first marathon, a running course of 26.2 miles.

No drug in current or prospective use holds as much promise for sustained health as a lifetime program of physical exercise.[1] Results of epidemiological research have established that a physically active lifestyle and participation in a lifetime exercise program greatly contribute to good health (see Chapter 6). Nonetheless, many individuals who are active and exercise regularly find that, when they take a battery of fitness tests, they are not as conditioned as they thought they were. Although these individuals may be exercising regularly, they most likely are not following the basic principles for exercise prescription and, therefore, are not reaping the full benefits of their activity and exercise programs.

A key to exercise prescription is that all programs must be individualized to obtain optimal results. Our bodies are not all alike, and fitness levels and needs vary among individuals. The information in this chapter provides the necessary guidelines to write a personalized cardiorespiratory endurance, muscular strength or endurance, and muscular flexibility exercise program that promotes and maintains good health and fitness. Information on weight control to achieve and maintain recommended body weight and body composition, a key component of good physical fitness, is presented in Chapters 9 and 10.

Lifestyle and Cardiorespiratory Health

Physical activity is no longer a natural part of our existence. If we need to go to a store only a couple of blocks away, most people drive their cars and then spend a couple of minutes driving around the parking lot to find a spot 10 yards closer to the store's entrance. Often, we do not even have to carry out the groceries; someone from the store offers to take them out and place them in our vehicle. During a visit to a multilevel shopping mall, almost everyone chooses to ride the escalators instead of taking the stairs—if stairs are accessible at all. Automobiles, elevators, escalators, cell phones, intercoms, remote controls, and electric garage door openers—all are modern-day commodities that minimize body movement and effort.

One of the most detrimental effects of modern-day technology has been an increase in chronic conditions related to this lack of physical activity. Some examples of these hypokinetic diseases ("hypo" means low or little, and "kinetic" denotes motion) are hypertension, heart disease, chronic low-back pain, and obesity.

Lack of adequate physical activity is a reality of modern life that most people no longer can avoid, but to enjoy modern-day commodities and still expect to live life to its fullest, a personalized lifetime exercise program must become part of daily living. Based on estimates in the 1996 Report of the Surgeon General, more than 60 percent of adults do not achieve the recommended amount of physical activity, and 25 percent are not physically active at all.[2]

Monitoring Daily Physical Activity

Almost half of all adults in the United States do not achieve the recommended daily amount of physical activity. The first step to become more active is to carefully monitor daily physical activity. An excellent tool to monitor daily physical activity is through the use of a pedometer, a small mechanical device that senses vertical body motion and is used to count footsteps. Wearing a pedometer throughout the day allows a person to determine the total steps taken in a day. Some pedometer brands also record distance, calories burned, speeds, and actual time of activity each day, but these vary in accuracy.

Pedometers tend to lose accuracy at very slow walking speeds (30 minutes per mile or less) because the vertical movement of the hip is too small to trigger the spring-mounted lever arm inside the pedometer to properly record the steps taken. The most accurate pedometer brands are Yamax, Kenz, New Lifestyles, and Walk4Life. To test the accuracy of a pedometer, follow these steps:

1. Clip the pedometer on the waist directly above the knee cap.
2. Reset the pedometer to zero
3. Carefully close the pedometer
4. Walk exactly 50 steps at your normal pace
5. Carefully open the pedometer, and look at the number of steps recorded. A reading within 10 percent of the actual steps taken (45 to 55 steps) is acceptable.

As you monitor daily physical activity with a pedometer, the general recommendation for adults is 10,000 steps per day. Table 1.2 in Chapter 1 (page 15) provides specific activity ratings based on the number of daily steps taken.

All daily steps count, but to meet national physical activity recommendations, some of your steps should occur in a timeframe of at least 10 minutes so you will accumulate 30 minutes of moderate-intensity physical activity in at least three 10-minute activity sessions most days of the week. A 10-minute brisk walk is approximately 1,300 steps (a distance of about a 1,200 yards). A brisk 1-mile walk

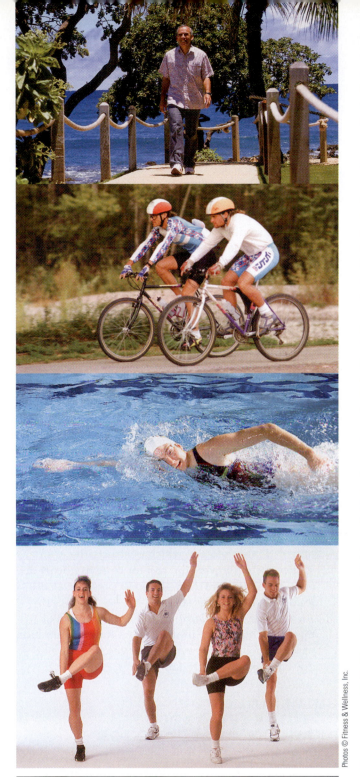

Aerobic exercise requires oxygen to supply the energy needed to carry out the activity.

Photos © Fitness & Wellness, Inc.

you do daily. On this log record the time of day, type and duration of the activity/exercise, and, if possible, steps taken while engaged in the activity. The results will provide an indication of how active you are and will serve to monitor changes in the months and years ahead.

Cardiorespiratory Endurance

Cardiorespiratory endurance refers to the body's ability to provide adequate amounts of oxygen to the cells to meet the demands of prolonged physical activity. Because the body uses oxygen to convert food (carbohydrates and fats) into energy, a greater capacity to deliver and utilize oxygen (oxygen uptake or VO_2) indicates a more efficient cardiorespiratory system.

Cardiorespiratory endurance activities also are referred to as aerobic activities. The word **aerobic** means "with oxygen." Whenever an activity requires oxygen to produce energy, it is considered an aerobic activity. Examples of cardiorespiratory or aerobic exercise are walking, jogging, swimming, cycling, cross-country skiing, water aerobics, rope skipping, and aerobic workouts.

Anaerobic activities, on the other hand, are carried out "without oxygen." The intensity of anaerobic exercise is so high that oxygen is not utilized to produce energy. Because energy production is limited without oxygen, these activities can be carried out for only 2 to 3 minutes. The higher the intensity of the activity, the shorter the duration of the anaerobic activity.

Good examples of anaerobic activities are the 100-, 200-, and 400-meter dash in track and field, the 100-meter in swimming, gymnastics routines, and weight training. Anaerobic activities will not contribute much to development of the cardiorespiratory system. Only aerobic activities will enhance cardiorespiratory endurance.

SIGNIFICANCE OF CARDIORESPIRATORY ENDURANCE

Aerobic exercise improves health and quality of life and is especially important in preventing diseases of the cardiovascular system. A poorly conditioned heart that has to pump more often just to keep a person alive is subject to more wear and tear than a well-conditioned heart. In situations that place strenuous demands on the heart, such as doing yardwork, lifting heavy objects or weights, or running to catch a train, the unconditioned heart may not be able to sustain the strain. In addition, regular participation in cardiorespiratory endurance activities helps achieve

(1,770 yards) is about 2,000 steps. To help users accomplish this amount of activity, new pedometer brands have an "aerobic steps" function that records steps taken in excess of 60 steps per minute over 10 minutes.

The first practical application you can perform in this course is to determine your current level of daily activity. You may want to use the log provided in Assessment 7.1 to help you keep a 4-day log of all physical activities that

> **Aerobic** Refers to an activity that requires oxygen to produce the necessary energy (ATP) to carry out the activity.
>
> **Anaerobic** Activity that does not require oxygen to produce the necessary energy (ATP) to carry out the activity.

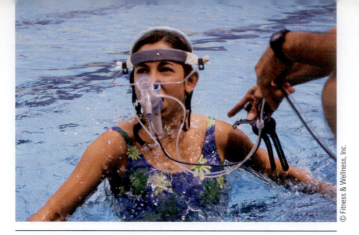

Physical work capacity, measured through an oxygen uptake test, increases with aerobic training.

and maintain recommended body weight, the fourth component of health-related physical fitness.

Everyone who initiates a cardiorespiratory or aerobic exercise program can expect a number of physiological adaptations from training. Among the most significant adaptations are:

1. *A higher maximal oxygen uptake (VO_{2max}).* The amount of oxygen the body is able to use during physical activity increases significantly, allowing the individual to exercise longer and at a higher rate before becoming fatigued.

    Small increases in VO_{2max} can be observed in as few as 2 to 3 weeks of aerobic training. Depending on the initial fitness level, VO_{2max} may rise as much as 30 percent, although higher increases have been reported in people with very low initial levels of fitness.

2. *An increase in the oxygen-carrying capacity of the blood.* As a result of training, the red blood cell count goes up. Red blood cells contain hemoglobin, which transports oxygen in the blood.

3. *A decrease in resting heart rate and an increase in cardiac muscle strength.* During resting conditions, the heart ejects between 5 and 6 liters of blood per minute (a liter is slightly larger than a quart). This amount of blood, also referred to as **cardiac output**, meets the energy demands in the resting state.

    Like any other muscle, the heart responds to training by gaining strength and size. As the heart gets stronger, the muscle can produce a more forceful contraction. A stronger contraction causes a greater ejection of blood with each beat (it increases the stroke volume), yielding a lower heart rate. This reduction in heart rate also allows the heart to rest longer between beats.

    The **resting heart rate** frequently decreases 10 to 20 beats per minute (bpm) after only 6 to 8 weeks of training. A reduction of 20 bpm saves the heart about 10,483,200 beats per year. The average heart beats between 70 and 80 bpm. Resting heart rates in highly trained athletes frequently are around 45 bpm.

4. *A lower heart rate at given workloads.* When compared with untrained individuals, a trained person has a lower heart rate response to a given task, because of higher efficiency of the cardiorespiratory system. Following several weeks of training, the heart's response to a given workload (let's say, a 10-minute mile) is a much lower heart rate compared to the response when training first started.

5. *An increase in the number and size of the mitochondria.* All energy necessary for cell function is produced in the mitochondria. As their size and number increase, so does the potential to produce energy for muscular work.

6. *An increase in the number of functional capillaries.* These smaller vessels allow for the exchange of oxygen and carbon dioxide between the blood and the cells. As more vessels open up, more gas exchange can take place, thereby decreasing the onset of fatigue during prolonged exercise. This increase in capillaries also speeds up the rate at which waste products of cell metabolism can be removed. Increased capillarization also is seen in the heart, which enhances the oxygen delivery capacity to the heart muscle itself.

7. *Faster recovery time.* Trained individuals have a faster recovery time following exercise. A fit system is able to more rapidly restore any internal equilibrium disrupted during exercise.

8. *A decrease in blood pressure and blood lipids.* A regular aerobic exercise program will result in lower blood pressure and reduced cholesterol and triglycerides (these two fats are linked to the formation of the atherosclerotic plaque, which obstructs the arteries). This reduction lowers the risk for coronary heart disease (see Chapter 11). High blood pressure also is a leading risk factor for strokes.

9. *An increase in fat-burning enzymes.* Fat is lost primarily by burning it in muscle. As the concentration of these enzymes increases with aerobic training, so does the ability to burn fat.

GUIDELINES FOR CARDIORESPIRATORY EXERCISE PRESCRIPTION

To develop the cardiorespiratory system, the heart muscle has to be overloaded like any other muscle in the human body. Just as the biceps muscle in the upper arm is developed through strength-training exercises, the heart muscle also has to be exercised to increase in size, strength, and efficiency. To better understand how the cardiorespiratory system can be developed, we have to be familiar with four basic principles: intensity, mode, duration, and frequency of exercise. Figure 7.1 summarizes the cardiorespiratory exercise prescription guidelines according to the American College of Sports Medicine (ACSM), the world's leading sports medicine organization.[3]

The ACSM recommends that a medical exam and a diagnostic exercise stress test or stress ECG be administered

FIGURE 7.1 Cardiorespiratory Exercise Prescription Guidelines

Activity:	Aerobic (examples: walking, jogging, cycling, swimming, aerobics, racquetball, soccer, stair climbing)
Intensity:	55/65%–90% of maximal heart rate
Duration:	20–60 minutes of continuous aerobic activity
Frequency:	3 to 5 days per week

Source: From American College of Sports Medicine, *ACSM's Guidelines for Exercise Testing and Prescription* (Baltimore: Williams & Wilkins, 2006).

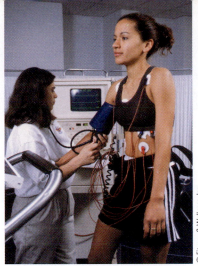

Exercise stress electrocardiogram test (stress ECG).

prior to vigorous exercise by apparently healthy men over age 45 and women over 55.[4] Vigorous exercise has been defined as an exercise intensity above 60 percent of VO_{2max}. This intensity is the equivalent of exercise that provides a "substantial challenge" to the participant or one that cannot be maintained for 20 continuous minutes.

Intensity of Exercise When people try to develop their cardiorespiratory system, the **intensity of exercise** perhaps is the most commonly ignored factor. This principle refers to how high the heart rate must be during exercise to improve cardiorespiratory endurance.

Muscles have to be overloaded to a given point for them to develop. Whereas the training stimulus to develop the biceps muscle can be accomplished with curl-up exercises, the stimulus for the cardiorespiratory system is provided by making the heart pump at a higher rate for a certain period of time. Research has shown that cardiorespiratory development occurs when you work at between 55/65 and 90 percent of your **maximal heart rate (MHR)**. The lower intensity, 55/65 percent, is recommended for beginners and people with health problems who have been cleared for exercise by a physician. The higher rate (up to 90 percent) is for healthy people who have completed the proper conditioning program.

Exercise intensity can be calculated easily and training can be monitored by checking your pulse. Use the following procedure to determine the intensity of exercise of your cardiorespiratory training zone.

1. Estimate the maximal heart rate (MHR). The maximal heart rate depends on the person's age and can be estimated according to the following formula:

   MHR = 220 minus age (220 – age)

2. Calculate the training intensities (TI) at 55 percent, 65 percent, and 90 percent. Multiply MHR by 55 percent, 65 percent, and 90 percent, respectively. For example, the 55 percent, 65 percent, and 90 percent training intensities for a 20-year-old person are:

   MHR: 220 – 20 = 200 beats per minute (bpm)
   55% TI   = (200 × .55) = 110 bpm

   65% TI   = (200 × .65) = 130 bpm
   90% TI   = (200 × .90) = 180 bpm

   Cardiorespiratory training zone: 110 to 180 bpm

According to your present age, you also may look up your cardiorespiratory training zone in Table 7.1. The training zone indicates that whenever you exercise to improve the cardiorespiratory system, you should maintain your heart rate between the 55 and 90 percent training intensities to obtain adequate development.

If you have been physically inactive and the objective is to attain the high physical fitness standard (see Chapter 6), you should train around the 55 to 65 percent intensity during the first 4 to 6 weeks of the exercise program. After the first few weeks, you may exercise between 65 and 90 percent training intensity.

Monitor your exercise heart rate regularly during exercise to make sure you are training in the correct zone. Wait until you are about 5 minutes into the exercise session before taking your first rate. When checking exercise heart rate, count your pulse for 10 seconds. Then multiply the 10-second count by 6 to obtain the rate in beats per minute. Exercise heart rate will remain at the same level for about 15 seconds following exercise. After 15 seconds, your heart rate will drop rapidly. Do not hesitate to stop during your exercise bout to check your pulse. If the rate is too low, increase the intensity of exercise. If the rate is too high, slow down.

Cardiac output Amount of blood ejected by the heart in one minute.

Resting heart rate Heart rate after a person has been sitting quietly for 15–20 minutes.

Intensity of exercise In cardiorespiratory exercise, how hard a person has to exercise to improve or maintain fitness.

Maximal heart rate (MHR) Highest heart rate for a person, primarily related to age.

TABLE 7.1 Recommended Cardiorespiratory Exercise Intensities

Age	Estimated Max HR*	55% HR Intensity	65% HR Intensity	90% HR Intensity
15	205	113	133	185
20	200	110	130	180
25	195	107	127	176
30	190	105	124	171
35	185	102	120	167
40	180	99	117	162
45	175	96	114	158
50	170	94	111	153
55	165	91	107	149
60	160	88	104	144
65	155	85	101	140
70	150	83	98	135
75	145	80	94	131

*HR = Heart Rate

FIGURE 7.2 Rate of Perceived Exertion Scale

6	
7	Very, very light
8	
9	Very light
10	
11	Fairly light
12	
13	Somewhat hard
14	
15	Hard
16	
17	Very hard
18	
19	Very, very hard
20	

From Gunnar Borg, "Perceived Exertion: A Note on History and Methods," *Medicine and Science in Sports and Exercise* (1983): 90–93.

To develop your cardiorespiratory system, you do not have to exercise above the 90 percent rate. From a fitness standpoint, training above this percentage will not yield extra benefits and actually may be unsafe for some people.

For unconditioned people and older adults, cardiorespiratory training should be conducted at about the 55 to 65 percent rate. This lower rate is recommended to reduce potential problems associated with high-intensity exercise.

Training benefits obtained by exercising at the 55 to 65 percent training intensity may place a person in an average or "moderately fit" category (see Table 6.2, page 114). Even though it is not an excellent cardiorespiratory fitness rating, exercising at this lower intensity does significantly decrease the risk for cardiovascular mortality (a health-fitness criterion) and other chronic diseases. An excellent fitness rating is obtained by exercising closer to the 90 percent threshold.

Many people do not check their heart rate during exercise, so an alternative method of prescribing intensity of exercise can be used. This method uses a **rate of perceived exertion (RPE)**, scale developed by Gunnar Borg.[5] Using the scale in Figure 7.2, a person subjectively rates the perceived exertion or difficulty of exercise when training in the appropriate target zone. The exercise heart rate then is associated with the corresponding RPE value.

If the training intensity requires a heart rate between 130 and 170 bpm, for example, this is associated with training between "somewhat hard" and "very hard" (13 and 17 on the scale). Some individuals, however, may perceive less exertion than others when training in the correct zone. You should associate your own inner perception of the task with the phrases given on the scale, then proceed to exercise at that rate of perceived exertion.

Whether you monitor the intensity of exercise by checking your pulse or using the rate of perceived exertion,

changes in normal exercise conditions affect the training zone. For example, exercising on a hot or humid day or at high altitude increases the heart rate response to a given task. Therefore, the intensity of your exercise may have to be adjusted.

Mode of Exercise The **mode of exercise** that develops the cardiorespiratory system has to be aerobic in nature. Once you have established your cardiorespiratory training zone, any activity or combination of activities that will get your heart rate up to that training zone and keep it there for as long as you exercise will produce adequate development.

Examples of aerobic activities are walking, jogging, aerobics, swimming, water aerobics, cross-country skiing, rope skipping, cycling, racquetball, stair climbing, and stationary running or cycling. Most of these activities can be used for either moderate- or high-intensity programs. Additional moderate-intensity activities include gardening; mowing the lawn (with a push mower); house cleaning; pushing a stroller; washing a car; raking leaves; or playing golf, tennis, or volleyball.

The activity you choose should be based on what you enjoy doing most and your physical limitations. Different activities may affect the amount of strength or flexibility you developed, but as far as the cardiorespiratory system is concerned, the heart doesn't know whether you are walking, swimming, or cycling. All the heart knows is that it has to pump at a certain rate, and as long as that rate is in the desired range, cardiorespiratory development will take place.

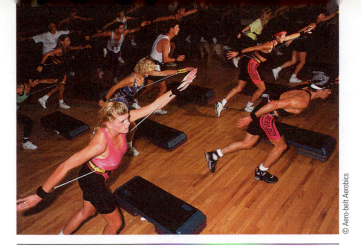
The more muscle groups involved during aerobic exercise, the greater the benefits.

Duration of Exercise In terms of **duration of exercise**, the general recommendation is that a person train between 20 and 60 minutes per session. For those who have been successful at losing weight, however, up to 90 minutes of daily moderate-intensity activity may be required to prevent weight regain.

The duration is based on how intensely a person trains. If the training is done around 85 percent, 20 minutes of exercise is sufficient. At 40 percent to 50 percent intensity, the individual should train at least 30 minutes. As mentioned in the discussion of intensity of exercise, unconditioned people and older adults should train at lower percentages and the activity should be carried out over a longer time.

Although most experts traditionally have recommended 20 to 60 minutes of continuous aerobic exercise per session, evidence suggests that accumulating 30 minutes or more of moderate-intensity physical activity can provide substantial health benefits. Research indicates that three 10-minute exercise sessions per day (separated by at least 4 hours), at approximately 70 percent of maximal heart rate, also produce fitness benefits.[6] Although the increases in VO_{2max} with this program were not as large (57 percent) as those in a group performing one continuous 30-minute bout of exercise per day, the researchers concluded that moderate-intensity exercise, conducted for 10 minutes three times per day, benefits the cardiorespiratory system significantly.

Results of this study are meaningful because people often mention lack of time as the reason for not taking part in an exercise program. Many people think they have to exercise at least 20 continuous minutes to get any benefits at all. Even though 20 to 60 minutes are recommended, short, intermittent exercise bouts also are helpful to the cardiorespiratory system.

From a weight management point of view, the Institute of Medicine of the National Academy of Sciences recommends an accumulation of 60 minutes of moderate-intensity physical activity per day,[7] whereas 60 to 90 minutes of daily moderate-intensity activity is necessary to prevent weight regain.[8] These recommendations are based on evidence that people who maintain healthy weight typically accumulate between 1 and 1½ hours of physical activity daily. The duration of exercise should be increased gradually to avoid undue fatigue and exercise-related injuries.

If lack of time is a concern, you should exercise daily at a high intensity for 30 minutes, which can burn as many calories as 60 minutes of moderate-intensity exercise (see "Low-Intensity Versus High-Intensity Exercise for Weight Loss," Chapter 10, page 243)—but only 15 percent of adults in the United States typically exercise at a high-intensity level. Novice and overweight exercisers also need proper conditioning prior to high-intensity exercise, to avoid injuries or cardiovascular-related problems.

Exercise sessions always should be preceded by a 5- to 10-minute **warm-up** and followed by a 10-minute cooldown (see Figure 7.3). The purpose of warm-up is to aid in the transition from rest to exercise. A good warm-up increases extensibility of muscle and connective tissue and range of motion around joints, and it enhances muscular activity. A warm-up consists of general, mild stretching exercises, and walking/jogging/cycling for a few minutes at a lower intensity level than the actual target zone. The concluding phase of the warm-up is a gradual increase in exercise intensity to the lower end of the target training zone.

In the cool-down, the intensity of exercise is decreased gradually to help the body return to near resting levels, followed by stretching and relaxation activities. Stopping abruptly causes blood to pool in the exercised body parts, which diminishes the return of blood to the heart. Less blood return can cause a sudden drop in blood pressure, dizziness and faintness, or even bring on cardiac abnormalities. The cool-down phase also helps dissipate body heat and aids in removing the lactid acid produced during high-intensity exercise.

Frequency of Exercise In terms of **frequency of exercise**, research indicates that a person should engage in aerobic exercise three to five times per week.[9] Any training beyond 5 days per week produces only minimal improvements in cardiorespiratory capacity (VO_{2max}).

For individuals on a weight-loss program, the recommendation is 60 to 90 minutes of low- to moderate-intensity activity on most days of the week. Longer exercise sessions increase caloric expenditure for faster weight reduction (see Chapter 10, "Exercise: The Key to Weight Management," page 241).

Rate of perceived exertion (RPE) A perception scale to monitor or interpret the intensity of aerobic exercise.

Mode of exercise Form of exercise.

Duration of exercise How long a person exercises.

Warm-up Starting a workout slowly.

Frequency of exercise How often a person engages in an exercise session.

FIGURE 7.3 Recommended Cardiorespiratory Training Pattern

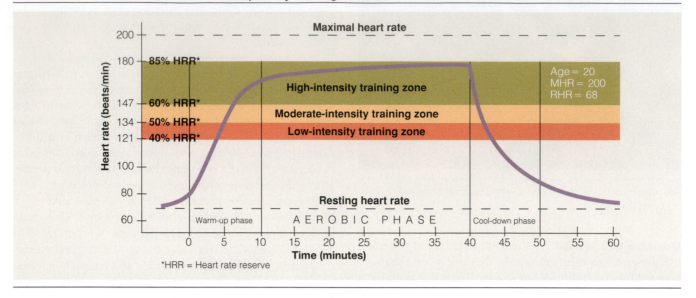

Ideally, a person should engage in physical activity six to seven times per week. To reap maximum benefits, a person needs to exercise a minimum of three times per week in the appropriate target zone for high fitness maintenance, and three to four additional times per week in moderate-intensity activities to enjoy the full benefits of health fitness. As indicated in the Surgeon General's report on physical activity and health,[10] people should strive to attain at least 30 minutes of physical activity per day most days of the week.

To enjoy better health and fitness, physical activity must be pursued regularly. According to Dr. William Haskell, from Stanford University: "Physical activity should be viewed as medication, and, therefore, should be taken on a daily basis." Many of the benefits of exercise and activity diminish within 2 weeks of substantially decreased physical activity. These benefits are completely lost within 2 to 8 months of inactivity.

Critical Thinking

Mary started an exercise program last year as a means to lose weight and enhance her body image. She now runs more than 6 miles every day, works out regularly on stairclimbers and elliptical machines, strength-trains daily, participates in step aerobics three times per week, and plays tennis or racquetball twice a week. Evaluate Mary's program. What suggestions do you have for improvements?

PHYSICAL ACTIVITY AND DIABETES

The Centers for Disease Control and Prevention report 18 million persons with diabetes in the United States and about 1 million new cases diagnosed each year. There are two types of diabetes:

Type 1, or insulin-dependent diabetes (IDDM), and
Type 2, or non-insulin-dependent diabetes (NIDDM).

In Type I, found primarily in young people, the pancreas produces little or no insulin. With Type 2, the pancreas may not produce enough insulin or the cells become insulin-resistant, thereby keeping glucose from entering the cells. Type 2 accounts for more than 90 percent of all cases of diabetes, and it occurs mainly in adults over age 40 who also are overweight.

If you are a diabetic, consult your physician before you start exercising. You may not be able to start until the diabetes is under control. Never exercise alone, and use a bracelet that identifies your condition. If you take insulin, the amount and timing of each dose may have to be regulated with your physician. If you inject insulin, inject it over a muscle that won't be exercised, then wait one hour before exercising. For Type I diabetics, it is recommended that you ingest 15 to 30 grams of carbohydrate during each 30 minutes of intense exercise and follow it with a carbohydrate snack after exercise.

Both types of diabetes improve with exercise, although the results are more notable in patients with Type 2 diabetes. Exercise usually lowers blood sugar and helps the body use food more effectively. The extent to which blood glucose level can be controlled in overweight Type 2 diabetics appears to be related directly to how long and how hard a person exercises. Normal or near-normal blood glucose levels can be achieved through a proper exercise program.

As with any fitness program, the exercise must be done regularly to be effective against diabetes. The benefit of a single exercise bout on blood glucose level is highest between 12 and 24 hours following exercise. These benefits are completely lost within 72 hours after exercise. Thus, regular participation is crucial to derive ongoing benefits. In terms of fitness, all diabetic patients can achieve higher fitness levels and reductions in weight, blood pressure, and total cholesterol and triglycerides.

According to the ACSM, diabetics should follow these guidelines to make the exercise program safe and derive the best benefits:[11]

- Burn a minimum of 1,000 calories per week through your exercise program.
- Exercise at a low–to-moderate intensity (55 to 65 percent of MHR). Start your program with 10 to 15 minutes per session, on at least three nonconsecutive days, but preferably exercise five days per week. Gradually increase the time you exercise to 30 minutes until you achieve your goal of at least 1,000 weekly calories. Diabetic individuals with a weight problem should build up to daily physical activity for 60 minutes per session.
- Choose an activity that you enjoy doing, and stay with it. As you select your activity, be aware of your condition. For example, if you have lost sensation in your feet, swimming or stationary cycling is better than walking or jogging from an injury prevention point of view.
- Check blood glucose levels before and after exercise. If you are on insulin or diabetes medication, monitor your blood glucose regularly and check it at least twice before exercising.
- Schedule your exercise 1 to 3 hours after a meal, and avoid exercise when your insulin is peaking.
- Be ready to treat low blood sugar with a fast-acting source of sugar, such as juice or raisins.
- Discontinue exercise immediately if you feel that a reaction is about to occur. Check your blood glucose level and treat the condition as needed.
- When you exercise outdoors, always do so with someone who knows what to do in a diabetes-related emergency.
- In addition, engage in strength training twice per week, using 8 to 10 exercises with a minimum of one set of 10 to 15 repetitions to near-fatigue.

MAINTAINING CARDIORESPIRATORY FITNESS

A decrease in cardiorespiratory fitness has been observed in as little as 2 weeks of nontraining. Depending on the duration of participation in the aerobic program, complete loss of training benefits is seen between 3 and 8 months after discontinuing the program. After an aerobic conditioning program, a person must continue a regular training program to maintain cardiorespiratory fitness.

The key to maintaining fitness seems to be the intensity of training.[12] Even though the duration and frequency of training may be reduced, VO_{2max} does not decline as long as the proper intensity is maintained. Three 20-minute training sessions per week, on non-consecutive days, maintains cardiorespiratory fitness as long as the heart rate is in the appropriate target zone.

PERSONAL CARDIORESPIRATORY EXERCISE PRESCRIPTION

Having learned the basic principles of cardiorespiratory exercise prescription, you can proceed to Assessment 7.2 at the end of this chapter and fill out your own prescription. If you have not been exercising regularly, you could go ahead and attempt to train five or six times a week for 30 minutes at a time. You may find this discouraging, however, and may drop out before getting too far because you probably will develop some muscle soreness and stiffness and possibly incur minor injuries. Muscle soreness and stiffness and the risk for injuries can be lessened or eliminated by progressively increasing the intensity, duration, and frequency of exercise.

Once you have determined your exercise prescription, the difficult part begins: starting and sticking to a lifetime exercise program. Although you may be motivated after reading the benefits to be gained from physical activity, lifelong dedication and perseverance are necessary to reap and maintain good fitness.

The first few weeks are probably the most difficult, but where there's a will, there's a way. Once you begin to see positive changes, it won't be as hard. Soon you will develop a habit for exercise that will be deeply satisfying and will bring about a sense of self-accomplishment.

Muscular Strength

An adequate level of strength is an important component of good physical fitness. The two forms of strength, as defined in Chapter 6, are muscular strength and muscular endurance. Muscular strength is the ability to exert maximum force against resistance. Muscular endurance is the ability of a muscle to exert submaximal force repeatedly over a period of time. For example, a person may have the muscular strength to lift 100 pounds once but may not have the muscular endurance to lift 60 pounds 20 times.

Over the years, it has been well-documented that the capacity of muscle cells to exert force increases and decreases according to the demands placed upon the muscular system. If muscle cells are overloaded beyond their normal use, such as in strength-training programs, the cells increase in size—**hypertrophy**—and strength. If the demands placed on the muscle cells decrease, such as in sedentary living or required rest because of illness or injury, the cells decrease in size—**atrophy**—and lose strength.

Hypertrophy An increase in the size of the cell (for example, muscle hypertrophy).

Atrophy Decrease in size of a cell, often stemming from non-use.

SIGNIFICANCE OF STRENGTH

Strength is important for optimal performance in daily tasks and recreational activities, to improve personal appearance and self-image, to lessen the risk of injury, and to cope with emergency situations in life. Adequate strength levels also contribute to weight control and enhanced overall health and well-being.

Perhaps one of the most significant benefits of maintaining a good strength level is its relationship to human **metabolism**, defined as all energy and material transformations that occur within living cells. A primary result of a strength-training program is an increase in muscle mass or size (lean body mass), known as muscle hypertrophy. Muscle tissue uses energy even at rest, whereas fatty tissue uses very little energy (that is, few calories) and may be considered metabolically inert.

As muscle size increases, so does the **resting metabolism**, or the amount of energy (expressed in calories) that an individual requires during resting conditions to sustain proper cell function. Even small increases in muscle mass may affect resting metabolism. In one study, a group of inactive older adults between ages 56 and 86 who participated in a 12-week strength-training program increased lean body mass by about 3 pounds, lost about 4 pounds of fat, and increased their resting metabolic rate by almost 7 percent.[13]

Loss of lean tissue is thought to be the main reason for the decrease in metabolism as people get older. Contrary to some beliefs, metabolism does not have to slow down significantly with aging. *We* slow down. Lean body mass declines with sedentary living, which in turn slows down the resting metabolic rate. If people continue eating at the same rate, body fat increases. The average decrease in resting metabolism for a 60-year-old individual is about 300 to 400 calories per day, compared to a 25-year-old person. Hence, participating in a strength-training program is a means of preventing and reducing obesity.

One of the most common misconceptions about physical fitness relates to women and strength training. Because of the increase in muscle mass commonly seen in men, some women avoid strength-training programs because they think they, too, will develop large muscles. Although the quality of muscle in men and women is the same, endocrinological differences will not allow women to achieve the same amount of muscle hypertrophy (size) as men. Men also have more muscle fibers, and because of the male sex-specific hormones, each fiber has a greater potential for hypertrophy.

As more women participate in sports, the myth that strength training for women leads to larger muscle size has waned. In recent years, better body appearance has become the rule rather than the exception for women who participate in strength-training programs. Some of the most attractive female movie stars and many beauty pageant participants train with weights to enhance their personal image.

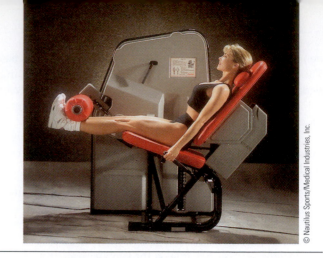

A regular strength-training program helps to increase and maintain a higher resting metabolic rate.

Another benefit of strength training, accentuated even more when combined with aerobic exercise, is a decrease in adipose (fatty) tissue. Research has shown that the decrease in fatty tissue often is greater than the amount of muscle hypertrophy gained through strength training. Therefore, losing inches but not body weight is a typical outcome.

Because muscle tissue is more dense than fatty tissue, and despite the fact that inches are being lost, people, especially women, often become discouraged because they cannot readily see the results on the scale. This discouragement can be offset easily by determining body composition regularly to monitor changes in percent body fat rather than simply measuring total body weight changes.

Adequate strength levels are especially critical in older age. Functional independence—the physical capacity to meet ordinary and unexpected demands of daily life safely and effectively—is dependent to a large extent on a person's strength level.

Older adults with good strength enjoy greater freedom of movement and functionality than their inactive counterparts. Simple daily tasks such as getting out of bed, getting in and out of a tub, doing household chores, climbing a flight of stairs, and crossing a street safely are enhanced greatly through a strength-training program.

Research has shown that older adults can increase their strength levels, but the amount of muscle hypertrophy they achieve decreases with age. Strength gains as high as 200 percent have been found in previously inactive adults over age 90.[14] Suddenly, many of these individuals who previously were dependent on others can perform most of life's daily tasks without restrictions or functional dependence.

Strength gains are achieved in two ways: (a) through greater ability of individual muscle fibers to get a stronger contraction, and (b) by recruiting a greater proportion of the total available fibers for each contraction. These two factors combine in the **progressive overload principle**. This principle states that, for strength to improve, the demands placed on the muscle must be increased systematically and progressively over time, and the resistance must be of a magnitude significant enough to cause physiologic adaptation. In simpler terms, just like all other organs and systems of the human body, muscles have to be taxed beyond their accustomed loads to increase in physical capacity.

GUIDELINES FOR STRENGTH DEVELOPMENT PRESCRIPTION

As in cardiorespiratory exercise, some guidelines are involved in developing a strength-training program. These relate to mode, resistance, sets, and frequency of training.

Mode of Training The principle of **specificity of training** states that, for a muscle to increase in strength or endurance, only a training program for that expressed purpose will obtain the desired effects. Two basic types of training methods are used to improve strength: **isometric** and **dynamic** (previously known as isotonic). Isometric training refers to a muscle contraction producing little or no movement, such as pushing or pulling against immovable objects. Dynamic training refers to a muscle contraction with movement, such as lifting an object over the head. Generally, the mode of training an individual uses depends mainly on the type of equipment available and the specific objective the training program is attempting to accomplish.

Isometric training was used commonly several years ago, but its popularity has waned. Because strength gains with isometric training are specific to the angle of muscle contraction, this type of training is most beneficial in a sport such as gymnastics, which requires static contractions during routines. Thus it has limited applications for overall health fitness.

Dynamic training is the most popular mode for strength training. Its main advantage is that strength is gained through the full range of motion. Most daily activities are dynamic in nature. We are constantly lifting, pushing, and pulling objects, and strength is needed through a complete range of motion. Another advantage is that improvements are easily measured by the amount lifted.

Dynamic training programs can be conducted without weights or with free weights (barbells and dumbbells) or on fixed resistance machines, variable-resistance machines, and **isokinetic** equipment. When you perform dynamic exercises without weights (for example, pull-ups, push-ups), with free weights, or with fixed-resistance machines, you move a constant resistance (weight) through a joint's full range of motion.

A limitation of dynamic training is that the greatest resistance that can be lifted equals the maximum weight that can be moved at the weakest angle of the joint. This is because of changes in muscle length and angle of pull as the joint moves through its range of motion.

As strength training became more popular, new strength-training machines were developed. This technology brought about isokinetic and variable-resistance

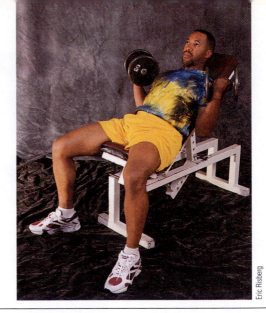

Eric Risberg

Example of dynamic training.

training. These training programs require special machines equipped with mechanical devices that provide varying amounts of resistance, with the intent of overloading the muscle group maximally through the entire range of motion.

A distinction of isokinetic training is that the speed of the muscle contraction is kept constant because the machine provides resistance to match the user's force through the range of motion. Another possible advantage of isokinetic training is that specific speeds in various sport skills can be duplicated more closely with this type of training, which may enhance performance (specificity of training). A disadvantage is that the equipment is not readily available to many people.

Metabolism All energy and material transformations that occur within living cells; necessary to sustain life.

Resting metabolism The amount of energy (expressed in milliliters of oxygen per minute or in total calories per day) an individual requires during resting conditions to sustain proper body function.

Progressive overload principle Training concept stating that the demands placed on a system (for example, cardio-respiratory or muscular) must be increased systematically and progressively over time to cause physiological adaptation (development or improvement).

Specificity of training Targeting the specific body system or area the person is attempting to improve (aerobic endurance, anaerobic capacity, strength, flexibility).

Isometric Strength-training method that uses muscle contractions that produce little or no movement, such as pushing or pulling against immovable objects.

Dynamic Strength-training method that uses muscle contractions with movement.

Isokinetic Strength-training method in which the speed of the muscle contraction is kept constant because the equipment (machine) provides an accommodating resistance to match the user's force through the range of motion.

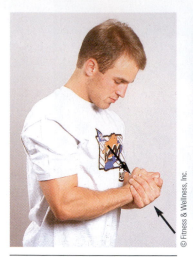

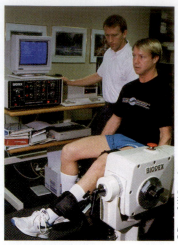

Example of isometric training.   Example of isokinetic training.

The benefits of isokinetic and variable-resistance training are similar to the other dynamic training methods. Theoretically, strength gains should be better because maximum resistance is applied at all angles. Research, however, has not shown this type of training to be more effective than other modes of dynamic training.

Resistance **Resistance** in strength training is the equivalent of intensity in cardiorespiratory exercise prescription. To stimulate strength development, the general recommendation has been to use a resistance of approximately 80 percent of the maximum capacity (1 RM). For example, a person with a 1 RM of 150 pounds should work with about 120 pounds (150 × .80).

The number of repetitions that one can perform at 80 percent of the 1 RM varies among exercises. Data indicate that the total number of repetitions performed at a certain percentage of the 1 RM depends on the amount of muscle mass involved (bench press versus triceps extension) and whether it is a single or multi-joint exercise (leg press versus leg curl). In both trained and untrained subjects, the number of repetitions is greater with larger muscle mass involvement and multi-joint exercises.[15]

Because of the time factor involved in constantly determining the 1 RM on each lift to ensure that the person is indeed working around 80 percent, the accepted rule for many years has been that individuals perform between 3 and 12 repetitions maximum (3 to 12 RM) for adequate strength gains. For example, if a person is training with a resistance of 120 pounds and cannot lift it more than 12 times—that is, the person reaches volitional fatigue at or before 12 repetitions—the training stimulus (weight used) is adequate for strength development. Once the person can lift the resistance more than 12 times, the resistance is increased by 5 to 10 pounds and the person again should build up to 12 repetitions. This is referred to as **progressive resistance training**.

Strength development, however, can also occur when working with less than 80 percent of the 1 RM. Although 3 to 12 RM is the most commonly prescribed resistance, benefits do occur when working below 3 or above 12 RM.

At least in the health-fitness area, little evidence presently supports the notion that working with a given number of repetitions elicits specific or greater strength, muscular endurance, or muscular hypertrophy.[16] Although not precisely to the same extent, muscular strength and endurance are both increased when using a reasonable number of repetitions. Thus, the American College of Sports Medicine recommends a range between 3 and 20 RM. The individual may choose the number of repetitions based on personal preference.

Elite strength athletes typically work between 1 and 6 RM but often shuffle training with different number of repetitions for selected periods (weeks) of time. Body builders tend to work with moderate resistance levels (60 to 85 percent of the 1 RM) and perform 8 to 20 repetitions to near fatigue. A foremost objective of body building is to increase muscle size. Moderate resistance promotes blood flow to the muscles, "pumping up the muscles" (also known as "the pump") and making them look much larger than they do in a resting state.

From a general fitness point of view, working near a 10-repetition threshold seems to improve overall performance most effectively. We live in a dynamic world in which muscular strength and endurance are both required to lead an enjoyable life. Working around 10 RM produces good results in terms of strength, endurance, and hypertrophy. For older and more frail individuals (50–60 years of age and older), 10 to 15 repetitions to near fatigue may be more appropriate.

We should mention here that a certain resistance (say, 50 pounds) is seldom the same on two different weight machines, or between free weights and weight machines. The industry has no standard calibration procedure for strength equipment. Consequently, if you lift a certain weight with free weights or a given machine, you may or may not be able to lift the same amount on a different piece of equipment.

Sets Strength training is done in **sets**. For example, a person lifting 120 pounds eight times performs one set of eight repetitions (1/8/120). For general fitness, the recommendation is one to three sets per exercise. Some evidence suggests that strength gains are greater when using multiple sets rather than a single set for a given exercise. Other research concludes that similar increases in strength, endurance, and hypertrophy are derived between single- and multiple-set strength training, as long as the single set, or at least one of the multiple sets, is performed to volitional exhaustion (heavy set).[17] Strength gains may be lessened by performing too many sets.

A recommended program for beginners in their first year of training is one or two light warm-up sets per exercise using about 50 percent of the 1 RM (no warm-up sets are necessary for subsequent exercises that use the same muscle group), followed by one to three sets per exercise. Maintaining a resistance and effort that will fatigue the muscle temporarily (volitional exhaustion) in the number of repetitions selected in at least one of the sets is critical to achieve optimal progress. Because of the lower resistances used in body building, four to eight sets can be done for each exercise.

To make the exercise program more time-effective, two or three exercises that require different muscle groups may be alternated. In this way, a person will not have to wait 2 to 3 minutes before proceeding to a new set on a different exercise. For example, the bench press, leg extension, and abdominal curl-up exercises may be combined so the person can go almost directly from one set to the next. Body builders should rest no more than a minute to maximize the "pumping" effect.

To avoid muscle soreness and stiffness, new participants ought to build up gradually to the three sets of maximal repetitions. This can be done by performing only one set of each exercise with a lighter resistance on the first day. During the second session, two sets of each exercise can be done—one light and the second with the regular resistance. During the third session, three sets could be performed—one light and two heavy sets. After that, a person should be able to do all three heavy sets.

Frequency of Training Strength training should be done either with a total-body workout two or three times per week, or more frequently if using a split-body routine (upper body one day, lower body the next). After a maximum strength workout, the muscles should be rested for about 48 hours to allow adequate recovery.

People who are not completely recovered in 2 or 3 days most likely are overtraining and, therefore, not reaping the full benefits of their program. In that case, decreasing the total number of sets or exercises performed during the previous workout is recommended.

To achieve significant strength gains, a minimum of 8 weeks of consecutive training is needed. Once an adequate level of strength is achieved, one training session per week will be sufficient to maintain the new strength level.

As you prepare to design your strength training program, keep the following guidelines in mind.

1. Select exercises that will involve all major muscle groups: chest, shoulders, back, legs, arms, hip, and trunk.

2. Never lift weights alone. Always have someone work out with you in case you need a spotter or help with an injury. When you use free weights, you should have one or two spotters for certain exercises (bench press, squats, overhead press).

3. Prior to lifting weights, warm up properly by performing a light- to moderate-intensity aerobic activity for 5 to 7 minutes, and some gentle stretches for a few minutes.

4. Exercise larger muscle groups first—such as those in the chest, back, and legs—before exercising smaller muscle groups (arms, abdominals, ankles, neck). The bench press exercise works the chest, shoulders, and back of the upper arms (triceps), whereas the triceps extension works the back of the upper arms only.

5. Exercise opposing muscle groups for a balanced workout. After you work the chest (bench press), work the back (rowing torso). If you work the biceps (arm curl), work the triceps (triceps extension).

6. Perform all exercises in a controlled manner. Avoid fast and jerky movements, and do not throw the entire body into the lifting motion. Failing to do so increases the risk for injury and decreases the effectiveness of the exercise. When lifting a weight, do not arch the back.

7. Perform each exercise through the entire possible range of motion.

8. Breathe naturally, and do not hold your breath as you lift the resistance (weight). Inhale during the eccentric phase (bringing the weight down), and exhale during the concentric phase (lifting or pushing the weight up). When you are learning a new exercise, practice proper breathing with lighter weights.

9. Avoid holding your breath while straining to lift a weight. Holding your breath greatly increases the pressure inside the chest and abdominal cavity, making it nearly impossible for the blood in the veins to return to the heart. Although rare, a sudden high intrathoracic pressure may lead to dizziness, a blackout, a stroke, a heart attack, or a hernia.

10. If you experience unusual discomfort or pain, discontinue training. The high tension (heavy resistance) loads used in strength training can exacerbate potential injuries. Discomfort and pain are signals to stop and determine what's wrong. Before you continue training, be sure to properly evaluate your condition.

11. At the end of each strength-training workout, stretch out for a few minutes to help muscles return to their normal resting length and to minimize muscle soreness and risk of injury.

Resistance Amount of weight lifted in strength training.

Progressive resistance training A gradual increase in resistance lifted over a period of time when training with weights.

Set Number of repetitions in strength training (e.g., one set of 12 repetitions).

DESIGNING A STRENGTH-TRAINING PROGRAM

Two strength-training programs are illustrated at the end of this chapter (pages 154–160). Only a minimum of equipment is required for the first program, "Strength-Training Exercises without Weights." (Exercises 1 through 11). This program can be done within the walls of your own home. Your body weight is used as the primary resistance for most exercises. A few exercises call for a friend's help or some basic implements from around the house to provide more resistance.

"Strength-Training Exercises with Weights" (Exercises 12 through 20) require machines such as those shown in the photographs. Some of these machines use fixed resistance; others use variable resistance. Many of these exercises also can be done with free weights.

Depending on the facilities available to you, you should be able to choose one of the two training programs outlined in this chapter. The resistance and the number of repetitions you use should be based on whether you want to increase your muscular strength or your muscular endurance. Do up to 10–12 repetitions maximum for strength gains and muscle hypertrophy, and more than 12 for muscular endurance.

As pointed out, three training sessions per week on nonconsecutive days is an ideal arrangement for proper development. Because both strength and endurance are required in daily activities, 3 sets of about 8 to 12 repetitions maximum for each exercise are enough. In doing this, you will obtain good strength gains and yet be close to the endurance threshold.

Perhaps the only exercises that call for more repetitions are abdominal exercises. The abdominal muscles are considered primarily antigravity or postural muscles. Hence, a little more endurance may be required. When doing abdominal work, most people do about 20 repetitions.

If time is a concern in completing a strength-training exercise program, the American College of Sports Medicine recommends as a minimum: (a) 1 set of 3 to 20 repetitions performed to near-fatigue and (b) 8 to 10 exercises involving the major muscle groups of the body, conducted twice a week[18] (see Figure 7.4). This recommendation is based on research showing that this training generates 70 to 80 percent of the improvements reported in other programs using 3 sets of about 10 RM. You are now ready to write your own strength-training prescription using Assessment 7.3.

Muscular Flexibility

Flexibility refers to the achievable range of motion at a joint or group of joints without causing injury. Healthcare professionals and practitioners have generally underestimated and overlooked the contribution of good muscular flexibility to overall fitness and preventive health care.

FIGURE 7.4 Strength-Training Guidelines

Mode:	8 to 10 dynamic strength-training exercises involving the body's major muscle groups
Resistance:	Sufficient resistance to perform 3 to 20 repetitions to complete or near-complete fatigue (the number of repetitions is optional; you may use 3 to 6, 8 to 12, 12 to 15, or 16 to 20 repetitions)
Sets:	A minimum of 1 set
Frequency:	2 to 3 days per week on nonconsecutive days

Adapted from: American College of Sports Medicine, *Guidelines for Exercise Testing and Prescription* (Baltimore: Williams & Wilkins, 2006).

SIGNIFICANCE OF FLEXIBILITY

We often have to make rapid or strenuous movements we are not accustomed to making, and this may cause injury. And physical therapists have indicated that improper body mechanics are often the result of poor flexibility.

A decline in flexibility can cause poor posture and subsequent aches and pains that lead to limited and painful movement of the joints. Inordinate tightness is uncomfortable and debilitating. Approximately 80 percent of all low-back problems in the United States are attributable to improper alignment of the vertebral column and pelvic girdle, a direct result of inflexible and weak muscles. This backache syndrome costs American industry billions of dollars each year in lost productivity, health services, and worker's compensation.[19]

Participating in a regular flexibility program helps a person maintain good joint mobility, increases resistance to muscle injury and soreness, prevents low-back and other spinal column problems, improves and maintains good postural alignment, promotes proper and graceful body movement, improves personal appearance and self-image, and helps to develop and maintain motor skills throughout life. Adequate flexibility also makes activities of daily living such as turning, lifting, and bending much easier to do. In addition, flexibility exercises have been prescribed successfully to treat dysmenorrhea[20] (painful menstruation) and general neuromuscular tension (stress). Regular stretching helps decrease the aches and pains caused by psychological stress and contributes to a decrease in anxiety, blood pressure, and breathing rate.[21]

Furthermore, stretching exercises in conjunction with calisthenics are helpful in warm-up routines to prepare the human body for more vigorous aerobic or strength-training exercises, as well as in cool-down routines following exercise to help the person return to a normal resting state. Fatigued muscles tend to contract to a shorter-than-average resting length, and stretching exercises help fatigued muscles reestablish their normal resting length.

Total range of motion around a joint is highly specific and varies from one joint to the other (hip, trunk, shoulder), as well as from one individual to the next. The

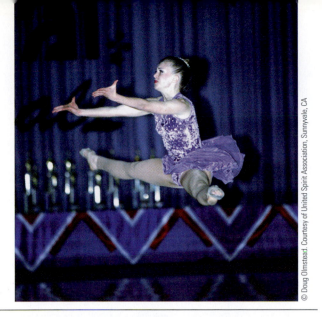
Adequate flexibility helps to develop and maintain sports skill throughout life.

amount of muscular flexibility relates primarily to genetic factors and frequency of physical activity. Other factors that influence range of motion about a joint include joint structure, ligaments, tendons, muscles, skin, tissue injury, adipose tissue (fat), body temperature, age, and gender.

Because of the specificity of flexibility, determining an ideal level of flexibility is difficult. Nevertheless, flexibility is important to everyone's health, and even more so as we age.

GUIDELINES FOR FLEXIBILITY DEVELOPMENT

Although genetics play a crucial role in body flexibility, range of joint mobility can be increased and maintained through a regular flexibility exercise program. Because range of motion is highly specific to each body part, a comprehensive stretching program, which includes all body parts and adheres to the basic guidelines for flexibility development, should be followed to obtain optimal results.

The progressive overload and specificity of training principles discussed in conjunction with strength development also apply to the development of muscular flexibility. To increase the total range of motion of a joint, the specific muscles surrounding that joint have to be stretched progressively beyond their accustomed length. The principles of mode, intensity, repetitions, and frequency of exercise can be applied to flexibility programs.

Mode of Exercise Three modes of stretching exercises can be used to increase flexibility: (a) ballistic stretching, (b) slow-sustained stretching, and (c) proprioceptive neuromuscular facilitation stretching. Although research has indicated that all three types of stretching are effective in developing better flexibility, each technique has certain advantages.

Ballistic (or dynamic) **stretching** exercises are most often performed using jerky, rapid, and bouncy movements that provide the necessary force to lengthen the muscles. Studies have shown that this type of stretching helps to develop flexibility, but the ballistic actions may cause muscle soreness and injury because of small tears to the soft tissue. Slow, gentle, and controlled ballistic stretching (instead of jerky, rapid, and bouncy movements), however, is quite effective in developing flexibility, and most individuals can perform this safely.

Precautions must be taken not to overstretch ligaments, because they will undergo plastic or permanent elongation. If the stretching force cannot be controlled, as in fast, jerky movements, ligaments easily can be overstretched. This, in turn, leads to excessively loose joints, which increases the risk for injuries, including joint dislocation and **subluxation**. Slow, gentle, and controlled ballistic stretching (instead of jerky, rapid, and bouncy movements), however, is quite effective in developing flexibility, and most people can perform these safely.

With **slow-sustained stretching**, muscles are lengthened gradually through a joint's complete range of motion and the final position is held for a few seconds. Using a slow-sustained stretch causes the muscles to relax so greater length can be achieved. This type of stretch causes little pain and has a low risk for injury. Slow-sustained stretching exercises are used most frequently in, and are recommended for, flexibility development programs.

Proprioceptive neuromuscular facilitation (PNF) stretching has become more popular in the last few years. This technique is based on a "contract and relax" method and requires the assistance of another person. The procedure is as follows:

1. The person assisting with the exercise provides an initial force by slowly pushing in the direction of the desired stretch. The initial stretch does not cover the entire range of motion.
2. The person being stretched then applies force in the direction opposite of the stretch, against the assistant, who tries to hold the initial degree of stretch as closely as possible. This creates an isometric contraction at that angle.

Flexibility Refers to the achievable range of motion at a joint or group of joints without causing injury.

Ballistic stretching Exercises performed using jerky, rapid, and bouncy movements.

Subluxation Partial dislocation of a joint.

Slow-sustained stretching Technique whereby the muscles are lengthened gradually through a joint's complete range of motion and the final position is held for a few seconds.

Proprioceptive neuromuscular facilitation (PNF) Stretching technique in which muscles are stretched out progressively with intermittent isometric contractions.

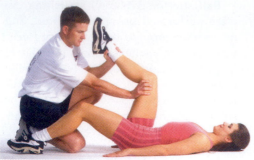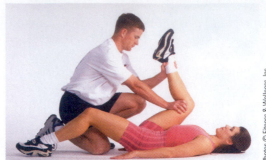

Photos © Fitness & Wellness, Inc.

Proprioceptive neuromuscular facilitation (PNF) stretching technique.

3. After 4 or 5 seconds of isometric contraction, the muscle(s) being stretched are relaxed completely. The assistant then slowly increases the degree of stretch to a greater angle.

4. The isometric contraction then is repeated for another 4 or 5 seconds, after which the muscle is relaxed again. The assistant then can increase the degree of stretch slowly one more time. This procedure is repeated two to five times, until the exerciser feels mild discomfort. On the last trial, the final stretched position should be held for several seconds.

Theoretically, with the PNF technique, the isometric contraction helps relax the muscle(s) being stretched, which results in greater muscle length. Some fitness leaders believe that PNF is more effective than slow-sustained stretching. Another benefit of PNF is an increase in strength of the muscle(s) being stretched. Research has shown an approximate 17 percent and 35 percent increase in absolute strength and muscular endurance, respectively, in the hamstring muscle group after 12 weeks of PNF stretching.[22] The results were consistent in men and women alike. These increases are attributed to the isometric contractions performed during PNF. The disadvantages are more pain with PNF, need for a second person to assist, and more time necessary to conduct each session.

Intensity of Exercise Before you start any flexibility exercises, the muscles always should be warmed up using some calisthenic exercises. Failing to do a proper warm-up increases the risk for muscle pulls and tears. For this reason, a good time to do flexibility exercises is after aerobic workouts. The higher body temperature can increase joint range of motion significantly.

When you do flexibility exercises, the intensity or degree of stretch should be only to a point of mild discomfort. Pain should not be a part of the stretching routine.

Excessive pain is an indication that the load is too high and may lead to injury. Stretching should be done to slightly below the pain threshold. As participants reach this point, they should try to relax the muscle or muscles being stretched as much as possible. After completing the stretch, gradually bring the body part back to the starting point.

FIGURE 7.5 Guidelines for Development of Flexibility

Mode:	Static or dynamic (slow ballistic or proprioceptive neuromuscular facilitation) stretching to include all major muscle groups
Intensity:	Stretch to tightness at the end of the range of motion
Repetitions:	Repeat each exercise 2 to 4 times and hold the final stretched position for 15 to 30 seconds
Frequency:	Minimal, 2 or 3 days per week. Ideal, 5 to 7 days per week

Adapted from American College of Sports Medicine, *Guidelines for Exercise Testing and Prescription* (Baltimore: Williams & Wilkins, 2006).

Repetitions In an exercise session, the time required for flexibility development is based on the number of repetitions performed and the length of time each repetition (the final stretched position) is held. The general recommendation is that each exercise be done four or five times, and that the final position be held each time for about 15 to 30 seconds.

As flexibility increases, the individual can gradually increase the time each repetition is held, to a maximum of a minute. Individuals who are susceptible to flexibility injuries should limit each stretch to 20 seconds.

Frequency of Training Flexibility exercises should be conducted five to six times a week in the initial stages of the program. After a minimum of 6 to 8 weeks of almost daily stretching, flexibility levels can be maintained with only two or three sessions per week, using about three repetitions of 15 to 30 seconds each. Figure 7.5 provides a summary of flexibility development guidelines.

DESIGNING A FLEXIBILITY PROGRAM

To improve body flexibility, each major muscle group should be subjected to at least one stretching exercise. A complete set of exercises for developing muscular flexibility is presented at the end of this chapter (Exercises 21 through 33). With some of the exercises, you may not be able to hold a final stretched position (examples are lateral head tilts and arm circles), but you still should perform the exercise through the joint's full range of motion. Depending on the number and the length of the repetitions, a complete workout will last between 15 and 30 minutes. You can use Assessment 7.4 at the end of this chapter to design your own stretching program.

Preventing and Rehabilitating Low-Back Pain

Few people make it through life without having low-back pain at some point. An estimated 60 percent to 90 percent of all Americans will suffer from chronic back pain in their lives.[23] On a yearly basis, more than 75 million people report having chronic low-back pain.

Back pain is considered chronic if it persists longer than 3 months. About 80 percent of the time, backache syndrome is preventable and is caused by: (a) physical inactivity, (b) poor postural habits and body mechanics, (3) excessive body weight, and/or (d) psychological stress.

Although people tend to think of back pain as a skeletal problem, the spine's curvature, alignment, and movement are controlled by surrounding muscles. The most common reason for chronic low-back pain is a lack of physical activity. A major contributor to back pain is sitting for long periods, which causes back muscles to shorten, stiffen, and become weaker.

Deterioration or weakening of the abdominal and gluteal muscles, along with tightening of the lower back (erector spinae) muscles, brings about an unnatural forward tilt of the pelvis (Figure 7.6). This tilt puts extra pressure on the spinal vertebrae, causing pain in the lower back. Accumulation of fat around the midsection of the body contributes to the forward tilt of the pelvis, which further aggravates the condition.

Low-back pain frequently is associated with faulty posture and improper body mechanics or body positions in all of life's daily activities, including sleeping, sitting, standing, walking, driving, working, and exercising. Incorrect posture and poor mechanics, as explained in Figure 7.7, increase strain on the lower back as well as many other bones, joints, muscles, and ligaments.

Back pain can be reduced greatly by including some specific stretching and strengthening exercises in the regular fitness program. In most cases, back pain is present only with movement and physical activity. If the pain is severe and persists even at rest, the first step is to consult a physician, who can rule out any disk damage and may prescribe proper bed rest using several pillows under the knees for leg support (see Figure 7.7). This position helps release muscle spasms by stretching the muscles involved. In addition, a physician may prescribe a muscle relaxant or anti-inflammatory medication (or both) and some type of physical therapy.

FIGURE 7.6 Incorrect (left) and Correct (right) Pelvic Alignment

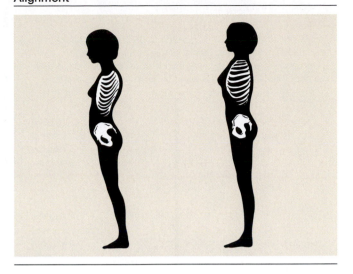

In most cases of low-back pain, even with severe pain, people feel better within days or weeks without treatment from health-care professionals.[24] To relieve symptoms, you may use over-the-counter pain relievers and hot or cold packs. You also should stay active to avoid further weakening of the back muscles. Low-impact activities such as walking, swimming, water aerobics, and cycling are recommended. Once you are pain-free in the resting state, you need to start correcting the muscular imbalance by stretching the tight muscles and strengthening the weak ones. Stretching exercises always are performed first.

If there is no indication of disease or injury, such as leg numbness or pain, a herniated disk, or fractures, spinal manipulation by a chiropractor or other health care professional can provide pain relief. Spinal manipulation as a treatment modality for low-back pain has been endorsed by the Federal Agency for Health Care Policy and Research. The guidelines suggest that spinal manipulation may help to alleviate discomfort and pain during the first few weeks of an acute episode of low-back pain. Generally, benefits are seen within 10 treatments. People who have had chronic pain for more than 6 months should avoid spinal manipulation until they have been thoroughly examined by a physician.

Several exercises for preventing and rehabilitating the backache syndrome are given at the end of the chapter on pages 162–164. These exercises can be done twice or more daily when a person has back pain. Under normal circumstances, doing these exercises three to four times a week is enough to prevent the syndrome.

Psychological stress may also lead to back pain.[25] Excessive stress causes muscles to contract. In the case of the lower back, frequent tightening of the muscles can throw the back out of alignment and constrict blood vessels that supply oxygen and nutrients to the back. If you suffer from excessive stress and back pain at the same time, proper stress management (see Chapter 3) should be a part of your comprehensive back-care program.

FIGURE 7.7 Your Back and How to Care For It

HOW TO STAY ON YOUR FEET WITHOUT TIRING YOUR BACK

To prevent strain and pain in everyday activities, it is restful to change from one task to another before fatigue sets in. You can lie down between chores; you should check body position frequently, drawing in the abdomen, flattening the back, bending the knees slightly.

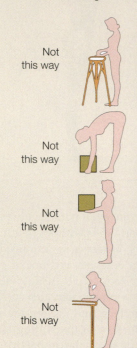
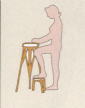
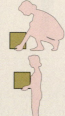

Not this way

Not this way

Not this way

Not this way

Use of a footrest relieves swayback.

Bend the knees and hips, not the waist.

Hold heavy objects close to you.

Never bend over without bending the knees.

HOW TO PUT YOUR BACK TO BED

For proper bed posture, a firm mattress is essential. Bedboards, sold commercially, or devised at home, may be used with soft mattresses. Bedboards, preferably, should be made of 3/4 inch plywood. Faulty sleeping positions intensify swayback and result not only in backache but in numbness, tingling, and pain in arms and legs.

Incorrect:

Lying flat on back makes swayback worse.
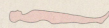

Use of high pillow strains neck, arms, shoulders.

Sleeping face down exaggerates swayback, strains neck and shoulders.
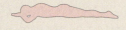

Bending one hip and knee does not relieve swayback.
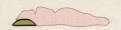

Correct:

Lying on side with knees bent effectively flattens the back. Flat pillow may be used to support neck, especially when shoulders are broad.

Sleeping on back is restful and correct when knees are properly supported.
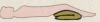

Raise the foot of the mattress eight inches to discourage sleeping on the abdomen.
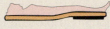

Proper arrangement of pillows for resting or reading in bed.

HOW TO SIT CORRECTLY

A back's best friend is a straight, hard chair. If you can't get the chair you prefer, learn to sit properly on whatever chair you get. To correct sitting position from forward slump: Throw head well back, then bend it forward to pull in the chin. This will straighten the back. Now tighten abdominal muscles to raise the chest. Check position frequently.

Use of footrest relieves swayback. Aim is to have knees higher than hips.

Correct way to sit while driving, close to pedals. Use seatbelt or hard backrest, available commercially.
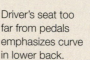

TV slump leads to "dowager's hump," strains neck and shoulders.

If chair is too high, swayback is increased.
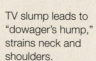

Keep neck and back in as straight a line as possible with the spine. Bend forward from hips.

Driver's seat too far from pedals emphasizes curve in lower back.
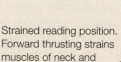

Strained reading position. Forward thrusting strains muscles of neck and head.

Managing Exercise-Related Injuries

To enjoy and maintain physical fitness, preventing injury during a conditioning program is essential. Exercise-related injuries, nonetheless, are common in individuals who participate in exercise programs. Surveys show that more than half of all new exercise participants will incur injuries during the first 6 months of the conditioning program.

The four most common causes of injuries are

1. high-impact activities,
2. rapid conditioning programs—doing too much too quickly,

TABLE 7.2 Reference Guide For Exercise-Related Problems

Injury	Signs/Symptoms	Treatment*
Bruise (contusion)	Pain, swelling, discoloration	Cold application, compression, rest
Dislocations/Fractures	Pain, swelling, deformity	Splinting, cold application, seek medical attention
Heat cramps	Cramps, spasms, and muscle twitching in the legs, arms, and abdomen	Stop activity, get out of the heat, stretch, massage the painful area, drink plenty of fluids
Heat exhaustion	Fainting, profuse sweating, cold/clammy skin, weak/rapid pulse, weakness, headache	Stop activity, rest in a cool place, loosen clothing, rub body with cool/wet towel, drink plenty of fluids, stay out of heat for 2–3 days
Heat stroke	Hot/dry skin, no sweating, serious disorientation, rapid/full pulse, vomiting, diarrhea, unconsciousness, high body temperature	*Seek immediate medical attention,* request help and get out of the sun, bathe in cold water / spray with cold water / rub body with cold towels, drink plenty of cold fluids
Joint sprains	Pain, tenderness, swelling, loss of use, discoloration	Cold application, compression, elevation, rest, heat after 36 to 48 hours (if no further swelling)
Muscle cramps	Pain, spasm	Stretch muscle(s), use mild exercises for involved area
Muscle soreness and stiffness	Tenderness, pain	Mild stretching, low-intensity exercise, warm bath
Muscle strains	Pain, tenderness, swelling, loss of use	Cold application, compression, elevation, rest, heat after 36 to 48 hours (if no further swelling)
Shin splints	Pain, tenderness	Cold application prior to and following any physical activity, rest, heat (if no activity is carried out)
Side stitch	Pain on the side of the abdomen below the rib cage	Decrease level of physical activity or stop altogether, gradually increase level of fitness
Tendonitis	Pain, tenderness, loss of use	Rest, cold application, heat after 48 hours

* Cold should be applied 3 to 4 times a day for 15 minutes. Heat can be applied 3 times a day for 15 to 20 minutes.

3. improper shoes or training surfaces, and
4. anatomical predisposition (body propensity).

The most common causes of injuries, by far, are high-impact activities and a substantial increase in quantity, intensity, and duration of activities. The body requires time to adapt to more intense activities. Most of these injuries could be prevented through a more gradual and proper conditioning program.

The best treatment always has been prevention itself. If an activity is causing unusual discomfort or chronic irritation, you need to treat the cause by decreasing the intensity, switching activities, improving technique, or using better equipment and clothing, such as proper-fitting shoes.

In cases of acute injury, the standard treatment is rest, cold application, compression or splinting (or both), and elevation of the affected body part. This commonly is referred to as RICE:

R = Rest
I = Ice application
C = Compression, and
E = Elevation.

Providing proper rest for the injured area is critical during the recovery process. Cold should be applied three to five times a day for 15 to 20 minutes at a time during the first 24 to 36 hours by submerging the injured area in cold water, using an ice bag, or applying ice massage to the affected part. An elastic bandage or wrap can be used for compression. Elevating the body part decreases blood flow to it.

The purpose of these four types of treatment is to minimize swelling in the area, which hastens recovery time. After the first 36 to 48 hours, heat can be used if there is no further swelling or inflammation. If you have doubts regarding the nature or seriousness of the injury (such as suspected fracture), you should seek a medical evaluation.

Obvious deformities (such as in fractures, dislocations, or partial dislocations) call for splinting, cold application with an ice bag, and medical attention. Never try to reset any of these conditions by yourself, because muscles, ligaments, and nerves could be further damaged. Treatment of these injuries always should be in the hands of specialized medical personnel. A quick reference guide for the signs or symptoms and treatment of exercise-related problems is provided in Table 7.2.

Exercise Intolerance

As you start your exercise program, be sure to stay within the safe limits for participation in exercise. The best method to determine whether you are exercising too strenuously is to check your heart rate and make sure it does not exceed the limits of your target zone. Exercising above this target zone may not be safe for unconditioned or high-risk individuals. You do not have to exercise beyond your target zone to gain the desired benefits for the cardiorespiratory system.

In addition, several physical signs will tell you when you are exceeding functional limitations. These include a rapid or irregular heart rate, difficult breathing, nausea, vomiting, lightheadedness, headaches, dizziness, pale or flushed skin, extreme weakness, lack of energy, shakiness, sore muscles, cramps, and tightness in the chest. If you notice any of these symptoms, you should seek medical attention before continuing your exercise program. When exercising, one of the most important things you need to learn is to listen to your body.

In addition, your recovery heart rate can be an indicator of overexertion. To a certain extent, recovery heart rate is related to fitness level. The higher your cardiorespiratory fitness level, the faster your heart rate will decrease following exercise. As a general rule, heart rate should be below 120 beats per minute 5 minutes into recovery. If your heart rate is above 120, you most likely have overexerted yourself or possibly could have some cardiac abnormality. If you decrease the intensity or duration of exercise and you still have a fast heart rate 5 minutes into recovery, consult your physician.

Leisure-Time Physical Activity

Leisure-time physical activity usually is considered to be any activity undertaken during an individual's discretionary time that helps increase resting energy or caloric expenditure. Although individuals have notable differences, the average person in developed countries has about 3.5 hours of "free" or leisure-time daily. Unfortunately, in the current automated society, many people spend their leisure time in sedentary living.

Leisure-time activities are selected based on personal interests. Typical leisure-time activities are walking, hiking, gardening, yardwork, and moderate sports such as tennis, table tennis, badminton, golf, and croquet. Motivational factors for participation include health, aesthetics, weight control, competition and challenge, fun, social interaction, mental arousal, relaxation, and stress management.

Every small increase in daily physical activity contributes to the development of health and wellness. Small increases in physical activity produce large decreases in the risk for disease and premature death. Therefore, health-conscious people will make a concerted effort to spend their leisure time in activities that promote energy expenditure, provide a break from daily tasks, and contribute to health-related fitness.

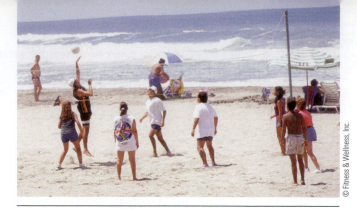

Leisure-time activities should promote energy expenditure and enhance overall health and fitness.

© Fitness & Wellness, Inc.

Behavior Change and Motivation

Scientific evidence of the benefits derived from living a healthy lifestyle continues to mount each day. Notwithstanding the impressive data, most people still do not adhere to a healthy lifestyle. To understand why people do not live a healthy lifestyle, we would do well to examine what motivates people and what actions are required to make permanent changes in behavior. The transtheoretical model presents a series of stages necessary to make lifestyle changes.

TRANSTHEORETICAL MODEL

For most people, changing chronic/unhealthy behaviors to stable/healthy behaviors is a challenge. Change usually does not occur all at once but, rather, is a lengthy process that involves several stages. To aid in this process, psychologists James Prochaska, John Norcross, and Carlo DiClemente developed the **transtheoretical model** for behavior change.[26] This model recognizes six stages in the process of willful change. Most frequently, the model is used to change health-related behaviors such as physical inactivity, smoking, nutrition, weight problems, stress, and alcohol abuse.

The five stages of change in the transtheoretical model are precontemplation, contemplation, preparation, action, and maintenance. A sixth stage was subsequently added —the termination/adoption stage. After years of study, researchers found that applying specific behavioral-change techniques during each stage of the model increases the success rate for change. Understanding each stage of this model will help you determine where you are in relation to your personal healthy-lifestyle behaviors. It also will help you identify techniques to make successful changes.

Precontemplation People in the precontemplation stage are not considering change or do not want to change a given behavior. They typically deny having a problem and have no intent to change. These people usually are unaware or underaware of the problem although people around them—family, friends, health-care practitioners, and co-workers—identify the problem clearly.

Precontemplators do not care about the problem behavior and may even avoid information and materials that address the issue. They tend to avoid free screenings and workshops that could help identify and change the problem. These people frequently have an active resistance to change and seem resigned to accept the unhealthy behavior as "their fate."

These are the most difficult people to reach for behavioral change. They often think that change isn't even a possibility. Educating them about the problem behavior is vital to help them start the process of change. Knowledge is power, and the challenge is to find ways to help them realize that they ultimately will be responsible for the consequences of their behavior. Frequently, they may initiate change only when they are under pressure from others.

Contemplation In the contemplation stage, people acknowledge that they have a problem and begin to seriously think about overcoming it. Although they are not quite ready for change, they are weighing the pros and cons. People may remain in this stage for years, but in their minds they are planning to take some action within the next six months. Education and peer support are valuable during this stage.

Preparation In the preparation stage, people are seriously considering and planning to change a behavior within the next month. They are taking initial steps for change and may even try it for a short while, such as stopping smoking for a day or exercising a few times during this month. In this stage, the person sets a general goal for behavioral change (for example, to quit smoking by the last day of the month) and write specific objectives necessary to accomplish this goal (see Goal Setting, page 150). Continued peer and environmental support are recommended during the preparation phase.

Action The action stage, as the name suggests, requires the greatest commitment of time and energy. Here, the person is actively doing things to change or modify their problem behavior or to adopt a new health behavior. The person is required to follow the specific guidelines set forth for that specific behavior. For example, a person actually has stopped smoking, or is exercising aerobically three times per week according to exercise prescription guidelines, or is maintaining a diet that derives less than 30 percent of its calories from fat. During this stage, relapse is common and the individual may regress to the previous stage. If the individual maintains the action stage for 6 consecutive months, he or she moves into the maintenance stage.

Maintenance During the maintenance stage, the person continues to maintain the behavioral change for up to 5 years. The maintenance phase requires continued adherence to the specific guidelines that govern the behavior (no smoking, exercising aerobically three times per week, or adhering to the healthy diet plan). During this stage the person works to reinforce the gains made through the various stages of change and strives to prevent lapses and **relapse**.

Termination/Adoption Once a behavior has been maintained for at least 5 years, the person is said to be in the termination or adoption phase and exits from the cycle of change without fear of relapse. In the case of negative behaviors that have stopped, the stage of change is referred to as termination. If a positive behavior has been maintained for more than 5 years, this stage is designated as the adoption stage. Many experts believe that after this length of time, any former addictions, problems, or lack of compliance with healthy behaviors no longer present an obstacle in the quest for wellness. The change, now a part of one's lifestyle, is the ultimate goal for everyone searching for a healthier lifestyle.

You may use the form provided in Figure 7.8 to determine where you stand in respect to old behaviors you want to change or new behaviors you wish to adopt. As you use this form, you will realize that you are at different stages for different behaviors. For instance, you may be in the termination stage for aerobic exercise and smoking, in the action stage for strength training, but only in the contemplation stage for a healthy diet. Realizing where you are with respect to different behaviors will help you design a better action plan for a healthy lifestyle.

MOTIVATION AND LOCUS OF CONTROL

Motivation is often set forth as an explanation for why some people succeed and others don't. Although motivation comes from within, external factors trigger the inner desire to accomplish a given task. These external factors, then, control behavior.

When studying motivation, you'll find it helpful to understand people's locus of control. People who believe they have control over events in their lives are said to have an internal locus of control. People with an external locus of control believe that what happens to them is a result of chance—the environment—and is unrelated to their behavior.

Transtheoretical model Behavioral modification model proposing that change is accomplished through a series of progressive stages in keeping with a person's readiness to change.

Relapse To slip or fall back into unhealthy behavior(s) or fail to maintain healthy behaviors.

Motivation The desire and will to do something.

FIGURE 7.8 Identifying Your Current Stage of Change for Behavior Modification

Please indicate which response most accurately describes your current _____ behavior (in the blank space identify the behavior: smoking, physical activity, stress, nutrition, weight control). Next, select the statement below (select only one) that best represents your current behavior pattern. To select the most appropriate statement, fill in the blank for one of the first three statements if your current behavior is a problem behavior. (For example, you may say, "I currently smoke and I do not intend to change in the foreseeable future," or "I currently do not exercise but I am contemplating changing in the next 6 months.") If you have already started to make changes, fill in the blank in one of the last three statements. (In this case, you may say: "I currently eat a low-fat diet but I have only done so within the last 6 months," or "I currently practice adequate stress management techniques and I have done so for over 6 months.") As you can see, you may use this form to identify your stage of change for any type of health-related behavior.

☐ 1. I currently_____ and I do not intend to change in the foreseeable future.

☐ 2. I currently_____ but I am contemplating changing in the next 6 months.

☐ 3. I currently _____ regularly but I intend to change in the next month.

☐ 4. I currently _____ but I have done so only within the last 6 months.

☐ 5. I currently _____ and I have done so for more than 6 months.

☐ 6. I currently _____ and I have done so for more than 5 years.

Stages of Change

1 =	Precontemplation	4 =	Action
2 =	Contemplation	5 =	Maintenance
3 =	Preparation	6 =	Termination/Adoption

People with an internal locus of control are healthier and have an easier time initiating and adhering to a wellness program. In contrast, those who perceive that they have no control think of themselves as powerless and vulnerable. Becoming motivated is often a challenge. These people are also at greater risk for illness. When illness strikes, restoring a sense of control is vital to regain health.

Few people have either a completely external or a completely internal locus of control. They fall somewhere along a continuum, and their location along the continuum relates to their health. Also, the more external the locus of control, the harder it is to adhere to exercise and maintain other healthy lifestyle behaviors.

Fortunately, one can develop a more internal locus of control. Understanding that most events in life are not controlled genetically or environmentally helps people pursue goals and gain control over their lives. Three impediments, however, can keep people from taking action: problems of competence, confidence, and motivation.[27]

1. *Problems of competence.* Lacking the skills to get a given task done leads to less competence. If your friends play basketball regularly but you don't know how to play, you might not be inclined to participate. The solution to the problem of competence is to master the skills needed to participate.

   A college professor continuously watched a group of students play an entertaining game of basketball every Friday at noon. Having no basketball skills, he was reluctant to play. The desire to join in the fun was strong enough that he enrolled in a beginning course at the college to learn to play the game. To his surprise, most students were impressed that he was willing to do this. Now, with greater competence, he is able to join Friday's "pick-up" games.

   Another alternative is to select an activity in which you are skilled. It may not be basketball, but it could well be aerobics. Don't be afraid to try new activities. Similarly, if your body weight is a problem, you could learn to cook low-fat meals. Try different recipes until you find some you like.

2. *Problems of confidence.* When the skills are there but you don't believe you can get it done, problems with confidence arise. Fear and feelings of inadequacy often interfere with the ability to perform the task.

   You should not talk yourself out of something until you have given it a fair try. If you have the skills, the sky is the limit. Initially, try to visualize yourself doing the task and getting it done. Repeat this several times, then give it a try. You will surprise yourself.

   Sometimes, lack of confidence develops when the task appears to be insurmountable. In these situations, dividing a goal into smaller, realistic objectives helps to accomplish the task. You may know how to swim, but swimming a continuous mile may take several weeks to accomplish. Set up your training program so that each day you swim a little farther until you are able to swim the entire mile. If on a given day you don't meet your objective, try it again, reevaluate, cut back a little, and, most important, don't give up.

3. *Problems of motivation.* With problems of motivation, the person has both the competence and the confidence but is unwilling to change because the reasons for change are not important to him or her. For example, people begin contemplating a smoking cessation program only when the reasons for quitting outweigh the reasons for smoking.

When it comes to quality of life, the primary causes of unwillingness to change are a lack of knowledge and lack of goals. Knowledge often determines goals, and goals determine motivation. How badly you want it dictates how hard you'll work at it. Many people are unaware of the magnitude of the benefits of a wellness program. Unfortunately, when it comes to a healthy lifestyle, you may not get a second chance. A stroke, a heart attack, or cancer can lead to irreparable or fatal consequences. Greater understanding of what leads to disease may be all that is needed to initiate change.

Also, feeling physically fit is difficult to explain unless you have experienced it yourself. Feelings of fitness, self-esteem, confidence, health, and quality of life cannot be conveyed to someone who is accustomed to sedentary living. In a way, wellness is like reaching the top of a mountain. The quietness, the clean air, the lush vegetation, the flowing water in the river, the wildlife, and the majestic valley below are difficult to explain to someone who has spent a lifetime within city limits.

Behavior Modification

Over the course of many years, we all develop habits that at some point in time we would like to change. Old habits die hard. **Behavior modification** requires continual effort. The sooner we implement a healthy lifestyle program, the greater the health benefits and quality of life that lie ahead. The following steps provide a pathway to changing behavior.

1. *Self-analysis.* The first step in behavior modification is a decisive desire to do so. If you have no interest in changing a behavior, you won't do it. A person who has no intention of quitting smoking will not quit, regardless of what anyone may say or how strong the evidence is against smoking. In your self-analysis, you may want to prepare a list of reasons for continuing or discontinuing a certain behavior. When the reasons for change outweigh the reasons for not changing, you are ready for the next step.
2. *Behavior analysis.* This means determining the frequency, circumstances, and consequences of the behavior to be altered or implemented. If the desired outcome is to decrease your consumption of fat, you first must find out what foods in your diet are high in fat, when you eat them, and when you don't eat them. Knowing when you don't eat them points to circumstances under which you exert control of your diet and will help as you set goals.

3. *Goal setting.* Goals motivate change in behavior. The stronger the goal (desire), the more motivated you'll be to either change unwanted behaviors or implement new, healthy behaviors. The discussion on goal setting that follows will help you write goals and prepare an action plan to achieve those goals.
4. *Social support.* Surrounding yourself with people who will work with you toward a common goal or will encourage you along the way is immensely helpful. If attempting to quit smoking, for example, you should try to do this with others who also are trying to quit or friends who already have done so. Peer support is a strong incentive for behavioral change.

   During this process, it's equally important to avoid people who will not support you. Friends who have no desire to quit smoking actually may tempt you to smoke and encourage relapse to unwanted behaviors. People who are beyond the goal you are trying to reach may not be supportive either. For instance, someone may say: "I can do six consecutive miles." Your response should be: "I'm proud that I can jog three consecutive miles."
5. *Monitoring.* Sometimes monitoring by itself is sufficient to cause change, because continuous behavior monitoring increases awareness of the desired outcome. For example, keeping track of daily food intake reveals sources of fat in the diet, which can motivate you to cut down gradually or completely eliminate high-fat foods before consuming them. If the goal is to increase the intake of fruit and vegetables, keeping track of the number of servings you eat each day will raise awareness and may help increase their intake.
6. *Positive outlook.* A belief in yourself and your ability to change will aid actual behavior change. Following the guidelines set out in this chapter will help you pace yourself so you can work toward change. Also look at the outcomes—how much healthier you will be, how much better you will look, or how far you will be able to jog, for instance.
7. *Reinforcement.* People tend to repeat behaviors that are rewarded and disregard those that are not rewarded or are punished. For example, if you have been successful in cutting down your fat intake during the week, reward yourself by going to a movie or buying a new pair of shoes. Do not reinforce yourself with destructive behaviors such as eating a high-fat dinner. If you fail to change a desired behavior (or to implement a new one), you may want to put off buying those new shoes. When a positive behavior becomes habitual, give yourself an even better reward. Treat yourself to a vacation weekend, buy a new bike, or get new clothing.

Behavior modification A process to permanently change destructive or negative behaviors and replace them with positive behaviors.

GOAL SETTING

Goals are essential in initiating change. Goals motivate behavioral change and provide a plan of action. Goals are most effective when they are:

- *Well planned.* Only a well-conceived action plan will help you attain your goal. The suggestions concluding this chapter will help you design your plan of action. Your objectives should be both general and specific objectives. The general objective is the ultimate goal you intend to achieve. The specific objectives are the steps required to reach this general objective. For example, a general objective might be to achieve recommended body weight. Several specific objectives could be to (a) lose an average of 1 pound (or 1 fat percentage point) per week; (b) monitor body weight before breakfast every morning; (c) assess body composition every 2 weeks; (d) limit fat intake to less than 25 percent of total calories; (e) eliminate all pastries from the diet during this time; and (f) exercise in the proper target zone for 45 minutes, five times per week.
- *Personalized.* Goals that you set for yourself are more motivational than goals that someone else sets for you.
- *Written.* An unwritten goal is simply a wish. A written goal, in essence, becomes a contract with yourself. Show this goal to a friend or an instructor and have him or her witness, by way of a signature, the contract you made with yourself.
- *Realistic.* Goals should be within reach. If you have not exercised regularly, for example, it would be unrealistic to start a daily exercise program consisting of 45 minutes of step aerobics at a vigorous intensity level. Unattainable goals lead to discouragement and loss of interest. Setting smaller, attainable goals is better.

  At times, even with realistic goals, problems arise. Try to anticipate potential difficulties as much as possible and plan for ways to deal with them. If your goal is to jog 30 minutes on six consecutive days, what are your alternatives if the weather turns bad? Possible solutions are to jog in the rain, find an indoor track, jog at a different time of day when the weather improves, or participate in a different aerobic activity, such as stationary cycling, swimming, or step aerobics.
- *Measurable.* Write your goals so they are clear and state specifically the objective to accomplish. "I will lose weight" is not clear enough and is not measurable. A better example is: "I will decrease my body fat to 17 percent."
- *Time-specific.* A goal always should have a specific date set for completion. This date should be realistic but not too distant in the future.
- *Monitored.* Monitoring your progress as you move toward a goal reinforces behavior. Keeping a physical activity log or doing a body composition assessment periodically determines where you are at any given time.
- *Evaluated.* Periodic reevaluations are vital for success. You may find that a given goal is unreachable. If so,

reassess the goal. Or, if a goal is too easy, you will lose interest and may stop working toward it. Once you achieve a goal, set a new one to improve or maintain what you have achieved. Goals keep you motivated.

Suggestions to Enhance Adherence to Exercise

Different things motivate different people to join and remain in a fitness program. Regardless of the initial reason for beginning a physical activity or an exercise program, you now need to plan for ways to make your workout fun. The psychology behind it is simple: If you enjoy an activity, you will continue to do it. If you don't, you will quit. Some of the following suggestions may help:

- Start your exercise program slowly. Adhering to new behaviors takes time. Don't be discouraged if you can exercise only a few minutes or if you miss one or more exercise sessions. The key to success is perseverance.
- Select aerobic activities you enjoy doing. Choosing an activity you don't enjoy makes you less likely to keep exercising. Don't be afraid to try a new activity, even if that means learning new skills.
- Combine activities. You can train by doing two or three different activities during the same week. Some people find that this counteracts the monotony of repeating the same activity every day. Try **lifetime sports**. Many endurance sports, such as racquetball, basketball, soccer, badminton, in-line skating, cross-country skiing, and surfing (paddling the board), provide a nice break from regular workouts.
- Set aside a regular time for exercise. If you don't plan ahead, exercise is a lot easier to skip. Holding your exercise hour "sacred" will help you adhere to the program.
- Obtain the proper equipment for exercise. A poor pair of shoes, for example, can increase the risk for injury, discouraging you from the very beginning.
- Find a friend or a group of friends to exercise with. Social interaction makes exercise more fulfilling. Besides, exercise is harder to skip if someone else is waiting for you.
- Set goals and share them with others. Quitting is tougher when someone else knows what you are trying to accomplish. When you reach a specific goal, reward yourself with a new pair of shoes or a jogging suit.
- Don't become a chronic exerciser. Learn to listen to your body. Overexercising can lead to chronic fatigue and injuries. Exercise should be enjoyable, and in the process you should "stop and smell the roses."
- Exercise in different places and facilities. This practice adds variety to your workouts.
- Exercise to music. People who listen to fast-tempo music tend to exercise more vigorously and longer.

Using headphones when exercising outdoors, however, can be dangerous. Even indoors, it is preferable not to use headphones so you can still be aware of your surroundings.

- Keep a regular record of your activities so you can monitor your progress and compare it against previous months and years.
- Conduct periodic assessments. Improving to a higher fitness category is a reward in itself.
- If health problems arise, see a physician. When in doubt, "better safe than sorry."
- Exercise for a lifetime. To stay fit, you must maintain a regular exercise program, even during vacations. If you have to interrupt your program for reasons beyond your control, do not attempt to resume your training at the same level you left off. Rather, build up gradually again.

The real challenge will come now: a lifetime commitment to physical activity and exercise. To make the commitment easier, enjoy yourself and have fun along the way. If you base your program on your interests and what you enjoy doing most, adhering to your new, active lifestyle will not be difficult.

Your activities over the next few weeks or months should help you develop positive behaviors that will carry on throughout life. If you truly commit to an active lifestyle and experience the feeling of being physically fit, there will be no looking back. If you don't get there, you won't know what it's like. Fitness and wellness is a process, and you must put forth a constant and deliberate effort to achieve and maintain a higher quality of life. Improving the quality of your life, and most likely your longevity, is in your hands. Only you can take control of your lifestyle and thereby reap the benefits of wellness.

Lifetime sports Activities that a person can do throughout the lifespan.

WEB Interactive

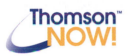

Don't forget to check out the wealth of resources on the ThomsonNOW website at **www.thomsonedu.com/ ThomsonNOW** that will:

- Coach you through identifying target goals for behavior change and monitoring your personal change plan throughout the semester
- Help you evaluate your knowledge of the material
- Allow you to take an exam-prep quiz
- Provide a Personalized Learning Plan targeting resources that address areas you should study.

WEB ACTIVITIES

Muscles Tutorial The following tutorials will allow you to review the names and location of the major superficial muscles.

http://www.gwc.maricopa.edu/class/bio201/muscle/mustut.htm

Sport Specific Exercises Use this helpful site to find exercise programs to increase speed, strength, agility, and power as required for different activities.

http://www.sportspecific.com/

Virtual Fitness Trainer Online personal training without the cost of a one-on-one session. Browse the free articles and create an exercise regimen for any fitness goal.

http://www.virtualfitnesstrainer.com/

InfoTrac®

You can find additional readings related to wellness via InfoTrac® College Edition, an online library of more than 900 journals and publications. Follow the instructions for accessing InfoTrac® that came packaged with your textbook, then search for articles using a key word search.

Suggested Reading Harne, Amanda and Bixby, Walter. "The benefits of and barries to strength training among college-age women," *Journal of Sport Behavior*, June 2005 v28 i2 p151 (16).

1. What are some of the benefits of strength training for women?
2. Do women who do strength training differ from those who don't in their perceptions of these benefits?
3. What do women in this study see as the biggest barrier to strength training? How do you think they can overcome it?

Web Activity

Phys.com calculators

http://www.self.com/fitness/calculators

Sponsor CondéNet, a division of Advance Internet Inc., is the site for the popular *Self* magazine. Consultants for this site include physicians, registered dietitians, exercise specialists, and others.

Description This site features 10 personal assessments in a fun interactive site. Also included are quizzes, exercise slide slows with color photographs and diagrams, a search engine, and an "Ask the Professionals" section.

Available Activities Investigate the many activities at this site, including

1. Personal assessments for your body, including body fat, ideal weight, health risk, fitness, and nutrition (caloric needs, fat needs, protein needs)
2. The Ideal Sport Finder
3. Workouts
4. Motivation Quiz
5. Personal Nutritionist
6. Sports Injury Center

Web Work

1. From the home page, click on each of the links under "Your body."
2. Complete each of the following personal assessments:
   • body mass
   • body fat percentage
   • ideal weight
   • health risk
3. Next, click on the links under the "Nutrition" section and complete each of these personal assessments:
   • caloric needs
   • fat needs
   • protein needs
   • carbohydrate needs
4. Using these directions, complete the other personal assessments.

Helpful Hints

Completion of each of the above interactive links will provide you with a valuable self-assessment on your physical dimension of wellness.

For additional Web activities, links, and suggested readings, visit our Health, Fitness, and Wellness Resource Center at http://health.wadsworth.com.

Notes

1. W. M. Bortz, II, "Disuse and Aging," *Journal of the American Medical Association* 248 (1982): 1203–1208.
2. U.S. Department of Health and Human Services, *Physical Activity and Health: A Report of the Surgeon General* (Atlanta: U.S. Department of Health and Human Services, Centers for Disease Control and Prevention, National Center for Chronic Disease Prevention and Health Promotion, 1996).
3. American College of Sports Medicine, *Guidelines for Exercise Testing and Prescription* (Baltimore: Williams & Wilkins, 2006).
4. See Note 3.
5. G. Borg, "Perceived Exertion: A Note on History and Methods," *Medicine and Science in Sports and Exercise* 5 (1983): 90–93.
6. R. F. DeBusk, U. Stenestrand, M. Sheehan, and W. L. Haskell, "Training Effects of Long Versus Short Bouts of Exercise in Healthy Subjects," *American Journal of Cardiology* 65 (1990): 1010–1013.
7. National Academy of Sciences, Institute of Medicine, *Dietary Reference Intakes for Energy, Carbohydrates, Fiber, Fat, Protein and Amino Acids (Macronutrients)* (Washington, DC: National Academy Press, 2002).
8. U.S. Department of Health and Human Services, Department of Agriculture, *Dietary Guidelines for Americans 2005.* (Washington, DC: DHHS, 2005).
9. American College of Sports Medicine, "Position Stand: The Recommended Quantity and Quality of Exercise for Developing and Maintaining Cardiorespiratory and Muscular Fitness, and Flexibility in Healthy Adults," *Medicine and Science in Sports and Exercise* 30 (1998): 975–991.
10. See Note 2.
11. American College of Sports Medicine, "Position Stand: Exercise and Type 2 Diabetes," *Medicine and Science in Sports and Exercise* 32 (2000): 1345–1360.
12. See Note 9.
13. W. Campbell, M. Crim, V. Young, and W. J. Evans, "Increased Energy Requirements and Changes in Body Composition with Resistance Training in Older Adults," *Journal of Clinical Nutrition* 60 (1994): 167–175.
14. W. S. Evans, "Exercise, Nutrition and Aging," *Journal of Nutrition* 122 (1992): 796–801.
15. W. W. K. Hoeger, D. R. Hopkins, S. L. Barette, and D. F. Hale, "Relationship Between Repetitions and Selected Percentages of One Repetition Maximum: A Comparison Between Untrained and Trained Males and Females," *Journal of Applied Sport Science Research* 4, no. 2 (1990): 47–51.
16. See Note 3.
17. See Note 3.
18. See Note 3.
19. S. A. Plowman, "Physical Fitness and Healthy Low Back Function," *President's Council on Physical Fitness and Sports: Physical Activity and Fitness Research Digest*, Series 1, no. 3 (1993): 3.
20. University of California at Berkeley, *The Wellness Guide to Lifelong Fitness* (New York: Random House, 1993), p. 198.
21. "Stretch Yourself Younger," *Consumer Reports on Health*, 11 (August 1999): 6–7.
22. J. Kokkonen and S. Lauritzen, "Isotonic Strength and Endurance Gains Through PNF Stretching," *Medicine and Science in Sports and Exercise* 27 (1995): S22:127.
23. "Minimizing Back Pain," *Tufts University Health and Nutrition Letter* (New York: The Editors, May 1998).
24. R. Deyo, "Chiropractic Care for Back Pain: The Physician's Perspective," *HealthNews* 4 (September 10, 1998).
25. A. Brownstein, "Chronic Back Pain Can Be Beaten," *Bottom Line/Health* 13 (October 1999): 3–4.
26. J. O. Prochaska, J. C. Norcross, and C. C. DiClemente, *Changing for Good* (New York: William Morrow and Co., 1994).
27. G. S. Howard, D. W. Nance, and P. Myers, *Adaptive Counseling and Therapy* (San Francisco: Jossey-Bass, 1987).

Assess Your Behavior

1. Do you exercise aerobically for 20 to 30 minutes at least three times per week in the appropriate target training zone?
2. Are progressive resistance strength training and stretching included in your weekly exercise program?
3. Do you accumulate 10,000 steps on most days of the week?
4. Do you set goals and regularly evaluate your progress toward these goals in your quest for a healthier lifestyle?

Evaluate how well you understand the concepts presented in this chapter by answering the following questions.

1. Which of the following adaptations occurs with aerobic training?
   a. a higher maximal oxygen uptake.
   b. a lower heart rate at given workloads.
   c. an increase in the number and size of the mitochondria.
   d. All of the above occur with aerobic training.
   e. Only choices a and c occur with aerobic training.

2. Which of the following activities does not contribute to the development of cardiorespiratory endurance?
   a. low-impact aerobics
   b. jogging
   c. 400-yard dash
   d. racquetball
   e. All of the activities contribute to its development.

3. The recommended cardiorespiratory training zone for a 22-year-old person is between
   a. 98 and 152 beats per minute.
   b. 102 and 160 beats per minute.
   c. 106 and 172 beats per minute.
   d. 109 and 178 beats per minute.
   e. 118 and 182 beats per minute.

4. The recommended duration for each cardiorespiratory endurance training session is
   a. 10 to 20 minutes.
   b. 15 to 30 minutes.
   c. 20 to 60 minutes.
   d. 45 to 70 minutes.
   e. 60 to 120 minutes.

5. The training concept that states that the demands placed on a system must be increased systematically and progressively over time to cause physiological adaptation is referred to as
   a. the overload principle.
   b. positive resistance training.
   c. specificity of training.
   d. variable-resistance training.
   e. progressive resistance.

6. General strength-training guidelines state that sufficient resistance should be used to perform each set between
   a. 1 and 3 reps to complete or near complete fatigue.
   b. 2 and 10 reps to complete or near complete fatigue.
   c. 3 and 20 reps to complete or near complete fatigue.
   d. 10 and 30 reps to complete or near complete fatigue.
   e. 15 and 40 reps to complete or near complete fatigue.

7. Which of the following is not a mode of stretching?
   a. elastic elongation
   b. proprioceptive neuromuscular facilitation
   c. ballistic stretching
   d. slow-sustained stretching
   e. All are modes of stretching.

8. When you perform stretching exercises, the degree of stretch should be
   a. to tightness at the end of the range of motion.
   b. to 80 percent of capacity.
   c. to the point of significant discomfort.
   d. applied until the muscle(s) start shaking.
   e. progressively increased until the muscle(s) fatigue.

9. Low-back pain is associated with
   a. physical inactivity.
   b. faulty posture.
   c. excessive body weight.
   d. improper body mechanics.
   e. All are correct choices.

10. A goal is effective when it is
    a. written.
    b. measurable.
    c. time-specific.
    d. monitored.
    e. All are correct choices.

Correct answers can be found on page 369.

Exercise 1 Step-up

Action

Step up and down using a box or chair approximately 12 to 15 inches high (A). Conduct one set using the same leg each time you step up, and then conduct a second set using the other leg. You also could alternate legs on each step-up cycle. You may increase the resistance by holding an object in your arms (B). Hold the object close to the body to avoid increased strain in the lower back.

Muscles Developed

Gluteal muscles, quadriceps, gastrocnemius, and soleus

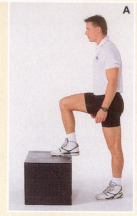
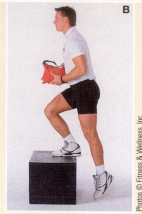

Exercise 2 Rowing Torso

Action

Raise your arms laterally (abduction) to a horizontal position and bend your elbows to 90°. Have a partner apply enough pressure on your elbows to gradually force your arms forward (horizontal flexion) while you try to resist the pressure. Next, reverse the action, horizontally forcing the arms backward as your partner applies sufficient forward pressure to create resistance.

Muscles Developed

Posterior deltoid, rhomboids, and trapezius

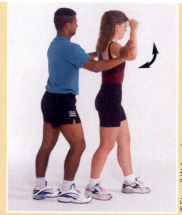

Exercise 3 Push-up

Action

Maintaining your body as straight as possible (A), flex the elbows, lowering the body until you almost touch the floor (B), then raise yourself back up to the starting position. If you are unable to perform the push-up as indicated, decrease the resistance by supporting the lower body with the knees rather than the feet (C) or using an incline plane and supporting your hands at a higher point than the floor (D). If you wish to increase the resistance, have someone else add resistance to your shoulders as you are coming back up (E).

Muscles Developed

Triceps, deltoid, pectoralis major, abdominals, and erector spinae

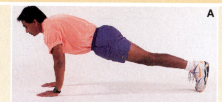
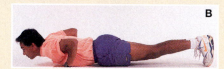
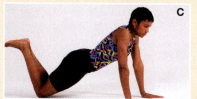
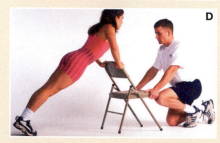
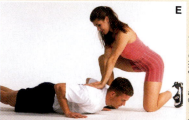

Exercise 4 Abdominal Crunch and Bent-leg Curl-up

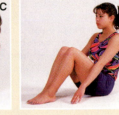

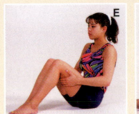

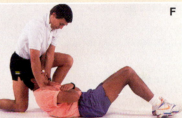

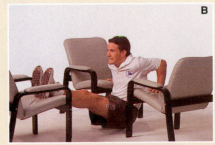

Action

Start with your head and shoulders off the floor, arms crossed on your chest, and knees slightly bent (A). The greater the flexion of the knee, the more difficult the curl-up. Now curl up to about 30°—abdominal crunch (illustration B)—or curl up all the way—abdominal curl-up (illustration C), then return to the starting position without letting the head or shoulders touch the floor or allowing the hips to come off the floor. If you allow the hips to raise off the floor and the head and shoulders to touch the floor, you most likely will "swing up" on the next crunch or curl-up, which minimizes the work of the abdominal muscles. If you cannot curl up with the arms on the chest, place the hands by the side of the hips or even help yourself up by holding on to your thighs (illustrations D and E). Do not perform the sit-up exercise with your legs completely extended, because this will strain the lower back. For additional resistance during the abdominal crunch, have a partner add slight resistance to your shoulders as you "crunch up" (illustration F).

Muscles Developed

Abdominal muscles and hip flexors

Note

The abdominal curl-up exercise should be used only by individuals of at least average fitness without a history of lower back problems. New participants and those with a history of lower back problems should use the abdominal crunch exercise in its place.

Exercise 5 Leg Curl

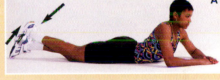

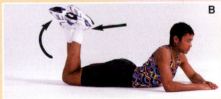

Action

Lie on the floor face down. Cross the right ankle over the left heel (A). Apply resistance with your right foot while you bring the left foot up to 90° at the knee joint (B). Apply enough resistance so the left foot can only be brought up slowly. Repeat the exercise, crossing the left ankle over the right heel.

Muscles Developed

Hamstrings (and quadriceps)

Exercise 6 Modified Dip

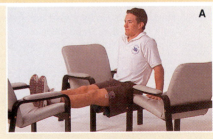

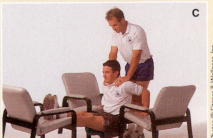

Action

Place your hands on opposite chairs; feet on a third chair with knees slightly bent (make sure that the chairs are well stabilized—see illustration A). Dip down at least to a 90° angle at the elbow joint (see illustration B), then return to the initial position. To increase the resistance, have someone else hold you down by the shoulders on the way up (see illustration C). You may also perform this exercise using a gymnasium bleacher or box and with the help of a partner.

Muscles Developed

Triceps, deltoid, and pectoralis major

Exercise 7   Pull-Up

Action

Suspend yourself from a bar with a pronated (thumbs-in) grip (A). Pull your body up until your chin is above the bar (B), then lower the body slowly to the starting position. If you are unable to perform the pull-up as described, either have a partner hold your feet to push off and facilitate the movement upward (illustrations C and D) or use a lower bar and support your feet on the floor (E).

Muscles Developed

Biceps, brachioradialis, brachialis, trapezius, and latissimus dorsi

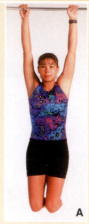
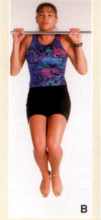
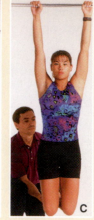
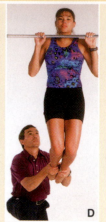
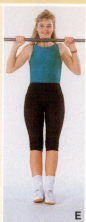

A   B   C   D   E

Photos © Fitness & Wellness, Inc.

Exercise 8   Arm Curl

Action

Using a palms-up grip, start with the arm completely extended and, with the aid of a sandbag or bucket filled (as needed) with sand or rocks (A), curl up as far as possible (B), then return to the initial position. Repeat the exercise with the other arm.

Muscles Developed

Biceps, brachioradialis, and brachialis

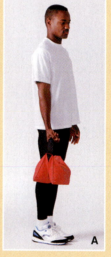
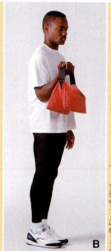

A   B

Photos © Fitness & Wellness, Inc.

Exercise 9   Heel Raise

Action

From a standing position with feet flat on the floor (A), raise and lower your body weight by moving at the ankle joint only (B). For added resistance, have someone else hold your shoulders down as you perform the exercise.

Muscles Developed

Gastrocnemius and soleus

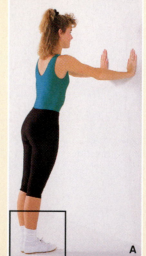
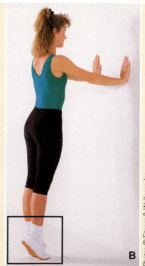

A   B

Photos © Fitness & Wellness, Inc.

Exercise 10   Leg Abduction and Adduction

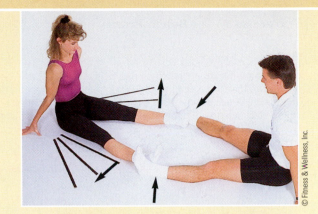

Action

Both participants sit on the floor. The person on the left places the feet on the inside of the other person's feet. Simultaneously, the person on the left presses the legs laterally (to the outside—abduction), while the person on the right presses the legs medially (adduction). Hold the contraction for 5 to 10 seconds. Repeat the exercise at all three angles, and then reverse the pressing sequence. The person on the left places the feet on the outside and presses inward, while the person on the right presses outward.

Muscles Developed

Hip abductors (rectus femoris, sartori, gluteus medius and minimus) and adductors (pectineus, gracilis, adductor magnus, adductor longus, and adductor brevis)

© Fitness & Wellness, Inc.

Exercise 11   Pelvic Tilt

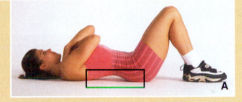
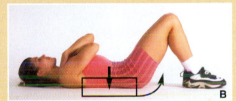
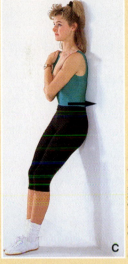

Action

Lie flat on the floor with the knees bent at about a 90° angle (A). Tilt the pelvis by tightening the abdominal muscles, flattening your back against the floor, and raising the lower gluteal area ever so slightly off the floor (B). Hold the final position for several seconds. The exercise can also be performed against a wall (C).

Areas Stretched

Low back muscles and ligaments

Areas Strengthened

Abdominal and gluteal muscles

Photos © Fitness & Wellness, Inc.

EXERCISES   Strength-Training with Weights

Exercise 12   Arm Curl

Action

Using a supinated (palms-up) grip, start with the arms almost completely extended (A). Curl up as far as possible (B), then return to the starting position.

Muscles Developed

Biceps, brachioradialis, and brachialis

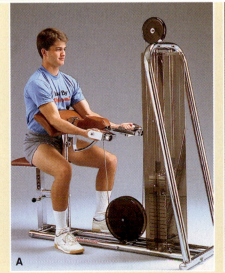
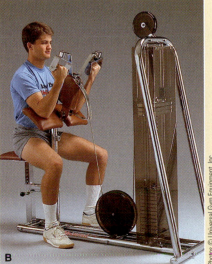

Photos © Universal Gym Equipment, Inc.

Exercise 13   Bench Press

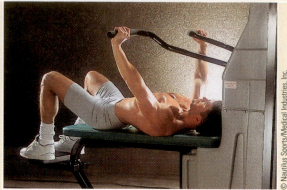

Action

Lie down on the bench with the head by the weight stack, the bench press bar above the chest, and the knees bent so the feet rest on the far end of the bench. Grasp the bar handles and press upward until the arms are completely extended, then return to the original position. Do not arch the back during this exercise.

Muscles Developed

Pectoralis major, triceps, and deltoid

Exercise 14   Abdominal Crunch and Bent-leg Curl-up

See Exercise 4 in this chapter.

Exercise 15   Leg Extension

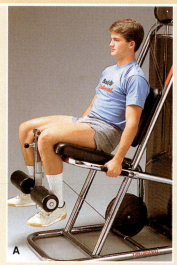
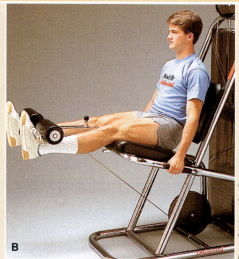

Action

Sit in an upright position with the feet under the padded bar and grasp the handles at the sides (A). Extend the legs until they are completely straight (B), then return to the starting position.

Muscles Developed

Quadriceps

A   B

Exercise 16   Leg Curl

Action

Lie with the face down on the bench, legs straight, and place the back of the feet under the padded bar (A). Curl up to at least 90° (B), and return to the original position.

Muscles Developed

Hamstrings

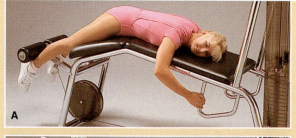

A

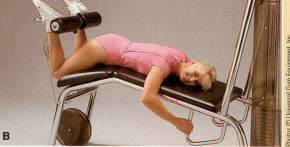

B

Exercise 17   Lat Pull-Down

Action

Starting from a sitting position, hold the exercise bar with a wide grip (A). Pull the bar down until it reaches the base of the neck (B), then return to the starting position. (If heavy resistance is used, stabilization of the body may be required either by using equipment as shown or by having someone else hold you down by the waist or shoulders.)

Muscles Developed

Latissimus dorsi, pectoralis major, and biceps

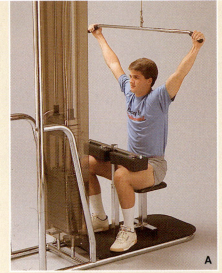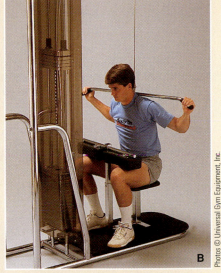

Photos © Universal Gym Equipment, Inc.

Exercise 18   Heel Raise

Action

Start with your feet either flat on the floor or the front of the feet on an elevated block (A), then raise and lower yourself by moving at the ankle joint only (B). If additional resistance is needed, you can use a squat strength-training machine.

Muscles Developed

Gastrocnemius, soleus

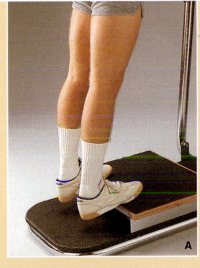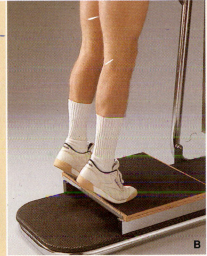

Photos © Universal Gym Equipment, Inc.

Exercise 19   Rowing Torso

Action

Sit in the machine with your arms in front of you, elbows bent and resting against the padded bars (A). Press back as far as possible, drawing the shoulder blades together (B). Return to the original position.

Muscles Developed

Posterior deltoid, rhomboids, and trapezius

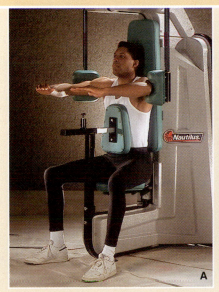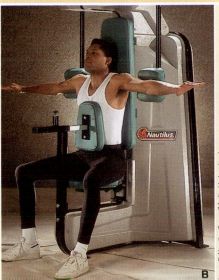

Photos © Nautilus Sports/Medical Industries, Inc.

Exercise 20 · Bent-Arm Pull-Over

Action

Sit back into the chair and grasp the bar behind your head (A). Pull the bar over your head all the way down to your abdomen (B), and slowly return to the original position.

Muscles Developed

Latissimus dorsi, pectoral muscles, deltoid, and serratus anterior

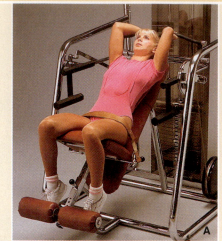
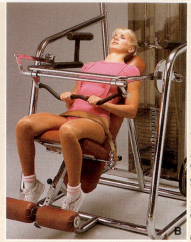

A

B

Photos © Universal Gym Equipment, Inc.

EXERCISES Flexibility

Exercise 21 · Lateral Head Tilt

Action

Slowly and gently tilt the head laterally. Repeat several times to each side.

Areas Stretched

Neck flexors and extensors and ligaments of the cervical spine

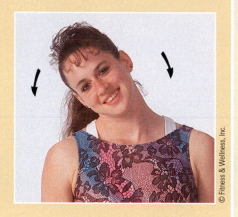

© Fitness & Wellness, Inc.

Exercise 22 · Arm Circles

Action

Gently circle your arms all the way around. Conduct the exercise in both directions.

Areas Stretched

Shoulder muscles and ligaments

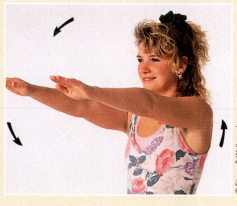

© Fitness & Wellness, Inc.

Exercise 23 · Side Stretch

Action

Stand straight up, feet separated to shoulder width, and place your hands on your waist. Now move the upper body to one side and hold the final stretch for a few seconds. Repeat on the other side.

Areas Stretched

Muscles and ligaments in the pelvic region

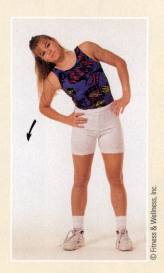

© Fitness & Wellness, Inc.

Exercise 24 · Body Rotation

Action

Place your arms slightly away from your body, and rotate the trunk as far as possible, holding the final position for several seconds. Conduct the exercise for both the right and left sides of the body. You also can perform this exercise by standing about 2 feet away from the wall (back toward the wall) and then rotating the trunk, placing the hands against the wall.

Areas Stretched

Hip, abdominal, chest, back, neck, and shoulder muscles; hip and spinal ligaments

© Fitness & Wellness, Inc.

Exercise 25   Chest Stretch

Action

Place your hand on the shoulder of your partner who will in turn push you down by your shoulders. Hold the final position for a few seconds.

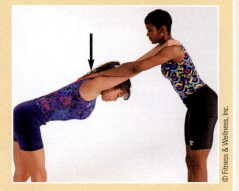

Areas Stretched

Chest (pectoral) muscles; shoulder ligaments

Exercise 26   Shoulder Hyperextension Stretch

Action

Have a partner grasp your arms from behind by the wrists and slowly push them upward. Hold the final position for a few seconds.

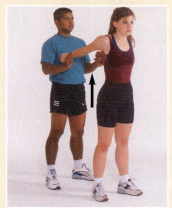

Areas Stretched

Deltoid and pectoral muscles; ligaments of the shoulder joint

---

Exercise 27   Shoulder Rotation Stretch

Action

With the aid of surgical tubing or an aluminum or wood stick, place the tubing or stick behind your back and grasp the two ends using a reverse (thumbs-out) grip. Slowly bring the tubing or stick over your head, keeping the elbows straight. Repeat several times (bring the hands closer together for additional stretch).

Areas Stretched

Deltoid, latissimus dorsi, and pectoral muscles; shoulder ligaments

---

Exercise 28   Quad Stretch

Action

Lie on your side and move one foot back by flexing the knee. Grasp the front of the ankle and pull the ankle toward the gluteal region. Hold for several seconds. Repeat with the other leg.

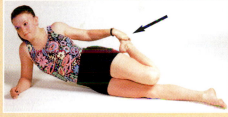

Areas Stretched

Quadriceps muscle; knee and ankle ligaments

Exercise 29   Heel Cord Stretch

Action

Stand against the wall or at the edge of a step, and stretch the heel downward, alternating legs. Hold the stretched position for a few seconds.

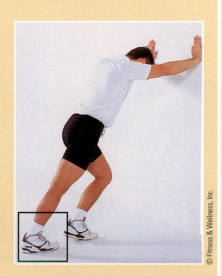

Areas Stretched

Heel cord (Achilles tendon), gastrocnemius and soleus muscles

---

Exercise 30   Adductor Stretch

Action

Stand with your feet about twice shoulder width and place your hands slightly above the knee. Flex one knee and slowly go down, holding the final position for a few seconds. Repeat with the other leg.

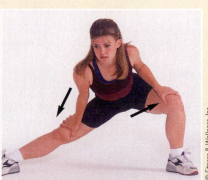

Areas Stretched

Hip adductor muscles

Exercise 31   Sitting Adductor Stretch

Action

Sit on the floor and bring your feet in close to you, allowing the soles of the feet to touch each other. Now place your forearms (or elbows) on the inner part of the thigh and push the legs downward, holding the final stretch for several seconds.

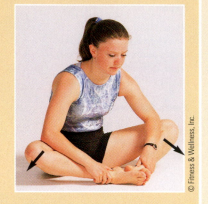

Areas Stretched

Hip adductor muscles

Exercise 32   Sit-and-Reach Stretch

Action

Sit on the floor with legs together and gradually reach forward as far as possible. Hold the final position for a few seconds. This exercise also may be performed with the legs separated, reaching to each side as well as to the middle.

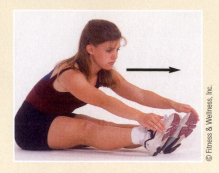

Areas Stretched

Hamstrings and lower back muscles; lumbar spine ligaments

Exercise 33   Triceps Stretch

Action

Place the right hand behind your neck. Grasp the right arm above the elbow with the left hand. Gently pull the elbow backward. Repeat the exercise with the opposite arm.

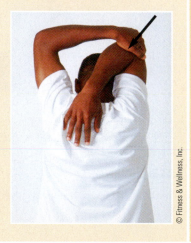

Areas Stretched

Back of upper arm (triceps muscle); shoulder joint

NOTE

Exercises 34 through 41 are also flexibility exercises and can be added to your stretching program.

EXERCISES   For the Prevention and Rehabilitation of Low-Back Pain

Exercise 34   Single-Knee-to-Chest Stretch

Action

Lie down flat on the floor. Bend one leg at approximately 100° and gradually pull the opposite leg toward your chest. Hold the final stretch for a few seconds. Switch legs and repeat the exercise.

Areas Stretched

Lower back and hamstring muscles; lumbar spine ligaments

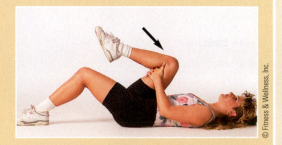

Exercise 35   Double-Knee-to-Chest Stretch

Action

Lie flat on the floor and then curl up slowly into a fetal position. Hold for a few seconds.

Areas Stretched

Upper and lower back and hamstring muscles; spinal ligaments

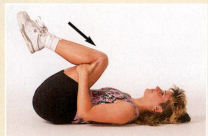

Exercise 36   Upper and Lower Back

Action

Sit on the floor and bring your feet in close to you, allowing the soles of the feet to touch each other. Holding on to your feet, bring your head and upper chest gently toward your feet.

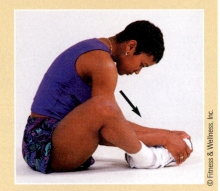

Areas Stretched

Upper and lower back muscles and ligaments

Exercise 37   Sit-and-Reach Stretch

See Exercise 32 in this chapter.

Exercise 38   Back Extension Stretch

Action

Lie face down on the floor with the elbows by the chest, forearms on the floor, and the hands beneath the chin. Gently raise the trunk by extending the elbows until you reach an approximate 90° angle at the elbow joint. Be sure the forearms remain in contact with the floor at all times. *Do not* extend the back beyond this point. Hyperextension of the lower back may lead to or aggravate an existing back problem. Hold the stretched position for about 10 seconds.

Areas Stretched

Abdominal region

Additional Benefits

Restore lower back curvature

Exercise 39   Gluteal Stretch

Action

Sit on the floor, bend your right leg and place your right ankle slightly above the left knee. Grasp the left thigh with both hands and gently pull the leg toward your chest. Repeat the exercise with the opposite leg.

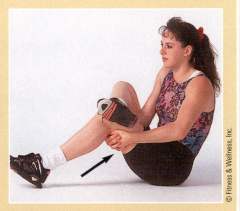

Areas Stretched

Buttock area (gluteal muscles)

Exercise 40   Trunk Rotation and Lower Back Stretch

Action

Sit on the floor and bend the right leg, placing the right foot on the outside of the left knee. Place the left elbow on the right knee and push against it. At the same time, try to rotate the trunk to the right (clockwise). Hold the final position for a few seconds. Repeat the exercise with the other side.

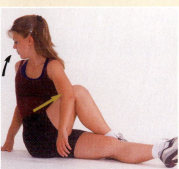

Areas Stretched

Lateral side of the hip and thigh; trunk and lower back

Exercise 41   Hip Flexors Stretch

Action

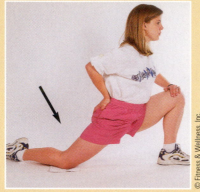

Kneel down on an exercise mat, a soft surface, or a folded towel under your knees. Raise the left knee off the floor and place the left foot about 3 feet in front of you. Place your left hand over your left knee and the right hand over the back of the right hip. Keeping the lower back flat, slowly move forward and downward as you apply gentle pressure over the right hip. Repeat the exercise with the opposite leg forward.

Areas Stretched

Flexor muscles in front of the hip joint

Exercise 42   Pelvic Tilt

See Exercise 11 in this chapter.

NOTE:

This is the most important exercise for use in prevention and treatment of low-back pain. This exercise should be incorporated as a part of your daily physical activity and exercise program.

Exercise 43   Abdominal Crunch and Bent-leg Curl-up

See Exercise 4 in this chapter.

NOTE:

It is important that you do not stabilize your feet when performing either of these exercises, because doing so decreases the work of the abdominal muscles. Also, remember not to "swing up" but rather to curl up as you perform these exercises.

Exercise 44   Back Extension

Action

Place your feet under the ankle rollers and the hips over the padded seat. Start with the trunk in a flexed position and the arms crossed over the chest (A). Slowly extend the trunk to a horizontal position (B), hold the extension for 2 to 5 seconds, then slowly flex (lower) the trunk to the original position.

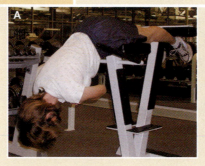
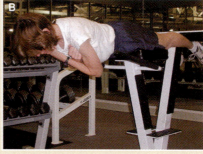

Muscles Developed

Erector spinae, gluteus maximus, and quadratus lumborum (lower back)

Exercise 45   Supine Bridge

Action

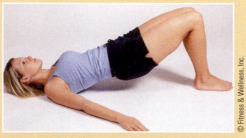

Lie face up on the floor with the knees bent at about 120°. Do a pelvic tilt (Exercise 11) and maintain the pelvic tilt while you raise the hips off the floor until the upper body and upper legs are in a straight line. Hold this position for up to 5 seconds.

Areas Strengthened

Gluteal and abdominal flexor muscles

Exercise 46   Pelvic Clock

Action

Lie face up on the floor with the knees bent at about 120°. Fully extend the hips as in the supine bridge (Exercise 45). Now progressively rotate the hips in a clockwise manner (2 o'clock, 4 o'clock, 6 o'clock, 8 o'clock, 10 o'clock, and 12 o'clock), holding each position in an isometric contraction for about 1 second. Repeat the exercise counter-clockwise.

Areas Strengthened

Gluteal, abdominal, and hip flexor muscles

Daily Physical Activity Log

Name: _____   Date: _____   Grade: _____

Instructor: _____   Course: _____   Section: _____

Date: [_____]   Day of the Week: [_____]

Time of Day	Exercise/Activity	Duration	Number of Steps	Comments

Totals: [_____] [_____] 🚶

Activity category based on steps per day (use Table 1.2, page 15): [_____]

Date: [_____]   Day of the Week: [_____]

Time of Day	Exercise/Activity	Duration	Number of Steps	Comments

Totals: [_____] [_____] 🚶

Activity category based on steps per day (use Table 1.2, page 15): [_____]

Date: _____   Day of the Week: _____

Time of Day	Exercise/Activity	Duration	Number of Steps	Comments

Totals: _____   _____ 🚶

Activity category based on steps per day (use Table 1.2, page 15): _____

Date: _____   Day of the Week: _____

Time of Day	Exercise/Activity	Duration	Number of Steps	Comments

Totals: _____   _____ 🚶

Activity category based on steps per day (use Table 1.2, page 15): _____

Briefly evaluate your current activity patterns, discuss your feelings about the results, and provide a goal for the weeks ahead.

_____
_____
_____
_____
_____
_____
_____

Cardiorespiratory Exercise Prescription

Name: _____   **Date:** _____   **Grade:** _____

Instructor: _____   **Course:** _____   **Section:** _____

Intensity of exercise

1. Estimate your own maximal heart rate (MHR)

$$MHR = 220 \text{ minus age } (220 - \text{age})$$

MHR = 220 − [_____] = [_____] bpm

2. Training intensities (TI) = MHR × TI

55% TI = [_____] × .55 = [_____] bpm

65% TI = [_____] × .65 = [_____] bpm

90% TI = [_____] × .90 = [_____] bpm

3. Cardiorespiratory Training Zone. The recommended cardiorespiratory training zone is found between the 55% and 90% training intensities. Individuals who have been physically inactive or are in the poor or fair cardiorespiratory fitness categories should use the 55% training intensity during the first few weeks of the exercise program.

Recommended Cardiorespiratory Training Zone:

Moderate Intensity = [_____] bpm (55%TI) to [_____] bpm (65% TI)

High Intensity = [_____] bpm (65%TI) to [_____] bpm (90% TI)

Rate of Perceived Exertion (see Figure 7.2, page 132):

[_____] to [_____]

Mode of Exercise

Select any activity or combination of activities that you enjoy doing. The activity has to be continuous in nature and must get your heart rate up to your recommended cardiorespiratory training zone and keep it there for as long as you exercise. Indicate your preferred mode(s) of exercise:

1. [_____]   **2.** [_____]   **3.** [_____]

4. [_____]   **5.** [_____]   **6.** [_____]

Duration and Frequency of Exercise

Please indicate how long each exercise session will last, the days of the week, and the time of day that you will exercise.

Duration: [_____] minutes

Select the days of the week and time of day that you will exercise.

☐ Monday [___:___]   ☐ Tuesday [___:___]   ☐ Wednesday [___:___]   ☐ Thursday [___:___]

☐ Friday [___:___]   ☐ Saturday [___:___]   ☐ Sunday [___:___]

Exercise Site(s) and Friends

Indicate place(s) where you will exercise:

_____

_____

_____

List the friends that will exercise with you

_____

_____

_____

Cardiorespiratory Exercise Training and Rate of Perceived Exertion

Perform an aerobic exercise workout and exercise at the perceived exertion intensities listed below. Following 5 minutes of exercise at those perceived exertion intensities, check your pulse and determine your exercise heart rate.

Physical activity performed: _____

Perceived Exertion	10-second pulse	Exercise Heart Rate (bpm)
Fairly light		
Somewhat hard		
Hard		

Indicate how your own perceived exertion during this activity relates to the RPE scale. Were your exercise heart rates as expected on the RPE scale? If not, what conclusion can you draw from your perceived exertion and your recommended exercise intensity computed in this assessment?

_____

_____

_____

_____

_____

_____

_____

_____

_____

_____

_____

_____

_____

Muscular Strength / Endurance Prescription

Name: _____   Date: _____   Grade: _____

Instructor: _____   Course: _____   Section: _____

Necessary Lab Equipment

No equipment if the "Strength-Training Exercises without Weights" program is selected. Strength-training machines or free weights if "Strength-Training Exercises with Weights" are used.

Objective

Write a strength-training exercise program that may be carried out throughout life.

Lab Preparation

Wear exercise clothing and prepare to participate in a sample strength-training exercise session. All of the strength-training exercises are illustrated in this chapter on pages 154–160.

Instructions

Select one of the two strength-training exercise programs. Perform all of the recommended exercises and, with the exception of the bent-leg curl-up or abdominal crunch exercises, determine the resistance required to do approximately 10 repetitions maximum (for "Strength Training Exercises without Weights," simply indicate the total number of repetitions performed). For the bent-leg curl-up and abdominal crunch exercises, perform or build up to about 20 repetitions.

I. Strength-Training without Weights

Exercise	Repetitions	Sets
Step-up		
Rowing torso		
Push-up		
Abdominal crunch or Bent-leg curl-up (select one)		
Leg curl		
Modified dip		
Pull-up or Arm curl (select one)		
Heel raise		
Leg abduction and adduction		
Pelvic tilt		
Supine bridge		
Pelvic clock		

II. Strength-Training with Weights*

Exercise	Repetitions	Resistance
Arm curl		
Bench press		
Abdominal crunch or Bent-leg curl-up (select one)		
Leg extension		
Leg curl		
Lat pull-down		
Heel raise		
Rowing torso		
Bent-arm pullover		
Back extension		

*Most of these exercises can also be performed with free weights.

III. Days of the week that you will strength-train:

☐ M   ☐ T   ☐ W   ☐ TH   ☐ F   ☐ S   ☐ SU

IV. Muscular Strength Workout

Perform a strength-training workout according to the program you have developed. If you are not strength-training regularly, be sure to perform only one set of each exercise using light resistances only. Briefly explain your experience and indicate the exercise, resistances, repetitions, and number of sets performed. Also indicate how you felt during the workout, a few hours later, and the day thereafter.

Muscular Flexibility Prescription

Name: _____ **Date:** _____ **Grade:** _____

Instructor: _____ **Course:** _____ **Section:** _____

Necessary Lab Equipment

Minor implements such as a chair, a table, an elastic band (surgical tubing or a wood or aluminum stick), and a stool or steps.

Objective

To introduce the participant to a sample stretching exercise program that may be carried out throughout life.

Instructions

Wear exercise clothing and prepare to participate in a sample stretching exercise session. All of the flexibility exercises are illustrated in this chapter on pages 160–162).

Introduction

Perform all of the recommended flexibility exercises given in Chapter 7. Use a combination of slow-sustained and proprioceptive neuromuscular facilitation stretching techniques. Indicate the technique(s) used for each exercise, and, where applicable, the number of repetitions performed and the length of time that the final degree of stretch was held.

I. Stretching Exercises

Exercise	Stretching Technique[1]	Repetitions	Length of Final Stretch
Lateral head tilt			NA[2]
Arm circles			NA
Side stretch			NA
Body rotation			
Chest stretch			
Shoulder hyperextension stretch			
Shoulder rotation stretch			NA
Quad stretch			
Heel cord stretch			
Adductor stretch			
Sitting adductor stretch			
Sit-and-reach stretch			
Triceps stretch			
Single-knee-to-chest stretch			

[1]SSS = Slow-sustained stretching, PNF = Proprioceptive neuromuscular facilitation
[2]Not Applicable

Exercise	Stretching Technique[1]	Repetitions	Length of Final Stretch
Double-knee-to-chest stretch			
Upper and lower back stretch			
Back extension stretch			
Gluteal stretch			
Trunk rotation and lower back stretch			
Hip flexors stretch			

II. Days of the week that you will strength train:

☐ M   ☐ T   ☐ W   ☐ TH   ☐ F   ☐ S   ☐ SU

III. Stretching Program

Using the flexibility program that you have designed, perform a stretching exercise session. Briefly explain your experience with this program and your feelings about your present flexibility level and potential implications for your future fitness and health.

_____
_____
_____
_____
_____
_____
_____
_____
_____
_____
_____
_____
_____
_____
_____
_____

8

CHAPTER

Nutrition and Wellness

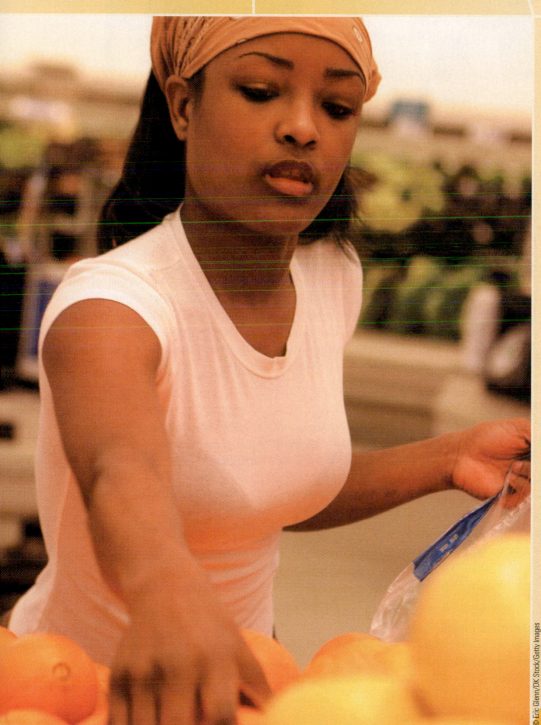

© Eric Glenn/DK Stock/Getty Images

OBJECTIVES

Identify the trends and eating habits of the average American and discuss why we choose to eat the foods we do.

List the six basic elements of nutrition and define their functions and sources.

Identify the types of fat and the roles of fat in the body.

Differentiate the types of carbohydrates and the role of fiber in the body.

Identify the types of vitamins and their sources and functions.

Identify the minerals the body needs, their sources, and their functions.

Describe the DRI and its four values: estimated average requirement, recommended dietary allowance, adequate intake, and tolerable upper intake.

Discuss consumer concerns about the quality and safety of foods, including additives, irradiation, and food-borne illnesses.

Describe the Food Guide and MyPyramid.

FIGURE 8.1 Living Large: U.S. Trend Toward Colossal Cuisine

Food	Typical 1970s	Today's Colossal
Cola	10 oz bottle, 120 cal	40–60 oz fountain, 580 cal
French fries	about 30, 475 cal	about 50, 790 cal
Hamburger	3–4 oz meat, 330 cal	6–12 oz meat, 1,000 cal
Bagel	2–3 oz, 230 cal	5–7 oz, 550 cal
Steak	8–12 oz, 690 cal	16–22 oz, 1,260 cal
Pasta	1 c, 200 cal	2–3 c, 600 cal
Baked potato	5–7 oz, 180 cal	1 lb, 420 cal
Candy bar	1½ oz, 220 cal	3–4 oz, 580 cal
Popcorn	1 c, 80 cal	8–16 c tub, 880 cal

NOTE: Calories are rounded values for the largest portions in a given range.

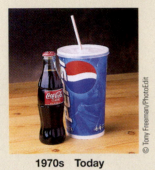
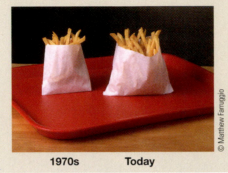
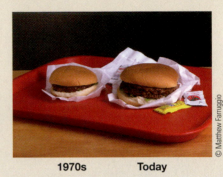

1970s   Today   1970s   Today   1970s   Today

Eating is so habitual that people hardly give it any thought, yet you choose when to eat, what to eat, and how much to eat about 1,000 times a year and 70,000 times in a lifetime. A single day's intake of nutrients may affect body organs and their functions only slightly, but over years and decades, the effects of those intakes are cumulative. Sound **nutrition** contributes to a long and healthy life.

Nutrition and Nutrients

Your body renews its structures continuously. Each day it replaces some old muscle, bone, skin, and blood with new tissues. In this way, the food you eat today becomes part of your body tomorrow. The best foods for you, then, are those that support growth and maintenance of strong muscles, sound bones, and healthy skin, and produce sufficient blood to cleanse and nourish all parts of your body.

Your food choices combine with other life choices to create a pattern that raises or lowers your chances of developing diseases and determining how long you will live. Good nutrition has the twofold effect of promoting health and helping prevent disease. To manage nutrition to your benefit, you have to learn what foods to eat, as not all are equally nutritious. You will want to avoid undernutrition—reducing your intake of food severely enough to cause disease or to make you more susceptible to disease.[1] For example, a condition related to undernutrition is iron-deficiency anemia.

At the same time, overnutrition threatens people's health. Overnutrition is overconsuming food **energy** or

nutrients sufficiently to cause disease or susceptibility to disease. An obvious example is obesity, and more subtle manifestations result from eating so much that you consistently gain weight each year without noticing it, rather than maintaining a healthy body weight.

Overeating is easy these days, in part because portions of many foods and beverages are substantially larger than they used to be and most of us are not active enough to burn the extra calories.[2] A portion (the amount of food actually served or taken) may have little in common with the food's serving size as listed on the label or recommended by Registered Dietitians. In addition, about one-third of our calories are consumed away from home, where servings are large.[3] Figure 8.1 displays the trend in the United States toward consuming larger food portions, especially of foods high in sugar and fat.

Another form of overnutrition is excessive intakes of vitamins and minerals. A person is unlikely to take in excessive levels of vitamins and minerals through foods. This form of overnutrition usually occurs from uninformed intakes of vitamin or mineral supplements (see pages 195–196).

Some people consume too few vegetables and fruits and too much meat; other people consume inadequate servings of calcium-rich foods including dairy products.

Food Choices

Because your accumulated food choices profoundly influence your health, your time will be well spent in questioning why you eat when you do, why you choose the

Eating Healthy at Fast-food Restaurants

If much of your fare comes from fast-food restaurants or cafeterias, that's okay. Try to make healthy choices within those environments:

- Look for healthy alternatives such as whole-grain buns, salads, or baked potatoes.
- For breakfast, choose English muffins or pancakes. Limit hash browns, bacon, sausage, croissants, butter, and Danish rolls.
- At salad bars, select fat-free or low-fat dressing and heap on the vegetables.
- Drink water, juice, or low-fat milk; skip soda.
- Top baked potatoes with broccoli if available; go easy on the butter or sour cream.
- Un-super your hamburgers: select a single, plain burger; for condiments, choose mustard or catsup. Avoid or limit bacon and mayonnaise.
- Order skinless chicken, or take the skin off yourself. Be aware of nuggets and extra crispy because they are usually high in fat.
- Mexican: Choose soft flour tortillas instead of fried corn tortillas; select dishes with lots of beans and vegetables and little sour cream.
- Pizza: Choose vegetable toppings. Limit sausage, pepperoni, and hamburger.

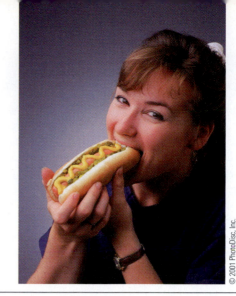

Fast foods should be limited in your diet.

foods you do, and, most important, whether they supply the nutrients you need.

To the question of what prompts you to eat, you may reply that you are hungry. Hunger is the physiological need to eat—a negative, unpleasant sensation. But the physiological need for food is not the only stimulus that triggers eating behavior. Another cue is appetite, the psychological desire to eat. This may arise in response to the sight, smell, or thought of food even when you do not physically need to eat. You may have an appetite when you are not hungry—or the reverse. That is, you may be hungry but have no appetite.

As for the question of why you choose the foods you do, several answers come to mind:[4]

- Personal preference (you like them).
- Habit or ethnic tradition (they are familiar; you always eat them).
- Social pressure (they are offered; you feel you can't refuse).
- Availability (they are there and ready to eat).
- Convenience (you are too rushed to prepare anything else).
- Economy (you can afford them).
- Emotional needs (some foods can make you feel better for a while).
- Values or beliefs (they fit your religious tradition or honor the environment).

- Nutritional value (you think they are good for you).

These are psychological and social reasons, with the exception of the last one, which suggests being conscious of the importance of nutrition to your wellness. This is not to say that your other reasons for choosing foods are invalid or will necessarily damage your health. Food sustains more than the body. It nourishes the mind and spirit. After you have learned about nutrition, you will be able to design a diet that meets your body's needs and honors your preferences, social values, and other needs.

The Six Basic Nutrients

Foods supply nutrients, fiber, and other substances that your body needs. **Nutrients** are substances obtained from food that promote growth, maintenance, or repair. Nutrients fall into six basic categories: proteins, fats, carbohydrates, vitamins, minerals, and water. They provide everything the body needs to continue healthy functioning, including

- growth and the formation of new tissue
- repair of damaged tissue
- production of energy
- conduction of nerve impulses
- reproduction.

Nutrition The science of foods, the nutrients and other substances they contain, and their actions within the body.

Energy The capacity to do work or produce heat.

Nutrients Substances obtained from food and used in the body to promote growth, maintenance, and repair. The essential nutrients are those the body cannot make for itself in sufficient quantity to meet physiological needs and, therefore, must be obtained from food.

1. *Adequate nutrients within calorie needs.* Consume a variety of nutrient-dense foods and beverages within and among the basic food groups while limiting intakes of saturated and *trans fats*, cholesterol, added sugars, salt and alcohol. Meet the recommended intakes within energy needs by adopting a balanced eating pattern, such as the USDA Food Guide or the DASH Eating Plan.
2. *Weight management.* To maintain body weight in a healthy range, balance calories from foods and beverages with calories expended. To prevent gradual weight gain over time, make small decreases in food and beverage calories and increase physical activity.
3. *Physical activity.* Engage in regular physical activity and reduce sedentary activities to promote healthy, psychological well-being, and a healthy body weight. Achieve physical fitness by including cardiovascular conditioning, stretching exercises for flexibility, and resistance exercises for muscle strength and endurance.
4. *Food groups to encourage.* Consume a sufficient amount of fruits and vegetables while staying within energy needs. Two cups of fruit and 2½ cups of vegetables per day are recommended for a reference 2,000 calorie intake, with higher or lower amounts depending on the calorie level. Choose a variety of fruits and vegetables each day. Selecting from all five subgroups: dark green, orange, legumes, starchy vegetables, and other vegetables several times a week. At least half of the grains should come from whole grains. Consume 3 cups per day of fat-free or low-fat milk or equivalent milk products.
5. *Fat.* Total fat intake should comprise 25 to 30 percent of total calories. Less than 10 percent should be from saturated; no more than 300 mg of cholesterol. *Trans fats* should be kept to a minimum. Select lean cuts of meats and bake or broil and limit sauces and gravies.
6. *Carbohydrates.* Choose fiber-rich fruits, vegetables, and whole grains often. Choose and prepare foods and beverages with minimal or no added sugar. Reduce the incidence of dental caries by practicing good oral hygiene and limiting sugary foods and beverages.
7. *Sodium and potassium.* Consume less than 2,300 mg (approximately 1 tsp of salt) of sodium per day. Choose and prepare foods with little salt. At the same time, consume potassium rich foods, such as fruits and vegetables.
8. *Alcoholic beverages.* If you choose to drink alcoholic beverages, do so sensibly and in moderation—defined as up to one drink per day for women and two drinks per day or men. People who should *not* drink alcohol include those who cannot restrict their alcohol intakes, women of childbearing age who may become pregnant, pregnant and lactating women, children and adolescents, individuals taking medicines that can interact with alcohol, and those with specific medical conditions. Avoid alcoholic beverages if you engage in activities that require attention, skill, or coordination such as driving or operating machinery.

Source: U. S. Department of Agriculture, U. S. Department of Health and Human Services, *Dietary Guidelines for Americans*, 2005.

Three classes of nutrients provide energy the body can use: protein, fat, and carbohydrate. The body uses energy from these nutrients to do its work and to generate heat. The units used to measure energy are **calories**, familiar to everyone as a reflection of how "fattening" a food is. Strictly speaking, the unit used to measure the energy in foods is a kilocalorie—the amount of heat necessary to raise the temperature of a kilogram (a liter) of water 1 degree Celsius. This book follows the common practice of using the abbreviated form (calorie) for kilocalorie.

Protein and carbohydrate each provide 4 calories per gram and fat provides 9 calories per gram. Figure 8.2 displays foods and the energy-yielding nutrients they contain.

One other energy-producing substance that some people ingest is the alcohol in alcoholic beverages. Alcohol is not a nutrient because it does not promote the body's growth, maintenance, or repair; but it is counted as an energy source because it provides 7 calories per gram. Although vitamins and minerals do not provide energy, they do assist in energy-processing reactions and other metabolic functions. Water provides a medium for these reactions to occur.

PROTEIN

Protein is an energy-yielding nutrient providing 4 calories per gram. Protein can be used as an energy source, but it is best utilized as the major structural and working material of cells. It provides the basic materials for cell growth and repair. Proteins are made of **amino acids**, each of which is composed of carbon, oxygen, hydrogen, and nitrogen. Protein helps build skin, blood, muscles, and bone; aids in the formation of hormones; regulates the body's chemical processes; forms enzymes; carries nutrients to all body cells; and is a major constituent of the immune system.

Sources of Protein Most Americans rely heavily on animal sources of protein, including milk and milk products, eggs, meat, poultry, and fish. Good plant sources of protein are

- legumes, such as dried beans, dried peas, dried lentils, peanuts, soybeans, and soy products.
- grains, such as oats, rice, barley, cornmeal, and whole-grain breads and pastas.

FIGURE 8.2 Some Foods and Their Energy-Yielding Nutrients

Foods contain carbohydrates, protein, fat, vitamins, minerals, and water. Portion sizes shown are useful for diet planning. The meat portion is moderate (3 ounces) and the vegetable portion, ample (1 cup), is consistent with recommended guidelines.

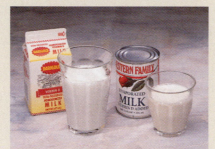

Milk = carbohydrate plus protein (plus vitamins, minerals, and water).

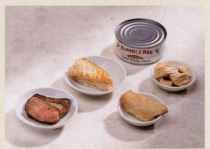

Meat = protein plus fat (plus vitamins, minerals, and water).

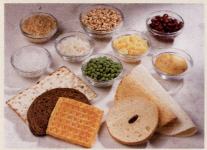

Bread (and starchy vegetables) = carbohydrate (plus protein, vitamins, and minerals).

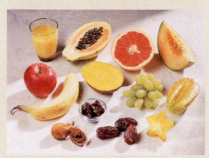

Fruit = carbohydrate (plus vitamins, minerals, and water).

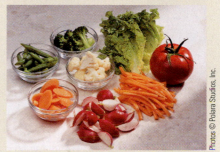

Vegetable (except starchy vegetables) = carbohydrate plus protein (plus vitamins, minerals, and water).

Photos © Polara Studios, Inc.

- nuts and seeds, such as walnuts, cashews, pecans, sunflower seeds, and sesame seeds.
- vegetables, such as broccoli and dark leafy green vegetables.

Proteins, whether derived from plant or animal sources, are made up of about 20 amino acids, of which the body can manufacture 11. The other 9, called **essential amino acids**, must be obtained from foods.

Complete proteins (such as chicken) contain all of the essential amino acids. **Incomplete proteins** (such as pinto beans and brown rice) may contain only some of the essential amino acids or may contain all of them but in insufficient amounts to allow humans to synthesize protein. An incomplete protein source, however, can be combined with another food that supplies the missing essential amino acids. One good combination is peanut butter on whole-grain bread; another is black beans and rice.

Only about 15 percent of total calories should come from protein. Most Americans eat more than twice the amount of protein they need. An American woman, for example, needs only about 46 to 48 grams of protein a day—the equivalent of a cup of low-fat yogurt, a cup of low-fat milk, and 4 ounces of chicken. Protein is essential for the body's growth and repair, but too much can be harmful. Contrary to popular belief, excess protein consumed beyond energy and physiological needs is not stored as muscle but, instead, is stored as fat.

Excessive protein causes the body to excrete calcium (needed for strengthening bones and teeth). If a person eats too much protein, the extra nitrogen is excreted in urine, which can strain the kidneys.

Vegetarians People who are **vegetarians** avoid some or all foods of animal origin. People who eat animal products sparingly usually realize several health benefits, including less risk for heart disease, lower levels of

Calories Units used to measure energy; determined from the heat food releases when burned; calories reflect the extent to which a food's energy can be stored in body fat.

Protein A nutrient composed of amino acids necessary for growth or tissue repair; protein also functions as enzymes, hormones, regulators of fluid and electrolyte balance, acid-base regulators, transporters, and antibodies.

Amino acids Building blocks of protein ("amino" means "containing nitrogen").

Essential amino acids Amino acids that the body cannot produce at all or produces in amounts insufficient to meet its needs; they must be provided by the diet.

Complete proteins Dietary proteins that contain all nine essential amino acids in the same relative amounts that humans require.

Incomplete proteins Dietary proteins that do not contain all the essential amino acids in sufficient quantities for human protein synthesis.

Vegetarians People who omit meat, fish, and poultry from their diet.

FIGURE 8.3 Protein Choices for Vegetarians

Choose from two or more of these columns to obtain balanced assortments of amino acids.

Grains	Legumes	Seeds and Nuts	Vegetables
Barley	Dried beans	Cashews	Broccoli
Bulgur	Dried lentils	Nut butters	Leafy greens
Cornmeal	Dried peas	Other nuts	Others
Oats	Peanuts	Sesame seeds	
Pasta	Soy products	Sunflower seeds	
Rice		Walnuts	
Whole-grain breads			

Beans and rice.

Peanut butter and bread.

Soybean curd (tofu) and rice.

Photos © Polara Studios, Inc.

cholesterol and other fats in the blood, lower blood pressure, and lower weight.

The wide array of available foods allows most vegetarians to get the proper balance of necessary nutrients. Strict vegetarians do need to make an extra effort to get essential amino acids, certain necessary minerals (especially calcium, iron, and zinc), and certain vitamins (such as vitamin B_{12} and vitamin D), because the best sources are milk, eggs, and meat. Good non-animal sources of these nutrients include fortified cereals and soy products, tofu, legumes, almonds, asparagus, dark green vegetables, and whole-grain breads.

If you are a vegetarian, consider these suggestions to help avoid nutritional deficiencies:

- Combine complementary proteins to make sure you get complete proteins. In essence, combine vegetables or legumes with grains—beans and corn (staples in Mexican cuisine), beans and rice, tofu and rice, black bean and rice soup.
- Eat at least one cup of dark green vegetables a day to boost your iron intake. Combine foods rich in vitamin C with foods rich in iron, as vitamin C helps the body absorb iron.
- If you don't drink milk, eat at least two cups of legumes (dried beans and peas) or calcium-fortified tofu daily to provide you with adequate calcium.
- Eat a wide range of foods to better your chances of getting balanced nutrients.
- Depending on how strict your diet is, you may need a nutritional supplement. Check with a nutrition expert or a registered dietitian for advice.

Figure 8.3 displays healthy protein choices for vegetarians.

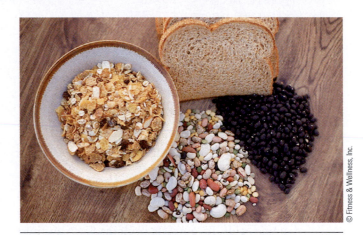

© Fitness & Wellness, Inc.

Legumes, grains, and nuts also provide protein.

FAT

Fat is another energy-yielding nutrient. The most concentrated form of food energy, fat provides 9 calories per gram, more than twice the calories in a gram of carbohydrate or protein. Fats provide valuable services: They transport fat-soluble vitamins in the body, insulate and protect body organs, regulate hormones, contribute to growth, provide a concentrated source of energy, and are essential for healthy skin. Fats give foods their flavor, texture, and palatability. Fats also provide foods with aromas that encourage people to eat them. Fat provides satiety, a feeling of fullness.

Although the proper amount of fat is essential for growth and functioning of the body, too much fat is harmful.[5] Excess dietary fat can lead to high blood pressure, stroke, heart disease, diabetes, and other diseases.

FIGURE 8.4 Fat and Calories

Fat hides calories in food. When you trim fat, you trim calories.

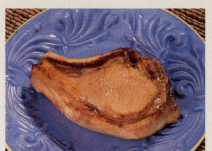

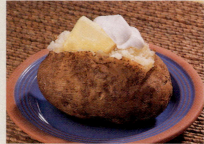

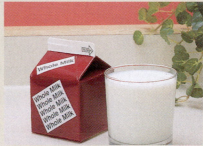

Small pork chop with ½ inch border of fat (25 grams fat) = 275 cal.

Large potato with 1 tbsp butter and 1 tbsp sour cream (14 grams fat) = 350 cal.

Whole milk, 1 c (8 grams fat) = 150 cal.

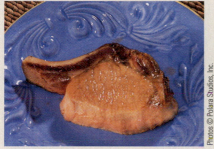

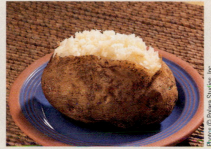

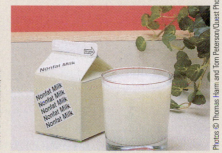

Small pork chop with fat trimmed off (13 grams fat) = 165 cal.

Plain large potato (less than 1 gram fat) = 220 cal.

Nonfat milk, 1 c (less than 1 gram fat) = 90 cal.

Excessive body fat is a leading factor in heart disease (see Chapter 11). It also has been linked to cancers of the colon, breast, uterus, and prostate.

The average American eats much more fat than is recommended or healthy. Experts recommend that no more than 30 percent of the total calories in the diet should come from fat. On a 30-percent fat diet, if you eat 1,600 calories a day, you should have no more than 53 grams of fat; for 2,000 calories a day, no more than 67 grams of fat.

To figure out the fat content of individual foods, multiply the grams of fat by 9 and divide this by the total calories in that food. Then multiply that number by 100 to get the percentage. For example, if a food label lists a total of 100 calories and 7 grams of fat, the fat content is 63 percent of total calories. This simple guideline can help you quickly assess the fat in your diet, and you can use this information to select foods that are lower in fat.

Reducing fat intake offers a fringe benefit to people who wish to cut calories. Remembering that fat contains more than twice as many calories as a spoonful of sugar or pure protein, you can drastically reduce the calorie count by removing the fat from a food. Figure 8.4 shows that the single most effective step you can take to reduce the energy value of a food is to eat it with less fat.

Types of Fats Fats can be categorized as saturated, monounsaturated, or polyunsaturated, based on their chemical structure. Each has health implications.

1. **Saturated fats** are solid at room temperature, and most come from animal sources. The only exceptions are coconut oil, palm oil, and palm kernel oil (the "tropical oils"), which are highly saturated but still liquid at room temperature. Saturated fats raise the level of low-density lipoproteins (the most harmful kind of cholesterol) in the bloodstream and have been linked to heart disease (see Chapter 11) and other degenerative diseases. Examples of foods high in saturated fats are butter, cream, lard, bacon, beef, veal, lamb, poultry skin, and many processed food items.

2. **Monounsaturated fats** are liquid at room temperature. They are found in peanuts, cashews, olives, and avocados, as well as olive oil, peanut oil, cottonseed oil, and canola oil.

3. **Polyunsaturated fats** are found in most vegetable oils and, with a few exceptions, are liquid at room

Fat Lipids in food or in the body that provide the body with a continuous fuel supply, protect it from mechanical shock, and carry fat-soluble vitamins.

Saturated fats Fats carrying the maximum possible numbers of hydrogen atoms; usually found in animal products such as butter and lard.

Monounsaturated fats Fatty acids that lack two hydrogen atoms and have one double bond between carbons; found in olive oil, canola oil, and peanut oil.

Polyunsaturated fats Fatty acids that lack four hydrogen atoms and have two or more double bonds between carbons; found in safflower, sunflower, corn, soybean, and cottonseed oils.

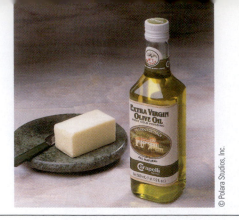

At room temperature unsaturated fats (such as those found in oil) are usually liquid, whereas saturated fats (such as those found in butter) are solid.

temperature. Foods containing polyunsaturated fats include fish, margarine, walnuts, almonds, pecans, corn oil, safflower oil, sunflower oil, sesame oil, and soybean oil.

Dietitians advise that people consume monounsaturated and polyunsaturated fats more often than saturated fats because of the negative effects of saturated fats on blood lipids. An even greater concern, though, is total dietary fat. The most important dietary steps you can take to prevent disease are to control total dietary fat and to control your body weight.

Some monounsaturated and polyunsaturated fats can undergo **hydrogenation** during manufacturing, creating trans fats. During this process, hydrogen is added to the fat to increase shelf life and to make the product harder or more spreadable. Hydrogenated fats are found in shortening, margarine, some crackers, and some nut butters. Eating a vegetable oil that has been hydrogenated may carry as many health risks as eating saturated fat. Many food products include labeling regarding the amount of trans fat in a product.

Cholesterol Cholesterol is another type of fat. Despite its negative publicity, cholesterol does play beneficial roles in the body. It aids in digestion, is a major component of the membranes that protect nerve fibers, aids in production of vitamin D, and helps the body produce sex hormones. Too much cholesterol in the bloodstream, however, places a person at significantly higher risk for developing heart disease. Cholesterol forms a major part of the deposits that accumulate along arteries and increase the risk of heart attacks and strokes.

Blood levels of cholesterol can increase by being overweight and consuming a high-fat diet. Cholesterol blood level is affected less by cholesterol intake than total fat intake. To test your knowledge about fat, see Assessment 8.1.

CARBOHYDRATES

The third energy-yielding nutrient is carbohydrate. **Carbohydrates** provide 4 calories per gram and supply the

Calorie Value of Nutrients

1 gram of carbohydrate	= 4 calories
1 gram of protein	= 4 calories
1 gram of fat	= 9 calories

body with the energy needed for daily activities. Because they are digested more easily and metabolized more efficiently and quickly than proteins, they are a preferred source of energy.

The two different kinds of carbohydrates are **simple carbohydrates** (sugars) and **complex carbohydrates** (starches). These terms refer to an important distinction among carbohydrates. Simply stated, the distinction is between starch and fiber (complex) versus sugars (simple). The simple carbohydrates (sugars) are found in both natural (dilute) and processed (concentrated) form—simply stated, fruit versus candy.

Simple Carbohydrates The simple carbohydrates are the sugars. All sugars are chemically similar to glucose and can be converted to glucose in the body. All of their names end in "-ose," which makes them easy to recognize as carbohydrates. The four sugars most important in human nutrition are

1. glucose (the body's fuel),
2. fructose (the sweet sugar of fruits, honey, and maple syrup),
3. sucrose (table sugar), and
4. lactose (milk sugar).

Simple carbohydrates are found mostly in fruits and milk and in concentrated forms such as sugar, honey, and other sweets.

Dietitians recommend that you consume abundant quantities of fruits and vegetables that contain sugars, but they urge you in the same breath to "avoid consuming too much sugar." What's the difference? Part of the answer lies in the concept of **empty calories**. When you eat an apple, you receive about 100 calories from the sugars, together with a little vitamin A, a bit of thiamin, some vitamin C, a moderate dose of fiber, a healthy bit of potassium, and several dozen other nutrients. By contrast, from a 12-ounce cola beverage, you get about 150 calories from sugar and no other nutrients. Actually, it creates a sort of debt, because to avoid overconsuming calories, you now have to derive all the nutrients you need in a day from food containing 150 fewer calories. Many people are surprised to learn about the number of calories and amount of sugar they consume from their beverage choices.

The same criticism applies to both honey and sugar. Some people believe that honey is an ideal substitute for sugar because they say it offers nutrients along with sugar. But honey contains only a trace of some nutrients, so relative to a person's daily need, these tiny amounts

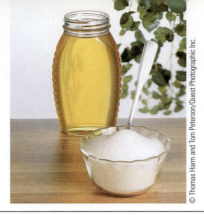

Pure fat = fat only. Pure sugar = carbohydrate only.

don't add up to much. Honey is almost identical to sugar chemically. In terms of nutrition, honey and sugar do not differ significantly.

The word "sugar" does not always appear on food labels. Instead, manufacturers often list the various kinds of sweeteners separately. The label may contain a long list of ingredients including corn syrup, corn starch, sucrose, and honey. These hidden sugars can be deceptive.

Sugar Substitutes Some people dream of calorie-less doughnuts, calorie-free candy, and ice cream having the calories of skim milk. At the same time, consumers insist that no risks to health must accompany calorie savings. The desire of most people to control body weight while retaining the taste of sugar has led to the introduction of sugar substitutes.

People can choose from two sets of substitutes: One is the sugar alcohols, which are energy-yielding sweeteners (sometimes referred to as "nutritive sweeteners"); the other is the artificial sweeteners, which provide virtually no energy or calories.

The sugar alcohols are familiar to people who use special dietary products. Among them are maltitol, mannitol, sorbitol, and xylitol. A benefit of sugar alcohols is that bacteria in the mouth cannot metabolize them as rapidly as they metabolize sugar, so sugar alcohols do not contribute to tooth decay.

Those who wish to reduce their energy intake should be aware that the sugar alcohols do provide as much energy (that is, calories) as sucrose, even though these products may be labeled "sugar-free." Thus, artificial sweeteners may offer a preferable alternative. Artificial sweeteners also make foods taste sweet without promoting tooth decay. Unlike sugar alcohols, though, they have the added advantages of being calorie-free. The most commonly used synthetic sweeteners are saccharin and aspartame.

Saccharin is used primarily in soft drinks and as a table sweetener. Because its safety has been questioned, these products must carry warnings. Saccharin has another disadvantage: It does not taste exactly like sugar.

Aspartame has been added to a variety of foods, including diet drinks, gum, cereals, gelatins, and puddings. Its popularity is related to its taste, which is almost like

Honey versus Sugar

Some people believe that honey is the ideal substitute for sugar because, they say, it offers nutrients along with its sweetness, rather than just empty calories. True, honey does contain traces of a few vitamins and minerals, but relative to a person's daily need, these nutrients don't add up to much.

A tablespoon of honey (65 calories) offers one-tenth of a milligram of iron, for example, but an adult's daily need for iron can be as high as 15 milligrams or more. Consequently, to meet the need for iron, an adult would need 150 tablespoons in a day—almost 10,000 calories of honey! (Most people can eat only 2,000 to 3,000 calories a day without getting fat.) The nutrients in honey just do not add up as fast as the calories do, so honey, like sugar, is a relatively empty-calorie food.

Chemically, honey is almost identical to sugar, too. And spoon for spoon, sugar contains fewer calories than honey because the sugar crystals take up more space.

sugar. Aspartame is FDA-approved and seems to be safe for everyone except those with a rare inherited disorder known as phenylketonuria.

As a sweet-toothed species, people often perceive sugar substitutes as a way to cheat the scales. Evidence seems to suggest that artificial sweeteners, used in moderation as part of a well-balanced diet, pose no health risks.

Complex Carbohydrates The complex carbohydrates are composed of long chains of glucose units. Starch, the principal complex carbohydrate in grains and vegetables, is the chief energy source for human beings throughout the world and is highly desirable in the diet. Starch provides the body with the glucose it needs in the form it uses best. And if the starchy foods you eat are wholesome—such as whole-grain breads (not refined white

Hydrogenation A chemical process by which hydrogens are added to monounsaturated or polyunsaturated fats to reduce the number of double bonds and make the product more saturated (solid) and more resistant to spoilage.

Cholesterol A type of fat called a "sterol"; necessary for synthesis of sex hormones, adrenal hormones, and vitamin D.

Carbohydrates Nutrients composed of carbon, oxygen, and hydrogen atoms; carbohydrates provide about half of all energy needed by muscles and other tissues and is the preferred fuel for the brain and nervous system.

Simple carbohydrates Sugars in the form of fruits and milk or honey, sucrose, corn syrup, and fructose.

Complex carbohydrates Polysaccharides composed of straight or branched chains of monosaccharides.

Empty calories A food or beverage that provides calories but little or no nutrients.

bread), potatoes (not potato chips), or whole-grain cereals (not the sugary kind)—your body obtains many of the other nutrients it needs, along with a steady supply of glucose. Most people would do well to boost their intakes of starchy foods like these.

Diets high in complex carbohydrates help to keep the blood sugar at a constant level and reduce the risks for heart disease, cancer, and other degenerative diseases. The best sources of complex carbohydrates are grains, such as wheat, rice, oats, corn, rye, barley, and millet; potatoes, sweet potatoes, and yams; fruits; vegetables; and legumes, such as soybeans, garbanzo beans, black-eyed peas, kidney beans, butter beans, and peanuts.

Because they are nutritionally dense, most complex-carbohydrate foods are rich in vitamins and minerals. Many contain a significant amount of protein. Complex carbohydrates provide a steady source of energy, making them an excellent choice for physically active people (especially endurance athletes). Complex carbohydrates also are stored in the muscles and the liver as **glycogen**, which fuels the body when it needs sudden bursts of energy.

Dietary fiber, another complex carbohydrate in food, is mostly indigestible by human beings and therefore yields no calories. Fiber holds water, so it provides the bulk inside the intestines that enables the muscle of the digestive tract walls to push their contents along. Foods that are high in fiber also make softer stools. The subject may be unglamorous, but it is of intense interest to anyone who suffers from the consequences of a lack of fiber: constipation (hard, sluggish stools), hemorrhoids (swollen, painful rectal veins that bulge out from straining to pass hard stools), or a host of other intestinal ills.

Fiber offers many health benefits.[6] Because fiber keeps the intestinal contents moving, it helps to prevent infection of the appendix (appendicitis). In addition, fiber helps to control blood cholesterol levels, a risk factor for heart disease. (Certain fibers bind cholesterol and keep it from being absorbed in the body; it is excreted with the feces instead.) Fiber also helps control the blood glucose concentration and so helps to prevent diabetes. Some fibers bind cancer-causing agents in the digestive tract and keep them from being absorbed by, or from touching, the intestinal walls.

Fiber also may help prevent obesity. The person who eats fiber-rich foods chews longer and fills up sooner on fewer calories. Consistently, foods that are high in fiber are often low in calories and vice versa, so it is hard to eat a diet high in fiber and also gain weight.

Plant foods, especially those with their skins intact, are high in fiber. Fiber breaks down when foods are refined or cooked. Apples have more fiber than applesauce, and apple juice has none. If you want to eat a diet high in fiber, choose whole grains, whole fruits, and whole vegetables. Most Americans eat about 15 grams of fiber a day. The National Cancer Institute recommends doubling that amount, to about 30 grams of fiber a day. Assessment 8.2 includes questions related to your fiber intake.

VITAMINS

Vitamins occur in foods in much smaller quantities than do the energy-yielding nutrients, and they make no contribution to energy themselves. Nor do they contribute building material, except for the minerals of bone. Instead they are mostly helpers, or facilitators, of body processes. They are, nonetheless, a powerful group of substances, as their absence attests. Vitamin A deficiency can cause blindness; a lack of niacin induces mental illness. The consequences of deficiencies are so dire and the effects of restoring the needed nutrients so dramatic that they make good fodder for faddists: Are you bald? Impotent? Do you have pimples? Are you nearsighted? The right vitamin will cure whatever ails you, they say.

Actually, a vitamin can cure only the disease caused by a deficiency of that vitamin. Also, an overdose of any vitamin can make people as sick as a deficiency can, and it can even cause death. For most healthy people, a balanced diet of ordinary foods supplies enough, but not too much, of each of the vitamins. The vitamins are listed, along with their sources, their more important roles, and deficiency symptoms, in Table 8.1.

The vitamins fall into two categories.

1. *Fat-soluble vitamins*, including vitamins A, D, E, and K, are stored in the body's fat cells. They are not excreted in the urine and are accumulated in the fat tissues of the body. If you consume too many, they can be toxic.

2. *Water-soluble vitamins*, including vitamin C and the B-complex vitamins, dissolve readily in water and are

TABLE 8.1 Vitamins: Sources, Major Functions, and Deficiency Symptoms

Nutrient	Good Sources	Major Functions	Deficiency Symptoms
Vitamin A	Milk, cheese, eggs, liver, yellow and dark green fruits and vegetables	Required for healthy bones, teeth, skin, gums, and hair; maintenance of inner mucous membranes, thus increasing resistance to infection; adequate vision in dim light.	Night blindness; decreased growth; decreased resistance to infection; rough, dry skin
Vitamin D	Fortified milk, cod liver oil, salmon, tuna, egg yolk	Necessary for bones and teeth; needed for calcium and phosphorus absorption.	Rickets (bone softening), fractures, muscle spasms
Vitamin E	Vegetable oils, yellow and green leafy vegetables, margarine, wheat germ, whole grain breads and cereals	Related to oxidation and normal muscle and red blood cell chemistry.	Leg cramps, breakdown of red blood cells
Vitamin K	Green leafy vegetables, cauliflower, cabbage, eggs, peas, potatoes	Essential for normal blood clotting.	Hemorrhaging
Vitamin B_1 (Thiamin)	Whole grain or enriched bread, lean meats and poultry, fish, liver, pork, poultry, organ meats, legumes, nuts, dried yeast	Assists in proper use of carbohydrates; normal functioning of nervous system; maintenance of good appetite.	Loss of appetite, nausea, confusion, cardiac abnormalities, muscle spasms
Vitamin B_2 (Riboflavin)	Eggs, milk, leafy green vegetables, whole grains, lean meats, dried beans and peas	Contributes to energy release from carbohydrates, fats, and proteins; needed for normal growth and development, good vision, and healthy skin.	Cracking of the corners of the mouth, inflammation of the skin, impaired vision
Vitamin B_6 (Pyridoxine)	Vegetables, meats, whole grain cereals, soybeans, peanuts, potatoes	Necessary for metabolism of protein and fatty acids and for formation of normal red blood cells.	Depression, irritability, muscle spasms, nausea
Vitamin B_{12}	Meat, poultry, fish, liver, organ meats, eggs, shellfish, milk, cheese	Required for normal growth, formation of red blood cells, nervous system, and digestive tract functioning.	Impaired balance, weakness, drop in red blood cell count
Niacin	Liver and organ meats, meat, fish, poultry, whole grains, enriched breads, nuts, green leafy vegetables, and dried beans and peas	Contributes to energy release from carbohydrates, fats, and proteins; normal growth and development; formation of hormones and nerve-regulating substances.	Confusion, depression, weakness, weight loss
Biotin	Liver, kidney, eggs, yeast, legumes, milk, nuts, dark green vegetables	Essential for carbohydrate metabolism and fatty acid synthesis.	Inflamed skin, muscle pain, depression, weight loss
Folate	Leafy green vegetables, organ meats, whole grains and cereals, dried beans	Needed for cell growth and reproduction and for red blood cell formation.	Decreased resistance to infection
Pantothenic Acid	All natural foods, especially liver, kidney, eggs, nuts, yeast, milk, dried peas and beans, green leafy vegetables	Related to carbohydrate and fat metabolism.	Depression, low blood sugar, leg cramps, nausea, headaches
Vitamin C (Ascorbic acid)	Fruits, vegetables	Helps protect against infection; required for formation of collagenous tissue, normal blood vessels, teeth, and bones.	Slow-healing wounds, loose teeth, hemorrhaging, rough scaly skin, irritability

excreted in the urine. Megadoses of these vitamins also can be toxic.

Vitamins C and E (and **beta-carotene**, a vitamin A precursor) function as **antioxidants**, preventing oxygen from combining with other body substances that it may damage. During normal **metabolism**, oxygen changes carbohydrates and fats into energy. In this process, oxygen is transformed into stable forms of water and carbon dioxide. A small amount of oxygen, however, ends up in an unstable form, referred to as oxygen free radicals, which can damage healthy tissue. Antioxidants protect cell membranes and DNA from this damage, which is

Glycogen A storage form of carbohydrate in the liver and muscle.

Dietary fiber Food substance that is not digested in the small intestine and provides the bulk needed to keep the digestive system running smoothly; found in vegetables, fruits, grains, and legumes.

Vitamins Organic, essential nutrients required in small amounts to perform specific functions that promote growth, maintenance, or repair.

Beta-carotene A vitamin A precursor made by plants; an orange pigment with antioxidant activity.

Antioxidant Compound that protects other compounds from oxidation by being oxidized itself, therefore protecting cell membranes and body fluids.

Metabolism All of the chemical reactions that occur within living cells.

TABLE 8.2 Minerals: Good Sources, Major Functions, and Deficiency Symptoms

Nutrient	Good Sources	Major Functions	Deficiency Symptoms
Calcium	Milk, yogurt, cheese, green leafy vegetables, dried beans, sardines and salmon with edible bones	Required for strong teeth and bone formation; maintenance of good muscle tone, heartbeat, and nerve function.	Bone pain and fractures, periodontal disease, muscle cramps
Copper	Seafood, meats, beans, nuts, whole grains	Helps with iron absorption and hemoglobin formation; required to synthesize the enzyme cytochrome oxidase.	Anemia (although deficiency is rare in humans)
Iron	Organ meats, lean meats, seafoods, eggs, dried peas and beans, nuts, whole and enriched grains, green leafy vegetables	Major component of hemoglobin; aids in energy utilization.	Nutritional anemia, overall weakness
Phosphorus	Meats, fish, milk, eggs, dried beans and peas, whole grains, processed foods	Required for bone and teeth formation; energy release regulation.	Bone pain and fracture, weight loss, weakness
Zinc	Milk, meat, seafood, whole grains, nuts, eggs, dried beans	Essential component of hormones, insulin, and enzymes; used in normal growth and development.	Loss of appetite, slow-healing wounds, skin problems
Magnesium	Green leafy vegetables, whole grains, nuts, soybeans, seafood, legumes	Needed for bone growth and maintenance; carbohydrate and protein utilization; nerve function; temperature regulation.	Irregular heartbeat, weakness, muscle spasms, sleeplessness
Sodium	Table salt, processed foods, meat	Needed for regulation of body fluids; transmission of nerve impulses; heart action.	Rarely seen
Potassium	Legumes, whole grains, bananas, orange juice, dried fruits, potatoes	Required for heart action; bone formation and maintenance; regulation of energy release; acid-base regulation.	Irregular heartbeat, nausea, weakness
Selenium	Seafood, meat, whole grains	Component of enzymes; functions in close association with vitamin E.	Muscle pain, possible heart muscle deterioration, possible hair and nail loss

believed to help prevent heart disease, cancer, and even emphysema.

MINERALS

Like vitamins, **minerals** occur in foods in much smaller quantities than do the energy-yielding nutrients, and they make no contribution of energy themselves. Nor do they contribute building material, except for the minerals of bone. They are mostly essential facilitators of body processes.

Minerals are the inorganic elements the body needs. According to how much the body needs, minerals are classified as

1. **major minerals**—essential nutrients found in the human body in amounts larger than 5 grams
2. **trace minerals**—minerals found in the body in amounts less than 5 grams.

Because they are needed in such small amounts, minerals can be extremely toxic if consumed in excess.

Table 8.2 lists selected minerals of both types, along with their sources, functions, and deficiency symptoms. Many people suffer from deficiencies of two important minerals—calcium and iron.

Calcium Calcium helps regulate the heart, maintain proper fluid balance in the cells, transmit nerve impulses,

and clot the blood. Among its other functions, calcium aids in the formation of bones, which is important to people of all ages. Low calcium intake during childhood and adolescence limits the bones' ability to achieve an optimal peak mass and density. Bone tissue is active. Bone cells are replaced throughout adulthood, so you need plenty of calcium to maintain bone strength and density. Women have smaller, less-dense bones than men and are about eight times more likely to develop osteoporosis, a disease characterized by weak and porous bones that are likely to fracture.

Unlike many diseases that make themselves known through symptoms such as pain, osteoporosis is silent. The body sends no signals that bone loss is occurring. For this reason, the disease is called "the silent thief." People need to take action when they are young to protect their bones and reduce the risk for osteoporosis. Assessment 8.3 can help you determine your risk for osteoporosis.

Bones respond to physical activity by becoming denser and stronger. If you walk a lot, for example, your leg bones will respond by developing more mass. If you use your arms regularly to lift weights or swing a tennis racket, the bones in your arms will become stronger.

Iron A deficiency of iron in the diet translates to too few red blood cells in the bloodstream. This can cause a condition called iron deficiency anemia, characterized by

For Optimal Bone Health

- Drink plenty of milk. Most adults get about half their calcium from milk. One cup of milk—whether whole milk, 2%, 1%, or skim milk—provides 300 milligrams of calcium.
- Eat foods rich in vitamin D, because they help your body absorb calcium. Primary sources are milk and dairy products.
- Avoid too much meat and other protein-rich foods, because they make your body excrete calcium.
- Cut down on alcohol, caffeine, and phosphates (found in soda), because they take the place of calcium-rich beverages in your diet.
- Be involved in weight-bearing physical activities.
- Maintain healthy body weight. The bones need the stimulation to grow dense by supporting a healthy body.
- If you smoke, stop.

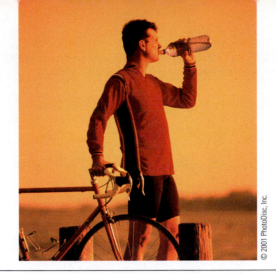

Water is the most vital nutrient.

weakness, pallor, shortness of breath, susceptibility to infection, shortened attention span, impaired learning abilities, loss of vision, and other serious physical problems. Women who are menstruating run a particular risk of iron deficiency. As many as 15 percent of American women of childbearing age may have an iron deficiency because of blood lost during menstruation.

As a note of caution: Too much iron can cause infections, tissue damage, and severe liver damage, and it also may increase the risk for heart disease. Because the proper balance is so important, you should consult your doctor before taking any iron supplement.

WATER

Next to air, water is the element most necessary for human survival. You could survive much longer without food than you could without water. Water is the major component of blood, which carries oxygen and nutrients to all cells in the body. It helps your body use the other nutrients in your diet, aids your body in getting rid of wastes, helps you digest foods, maintains the proper electrolyte balance in the body, lubricates joints, and regulates body temperature—to name just a few functions.

Water comprises approximately 60 percent of your body. You get some water from the foods you eat. Fruits, for example, are as much as 80 percent water. Especially good choices are melons and apples. Even foods you typically don't think of as containing much water, such as bread and meat, can be anywhere from 33 to 50 percent water. In addition to the foods you eat, you should drink eight to ten 8-ounce glasses of water a day—more if you are large, physically active, live in a hot climate, or perspire excessively.

You cannot always rely on thirst to indicate a water deficit. A rough indicator is the color of your urine. If it is a dark amber color or has a strong odor, you are not drinking enough water. Passing a full bladder of colorless

or pale yellow urine at least four times a day means you are getting enough water. The following—in addition to drinking plenty of water—will help you maintain the proper intake:

- Avoid caffeine. It increases the body's need for water while it increases the amount of water the body puts out.
- Avoid alcohol. You need 8 ounces of water to metabolize a single ounce of alcohol.
- Cut back protein to a healthy level. The wastes produced from proteins build up in the kidneys, and you need extra water to flush them out.
- Drink a steady amount of water throughout the day to keep your body well supplied.

Dietary Reference Intakes

The amounts of energy, nutrients, and other dietary components that best support health have been defined in the **Dietary Reference Intakes (DRIs)**, which offer four values:

1. **Estimated Average Requirement (EAR).** Nutrition experts have reviewed hundreds of research studies

Minerals Inorganic elements that the body needs to provide specific body functions.

Major minerals Essential mineral nutrients found in the human body in amounts larger than 5 grams; also called "macrominerals."

Trace minerals Essential mineral nutrients found in the human body in amounts less than 5 grams; also called "microminerals."

Dietary Reference Intakes (DRI) A set of nutrient values for the dietary nutrient intakes of healthy people; includes Estimated Average Requirements, Recommended Dietary Allowances, Adequate Intakes, and Tolerable Upper Intake Levels.

Estimated Average Requirement (EAR) The amount of a nutrient that will maintain a specific biochemical or physiological function in half of the population.

TABLE 8.3 Estimated Energy Requirements (EER), Recommended Dietary Allowances (RDA), and Adequate Intakes (AI) for Water, Energy, and the Energy Nutrients

Age(yr)	Reference BMI (kg/m²)	Reference height, cm (in)	Reference weight, kg (lb)	Water[a] AI (L/day)	Energy EER[b] (kcal/day)	Carbohydrate RDA (g/day)	Total fiber AI (g/day)	Total fat AI (g/day)	Linoleic acid AI (g/day)	Linolenic acid[c] AI (g/day)	Protein RDA (g/day)[d]	Protein RDA (g/kg/day)
Males												
0–0.5	—	62 (24)	6 (13)	0.7[e]	570	60	—	31	4.4	0.5	9.1	1.52
0.5–1	—	71 (28)	9 (20)	0.8[f]	743	95	—	30	4.6	0.5	13.5	1.5
1–3[g]	—	86 (34)	12 (27)	1.3	1046	130	19	—	7	0.7	13	1.1
4–8[g]	15.3	115 (45)	20 (44)	1.7	1742	130	25	—	10	0.9	19	0.95
9–13	17.2	144 (57)	36 (79)	2.4	2279	130	31	—	12	1.2	34	0.95
14–18	20.5	174 (68)	61 (134)	3.3	3152[h]	130	38	—	16	1.6	52	0.85
19–30	22.5	177 (70)	70 (154)	3.7	3067[h]	130	38	—	17	1.6	56	0.8
31–50				3.7	3067[h]	130	38	—	17	1.6	56	0.8
>50				3.7	3067[h]	130	30	—	14	1.6	56	0.8
Females												
0–0.5	—	62 (24)	6 (13)	0.7[e]	520	60	—	31	4.4	0.5	9.1	1.52
0.5–1	—	71 (28)	9 (20)	0.8[f]	676	95	—	30	4.6	0.5	13.5	1.5
1–3[g]	—	86 (34)	12 (27)	1.3	992	130	19	—	7	0.7	13	1.1
4–8[g]	15.3	115 (45)	20 (44)	1.7	1642	130	25	—	10	0.9	19	0.95
9–13	17.4	144 (57)	37 (81)	2.1	2071	130	26	—	10	1.0	34	0.95
14–18	20.4	163 (64)	54 (119)	2.3	2368	130	26	—	11	1.1	46	0.85
19–30	21.5	163 (64)	57 (126)	2.7	2403[i]	130	25	—	12	1.1	46	0.8
31–50				2.7	2403[i]	130	25	—	12	1.1	46	0.8
>50				2.7	2403[i]	130	21	—	11	1.1	46	0.8
Pregnancy												
1st trimester				3.0	10	175	28	—	13	1.4	125	1.1
2nd trimester				3.0	1340	175	28	—	13	1.4	125	1.1
3rd trimester				3.0	1452	175	28	—	13	1.4	125	1.1
Lactation												
1st 6 months				3.8	1330	210	29	—	13	1.3	125	1.1
2nd 6 months				3.8	1400	210	29	—	13	1.3	125	1.1

Note: For all nutrients, values for infants are AI. Dashes indicate that values have not been determined.

[a] The water AI includes drinking water, water in beverages, and water in foods; in general, drinking water and other beverages contribute about 70 to 80 percent, and foods, the remainder. Conversion factors: 1 L = 33.8 fluid oz; 1 L = 1.06 qt; 1 cup = 8 fluid oz.

[b] The Estimated Energy Requirement (EER) represents the average dietary energy intake that will maintain energy balance in a healthy person of a given gender, age, weight, height, and physical activity level. The values listed are based on an "active" person at the reference height and weight and at the midpoint ages for each group until age 19.

[c] The linolenic acid referred to in this table and text is the omega-3 fatty acid known as alpha-linolenic acid.

[d] The values listed are based on reference body weights.

[e] Assumed to be from human milk.

[f] Assumed to be from human milk and complementary foods and beverages. This includes approximately 0.6 L (~3 cups) as total fluid including formula, juices, and drinking water.

[g] For energy, the age groups for young children are 1–2 years and 3–8 years.

[h] For males, subtract 10 kcalories per day for each year of age above 19.

[i] For females, subtract 7 kcalories per day for each year of age above 19.

Source: Reprinted with permission from *Dietary Reference Intakes.* © 2005 by the National Academies of Sciences, courtesy of the National Academies Press, Washington, DC.

to determine how much of a nutrient is required in the diet to maintain a specific function, such as the amount of calcium needed to minimize bone loss in later life. Using a population-wide average, the Estimated Average Requirement is an amount that seems to be sufficient to maintain a specific body function.

2. **Recommended Dietary Allowance (RDA).** The RDA is the intake recommended for most healthy people. The RDAs are considered generous so they will meet the needs of most people, particularly for vitamins and minerals.

3. **Adequate Intake (AI).** For nutrients that lack enough scientific evidence to determine an Estimated Average Requirement, an Adequate Intake (AI) is established instead of an RDA. An AI reflects the average amount of a nutrient that a group of healthy people consumes.

(Table 8.3 displays the Dietary Reference Intakes for water, energy and the energy nutrients; Table 8.4

TABLE 8.4 Recommended Dietary Allowances (RDA) and Adequate Intakes (AI) for Vitamins

Age (yr)	Thiamin RDA (mg/day)	Riboflavin RDA (mg/day)	Niacin RDA (mg/day)[a]	Biotin AI (mg/day)	Pantothenic acid AI (mg/day)	Vitamin B₆ RDA (mg/day)	Folate RDA (µg/day)[b]	Vitamin B₁₂ RDA (µg/day)	Choline AI (mg/day)	Vitamin C RDA (mg/day)	Vitamin A RDA (µg/day)[c]	Vitamin D AI (µg/day)[d]	Vitamin E RDA (mg/day)[e]	Vitamin K AI (µg/day)
Infants														
0–0.5	0.2	0.3	2	5	1.7	0.1	65	0.4	125	40	400	5	4	2.0
0.5–1	0.3	0.4	4	6	1.8	0.3	80	0.5	150	50	500	5	5	2.5
Children														
1–3	0.5	0.5	6	8	2	0.5	150	0.9	200	15	300	5	6	30
4–8	0.6	0.6	8	12	3	0.6	200	1.2	250	25	400	5	7	55
Males														
9–13	0.9	0.9	12	20	4	1.0	300	1.8	375	45	600	5	11	60
14–18	1.2	1.3	16	25	5	1.3	400	2.4	550	75	900	5	15	75
19–30	1.2	1.3	16	30	5	1.3	400	2.4	550	90	900	5	15	120
31–50	1.2	1.3	16	30	5	1.3	400	2.4	550	90	900	5	15	120
51–70	1.2	1.3	16	30	5	1.7	400	2.4	550	90	900	10	15	120
>70	1.2	1.3	16	30	5	1.7	400	2.4	550	90	900	15	15	120
Females														
9–13	0.9	0.9	12	20	4	1.0	300	1.8	375	45	600	5	11	60
14–18	1.0	1.0	14	25	5	1.2	400	2.4	400	65	700	5	15	75
19–30	1.1	1.1	14	30	5	1.3	400	2.4	425	75	700	5	15	90
31–50	1.1	1.1	14	30	5	1.3	400	2.4	425	75	700	5	15	90
51–70	1.1	1.1	14	30	5	1.5	400	2.4	425	75	700	10	15	90
>70	1.1	1.1	14	30	5	1.5	400	2.4	425	75	700	15	15	90
Pregnancy														
≤18	1.4	1.4	18	30	6	1.9	600	2.6	450	80	750	5	15	75
19–30	1.4	1.4	18	30	6	1.9	600	2.6	450	85	770	5	15	90
31–50	1.4	1.4	18	30	6	1.9	600	2.6	450	85	770	5	15	90
Lactation														
≤18	1.4	1.6	17	35	7	2.0	500	2.8	550	115	1200	5	19	75
19–30	1.4	1.6	17	35	7	2.0	500	2.8	550	120	1300	5	19	90
31–50	1.4	1.6	17	35	7	2.0	500	2.8	550	120	1300	5	19	90

Note: For all nutrients, values for infants are AI.

[a] Niacin recommendations are expressed as niacin equivalents (NE), except for recommendations for infants younger than 6 months, which are expressed as preformed niacin.

[b] Folate recommendations are expressed as dietery folate equivalents (DFE).

[c] Vitamin A recommendations are expressed as retinol activity equivalents (RAE).

[d] Vitamin D recommendations are expressed as cholecalciferol and assume an absence of adequate exposure to sunlight.

[e] Vitamin E recommendations are expressed as α-tocopherol.

Source: Reprinted with permission from *Recommended Dietary Allowances (RDA) and Adequate Intakes (AI) for Vitamins*. © 2005 by the National Academies of Sciences, courtesy of the National Academies Press, Washington, DC.

lists the RDA and AI for vitamins, and Table 8.5 provides the RDA and AI for minerals.)

4. **Tolerable Upper Intake Level (TUIL).** This is the level at which a nutrient is likely to become toxic. People's tolerances for high doses of nutrients vary, and somewhere above the recommended intake is the Tolerable Upper Intake Level. Nutrient recommendations fall within a range, with marginal and danger zones both below and above it. Upper levels are useful in guarding against the overconsumption of nutrients, which is most likely to occur when people use supplements or fortified foods regularly. (Table 8.8 displays the Tolerable Upper Intake Levels.)

Recommended Dietary Allowances (RDA) The average daily amount of a nutrient considered adequate to meet the known nutrient needs of most healthy people—a goal for dietary intakes by individuals.

Adequate Intakes (AI) The average amount of a nutrient that appears to be sufficient to maintain a specific criteria; used as a guide for nutrient intake when an RDA cannot be determined.

Tolerable Upper Intake Level (TUIL) The maximum amount of a nutrient that seems to be safe for most healthy people and beyond which there is an increased risk of adverse effects.

TABLE 8.5 Recommended Dietary Allowances (RDA) and Adequate Intakes (AI) for Minerals

Age (yr)	Sodium AI (mg/day)	Chloride AI (mg/day)	Potassium AI (mg/day)a	Calcium AI (mg/day)	Phosphorus RDA (mg/day)	Magnesium RDA (mg/day)	Iron RDA (mg/day)	Zinc RDA (mg/day)	Iodine RDA (µg/day)	Selenium RDA (µg/day)	Copper RDA (µg/day)	Manganese AI (mg/day)	Fluoride AI (mg/day)	Chromium AI (µg/day)	Molybdenum RDA (µg/day)
Infants															
0–0.5	120	180	400	210	100	30	0.27	2	110	15	200	0.003	0.01	0.2	2
0.5–1	370	570	700	270	275	75	11	3	130	20	220	0.6	0.5	5.5	3
Children															
1–3	1000	1500	3000	500	460	80	7	3	90	20	340	1.2	0.7	11	17
4–8	1200	1900	3800	800	500	130	10	5	90	30	440	1.5	1.0	15	22
Males															
9–13	1500	2300	4500	1300	1250	240	8	8	120	40	700	1.9	2	25	34
14–18	1500	2300	4700	1300	1250	410	11	11	150	55	890	2.2	3	35	43
19–30	1500	2300	4700	1000	700	400	8	11	150	55	900	2.3	4	35	45
31–50	1500	2300	4700	1000	700	420	8	11	150	55	900	2.3	4	35	45
51–70	1300	2000	4700	1200	700	420	8	11	150	55	900	2.3	4	30	45
>70	1200	1800	4700	1200	700	420	8	11	150	55	900	2.3	4	30	45
Females															
9–13	1500	2300	4500	1300	1250	240	8	8	120	40	700	1.6	2	21	34
14–18	1500	2300	4700	1300	1250	360	15	9	150	55	890	1.6	3	24	43
19–30	1500	2300	4700	1000	700	310	18	8	150	55	900	1.8	3	25	45
31–50	1500	2300	4700	1000	700	320	18	8	150	55	900	1.8	3	25	45
51–70	1300	2000	4700	1200	700	320	8	8	150	55	900	1.8	3	20	45
>70	1200	1800	4700	1200	700	320	8	8	150	55	900	1.8	3	20	45
Pregnancy															
≤18	1500	2300	4700	1300	1250	400	27	12	220	60	1000	2.0	3	29	50
19–30	1500	2300	4700	1000	700	350	27	11	220	60	1000	2.0	3	30	50
31–50	1500	2300	4700	1000	700	360	27	11	220	60	1000	2.0	3	30	50
Lactation															
≤18	1500	2300	5100	1300	1250	360	10	14	290	70	1300	2.6	3	44	50
19–30	1500	2300	5100	1000	700	310	9	12	290	70	1300	2.6	3	45	50
31–50	1500	2300	5100	1000	700	320	9	12	290	70	1300	2.6	3	45	50

Source: Reprinted with permission from *Recommended Dietary Allowances (RDA) and Adequate Intakes (AI) for Minerals.* © 2005 by the National Academies of Sciences, courtesy of the National Academies Press, Washington, DC.

Daily Values and Food Labels

The U. S. Food and Drug Administration developed a system for food labeling, called **Daily Values (DV)**. Based on a 2,000 calorie diet, each nutrient contained in a serving of the product is expressed as a percent of that nutrient's daily recommended intake. Assuming that you consume a 2,000 calorie diet, then, you will obtain that percent of the daily value from one serving of the product. These percentages, of course, require adjustments depending on an individual's daily caloric needs. Both the RDA and the Daily Values apply only to healthy people. They are not intended for people who are ill and who may require additional nutrients.

Reading the Food Label (Figure 8.5) can help you make wise food choices. By law, the FDA requires that all the nutrients in a food must be listed on the label in language the consumer can understand. By law, every food label also must include the following:

- Common name of the product
- Name and address of the manufacturer, distributor, or packer
- Net contents of the package (count, measure, or weight)
- Ingredients listed in descending order, with the most plentiful ingredient listed first

If the product makes any nutritional claims, the law requires that the following nutritional information be listed on the label under the heading "Nutritional Information":

- Serving or portion size
- Servings per container

Daily Values (DV) Reference values of daily requirements developed by the Food and Drug Administration (FDA) specifically for use on food labels.

FIGURE 8.5   Information on a Food Label

Nutrition Facts

Serving Size 1 cup (228g)
Servings Per Container 2

Amount Per Serving

Calories 90	Calories from Fat 30

	% Daily Value*
Total Fat 3g	**5%**
Saturated Fat 0g	**0%**
Cholesterol 0mg	**0%**
Sodium 300mg	**13%**
Total Carbohydrate 13g	**4%**
Dietary Fiber 3g	**12%**
Sugars 3g	
Protein 3g	

Vitamin A	80%	•	Vitamin C	60%
Calcium	4%	•	Iron	4%

*% Daily Values are based on a 2000 calorie diet. Your daily values may be higher or lower depending on your calorie needs:

		Calories	2000	2500
Total Fat	Less than		65g	80g
Sat Fat	Less than		20g	25g
Cholesterol	Less than		300mg	300mg
Sodium	Less than		2400mg	2400mg
Total Carbohydrate			300g	375g
Dietary Fiber			25g	30g

Calories per gram:
Fat 9   •   Carbohydrates 4   •   Protein 4

Serving Size

Similar food products now have similar serving sizes. This makes it easier to compare foods. Serving sizes are based on amounts people actually eat.

New Label Information

Some label information may be new to you. The new nutrient list covers those most important to your health. You may have seen this information on some old labels, but it is now required.

Vitamins and Minerals

Only two vitamins, A and C, and two minerals, calcium and iron, are required on the food label. A food company can voluntarily list other vitamins and minerals in the food.

Label Numbers

Numbers on the nutrition label may be rounded for labeling.

Foods that have only a few of the nutrients required on the standard label can use a short label format. What's on the label depends on what's in the food. Small- and medium-sized packages with very little label space also can use a short label.

% Daily Value

% Daily Value shows how a food fits into a 2,000-calorie reference diet.

You can use % Daily Value to compare foods and see how the amount of a nutrient in a serving of food fits in a 2,000-calorie reference diet.

Daily Values Footnote

Daily Values are the new label reference numbers. These numbers are set by the government and are based on current nutrition recommendations.

Some labels list the daily values for a daily diet of 2,000 and 2,500 calories. Your own nutrient needs may be less than or more than the Daily Values on the label.

Calories Per Gram Footnote

Some labels tell the approximate number of calories in a gram of fat, carbohydrate, and protein.

Some food packages make claims such as "light," "low-fat," and "cholesterol-free." These claims can be used only if a food meets strict government definitions. Here are some of the meanings:

Label claim	Definition*
Calorie-Free	Less than 5 calories
Light or Lite	1/3 fewer calories or 50% less fat; if more than half the calories are from fat, fat content must be reduced by 50% or more
Light in Sodium	50% less sodium
Fat-Free	Less than 1/2 gram fat
Low-Fat	3 grams or less fat**
Cholesterol-Free	Less than 2 milligrams cholesterol and 2 grams or less saturated fat**
Low Cholesterol	20 milligrams or less cholesterol and 2 grams or less saturated fat**
Sodium-Free	Less than 5 milligrams sodium**
Very Low Sodium	35 milligrams or less sodium**
Low-Sodium	140 milligrams or less sodium**
High Fiber	5 grams or more fiber

*Per Reference Amount (standard serving size). Some claims have higher nutrient levels for main dish products and meal products, such as frozen entrees and dinners.

**Also per 50 g for products with small serving sizes (reference amount is 30 g or less or 2 tbsp or less).

Some food packages may now carry health claims. A health claim is a label statement that describes the relationship between a nutrient and a disease or health-related condition. A food must meet certain nutrient levels to make a health claim. Seven types of health claims are allowed. These nutrient-disease relationships include

A diet:	And:
High in calcium	Osteoporosis (brittle bone disease)
High in fiber-containing grain products, fruits, and vegetables	Cancer
High in fruits or vegetables (high in dietary fiber or vitamins A or C)	Cancer
High in fiber from fruits, vegetables, and grain products	Heart disease
Low in fat	Cancer
Low in saturated fat and cholesterol	Heart disease
Low in sodium	High blood pressure

- Calories per serving
- Carbohydrates (in grams) per serving
- Fats (in grams) per serving
- Vitamins, minerals, and proteins (as percentages of the RDA) per serving
- Amount of eight "indicator nutrients"—protein, vitamin A, niacin, thiamine, riboflavin, vitamin C, calcium, and iron

Consumer Concerns about Foods

From time to time, people raise concerns regarding food safety issues. Primary among these are additives, **irradiation**, and food-borne illness.

Food additives are chemical agents added to processed foods to help preserve them or to change their appearance or enhance their flavor. Food additives fall into the general categories of antioxidants, emulsifiers, flavorings, preservatives, and sweeteners.

Antioxidants, such as BA and BHT, are synthetic chemicals used to keep oils and fats from becoming rancid. Emulsifiers suspend the flavor oils throughout the product, improving both flavor and appearance. A number of artificial agents are used in processed foods to enhance flavor. Some—such as sodium nitrate, used in corned beef and bacon as well as other red meats—are also used as coloring agents or preservatives. Preservatives inhibit bacterial growth, giving processed foods a longer shelf life.

In an attempt to improve the quality of food, some manufacturers use radiation to treat both fresh and processed foods. Essentially, foods are exposed to gamma radiation, which increases the shelf life of the product and destroys any microorganisms that might have contaminated the food. The process of irradiation does not make food radioactive. The FDA has approved irradiation to enhance food safety.

Food contaminated with bacteria or parasites can cause food-borne illness, characterized by nausea, vomiting, abdominal pain, bloating, gas, and diarrhea. The symptoms of food-borne illness most often begin within 5 to 8 hours after eating the contaminated food. Symptoms, however, depend on the type of organism that causes the illness: they may begin as soon as 30 minutes after eating the food or as long as several weeks afterward. When symptoms do not develop for days or weeks, the problem often is misdiagnosed because it cannot be related readily to a specific food.

Although many cases of food-borne illness can be traced to food served at restaurants, approximately one-third can be traced to careless or unsafe handling and preparation of food in the home. To protect yourself from food-borne illness at home, do the following:

- When you shop, put meat, poultry, and fish in separate plastic bags so their drippings don't contaminate your other groceries.

- Check the expiration date on all meat, poultry, and fish before you buy it. When possible, get meat that was put in the cooler that day. Buy only what you can use within the next few days unless you are planning to freeze it. Keep meat, poultry, and fish in the refrigerator (that is, unfrozen) no longer than 3 days.
- Never buy meat, poultry, fish, or fresh produce from counters that are not clean.
- Refrigerate perishable foods (including fresh produce) as soon as you get home from the store. Make sure that your refrigerator keeps foods at 40°F or cooler, as bacteria thrive at temperatures as low as 45°F.
- Never thaw foods on the counter. Foods should be thawed in the refrigerator, in the microwave, or submerged in cold water. Cook food as soon as it is defrosted.
- After you've touched any raw meat (including poultry and fish), and before you handle any other food or eat, wash your hands thoroughly with soap and running hot water.
- Use paper towels to wipe up meat juices, then discard the paper towels. Wash sponges in the dishwasher at least every other day. Wash dishcloths and kitchen towels in hot water and machine-dry. Hang kitchen towels promptly after each use to air-dry and discourage growth of bacteria.
- Wash utensils and cutting boards thoroughly with hot, soapy water after preparing raw meat, poultry, or fish and before using them to prepare other uncooked foods, such as salad ingredients. When possible, use separate cutting boards.
- If you use a wood cutting board for meat or poultry, never use it to prepare other foods, regardless of how well you wash it. Wood can absorb bacteria, and it is difficult to clean thoroughly.
- Wash cutting boards with soap and hot water after each use, and allow them to air-dry. Wash glass, solid wood, and plastic cutting boards in the dishwasher. Discard a plastic cutting board when it gets excessively cut up.
- Sanitize cutting boards at least once a week with a solution of 2 teaspoons of chlorine (household) bleach in 1 quart of water. Leave the bleach solution standing on the surface of the cutting board for 5 minutes, rinse well, and allow to air-dry.
- Avoid eating raw eggs (common in homemade ice cream, homemade mayonnaise, Caesar salad, hollandaise sauce, and homemade "energy drinks"). Cook eggs until both the yolks and whites are set (not runny).
- Cook all meat, poultry, and fish thoroughly. An estimated 5 percent of all meat is contaminated with *E. coli* bacteria, and these bacteria are not destroyed by refrigeration or freezing. Approximately 25 percent of all chicken marketed in the United States is contaminated with salmonella bacteria. The only way to destroy any bacteria in meat is to cook it thoroughly. The juices of pork and chicken should run clear, with no trace of pink in the meat. Cook beef until it is at least medium

rare; the more rare the beef, the greater the risk for food-borne illness. Cook fish until the thickest part is opaque and flakes easily with a fork. Ground meat and poultry pose the highest risk for contamination, because bacteria on the surface can be mixed into the meat during grinding. Make sure that all ground meat is cooked thoroughly, with no traces of pink.

- Never place cooked meat on the same plate that held the raw meat.
- Do not leave cooked foods standing at room temperature for longer than 2 hours, and refrigerate leftovers immediately.
- If you have any question regarding the safety of a food item, do not eat it. The rule of thumb is, "When in doubt, throw it out."

How to Choose Nutritious Foods

Altogether, people need about 40 vitamins and minerals. How can we meet our needs for all these nutrients? Eating wisely usually does not mean making drastic changes. More often it means fine-tuning your current diet: Eat this food more often, and eat that food a little less often. For many people, a helpful way to plan adequate, balanced diets is offered by the USDA Food Guide.

USDA FOOD GUIDE

The **USDA Food Guide**, shown in Figure 8.7, can help a diet planner design an adequate and balanced diet. This food group plan defines the major food groups and their subgroups and suggests portions of foods from each group. One goal is to convey the key nutrients provided by foods within the groups. These are listed in the figure. This figure also categorized foods within each group according to nutrient density. To control calories and prevent overweight or obesity, the most nutrient-dense foods from each group are recommended.

The USDA recommends eating fresh fruits or fruit juices each day. Fruits supply carbohydrates, vitamins A and C, potassium, and other nutrients. A serving is considered to be one whole fresh fruit (such as a medium banana or medium apple); ½ cup of raw, cooked, or canned fruit; ¼ cup of dried fruit; or ¾ cup of fruit juice (fresh, frozen, or canned).

Most vegetables and fruits are naturally low in calories and rich in nutrients. Vegetables supply carbohydrate, vitamin A, folate, and other nutrients. A serving of vegetables is considered to be ½ cup of chopped fresh, frozen, or canned vegetables; ¼ cup of dried vegetables; 1 cup of raw leafy vegetables; or ¾ cup of vegetable juice (fresh, frozen, or canned). To save the nutrients in vegetables, they should not be cooked in water or overcooked. Baking, steaming, and microwaving vegetables best preserves the nutrients. Eating them raw, when possible, is

Selecting Nutritious Foods

To select nutritious foods:

1. Given the choice between whole foods and refined, processed foods, choose the former (apples rather than apple pie, potatoes rather than potato chips). Fewer nutrients have been refined out of the whole foods; less fat, salt, and sugar have been added.
2. Choose the leaner cuts of meat. Select fish or poultry often, beef seldom. Ask for broiled, not fried, to control your fat intake.
3. Use both raw and cooked vegetables and fruits. Raw foods offer more fiber and vitamins, such as folate and thiamin, that are destroyed by cooking. Cooking foods frees other vitamins and minerals for absorption.
4. Include milk, milk products, or other calcium sources for the calcium you need. Use low-fat or nonfat items to reduce fat and calories.
5. Learn to use margarine, butter, and oils sparingly. A little gives flavor; a lot overloads you with fat and calories.
6. Vary your choices. Eat broccoli today, carrots tomorrow, and corn the next day. Eat Chinese today, Italian tomorrow, and hot dogs and beans on Saturday.
7. Load your plate with vegetables and unrefined starchy foods. A small portion of meat or cheese is all you need for protein.
8. When choosing breads and cereals, choose the whole-grain varieties.

To select nutritious fast foods:

9. Choose the broiled sandwich with lettuce, tomatoes, and other goodies—and hold the mayo—rather than the fish or chicken patties coated with breadcrumbs and cooked in fat.
10. Select a salad—and use more plain vegetables than those mixed with oily or mayonnaise-based dressings.
11. Order chili with more beans than meat. Choose a soft bean burrito over tacos with fried shells.
12. Drink low-fat milk rather than a cola beverage.

When choosing from a vending machine:

13. Choose cracker sandwiches over chips and pork rinds (virtually pure fat). Choose peanuts, pretzels, and popcorn over cookies and candy.
14. Choose milk and juices over cola beverages.

Irradiation Sterilizing a food by exposure to energy waves; kills microorganisms and insects.

USDA Food Guide A food group plan that assigns foods to major food groups; developed by U. S. Department of Agriculture.

FIGURE 8.7 USDA Food Guide

Key:

● Foods generally high in nutrient density (choose most often)

▲ Foods lower in nutrient density (limit selections)

GRAINS

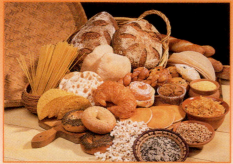

© Polara Studios, Inc.

Make at least half of the grain selections whole grains.

These foods contribute folate, niacin, riboflavin, thiamin, iron, magnesium, selenium, and fiber.

> **1 oz grains is equivalent to 1 slice bread; ½ c cooked rice, pasta, or cereal; 1 oz dry pasta or rice; 1 c ready-to-eat cereal; 3 c popped popcorn.**

● Whole grains (barley, brown rice, bulgur, millet, oats, rye, wheat) and whole-grain, low-fat breads, cereals, crackers, and pastas; popcorn.

● Enriched bagels, breads, cereals, pastas (couscous, macaroni, spaghetti), pretzels, rice, rolls, tortillas.

▲ Biscuits, cakes, cookies, cornbread, crackers, croissants, doughnuts, french toast, fried rice, granola, muffins, pancakes, pastries, pies, presweetened cereals, taco shells, waffles.

VEGETABLES

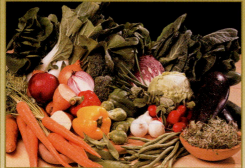

© Polara Studios, Inc.

Choose a variety of vegetables from all five subgroups several times a week.

These foods contribute folate, vitamin A, vitamin C, vitamin E, magnesium, potassium, and fiber.

> **½ c vegetables is equivalent to ½ c cut-up raw or cooked vegetables; ½ c cooked legumes; ½ c vegetable juice; 1 c raw, leafy greens.**

● Dark green vegetables: Broccoli and leafy greens such as arugula, beet greens, bok choy, collard greens, kale, mustard greens, romaine lettuce, spinach, and turnip greens.

● Orange and deep yellow vegetables: Carrots, carrot juice, pumpkin, sweet potatoes, and winter squash (acorn, butternut).

● Legumes: Black beans, black-eyed peas, garbanzo beans (chickpeas), kidney beans, lentils, navy beans, pinto beans, soybeans and soy products such as tofu, and split peas.

● Starchy vegetables: Cassava, corn, green peas, hominy, lima beans, and potatoes.

● Other vegetables: Artichokes, asparagus, bamboo shoots, bean sprouts, beets, Brussels sprouts, cabbages, cactus, cauliflower, celery, cucumbers, eggplant, green beans, iceberg lettuce, mushrooms, okra, onions, peppers, seaweed, snow peas, tomatoes, vegetable juices, zucchini.

▲ Baked beans, candied sweet potatoes, coleslaw, french fries, potato salad, refried beans, scalloped potatoes, tempura vegetables.

FRUITS

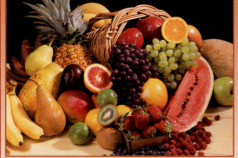

© Polara Studios, Inc.

Consume a variety of fruits and no more than one-third of the recommended intake as fruit juice.

These foods contribute folate, vitamin A, vitamin C, potassium, and fiber.

> **½ c fruit is equivalent to ½ c fresh, frozen, or canned fruit; 1 small fruit; ¼ c dried fruit; ½ c fruit juice.**

● Apples, apricots, avocados, bananas, blueberries, cantaloupe, cherries, grapefruit, grapes, guava, kiwi, mango, oranges, papaya, peaches, pears, pineapples, plums, raspberries, strawberries, watermelon; dried fruit; unsweetened juices.

▲ Canned or frozen fruit in syrup; juices, punches, ades, and fruit drinks with added sugars; fried plantains.

MEAT, POULTRY, FISH, LEGUMES, BEANS, EGGS, AND NUTS

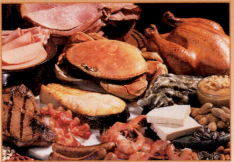

© Polara Studios, Inc.

Make lean or low-fat choices. Prepare them with little, or no, added fat.

Meat, poultry, fish, and eggs contribute protein, niacin, thiamin, vitamin B_6, vitamin B_{12}, iron, magnesium, potassium, and zinc; legumes and nuts are notable for their protein, folate, thiamin, vitamin E, iron, magnesium, potassium, zinc, and fiber.

> 1 oz meat is equivalent to 1 oz cooked lean meat, poultry, or fish; 1 egg;
> $\frac{1}{4}$ c cooked legumes or tofu; 1 tbs peanut butter; $\frac{1}{2}$ oz nuts or seeds.

● Poultry (no skin), fish, shellfish, legumes, eggs, lean meat (fat-trimmed beef, game, ham, lamb, pork); low-fat tofu, tempeh, peanut butter, nuts or seeds.

▲ Bacon; baked beans; fried meat, fish, poultry, eggs, or tofu; refried beans; ground beef; hot dogs; luncheon meats; marbled steaks; poultry with skin; sausages; spare ribs.

MILK, YOGURT, AND CHEESE

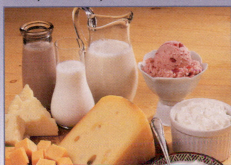

© Polara Studios, Inc.

Make fat-free or low-fat choices. Choose lactose-free products or other calcium-rich foods if you don't consume milk.

These foods contribute protein, riboflavin, vitamin B_{12}, calcium, magnesium, potassium, and, when fortified, vitamin A and vitamin D.

> 1 c milk is equivalent to 1 c fat-free milk or yogurt;
> $1\frac{1}{2}$ oz fat-free natural cheese; 2 oz fat-free processed cheese.

● Fat-free milk and fat-free milk products such as buttermilk, cheeses, cottage cheese, yogurt; fat-free fortified soy milk.

▲ 1% low-fat milk, 2% reduced-fat milk, and whole milk; low-fat, reduced-fat, and whole-milk products such as cheeses, cottage cheese, and yogurt; milk products with added sugars such as chocolate milk, custard, ice cream, ice milk, milk shakes, pudding, sherbet; fortified soy milk.

OILS

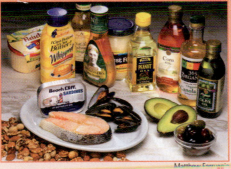

Matthew Farruggio

Select the recommended amounts of oils from among these sources.

These foods contribute vitamin E and essential fatty acids, along with abundant calories.

> 1 tsp oil is equivalent to 1 tbs low-fat mayonnaise; 2 tbs light salad
> dressing; 1 tsp vegetable oil; 1 tsp soft margarine.

● Liquid vegetable oils such as canola, corn, flaxseed, nut, olive, peanut, safflower, sesame, soybean, and sunflower oils; mayonnaise, oil-based salad dressing, soft *trans*-free margarine.

● Unsaturated oils that occur naturally in foods such as avocados, fatty fish, nuts, olives, and shellfish.

SOLID FATS AND ADDED SUGARS

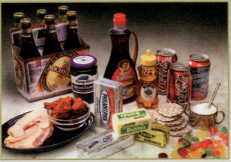

Matthew Farruggio

Limit intakes of food and beverages with solid fats and added sugars.

Solid fats deliver saturated fat and *trans* fat, and intake should be kept low. Solid fats and added sugars contribute abundant calories but few nutrients, and intakes should not exceed the discretionary calorie allowance—calories to meet energy needs after all nutrient needs have been met with nutrient-dense foods. Alcohol also contributes abundant calories but few nutrients, and its calories are counted among discretionary calories.

▲ Solid fats that occur in foods naturally such as milk fat and meat fat (see ▲ in previous lists).

▲ Solid fats that are often added to foods such as butter, cream cheese, hard margarine, lard, sour cream, and shortening.

▲ Added sugars such as brown sugar, candy, honey, jelly, molasses, soft drinks, sugar, and syrup.

▲ Alcoholic beverages include beer, wine, and liquor.

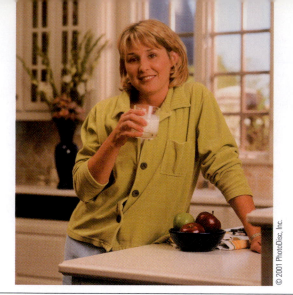

Consuming dairy foods today will help reduce your risk of osteoporosis tomorrow.

© 2001 PhotoDisc, Inc.

TABLE 8.6 Estimated Daily Calorie Needs for Adults

	Sedentary	Active
Women		
19–30 yr	2000	2400
31–50 yr	1800	2200
51 + yr	1600	2100
Men		
19–30 yr	2400	3000
31–50 yr	2200	2900
51 + yr	2000	2600

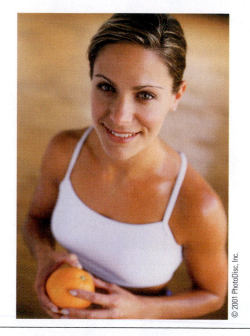

Once you are achieving the dietary behaviors you seek, congratulate yourself.

© 2001 PhotoDisc, Inc.

also beneficial. Eating skins (well-scrubbed)—of apples or potatoes, for instance—boosts fiber in the diet, as does eating the edible seeds of fruits, such as the seeds in strawberries, raspberries, and pomegranates.

Grains supply complex carbohydrate, riboflavin, thiamin, niacin, iron, and other nutrients. Within this group, you should focus on whole-grain foods that are lowest in fat and eat fewer refined foods from this group (white bread, white rice, and refined cereals).

Meats or meat alternatives supply protein, iron, niacin, folate, zinc, and other nutrients. The best sources are low in fat: fish, skinless poultry, lean cuts of meat, dried beans, and peas, for example. The key with meats is to serve smaller portions than you probably are accustomed to. A single serving of cooked protein is only 2 to 3 ounces, or about the size of a deck of playing cards. The following non-meat proteins can be substituted for 1 ounce of meat:

- 3 ounces of tofu
- 1 egg
- 2 tablespoons of peanut butter
- 1¼ cup of dried beans or peas, cooked
- 1¼ cup nuts

Milk, yogurt and cheese products provide carbohydrate, calcium, riboflavin, protein, vitamin D, and other nutrients. The wiser choices are those that are low in fat, such as low-fat or skim milk, 1% cottage cheese, and part-skim cheeses (such as ricotta and mozzarella). A single serving of dairy food consists of 1 cup of milk, 1 cup of yogurt, 2 ounces of processed cheese, 1½ ounces of natural cheese, ½ cup of cottage cheese, or 1½ cups of ice cream or frozen yogurt.

Oils, solid fat and sweets—should be eaten sparingly. People who consistently choose nutrient-dense foods, however, may be able to meet their nutrient needs without consuming their full allotment of calories. This difference between the calories needed to supply nutrients and

those needed for energy is known as the discretionary calorie allowance. Table 8.6 shows the estimated daily calorie needs for adults, and Table 8.7 gives the recommended daily amounts from each food group.

MYPYRAMID—STEPS TO A HEALTHIER YOU

The USDA created an educational tool called MyPyramid to illustrate the concepts of the Dietary Guidelines and USDA Food Guide. Figure 8.6 presents MyPyramid. People are able to create an individualized diet plan and utilize other valuable resources. On the Internet, this is available at MyPyramid.gov.

When you plan your meals, remember that your own body is unique. It responds to food in its own characteristic ways according to your genetic inheritance and current needs. For example, a sedentary young woman who tends to gain weight may need to take steps to reduce her intake of fat, but an active young man who tends to stay thin might have to consume more calorie-dense foods to

TABLE 8.7 Recommended Daily Amounts from Each Food Group

Food Group	1600 cal	1800 cal	2000 cal	2200 cal	2400 cal	2600 cal	2800 cal	3000 cal
Fruits	1½ c	1½ c	2 c	2 c	2 c	2 c	2½ c	2½ c
Vegetables	2 c	2½ c	2½ c	3 c	3 c	3½ c	3½ c	4 c
Grains	5 oz	6 oz	6 oz	7 oz	8 oz	9 oz	10 oz	10 oz
Meat and legumes	5 oz	5 oz	5½ oz	6 oz	6½ oz	6½ oz	7 oz	7 oz
Milk	3 c	3 c	3 c	3 c	3 c	3 c	3 c	3 c
Oils	5 tsp	5 tsp	6 tsp	6 tsp	7 tsp	8 tsp	8 tsp	10 tsp
Discretionary calorie allowance	132 cal	195 cal	267 cal	290 cal	362 cal	410 cal	426 cal	512 cal

FIGURE 8.6 MyPyramid

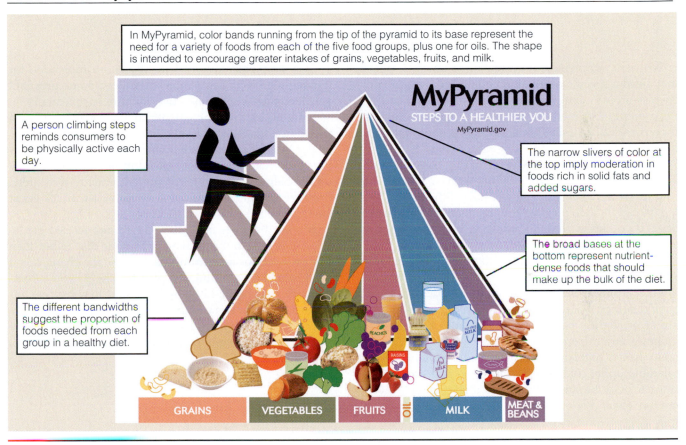

In MyPyramid, color bands running from the tip of the pyramid to its base represent the need for a variety of foods from each of the five food groups, plus one for oils. The shape is intended to encourage greater intakes of grains, vegetables, fruits, and milk.

A person climbing steps reminds consumers to be physically active each day.

The narrow slivers of color at the top imply moderation in foods rich in solid fats and added sugars.

The broad bases at the bottom represent nutrient-dense foods that should make up the bulk of the diet.

The different bandwidths suggest the proportion of foods needed from each group in a healthy diet.

MyPyramid
STEPS TO A HEALTHIER YOU
MyPyramid.gov

GRAINS VEGETABLES FRUITS OIL MILK MEAT & BEANS

add to his body weight. The point here is to think carefully about your own body and its needs before taking any dietary actions. Assessment 8.4 can help you evaluate the quality of your diet. If you have special concerns, see a nutrition expert, or a registered dietitian.

Nutrient Supplements

Billions of dollars are spent on vitamin/mineral supplements each year. Some people who haven't learned enough about nutrition think they need supplements as insurance against their own poor food choices. Indeed, their food choices may be poor, but taking supplements is no guarantee that they will obtain the nutrients they

need. It is just as likely that they will duplicate the nutrients their food supply provides and still lack the ones they need. The only way to be sure to get the needed assortment of nutrients is to construct a balanced diet from a variety of foods. Besides, no supplement can give you all the nutrients you get from food.

No one supplement can match a balanced diet, and no combination of supplements can, either. No one knows enough yet to construct a synthetic substitute for food. Even in hospitals where the most advanced technology is available and advanced formulas are supplied for patients who cannot eat, these formulas only enable patients to survive. The patients do not thrive until they are consuming food again.

TABLE 8.8 Tolerable Upper Intake Levels

Adults	Vitamins								Minerals			
	Niacin (mg/day)[a]	Vitamin B₆ (mg/day)	Folate (mg/day)[b]	Choline (mg/day)	Vitamin C (mg/day)	Vitamin A (mg/day)[c]	Vitamin D (mg/day)[d]	Vitamin E (mg/day)[e]	Calcium (mg/day)	Phosporus (mg/day)	Magnesium (mg/day)	Iron (mg/day)
19–70	35	100	1000	3500	2000	3000	50	1000	2500	4000	350	45
>70	35	100	1000	3500	2000	3000	50	1000	2500	3000	350	45

[a] The UL for niacin and folate apply to synthetic forms obtained from supplements, fortified foods, or a combination of the two.

[b] The UL for vitamin A applies to the preformed vitamin only.

[c] The UL for vitamin E applies to any form of supplemental α-tocopherol, fortified foods, or a combination of the two.

[d] The UL for magnesium applies to synthetic forms obtained from supplements or drugs only.

Source: Reprinted with permission from *Tolerable Upper Intake Levels.* © 2005 by the National Academies of Sciences, courtesy of the National Academies Press, Washington, DC.

Nutrient supplements are useful at times. A person may need a specific nutrient to counteract a specific deficiency—iron to compensate for iron-deficiency anemia, for example. But medical training and tests are required for a correct diagnosis. People cannot diagnose their own deficiencies.

Other circumstances in which you may consider taking a supplement are (1) if your energy intake is below 1,500 calories per day, because you will have difficulty consuming enough food to meet your vitamin and mineral needs; or (2) if you know that, for whatever reason, you will be eating irregularly for a limited time.

Whenever a health care provider has recommended a supplement, follow directions carefully as to the type and dosage. A single, balanced, vitamin/mineral supplement should suffice. Look for one in which the nutrient levels are at or slightly below the RDA. Avoid high doses of vitamins and minerals, as excessive intakes can cause as many health problems as deficient intakes. Table 8.8 lists tolerable upper intake levels or levels that are likely to cause toxicity. Be sure to keep your intake at a safe level—not too low and not too high.

Iron supplementation frequently is recommended for women who have heavy menstrual flow. Some pregnant and lactating women also may require supplements. In specific instances, supplements should be selected with the advice of a registered dietitian.

For healthy people with a balanced diet, most supplements do not seem to provide additional benefits. They do not help people run faster, jump higher, relieve stress, improve sexual prowess, cure a common cold, or boost energy levels.

If your diet does not follow the recommended guidelines, it is best to make changes in your diet rather than rely on a pill for nutrient needs. Outline the changes you need to make, then design a plan that helps you accomplish those changes. Little by little, start to substitute nutritious foods for some empty-calorie foods. Once you are achieving the dietary behaviors you desire, congratulate yourself. You'll begin to feel better and your body will appreciate it!

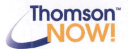

Don't forget to check out the wealth of resources on the ThomsonNOW website at **www.thomsonedu.com/ThomsonNOW** that will:

- Coach you through identifying target goals for behavior change and monitoring your personal change plan throughout the semester
- Help you evaluate your knowledge of the material
- Allow you to take an exam-prep quiz
- Provide a Personalized Learning Plan targeting resources that address areas you should study.

WEB ACTIVITIES

American Dietetic Association This comprehensive site features daily food tips, frequently asked questions, nutrition resources, and links to other reliable Web sites on nutrition.

http://www.eatright.org

Dietary Guidelines from the Food and Nutrition Information Center This site features the 2000 American Dietary guidelines and also has links to historical dietary guidelines (since 1894) and dietary guidelines from 20 countries.

http://www.nal.usda.gov/fnic/dga/index.html

InfoTrac®

You can find additional readings related to wellness via InfoTrac® College Edition, an online library of more than 900 journals and publications. Follow the instructions for accessing InfoTrac® that came packaged with your textbook, then search for articles using a key word search.

Suggested Reading "Dark Chocolate May Help Hypertension, but chocolate's no 'health food'—it's the flavenoids," *Tufts University Health & Nutrition Letter*, October 25, 2005, v23m i8 p1.

1. Why do chocolate and cocoa seem to possess antioxidant properties?
2. Physiologically, how do the antioxidants found in chocolate promote vascular health?
3. How does chocolate affect blood pressure?

Conklin, Martha et al. "College students' use of point of selection nutrition information," *Topics in Clinical Nutrition*, April–June 2005 v20 i2 p97 (12).

1. Which gender was more likely to use labels to make food choices? Why do you think this may occur?
2. What motivated women to select particular food items?
3. Which types of foods did men tend to select? What was their motive?

Web Activity

Nutrition Analysis Tool

http://www.ag.uiuc.edu/~food-lab/nat

Sponsor University of Illinois–Urbana/Champaign Council on Food and Agricultural Research.

Description This site features a personalized nutrition assessment tool that allows you to analyze the foods you eat for a variety of nutrients.

Available Activities This site consists of an interactive personalized diet analysis tool that will provide you with nutrient content of foods that you select from a comprehensive database.

- Nutrition Analysis
- Energy Calculator
- Soy Food Finder

Web Work

1. Click on the "Step by Step" button.
2. Enter your age and gender, then click the "Step 2" button.
3. Select the nutrient or nutrients that you would like to include in your analysis.
4. Go back to the home page and select the "Direct to NAT" link. Add the first food to your personal diet list by clicking in the white box above this list and typing the name of the food you wish to add. Then press Enter or click on "Add Food."
5. The Nutrient Analysis Tool now searches its extensive database. NAT will return a list of all the food items that match the word or words you typed. The personal diet list keeps track of all the foods you add, the serving size and number of servings for each food, and the total gram-weight of each food you add.
6. Scroll down the list of foods from the database that match your typed foods, and click on the radio button that best corresponds to it. Then click on the "Add Selected Food" button below this list.
7. Type the number of servings in the appropriate box and use the scroll-down menu to select your serving size. Click on the "Add this Amount" button.
8. This takes you back to the "Add New Food" page. Type in the name of the second food product that you would like analyzed and follow the instructions above. Repeat steps 4–8 for each new food you desire to add to your personal diet list.
9. Finally, click on the "Analyze Food" button to receive your results for the selected nutrients.

Helpful Hints

1. The database has almost every type of food, but some foods may be listed under a different name. http://www.eatright.org.
2. If you have trouble finding a specific food, try using other words that mean the same thing. It is best to start with general terms and then narrow the choices by using more specific terms that describe the food, its contents, or even how it is prepared.

For additional Web activities, links, and suggested readings, visit our Health, Fitness, and Wellness Resource Center at http://health.wadsworth.com.

Notes

1. E. Whitney et al., *Understanding Nutrition,* 10th edition (St. Paul: West Publishing, 2005).
2. J. Matthiessen, S. Fagt, A. Biltoft-Jensen, A. M. Beck, and L. Oversen, "Size Makes a Difference," *Public Health Nutrition* 6 (2003): 65–72.
3. R. R. Briefel, C. L. Johnson "Secular Trends in Dietary Intake in the United States," *Annual Review of Nutrition* 24 (2004): 401–431.
4. K. Glanz, M. Basil, E. Maibach, J. Goldberg, and D. Snyder, "Why Americans Eat What They Do: Taste, Nutrition, Cost, Convenience, and Weight Control Concerns as Influences on Food Consumption," *Journal of the American Dietetic Association*, 98 (1998): 1118–1126.
5. M. A. Pereira, A. I. Kartashov, D. B. Ebbeling, et al., "Fast-Food Habits, Weight Gain, and Insulin Resistance: (The CARDIA study): 15-year Prospective Analysis," *Lancet* 365 (2004): 36–42.
6. J. A. Marlatt, M. I. McBurney, J. L. Slavin, "Position of the American Dietetic Association: Health Implications of Dietary Fiber," *Journal of the American Dietetic Association* 102 (2002): 993–1000.

Assess Your Behavior

1. Thinking about reasons for food choices, which reasons guide your food selections?

2. Comparing your food intake to the food guide recommendations, which food groups are you including and which ones are you omitting? How can you improve the adequacy of your diet?

Assess Your Knowledge

Evaluate how well you understand the concepts presented in this chapter by answering the following questions.

1. The psychological desire to eat is called
   a. hunger.
   b. craving.
   c. appetite.
   d. bulimia.
   e. obesity.

2. The 6 basic nutrients include
   a. protein, vitamins, amino acids, carbohydrates, milk, grains.
   b. protein, fat, carbohydrates, fruits, vegetables, water.
   c. protein, vitamin supplements, carbohydrates, whole grains, water, meat.
   d. protein, fat, carbohydrate, vitamins, minerals, water.
   e. All of the above.

3. Most Americans consume too much
   a. complex carbohydrate.
   b. fiber.
   c. protein.
   d. water.

4. The nutrient that provides the most energy per gram is
   a. protein.
   b. fat.
   c. carbohydrate.
   d. vitamins.
   e. water.

5. The Dietary Reference Intake value that describes toxic levels is
   a. estimated average requirement.
   b. recommended dietary allowance.
   c. adequate intake.
   d. tolerable upper intake level.

6. Strategies for preventing food borne illnesses include
   a. never thawing foods on the counter.
   b. washing your hands thoroughly after handling raw meat.
   c. avoiding eating raw eggs.
   d. cooking all meat, poultry, and fish thoroughly.
   e. All of the above.

7. Guidelines for taking nutrient supplements include
   a. using them confidently with a poor diet.
   b. taking them to help you manage stress.
   c. selecting ones to enhance your sexual performance.
   d. avoiding high doses.

Correct answers can be found on page 369.

How Much Do You Know About Fat?

Name: _____   Date: _____   Grade: _____

Instructor: _____   Course: _____   Section: _____

True/False

1. Egg yolks contain the "bad" cholesterol called LDL.

2. Mayonnaise made from canola oil has less fat than regular mayonnaise, which usually is made from soybean oil.

3. The more unsaturated fat a food contains, the more it will raise blood-cholesterol levels.

4. Polyunsaturated fats are converted to saturated fats when heated, such as in deep-fat frying.

5. A jar of peanut butter labeled "cholesterol free" is better than "regular" peanut butter.

6. A label that reads "95% fat-free" means that the food derives only 5 percent of its calories from fat.

7. The best way to decrease blood-cholesterol levels is to eat less cholesterol.

8. A third of the average U.S. woman's fat intake comes from salad dressing, margarine, cheese, and beef.

9. A label that reads "low cholesterol" means the food has fewer calories than "regular" items and no saturated fat.

10. Veggie burgers are always a low-fat alternative to hamburgers.

Multiple Choice

Select the best answer to the following questions.

11. If a product's label says it contains only vegetable oils, it is:
    a. high in only saturated fat.
    b. high in only unsaturated fat.
    c. high in either saturated fat or unsaturated fat.
    d. high in unsaturated fat and might contain some cholesterol.

12. A woman has a total blood-cholesterol level of 220 mg/dl and an HDL level of 60 mg/dl. What is this person's ratio of total cholesterol to HDL cholesterol? Is she at high or low risk for heart disease?
    a. 3:7 ratio and low risk
    b. 2:7 ratio and low risk
    c. 7:2 ratio and low risk
    d. 4:5 ratio and high risk

13. A 5-ounce serving of ground beef has how much more fat than the same size serving of skinless chicken breast?
    a. 50 percent   c. 75 percent
    b. 65 percent   d. 95 percent

14. An avocado has 30 grams of fat and 309 calories. What is the percentage of fat calories?
    a. 42 percent   c. 87 percent
    b. 62 percent   d. 97 percent

15. A food is considered low-fat if it has how many grams of fat per 100 calories?
    a. 3   c. 10
    b. 5   d. 30

16. According to the American Heart Association, people ideally should adopt a low-fat diet that contains no more than 30 percent fat calories
    a. starting at birth.
    b. at 2 years of age.
    c. at puberty.
    d. in early adulthood.

17. An olive-oil label states that the product is "extra light." This means
    a. it has a lighter color and taste than other olive oils.
    b. it weighs less.
    c. it has fewer calories.
    d. it is lower in saturated fats.

18. In whole milk, 48 percent of the calories come from fat. What percentage of calories in 2% low-fat milk come from fat?
    a. 2 percent   c. 25 percent
    b. 15 percent   d. 30 percent

19. Experts recommend limiting your saturated-fat intake to no more than 10 percent of total calorie intake. If you eat 2,000 calories per day, your saturated-fat allowance would be
    a. 10 grams   c. 27 grams
    b. 22 grams   d. 36 grams

20. A Taco Bell taco salad contains how many teaspoons of fat?
    a. 9   c. 15
    b. 12   d. 25

From "Facing Fats," by Elizabeth Somer. *SHAPE* (January, 1994). Reprinted by permission.

Answers

1. **False.** LDL is a carrier of cholesterol in the blood. It is not found in food.

2. **False.** They contain similar amounts of fat and calories.

3. **False.** The more *saturated* fat in your diet, the more your blood-cholesterol level will be raised.

4. **False.** But frying does expose these fats to oxygen, and once oxidized, they can increase the risk for heart disease.

5. **False.** Cholesterol is found only in animal products.

6. **False.** The label refers only to fat content by weight. The percentage of calories from fat would be much higher. For instance, a 95% fat-free Janet Lee Chopped Ham contains 60% fat calories (2 grams of fat per 30-calorie slice).

7. **False.** Reducing your saturated fat intake is the most important dietary factor for lowering blood cholesterol.

8. **True.** The average woman in the United States gets 9 percent of her fat from salad dressing, 8 percent from margarine, 8 percent from cheese, and 7 percent from beef, for a total of one-third.

9. **False.** A food can be cholesterol-free and still be high in calories and/or saturated fat.

10. **False.** Commercial veggie burgers get anywhere from 6 to 66 percent of their calories from fat.

11. **c.** Most vegetable oils are high in unsaturated fats, but manufacturers also use tropical oils, such as palm or coconut oils, which are as saturated as lard.

12. **a.**

13. **d.**

14. **c.**

15. **a.** Fat has 9 calories per gram, so a food that has 3 grams of fat per 100 calories is 27% fat; a food that is less than 30% fat is considered low-fat.

16. **b.**

17. **a.**

18. **d.**

19. **b.**

20. **c.**

To find your score, total your correct answers.

18 or more: All of that label reading has paid off! You are a bona-fide fat sleuth.

15 to 17: You put the average American to shame. If you practice what you know, your diet is probably within the low-fat zone.

12 to 14: You keep company with the majority of Americans and may be confused when it comes to fat. Review the answers and see if you can improve your score.

Fewer than 12: Oops. It's time for you to take the fat issue more seriously.

Personal Diet Quiz

Name: _____   Date: _____   Grade: _____

Instructor: _____   Course: _____   Section: _____

Are You Meeting Your Fiber Quota?

To find out how close you come to meeting your daily fiber quota, keep track of everything you eat for three days. Then, take the quiz below and add up your points.

1. What type of bread (including rolls and muffins) did you usually eat?

   a. whole-wheat or whole-grain   +4

   b. white or partial whole-wheat   +2

2. How many servings of oat products did you average daily? (1 serving = 1 cup cooked oatmeal or oat bran.)

   a. two or more   +4

   b. one   +3

   c. one-half   +2

   d. none   0

3. How many times during the last three days did you eat beans (legumes), such as kidney beans, pintos, garbanzos, soybeans, lentils, and split peas?

   a. three or more   +4

   b. two   +3

   c. one   +2

   d. none   0

4. How many times during the three-day period did you eat high-fiber breakfast cereals?

   a. three or more   +4

   b. two   +3

   c. one   +2

   d. none   0

5. How many times during the three-day period did you eat cooked whole-grain side dishes, such as brown rice or barley?

   a. three or more   +4

   b. two   +3

   c. one   +2

   d. none   0

6. Approximately how many servings of canned or fresh fruits and vegetables did you eat daily? (Use an average from the previous three days. 1 serving = 1/2 cup cooked or 1 cup or 1 piece raw.)

   a. seven or more   +5

   b. five or six   +4

   c. three or four   +2

   d. one or two   +1

   e. none   −2

Scoring: If your overall score is above 20, your fiber intake is probably adequate. If it is lower, try to increase your fiber intake using the foods mentioned above. Be sure to increase your water intake when you eat more fiber.

This quiz on fiber intake was developed with assistance from nutrition lecturer Liz Applegate and nutrition professor Judith Stern, both at the University of California, Davis.

Check Your Calcium Intake

If you are not a fan of dairy products, you may be coming up far short of your calcium needs. But even if you are a milk lover, how much calcium your body actually absorbs depends upon your genetic makeup and other factors. And how much you retain depends upon your intake of salt and protein. This duo may increase the elimination of calcium, causing your body to steal calcium it needs from your bones.

The quiz can tell you how close your diet comes to providing the appropriate amount of bone food. Just check the answer that applies to you.

1. I eat one serving of yogurt (8 ounces), drink milk (1 cup), or eat cheese (1 ounce) at least once a day.

   ____ True   +3

   ____ False   −1

2. Dairy products give me gas and bloating, so I avoid them.

   ____ True   −1

   ____ False   +1

This quiz on calcium was developed with the assistance of Robert P. Heaney, professor of medicine at Creighton University School of Medicine, Omaha, NE.

3. I make sure to eat one or more of the following nondairy sources of calcium at least three times a week: leafy green vegetables (kale or broccoli), shellfish (oysters or clams), or canned fish with edible bones (salmon or sardines).

____ True   +1

____ False   0

4. I make an effort to slip dairy foods into my diet whenever I can (grating cheese over salads, for example).

____ True   +1

____ False   0

5. I eat calcium-enriched forms of products (such as breakfast cereal or fruit juice) whenever I can.

____ True   +1

____ False   −1

6. When given a choice, I drink carbonated soft drinks over low-fat dairy drinks or water.

____ True   −1

____ False   0

Can You Find the Hidden Salt?

If you've already banned the saltshaker from the table and sworn off salty snacks—good for you! But to keep your intake at the recommended one-teaspoon-a-day limit takes a bit more vigilance. Three-fourths of your dietary sodium is hidden in already-prepared foods, experts say. And many salt-laced foods, such as cereal, diet soda, and instant pudding don't taste a bit salty.

Just how good are you at avoiding this hidden salt? If you're eating more potassium-rich fresh fruits and vegetables than packaged convenience foods, for example, you're probably doing great.

Take this quiz to find out where you stand on the hidden salt scale.

1. When barbecuing meat or fish, I'm more likely to brush on herbs or homemade marinara sauce than commercial ketchup, barbecue sauce, or soy sauce.

____ True   +1

____ False   −1

2. The fresh or frozen fruits and vegetables and lean meats in my grocery cart usually crowd out the canned, and processed foods.

____ True   +1

____ False   −1

3. I buy only the low-salt type of margarine.

____ True   +1

____ False   −1

4. I usually have dehydrated, instant versions of soups, sauces, salad dressings, oatmeal, or other foods on hand.

____ True   −1

____ False   +1

7. I tend to get my protein from meats.

____ True   −1

____ False   +1

8. I usually salt food automatically without tasting it.

____ True   −1

____ False   +1

Scoring: If you scored between 7 and 9, you are laying the dietary foundation for a rock-solid skeleton. (Remember, though, that even if you scored a perfect 9, you still may have a bone deficit if you are inactive, underweight or post-menopausal, have a family history of osteoporosis, or take aluminum-based antacids or other calcium-robbing drugs.) If you scored between 4 and 6, try to include more low-fat dairy products and go easy on the calcium bandits. If you scored below 4, your skeleton may be becoming perilously porous. Learn to love low-fat yogurt and make friends with skim milk. Ask your doctor about taking a calcium supplement.

5. I steam, microwave, broil, or stir-fry vegetables rather than boil them.

____ True   +1

____ False   −1

6. Processed cheese never passes my lips.

____ True   +1

____ False   −1

7. I rinse canned foods such as tuna, ham, and beans before preparing them.

____ True   +1

____ False   −1

8. I'm a sucker for deli food—cold cuts, prepared salads, pastrami, ham, smoked fish, and that sort of thing.

____ True   −1

____ False   +1

9. I usually order my hamburger with the works—pickles, ketchup, mustard, and special sauce.

____ True   −1

____ False   +1

10. When dining out, I usually order oil and vinegar dressing for my salad and ask for gravies and sauces on the side.

____ True   +1

____ False   −1

Scoring: 8–10: You're a top-notch salt sleuth. 5–7: There's room for improvement. Scan food labels closely for the key phrases "sodium-free" or "very low sodium." Below 5: You're probably relying on too many prepared condiments and packaged convenience foods. Try to cut down on these.

Is Osteoporosis in Your Future?

Name: _____   Date: _____   Grade: _____

Instructor: _____   Course: _____   Section: _____

Risk factors you CANNOT control:

		YES	NO
1.	Are you female?	☐	☐
2.	Do you have a family history of osteoporosis?	☐	☐
3.	Are your ancestors from the British Isles, northern Europe, China, or Japan?	☐	☐
4.	Are you very fair-skinned?	☐	☐
5.	Are you small-boned?	☐	☐
6.	Are you over age 35?	☐	☐
7.	Have you had your ovaries removed, or did you have an early menopause?	☐	☐
8.	Are you allergic to milk and milk products?	☐	☐
9.	Have you never been pregnant?	☐	☐
10.	Do you have cancer or kidney disease?	☐	☐
11.	Do you have to take chemotherapy, steroids, anticonvulsants, or anticoagulants?	☐	☐

Risk factors you CAN control:

		YES	NO
12.	Do you smoke?	☐	☐
13.	Do you drink alcohol?	☐	☐
14.	Do you avoid milk and cheese in your diet?	☐	☐
15.	Do you get very little exercise?	☐	☐
16.	Do you drink a lot of soft drinks?	☐	☐
17.	Is your diet high in protein?	☐	☐
18.	Do you consume a lot of caffeine (five or more cups of coffee per day or equivalent)?	☐	☐
19.	Are you amenorrheic (without a monthly period)?	☐	☐
20.	Do you get less than 1,000 mg of calcium a day?	☐	☐
21.	Is your body weight very low?	☐	☐
22.	Do you go on extreme or crash diets?	☐	☐
23.	Do you have a high sodium (salt) intake?	☐	☐

If you answered "yes" to three of the above questions, you are at risk for osteoporosis and may want to ask your doctor to schedule a bone density screening test. The more questions you answered "yes" to, the higher is your risk of developing osteoporosis in the future.

Many clinical studies suggest that osteoporosis is preventable. As you can see from the quiz, you can do several things right now to help prevent osteoporosis in your future.

Adapted from Marion Laboratories, Inc.

Rate Your Diet

Name: _____ **Date:** _____ **Grade:** _____

Instructor: _____ **Course:** _____ **Section:** _____

These 39 questions will give you a rough sketch of your typical eating habits. The + or − number for each answer either pats you on the back for good eating habits (+) or alerts you to problems you didn't even know you had (−). The quiz focuses on fat, saturated fat, cholesterol, sodium, sugar, fiber, fruits, and vegetables. It doesn't attempt to cover everything in your diet. Also, it doesn't try to measure precisely how much of the key nutrients you eat.

Instructions

Next to each answer is a number with a + or − sign in front of it. *Circle the number that corresponds to the answer you choose.* That's your score for the question. If two or more answers apply, circle each one. Then average them to get your score for the question.

How to average. In answering question 19, for example, if your sandwich-eating is equally divided among tuna salad (−2), roast beef (+1), and turkey breast (+3), add the three scores (which gives you +2) and then divide by 3. That gives you a score of + 2/3 for the question. Round it to +1.

Pay attention to serving sizes, which are included when needed. For example, a serving of vegetables is 1/2 cup. If you usually eat one cup of vegetables at a time, count it as two servings.

Fruits, Vegetables, Grains, and Beans

1. How many servings of fruit or 100% fruit juice do you eat/drink per day? (*Omit* fruit snacks such as Fruit Roll-Ups and fruit-on-the-bottom yogurt. One serving = one piece or 1/2 cup of fruit or 6 oz of fruit juice.)
   - (a) 0 ...−3
   - (b) less than 1 ...−2
   - (c) 1 ... 0
   - (d) 2 ...+1
   - (e) 3 ...+2
   - (f) 4 or more ...+3

2. How many servings of non-fried vegetables do you eat per day? (One serving = 1/2 cup. *Include* potatoes.)
   - (a) 0 ...−3
   - (b) less than 1 ...−2
   - (c) 1 ... 0
   - (d) 2 ...+1
   - (e) 3 ...+2
   - (f) 4 or more ...+3

3. How many servings of vitamin-rich vegetables do you eat per week? (One serving = 1/2 cup, count *only* broccoli, Brussels sprouts, carrots, collards, kale, red pepper, spinach, sweet potatoes, and winter squash.)
   - (a) 0 ...−3
   - (b) 1 to 3 ...+1
   - (c) 4 to 6 ...+2
   - (d) 7 or more ...+3

4. How many servings of leafy green vegetables do you eat per week? (One serving = 1/2 cup cooked or 1 cup raw. Count *only* collards, kale, mustard greens, romaine lettuce, spinach, or Swiss chard.)
   - (a) 0 ...−3
   - (b) less than 1 ...−2
   - (c) 1 to 2 ...+1
   - (d) 3 to 4 ...+2
   - (e) 5 or more ...+3

5. How many times per week does your lunch or dinner contain grains, vegetables, or beans, but little or no meat, poultry, fish, or eggs?
   - (a) 0 ...−1
   - (b) 1 to 2 ...+1
   - (c) 3 to 4 ...+2
   - (d) 5 or more ...+3

6. How many times per week do you eat dried beans, split peas, or lentils? (*Omit* green beans.)
   - (a) 0 ...−3
   - (b) less than 1 ...−1
   - (c) 1 ... 0
   - (d) 2 ...+1
   - (e) 3 ...+2
   - (f) 4 or more ...+3

Adapted from *Nutrition Action Healthletter*, May 1996. Reprinted with permission.

7. How many servings of grains do you eat per day? (1 serving = 1 slice of bread, 1 oz. of crackers, 1 large pancake, 1 cup pasta or cold cereal, or ½ cup granola, cooked cereal, rice, or bulgar. *Omit* heavily sweetened cold cereals.)

   (a) 0 . . . . –3
   (b) 1 to 2 0
   (c) 3 to 4 . . . . +1
   (d) 5 to 7 . . . . +2
   (e) 8 or more . . . . +3

8. What type of bread, rolls, etc., do you eat?

   (a) 100% whole-wheat as the only flour . . . . +3
   (b) whole-wheat flour as the 1st or 2nd flour . . . . +2
   (c) rye, pumpernickel, or oatmeal . . . . +1
   (d) white, French, or Italian 0

9. What kind of breakfast cereal do you eat?

   (a) whole-grain (like oatmeal or Wheaties) . . . . +3
   (b) low-fiber (such as Cream of Wheat or Corn Flakes) 0
   (c) sugary low-fiber (such as Frosted Flakes) or low-fat granola . . . . –1
   (d) regular granola . . . . –2

10. How many times per week do you eat high-fat red meats (hamburgers, pork chops, ribs, hot dogs, pot roast, sausage, bologna, steaks other than round steak, etc.)?

    (a) 0 . . . . +3
    (b) less than 1 . . . . +2
    (c) 1 . . . . –1
    (d) 2 . . . . –2
    (e) 3 . . . . –3
    (f) 4 or more . . . . –4

11. How many times per week do you eat lean red meats (hot dogs or luncheon meats with no more than 2 grams of fat per serving, round steak, or pork tenderloin)?

    (a) 0 . . . . +3
    (b) less than 1 . . . . +1
    (c) 1 0
    (d) 2–3 . . . . –1
    (e) 4–5 . . . . –2
    (f) 6 or more . . . . –3

12. After cooking, how large is the serving of red meat you eat? (To convert from raw to cooked, reduce by 25 percent. For example, 4 oz of raw meat shrinks to 3 oz after cooking. 16 oz = 1 pound.)

    (a) 6 oz or more . . . . –3
    (b) 4 to 5 oz . . . . –2
    (c) 3 oz or less 0
    (d) don't eat red meat . . . . +3

13. If you eat red meat, do you trim the visible fat when you cook or eat it?

    (a) yes . . . . +1
    (b) no . . . . –3

14. What kind of ground meat or poultry do you eat?

    (a) regular ground beef . . . . –4
    (b) ground beef that's 11% to 25% fat . . . . –3
    (c) ground chicken or 10%-fat ground beef . . . . –2
    (d) ground turkey . . . . –1
    (e) ground turkey breast . . . . +3
    (f) don't eat ground meat or poultry . . . . +3

15. What chicken parts do you eat?

    (a) breast . . . . +3
    (b) drumstick . . . . +1
    (c) thigh . . . . –1
    (d) wing . . . . –2
    (e) I don't eat poultry . . . . +3

16. If you eat poultry, do you remove the skin before eating?

    (a) yes . . . . +2
    (b) no . . . . –3

17. If you eat seafood, how many times per week? (Omit deep-fried foods, tuna packed in oil, and mayonnaise-laden tuna salad; low-fat mayo is okay.)

    (a) less than 1 0
    (b) 1 . . . . +1
    (c) 2 . . . . +2
    (d) 3 or more . . . . +3

Mixed Foods

18. What is your most typical breakfast? (*Subtract* an extra 3 points if you also eat sausage.)

    (a) biscuit sandwich or croissant sandwich . . . . –4
    (b) croissant, danish, or doughnut . . . . –3
    (c) don't eat breakfast . . . . –3
    (d) pancakes, French toast, or waffles . . . . –1
    (e) cereal, toast, or bagel . . . . +3
    (f) low-fat yogurt or low-fat cottage cheese . . . . +3

19. What sandwich fillings do you eat?

    (a) regular luncheon meat or bologna . . . . –3
    (b) tuna, egg, or chicken salad, or ham . . . . –2
    (c) peanut butter . . . . +1
    (d) roast beef . . . . +1
    (e) low-fat luncheon meat . . . . +1
    (f) tuna or chicken salad made with fat-free mayo . . . +3
    (g) turkey breast or hummus . . . . +3

20. What do you order on your pizza?

    (a)   at least one vegetable topping . . . .+3

    (b)   one lean meat topping 0

    (c)   one high-fat meat topping (sausage, pepperoni) . .–2

    (d)   more than 1 high-fat meat topping . . . .–3

21. What do you put on your pasta?

    (a)   sautéed vegetables . . . .+3

    (b)   tomato sauce or red clam sauce . . . .+2

    (c)   meat sauce or meat balls . . . .–1

    (d)   pesto or another oily sauce . . . .–2

    (e)   Alfredo or another creamy sauce . . . .–4

22. How many times per week do you eat deep-fried foods (fish, chicken, french fries, potato chips, etc.)?

    (a)   0 . . . .+3

    (b)   1 0

    (c)   2 . . . .–1

    (d)   3 . . . .–2

    (e)   4 or more . . . .–3

23. At a salad bar, what do you choose?

    (a)   no dressing, lemon, or vinegar . . . .+3

    (b)   fat-free dressing . . . .+2

    (c)   low- or reduced-calorie dressing . . . .+1

    (d)   oil and vinegar . . . .–1

    (e)   regular dressing . . . .–2

    (f)   cole slaw, pasta salad, or potato salad . . . .–2

24. How many servings of low-fat calcium-rich foods do you eat per day? (One serving = ⅔ cup low-fat or non-fat milk or yogurt, 1 oz low-fat cheese, 1½ oz sardines, 3½ oz canned salmon with bones, 1 oz tofu enriched with calcium, 1 cup collards or kale, or 200 mg of a calcium supplement.)

    (a)   0 . . . .–3

    (b)   less than 1 . . . .–1

    (c)   1 . . . .+1

    (d)   2 . . . .+2

    (e)   3 or more . . . .+3

Fats and Oils

25. What do you put on your bread, toast, bagel, or English muffin?

    (a)   stick butter or cream cheese . . . .–4

    (b)   stick margarine or whipped butter . . . .–3

    (c)   regular tub margarine . . . .–2

    (d)   light tub margarine or whipped light butter . . . . . .–1

    (e)   jam, fat-free margarine, or fat-free cream cheese . . . 0

    (f)   nothing . . . .+3

26. What do you spread on your sandwiches?

    (a)   mayonnaise . . . .–2

    (b)   light mayonnaise . . . .–1

    (c)   ketchup, mustard, or fat-free mayonnaise . . . .+1

    (d)   nothing . . . .+2

27. With what do you make tuna salad, pasta salad, chicken salad, etc.?

    (a)   mayonnaise . . . .–2

    (b)   light mayonnaise . . . .–1

    (c)   fat-free mayonnaise 0

    (d)   low-fat yogurt . . . .+2

28. What do you use to sauté vegetables or other foods? (Vegetable oil includes safflower, corn, sunflower, and soybean.)

    (a)   butter or lard . . . .–3

    (b)   margarine . . . .–2

    (c)   vegetable oil or light margarine . . . .–1

    (d)   olive or canola oil . . . .+1

    (e)   broth . . . .+2

    (f)   cooking spray . . . .+3

Beverages

29. What do you drink on a typical day?

    (a)   water, or low-fat or skim milk . . . .+3

    (b)   caffeine-free coffee or tea 0

    (c)   diet soda . . . .–1

    (d)   coffee or tea (up to 4 cups a day) . . . .–1

    (e)   regular soda (up to 2 cans or bottles a day) . . . . . .–2

    (f)   regular soda (3 or more cans or bottles a day) . . . .–3

    (g)   coffee or tea (5 or more cups a day) . . . .–3

30. What kind of "fruit" beverage do you drink?

    (a)   orange, grapefruit, prune, or pineapple juice . . . . .+3

    (b)   apple, grape, or pear juice . . . .+1

    (c)   cranberry juice blend or cocktail 0

    (d)   fruit "drink," "ade," or "punch" . . . .–3

31. What kind of milk do you drink?

    (a)   whole . . . .–3

    (b)   2% fat 0

    (c)   1% low-fat . . . .+2

    (d)   skim (no fat) . . . .+3

Desserts and Snacks

32. What do you eat as a snack?

    (a) fruits or vegetables . . . .+3

    (b) low-fat yogurt . . . .+2

    (c) low-fat crackers . . . .+1

    (d) cookies or fried chips . . . .–2

    (e) nuts or granola bar . . . .–2

    (f) candy bar or pastry . . . .–3

33. Which of the following "salty" snacks do you eat?
(*Average* two or more scores if necessary.)

    (a) potato chips, corn chips, or popcorn . . . .–3

    (b) tortilla chips . . . .–2

    (c) salted pretzels or light microwave popcorn . . . . . .–1

    (d) unsalted pretzels . . . .+2

    (e) baked tortilla or potato chips or homemade
         air-popped popcorn . . . .+3

    (f) I don't eat salty snacks . . . .+3

34. What kind of cookies do you usually eat?

    (a) fat-free cookies . . . .+2

    (b) graham crackers or reduced-fat cookies . . . .+1

    (c) oatmeal cookies . . . .–1

    (d) sandwich cookies (such as Oreos) . . . .–2

    (e) chocolate coated, chocolate chip,
         or peanut butter . . . .–3

    (f) I don't eat cookies . . . .+3

35. What kind of cake or pastry do you eat?

    (a) cheesecake . . . .–4

    (b) pie or doughnuts . . . .–3

    (c) cake with frosting . . . .–2

    (d) cake without frosting . . . .–1

    (e) muffins 0

    (f) angel food, fat-free cake, or fat-free pastry . . . . .+1

    (g) I don't eat cakes or pastries . . . .+3

36. What kind of frozen dessert do you usually eat? (*Subtract*
1 point for each of the following toppings: hot fudge, nuts,
or chocolate candy bars or pieces.)

    (a) gourmet ice cream . . . .–3

    (b) regular ice cream . . . .–2

    (c) frozen yogurt or light ice cream 0

    (d) sorbet, sherbet, or ices 0

    (e) non-fat frozen yogurt or fat-free ice cream . . . . . .+3

SCORING YOUR DIET

Add up your score for each question.

Score

0 or below	Oops!	There is much room for improvement. Work on one positive change at a time.
1 to 29	Hmmm.	Don't be discouraged. This eating business is tough.
30 to 59	Yesss!	Congratulations. You can invite us over to eat any day.
60 or above	C-o-o-o-l.	Our photographer should be at your door any second.

9

CHAPTER

Assessment of Body Composition

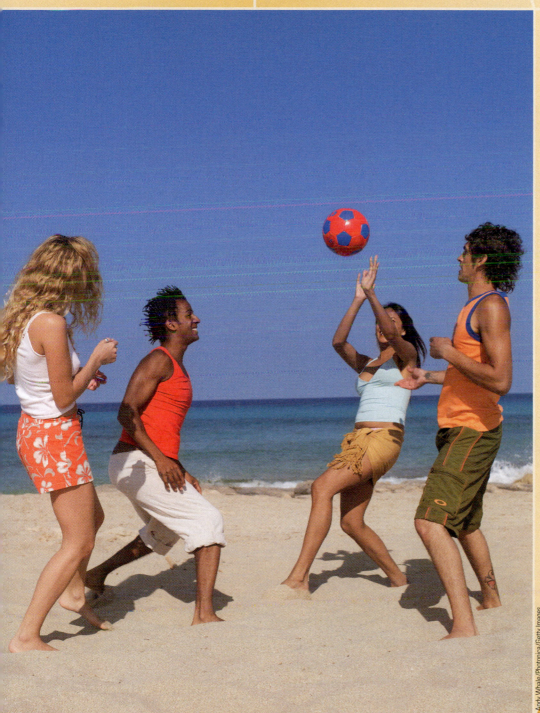

© Andy Whale/Photonica/Getty Images

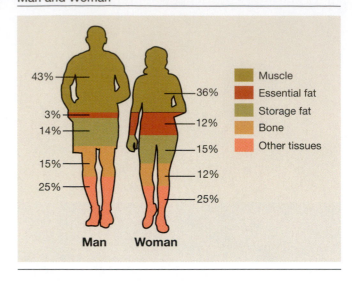

FIGURE 9.1 Typical Body Composition of an Adult Man and Woman

To understand **body composition**, we first must recognize that the human body consists of fat and non-fat components. The fat component is usually called fat mass or **percent body fat**. The non-fat component is termed **lean body mass**.

For years, people relied on simple height/weight charts to determine **recommended body weight**. First published in 1912, these charts were based on average weights (including shoes and clothing) for men and women who obtained life insurance policies between 1888 and 1905—a notably unrepresentative population. The recommended body weight on these tables was obtained according to sex, height, and frame size. Because no scientific guidelines were given to determine frame size, most people chose their frame size based on the column in which the weight comes closest to their own! These tables were shown to be highly inaccurate and failed to identify critical fat values associated with higher risk for disease.

A better approach to determine recommended weight is to find out what percent of total body weight is fat and what amount is lean tissue—to determine body composition. Body composition should be assessed by a well-trained technician who understands the procedure that is being used.

Once the fat percentage is known, recommended body weight can be calculated from recommended body fat. Recommended body weight, also called healthy weight, implies the absence of any medical condition that would improve with weight loss and a fat distribution pattern that is not associated with higher risk for illness.

The best procedure to determine whether people are truly overweight or falsely at recommended body weight, is through the assessment of body composition. **Overweight** and **obesity** are terms denoting an excess of body fat (discussed further in Chapter 10). If body weight is the only criterion, an individual might easily appear to be overweight according to height/weight charts, yet not have too much body fat. Typical examples are football players, body builders, weight lifters, and other athletes with large muscle size. Some athletes who appear to be 20 or 30 pounds overweight really have little body fat.

At the other end of the spectrum, some people who weigh very little (and may be viewed as skinny or underweight) actually can be classified as overweight because of their high body fat content. More people than you might think weigh as little as 120 pounds but are more than 30 percent fat (about one-third of their total body weight). These cases are found more readily in the sedentary population and among people who are always dieting. Physical inactivity and a constant negative caloric balance both lead to a loss in lean body mass (see Chapter 10). These examples illustrate that body weight alone clearly does not tell the whole story.

Essential and Storage Fat

Total fat in the human body is classified into two types: essential fat and storage fat. **Essential fat** is needed for normal physiological functions and without it, health and physical performance deteriorate. This type of fat is found within tissues such as muscles, nerves, bone marrow, intestines, heart, liver, and lungs. Essential fat constitutes about 3 percent of the total weight in men and 12 percent in women (see Figure 9.1). The percentage is higher in women because it includes sex-specific fat, such as that found in the breast tissue, the uterus, and other sex-related fat deposits.

Storage fat is the fat stored in adipose tissue, mostly just beneath the skin (subcutaneous fat) and around major organs in the body. This fat serves three basic functions:

1. As an insulator to retain body heat
2. As energy substrate for metabolism
3. As padding against physical trauma to the body

The amount of storage fat in men and women depends on individuals' lifestyle habits. When overweight, men tend to store fat around the waist and women are more likely to store fat around the hips and thighs.

Techniques to Assess Body Composition

Many exercise scientists consider **dual energy X-ray absorptiometry (DEXA)** as the standard technique to assess body composition. This procedure is used most frequently in research and by medical facilities. A radiographic technique, DEXA uses very low-dose beams of X-ray energy (hundreds of times lower than a typical body X-ray) to measure total body fat mass, fat distribution pattern (see waist circumference on page 220), and bone density. Bone density is measured to assess the risk for osteoporosis. The procedure itself is simple and takes less than 15 minutes to administer.

Because DEXA is not readily available to most fitness participants, other methods to estimate body composition are used. The most common of these are:

1. hydrostatic or underwater weighing
2. air displacement
3. skinfold thickness
4. girth measurements
5. bioelectrical impedance.

Because these procedures yield estimates of body fat, each technique may yield slightly different values. Therefore, when assessing changes in body composition, be sure to use the same technique for pre-test and post-test comparisons.

Hydrostatic weighing is the most accurate technique presently available in fitness laboratories. Although other techniques to assess body composition are available, the equipment is costly and not easily accessible to the general population. In addition to percentages of lean tissue and body fat, some of these methods also provide information on total body water and bone mass.

Besides DEXA, these techniques include air displacement, magnetic resonance imaging (MRI), computed tomography (CT), and total body electrical conductivity (TOBEC). In terms of predicting percent body fat, these techniques do not seem to be more accurate than hydrostatic weighing.

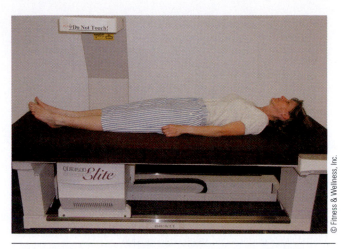

© Fitness & Wellness, Inc.

The dual energy X-ray absorptiometry (DEXA) technique used to assess body composition and bone density.

HYDROSTATIC WEIGHING

For decades, **hydrostatic weighing** has been the most accurate technique used in determining body composition in exercise physiology laboratories. In essence, a person's "regular" weight is compared with a weight taken underwater. Because fat is more buoyant than lean tissue, comparing the two weights can determine a person's percent of fat. The procedure requires time, skill, space, and equipment and must be administered by a well-trained technician.

Body composition The fat and non-fat components of the human body; important in assessing recommended body weight.

Percent body fat Proportional amount of fat in the body based on the person's total weight; includes both essential fat and storage fat; also termed fat mass.

Lean body mass Body weight without body fat.

Recommended body weight Body weight at which there seems to be no harm to human health; healthy weight.

Overweight An excess amount of weight against a given standard, such as recommended percent body fat.

Obesity An excessive accumulation of body fat, usually at least 30 percent above recommended body weight.

Essential fat Minimal amount of body fat needed for normal physiological functions; constitutes about 3 percent of total weight in men and 12 percent in women.

Storage fat Body fat in excess of essential fat; stored in adipose tissue.

Dual energy X-ray absorptiometry (DEXA) Method to assess body composition that uses very low-dose beams of X-ray energy to measure total body fat mass, fat distribution pattern, and bone density.

Hydrostatic weighing Underwater technique to assess body composition; considered the most accurate of the body composition assessment techniques.

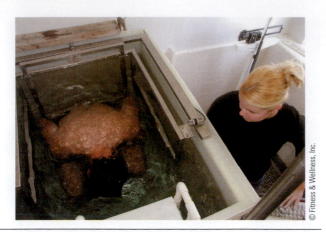

Hydrostatic or underwater weighing technique.

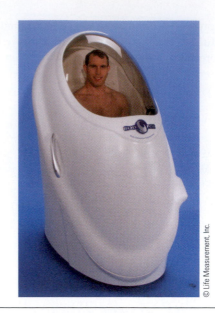

The BodPod, used for assessment of body composition.

This technique has several drawbacks. First, because each individual assessment can take as long as 30 minutes, hydrostatic weighing is not feasible when testing a lot of people. Furthermore, the person's residual lung volume (amount of air left in the lungs following complete forceful exhalation) should be measured before testing. If residual volume cannot be measured, as is the case in some laboratories and health/fitness centers, it is estimated using the predicting equations, which may decrease the accuracy of hydrostatic weighing. Also, the requirement of being weighed completely under water makes hydrostatic weighing difficult to administer to **aquaphobic** people. For accurate results, the individual must be able to perform the test properly.

For each underwater weighing trial, the person has to (a) force out all of the air in the lungs, (b) lean forward and completely submerge underwater for about 5 to 10 seconds (long enough to get the underwater weight), and (c) remain as calm as possible (chair movement makes reading the scale difficult). This procedure is repeated eight to ten times.

Forcing all of the air out of the lungs is not easy for everyone but is important for an accurate reading. Leaving additional air (beyond residual volume) in the lungs makes a person more buoyant. Because fat is less dense than water, overweight individuals weigh less in water. Additional air in the lungs makes a person lighter in water, yielding a false, higher body fat percentage.

AIR DISPLACEMENT

Air displacement (also known as air displacement plethysmography) is a newer technique. With this method, an individual sits inside a small chamber, commercially known as the **Bod Pod**. Computerized pressure sensors determine the amount of air displaced by the person inside the chamber. Body volume is calculated by subtracting the air volume with the person inside the chamber from the volume of the empty chamber. The amount of air in the person's lungs also is taken into consideration when determining the actual body volume. Body density

and percent body fat then are calculated from the obtained body volume.

Initial research has shown that this technique compares favorably with hydrostatic weighing and it is less cumbersome to administer. The procedure takes only about 5 minutes. Additional research is needed, however, to determine its accuracy among different age groups, ethnic backgrounds, and athletic populations. Administering this assessment is relatively easy, but because of the high cost, the Bod Pod is not readily available in fitness centers and exercise laboratories.

SKINFOLD THICKNESS

Because of the cost, time, and complexity of hydrostatic weighing and the expense of Bod Pod equipment, most health and fitness programs use **anthropometric measurement techniques**. These techniques, primarily skinfold thickness and girth measurements, allow quick, simple, and inexpensive estimates of body composition.

Assessing body composition using **skinfold thickness** is based on the principle that the amount of **subcutaneous fat** is proportional to total body fat. Valid and reliable measurements of this tissue give a good indication of percent body fat.

The skinfold test is done with the aid of pressure calipers. Several techniques requiring measurement of three to seven sites have been developed, of which the following three-site procedure is most common: The sites measured are (also see Figure 9.2):

women: triceps, suprailium, and thigh skinfolds
men: chest, abdomen, and thigh.

All measurements should be taken on the right side of the body.

FIGURE 9.2 Procedure and Anatomical Landmarks for Skinfold Measurements

Skinfold Measurement

1. Select the proper anatomical sites. For men, use chest, abdomen, and thigh skinfolds. For women, use triceps, suprailium, and thigh skinfolds. Take all measurements on the right side of the body with the person standing.

2. Measure each site by grasping a double thickness of skin firmly with the thumb and forefinger, pulling the fold slightly away from the muscular tissue. Hold the caliper perpendicular to the fold and take the measurement ½" below the finger hold. Measure each site three times and read the values to the nearest .1 to .5 mm. Record the average of the two closest readings as the final value for that site. Take the readings without delay to avoid excessive compression of the skinfold. Release and refold the skinfold between readings.

3. When doing pre- and post-assessments, conduct the measurement at the same time of day. The best time is early in the morning to avoid water hydration changes resulting from activity or exercise.

4. Obtain percent fat by adding the skinfold measurements from all three sites and looking up the respective values in Tables 9.1, 9.2, or 9.3.

For example, if the skinfold measurements for an 18-year-old female are (a) triceps = 16, (b) suprailium = 4, and (c) thigh = 30 (total = 50), the percent body fat is 20.6%.

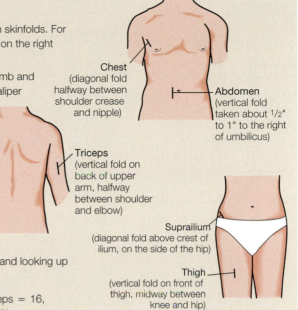

Chest (diagonal fold halfway between shoulder crease and nipple)

Abdomen (vertical fold taken about ½" to 1" to the right of umbilicus)

Triceps (vertical fold on back of upper arm, halfway between shoulder and elbow)

Suprailium (diagonal fold above crest of ilium, on the side of the hip)

Thigh (vertical fold on front of thigh, midway between knee and hip)

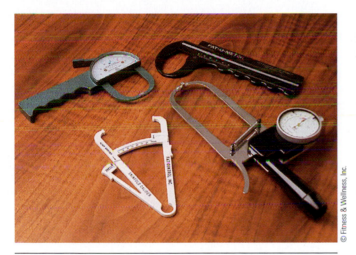

Various types of skinfold calipers can be used to assess skinfold thickness.

© Fitness & Wellness, Inc.

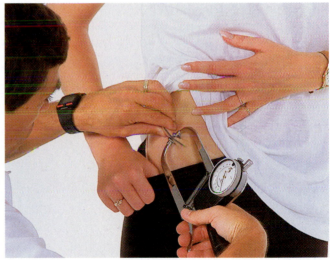

Skinfold thickness technique used for the assessment of body composition.

© Fitness & Wellness, Inc.

Even with the relatively simple skinfold technique, training is necessary to obtain accurate measurements. In addition, different technicians may produce slightly different measurements of the same person. Therefore, the same technician should take pre-test and post-test measurements.

Measurements should be done at the same time of the day—preferably in the morning, because changes in water hydration from activity and exercise can affect skinfold girth. The procedure is given in Figure 9.2. If skinfold calipers are available, you may assess your percent body fat with the help of your instructor or an experienced technician (also see Assessment 9.1). Then locate the percent fat estimates on the appropriate Table 9.1, 9.2, or 9.3.

Aquaphobic Having a fear of water.

Air displacement Technique to assess body composition by calculating the body volume from the air displaced by an individual sitting inside a small chamber.

Bod Pod Commercial name of the equipment used for assessing body composition through the air displacement technique.

Anthropometric measurement techniques Measurement of body girths at different sites.

Skinfold thickness Technique to assess body composition by measuring a double thickness of skin at specific body sites.

Subcutaneous fat Fat deposits directly under the skin.

TABLE 9.1 Skinfold Thickness Technique: Percent Fat Estimates for Women Calculated From Triceps, Suprailium, and Thigh

Sum of 3 Skinfolds	Age at Last Birthday								
	22 or Under	23 to 27	28 to 32	33 to 37	38 to 42	43 to 47	48 to 52	53 to 57	58 and Over
23– 25	9.7	9.9	10.2	10.4	10.7	10.9	11.2	11.4	11.7
26– 28	11.0	11.2	11.5	11.7	12.0	12.3	12.5	12.7	13.0
29– 31	12.3	12.5	12.8	13.0	13.3	13.5	13.8	14.0	14.3
32– 34	13.6	13.8	14.0	14.3	14.5	14.8	15.0	15.3	15.5
35– 37	14.8	15.0	15.3	15.5	15.8	16.0	16.3	16.5	16.8
38– 40	16.0	16.3	16.5	16.7	17.0	17.2	17.5	17.7	18.0
41– 43	17.2	17.4	17.7	17.9	18.2	18.4	18.7	18.9	19.2
44– 46	18.3	18.6	18.8	19.1	19.3	19.6	19.8	20.1	20.3
47– 49	19.5	19.7	20.0	20.2	20.5	20.7	21.0	21.2	21.5
50– 52	20.6	20.8	21.1	21.3	21.6	21.8	22.1	22.3	22.6
53– 55	21.7	21.9	22.1	22.4	22.6	22.9	23.1	23.4	23.6
56– 58	22.7	23.0	23.2	23.4	23.7	23.9	24.2	24.4	24.7
59– 61	23.7	24.0	24.2	24.5	24.7	25.0	25.2	25.5	25.7
62– 64	24.7	25.0	25.2	25.5	25.7	26.0	26.2	26.4	26.7
65– 67	25.7	25.9	26.2	26.4	26.7	26.9	27.2	27.4	27.7
68– 70	26.6	26.9	27.1	27.4	27.6	27.9	28.1	28.4	28.6
71– 73	27.5	27.8	28.0	28.3	28.5	28.8	29.0	29.3	29.5
74– 76	28.4	28.7	28.9	29.2	29.4	29.7	29.9	30.2	30.4
77– 79	29.3	29.5	29.8	30.0	30.3	30.5	30.8	31.0	31.3
80– 82	30.1	30.4	30.6	30.9	31.1	31.4	31.6	31.9	32.1
83– 85	30.9	31.2	31.4	31.7	31.9	32.2	32.4	32.7	32.9
86– 88	31.7	32.0	32.2	32.5	32.7	32.9	33.2	33.4	33.7
89– 91	32.5	32.7	33.0	33.2	33.5	33.7	33.9	34.2	34.4
92– 94	33.2	33.4	33.7	33.9	34.2	34.4	34.7	34.9	35.2
95– 97	33.9	34.1	34.4	34.6	34.9	35.1	35.4	35.6	35.9
98–100	34.6	34.8	35.1	35.3	35.5	35.8	36.0	36.3	36.5
101–103	35.2	35.4	35.7	35.9	36.2	36.4	36.7	36.9	37.2
104–106	35.8	36.1	36.3	36.6	36.8	37.1	37.3	37.5	37.8
107–109	36.4	36.7	36.9	37.1	37.4	37.6	37.9	38.1	38.4
110–112	37.0	37.2	37.5	37.7	38.0	38.2	38.5	38.7	38.9
113–115	37.5	37.8	38.0	38.2	38.5	38.7	39.0	39.2	39.5
116–118	38.0	38.3	38.5	38.8	39.0	39.3	39.5	39.7	40.0
119–121	38.5	38.7	39.0	39.2	39.5	39.7	40.0	40.2	40.5
122–124	39.0	39.2	39.4	39.7	39.9	40.2	40.4	40.7	40.9
125–127	39.4	39.6	39.9	40.1	40.4	40.6	40.9	41.1	41.4
128–130	39.8	40.0	40.3	40.5	40.8	41.0	41.3	41.5	41.8

Body density is calculated based on the "Generalized equation for predicting body density of women" developed by A. S. Jackson, M. L. Pollock, and A. Ward, *Medicine and Science in Sports and Exercise* 12 (1980): 175–182. Percent body fat is determined from the calculated body density using the Siri formula.

TABLE 9.2 Skinfold Thickness Technique: Percent Fat Estimates for Men Under Age 40 Calculated from Chest, Abdomen, and Thigh

Sum of 3 Skinfolds	Age at Last Birthday							
	Under 19	20 to 22	24 to 25	26 to 28	29 to 31	32 to 34	35 to 37	38 to 40
8– 10	.9	1.3	1.6	2.0	2.3	2.7	3.0	3.3
11– 13	1.9	2.3	2.6	3.0	3.3	3.7	4.0	4.3
14– 16	2.9	3.3	3.6	3.9	4.3	4.6	5.0	5.3
17– 19	3.9	4.2	4.6	4.9	5.3	5.6	6.0	6.3
20– 22	4.8	5.2	5.5	5.9	6.2	6.6	6.9	7.3
23– 25	5.8	6.2	6.5	6.8	7.2	7.5	7.9	8.2
26– 28	6.8	7.1	7.5	7.8	8.1	8.5	8.8	9.2
29– 31	7.7	8.0	8.4	8.7	9.1	9.4	9.8	10.1
32– 34	8.6	9.0	9.3	9.7	10.0	10.4	10.7	11.1
35– 37	9.5	9.9	10.2	10.6	10.9	11.3	11.6	12.0
38– 40	10.5	10.8	11.2	11.5	11.8	12.2	12.5	12.9
41– 43	11.4	11.7	12.1	12.4	12.7	13.1	13.4	13.8
44– 46	12.2	12.6	12.9	13.3	13.6	14.0	14.3	14.7
47– 49	13.1	13.5	13.8	14.2	14.5	14.9	15.2	15.5
50– 52	14.0	14.3	14.7	15.0	15.4	15.7	16.1	16.4
53– 55	14.8	15.2	15.5	15.9	16.2	16.6	16.9	17.3
56– 58	15.7	16.0	16.4	16.7	17.1	17.4	17.8	18.1
59– 61	16.5	16.9	17.2	17.6	17.9	18.3	18.6	19.0
62– 64	17.4	17.7	18.1	18.4	18.8	19.1	19.4	19.8
65– 67	18.2	18.5	18.9	19.2	19.6	19.9	20.3	20.6
68– 70	19.0	19.3	19.7	20.0	20.4	20.7	21.1	21.4
71– 73	19.8	20.1	20.5	20.8	21.2	21.5	21.9	22.2
74– 76	20.6	20.9	21.3	21.6	22.0	22.2	22.7	23.0
77– 79	21.4	21.7	22.1	22.4	22.8	23.1	23.4	23.8
80– 82	22.1	22.5	22.8	23.2	23.5	23.9	24.2	24.6
83– 85	22.9	23.2	23.6	23.9	24.3	24.6	25.0	25.3
86– 88	23.6	24.0	24.3	24.7	25.0	25.4	25.7	26.1
89– 91	24.4	24.7	25.1	25.4	25.8	26.1	26.5	26.8
92– 94	25.1	25.5	25.8	26.2	26.5	26.9	27.2	27.5
95– 97	25.8	26.2	26.5	26.9	27.2	27.6	27.9	28.3
98–100	26.6	26.9	27.3	27.6	27.9	28.3	28.6	29.0
101–103	27.3	27.6	28.0	28.3	28.6	29.0	29.3	29.7
104–106	27.9	28.3	28.6	29.0	29.3	29.7	30.0	30.4
107–109	28.6	29.0	29.3	29.7	30.0	30.4	30.7	31.1
110–112	29.3	29.6	30.0	30.3	30.7	31.0	31.4	31.7
113–115	30.0	30.3	30.7	31.0	31.3	31.7	32.0	32.4
116–118	30.6	31.0	31.3	31.6	32.0	32.3	32.7	33.0
119–121	31.3	31.6	32.0	32.3	32.6	33.0	33.3	33.7
122–124	31.9	32.2	32.6	32.9	33.3	33.6	34.0	34.3
125–127	32.5	32.9	33.2	33.5	33.9	34.2	34.6	34.9
128–130	33.1	33.5	33.8	34.2	34.5	34.9	35.2	35.5

Body density is calculated based on the "Generalized equation for predicting body density of men" developed by A. S. Jackson and M. L. Pollock, *British Journal of Nutrition* 40 (1978): 497–504. Percent body fat is determined from the calculated body density using the Siri formula.

TABLE 9.3 Skinfold Thickness Technique: Percent Fat Estimates for Men Over Age 40 Calculated from Chest, Abdomen, and Thigh

Sum of 3 Skinfolds	Age at Last Birthday							
	41 to 43	44 to 46	47 to 49	50 to 52	53 to 55	56 to 58	59 to 61	62 and Over
8– 10	3.7	4.0	4.4	4.7	5.1	5.4	5.8	6.1
11– 13	4.7	5.0	5.4	5.7	6.1	6.4	6.8	7.1
14– 16	5.7	6.0	6.4	6.7	7.1	7.4	7.8	8.1
17– 19	6.7	7.0	7.4	7.7	8.1	8.4	8.7	9.1
20– 22	7.6	8.0	8.3	8.7	9.0	9.4	9.7	10.1
23– 25	8.6	8.9	9.3	9.6	10.0	10.3	10.7	11.0
26– 28	9.5	9.9	10.2	10.6	10.9	11.3	11.6	12.0
29– 31	10.5	10.8	11.2	11.5	11.9	12.2	12.6	12.9
32– 34	11.4	11.8	12.1	12.4	12.8	13.1	13.5	13.8
35– 37	12.3	12.7	13.0	13.4	13.7	14.1	14.4	14.8
38– 40	13.2	13.6	13.9	14.3	14.6	15.0	15.3	15.7
41– 43	14.1	14.5	14.8	15.2	15.5	15.9	16.2	16.6
44– 46	15.0	15.4	15.7	16.1	16.4	16.8	17.1	17.5
47– 49	15.9	16.2	16.6	16.9	17.3	17.6	18.0	18.3
50– 52	16.8	17.1	17.5	17.8	18.2	18.5	18.8	19.2
53– 55	17.6	18.0	18.3	18.7	19.0	19.4	19.7	20.1
56– 58	18.5	18.8	19.2	19.5	19.9	20.2	20.6	20.9
59– 61	19.3	19.7	20.0	20.4	20.7	21.0	21.4	21.7
62– 64	20.1	20.5	20.8	21.2	21.5	21.9	22.2	22.6
65– 67	21.0	21.3	21.7	22.0	22.4	22.7	23.0	23.4
68– 70	21.8	22.1	22.5	22.8	23.2	23.5	23.9	24.2
71– 73	22.6	22.9	23.3	23.6	24.0	24.3	24.7	25.0
74– 76	23.4	23.7	24.1	24.4	24.8	25.1	25.4	25.8
77– 79	24.1	24.5	24.8	25.2	25.5	25.9	26.2	26.6
80– 82	24.9	25.3	25.6	26.0	26.3	26.6	27.0	27.3
83– 85	25.7	26.0	26.4	26.7	27.1	27.4	27.8	28.1
86– 88	26.4	26.8	27.1	27.5	27.8	28.2	28.5	28.9
89– 91	27.2	27.5	27.9	28.2	28.6	28.9	29.2	29.6
92– 94	27.9	28.2	28.6	28.9	29.3	29.6	30.0	30.3
95– 97	28.6	29.0	29.3	29.7	30.0	30.4	30.7	31.1
98–100	29.3	29.7	30.0	30.4	30.7	31.1	31.4	31.8
101–103	30.0	30.4	30.7	31.1	31.4	31.8	32.1	32.5
104–106	30.7	31.1	31.4	31.8	32.1	32.5	32.8	33.2
107–109	31.4	31.8	32.1	32.4	32.8	33.1	33.5	33.8
110–112	32.1	32.4	32.8	33.1	33.5	33.8	34.2	34.5
113–115	32.7	33.1	33.4	33.8	34.1	34.5	34.8	35.2
116–118	33.4	33.7	34.1	34.4	34.8	35.1	35.5	35.8
119–121	34.0	34.4	34.7	35.1	35.4	35.8	36.1	36.5
122–124	34.7	35.0	35.4	35.7	36.1	36.4	36.7	37.1
125–127	35.3	35.6	36.0	36.3	36.7	37.0	37.4	37.7
128–130	35.9	36.2	36.6	36.9	37.3	37.6	38.0	38.5

Body density is calculated based on the "Generalized equation for predicting body density of men" developed by A. S. Jackson and M. L. Pollock, *British Journal of Nutrition* 40 (1978): 497–504. Percent body fat is determined from the calculated body density using the Siri formula.

GIRTH MEASUREMENTS

A simpler method to determine body fat is by measuring circumferences at various body sites. This technique requires only a standard measuring tape, and good accuracy can be achieved with little practice. The limitation is that it may not be valid for athletic individuals (men or women) who participate actively in strenuous physical activity or people who can be classified visually as thin or obese.

The required procedure for **girth measurements** is given in Figure 9.3. Measurements for women include the upper arm, hip, and wrist; for men, the waist and wrist. Tables 9.4 and 9.5 translate these measurements into body density and percent fat estimates for women and men, respectively.

BIOELECTRICAL IMPEDANCE

The **bioelectrical impedance** technique is much simpler to administer, but its accuracy is questionable. In this technique, sensors are applied to the skin and a weak (totally painless) electrical current is run through the body to estimate body fat, lean body mass, and body water. The technique is based on the principle that fat tissue is a less efficient conductor of electrical current than lean tissue is. The easier the conductance, the leaner the individual. Body weight scales with sensors on the surface are also available to perform this procedure.

The accuracy of equations used to estimate percent body fat with this technique is questionable. A single equation cannot be used for everyone, but rather valid and accurate equations to estimate body fat for the specific population (age, gender, and ethnicity) being tested are required. Following all manufacturers' instructions will ensure the most accurate result, but even then percent body fat may be off by as much as 10 percentage points (or even more on some scales).

BODY MASS INDEX

The most common technique to determine thinness and excessive fatness is the **body mass index (BMI)**. BMI incorporates height and weight to estimate critical fat values at which the risk for disease increases.

BMI is calculated by either (a) dividing the weight in kilograms by the square of the height in meters or

Girth measurements Technique to assess body composition by measuring circumferences at specific body sites.

Bioelectrical impedance Technique to assess body composition by running a weak electrical current through the body.

Body mass index (BMI) A technique to determine thinness and excessive fatness that incorporates height and weight to estimate critical fat values at which the risk for disease increases.

Girth Measurements for Women*

1. Using a regular tape measure, determine the following girth measurements in centimeters (cm):

   Upper Arm: Measure halfway between the shoulder and the elbow.

   Hip: Measure at the point of largest circumference.

   Wrist: Take the girth in front of the bones where the wrist bends.

2. Obtain the person's age.

3. According to Table 9.4, use the girth measurement for each site and your age. Look up the corresponding constant values. These values will allow you to derive body density (BD) by substituting the constants in the following formula:

   $BD = A - B - C + D$

4. Using the derived body density, calculate percent body fat (%F) according to the following equation:

   $\%F = (495 \div BD) - 450**$

   Example: Jane is 20 years old, and the following girth measurements were taken: upper arm = 27 cm, hip = 99.5 cm, wrist = 15.4 cm.

Data		Constant
Upper Arm = 27 cm	A =	1.0813
Age = 20	B =	.0102
Hip = 99.5 cm	C =	.1206
Wrist = 15.4 cm	D =	.0971

$BD = A - B - C + D$
$BD = 1.0813 - .0102 - .1206 + .0971 = 1.0476$

$\%F = (495 \div BD) - 450$
$\%F = (495 \div 1.0476) - 450 = 22.5$

Girth Measurements for Men***

1. Using a regular tape measure, determine the following girth measurements in inches (the men's measurements are taken in inches as contrasted with centimeters for women):

   Waist: Measure at the umbilicus (belly button).

   Wrist: Measure in front of the bones where the wrist bends.

2. Subtract the wrist from the waist measurement.

3. Obtain the person's weight in pounds.

4. Look up the percent body fat (%F) in Table 9.5 by using the difference obtained in Step 2 above and the person's body weight.

Example: John weighs 160 pounds, and his waist and wrist girth measurements are 36.5 and 7.5 inches, respectively.

Waist girth = 36.5 inches
Wrist girth = 7.5 inches
Difference = 29.0 inches
Body weight = 160.0 lbs.
%F = 22

* Reproduced by permission from R. B. Lambson, "Generalized Body Density Prediction Equations for Women Using Simple Anthropometric Measurements." (Ph.D. diss. Brigham Young University, August 1987).

** From W. E. Siri, *Body Composition From Fluid Spaces and Density*, (Berkeley: University of California, Donner Laboratory of Medical Physics, 1956).

*** Table 9.5 reproduced by permission from A. G. Fisher, and P. E. Allsen, *Jogging* (Dubuque, IA: Wm. C. Brown, 1987). This table was developed according to the generalized body composition equation for men using simple measurement techniques by K. W. Penrouse, A. G Nelson, and A. G. Fisher, *Medicine and Science in Sports and Exercise* 17, no. 2 (1985): 189. © American College of Sports Medicine 1985.

TABLE 9.4 Conversion Constants from Girth Measurements to Calculate Body Density for Women

Upper Arm (cm)	Constant A	Age	Constant B	Hip (cm)	Constant C	Hip (cm)	Constant C	Wrist (cm)	Constant D
20.5	1.0966	17	.0086	79	.0957	114.5	.1388	13.0	.0819
21	1.0954	18	.0091	79.5	.0963	115	.1394	13.2	.0832
21.5	1.0942	19	.0096	80	.0970	115.5	.1400	13.4	.0845
22	1.0930	20	.0102	80.5	.0976	116	.1406	13.6	.0857
22.5	1.0919	21	.0107	81	.0982	116.5	.1412	13.8	.0870
23	1.0907	22	.0112	81.5	.0988	117	.1418	14.0	.0882
23.5	1.0895	23	.0117	82	.0994	117.5	.1424	14.2	.0895
24	1.0883	24	.0122	82.5	.1000	118	.1430	14.4	.0908
24.5	1.0871	25	.0127	83	.1006	118.5	.1436	14.6	.0920
25	1.0860	26	.0132	83.5	.1012	119	.1442	14.8	.0933
25.5	1.0848	27	.0137	84	.1018	119.5	.1448	15.0	.0946
26	1.0836	28	.0142	84.5	.1024	120	.1454	15.2	.0958
26.5	1.0824	29	.0147	85	.1030	120.5	.1460	15.4	.0971
27	1.0813	30	.0152	85.5	.1036	121	.1466	15.6	.0983
27.5	1.0801	31	.0157	86	.1042	121.5	.1472	15.8	.0996
28	1.0789	32	.0162	86.5	.1048	122	.1479	16.0	.1009
28.5	1.0777	33	.0168	87	.1054	122.5	.1485	16.2	.1021

Upper Arm (cm)	Constant A	Age	Constant B	Hip (cm)	Constant C	Hip (cm)	Constant C	Wrist (cm)	Constant D
29	1.0775	34	.0173	87.5	.1060	123	.1491	16.4	.1034
29.5	1.0754	35	.0178	88	.1066	123.5	.1497	16.6	.1046
30	1.0742	36	.0183	88.5	.1072	124	.1503	16.8	.1059
30.5	1.0730	37	.0188	89	.1079	124.5	.1509	17.0	.1072
31	1.0718	38	.0193	89.5	.1085	125	.1515	17.2	.1084
31.5	1.0707	39	.0198	90	.1091	125.5	.1521	17.4	.1097
32	1.0695	40	.0203	90.5	.1097	126	.1527	17.6	.1109
32.5	1.0683	41	.0208	91	.1103	126.5	.1533	17.8	.1122
33	1.0671	42	.0213	91.5	.1109	127	.1539	18.0	.1135
33.5	1.0666	43	.0218	92	.1115	127.5	.1545	18.2	.1147
34	1.0648	44	.0223	92.5	.1121	128	.1551	18.4	.1160
34.5	1.0636	45	.0228	93	.1127	128.5	.1558	18.6	.1172
35	1.0624	46	.0234	93.5	.1133	129	.1563		
35.5	1.0612	47	.0239	94	.1139	129.5	.1569		
36	1.0601	48	.0244	94.5	.1145	130	.1575		
36.5	1.0589	49	.0249	95	.1151	130.5	.1581		
37	1.0577	50	.0254	95.5	.1157	131	.1587		
37.5	1.0565	51	.0259	96	.1163	131.5	.1593		
38	1.0554	52	.0264	96.5	.1169	132	.1600		
38.5	1.0542	53	.0269	97	.1176	132.5	.1606		
39	1.0530	54	.0274	97.5	.1182	133	.1612		
39.5	1.0518	55	.0279	98	.1188	133.5	.1618		
40	1.0506	56	.0284	98.5	.1194	134	.1624		
40.5	1.0495	57	.0289	99	.1200	134.5	.1630		
41	1.0483	58	.0294	99.5	.1206	135	.1636		
41.5	1.0471	59	.0300	100	.1212	135.5	.1642		
42	1.0459	60	.0305	100.5	.1218	136	.1648		
42.5	1.0448	61	.0310	101	.1224	136.5	.1654		
43	1.0434	62	.0315	101.5	.1230	137	.1660		
43.5	1.0424	63	.0320	102	.1236	137.5	.1666		
44	1.0412	64	.0325	102.5	.1242	138	.1672		
		65	.0330	103	.1248	138.5	.1678		
		66	.0335	103.5	.1254	139	.1685		
		67	.0340	104	.1260	139.5	.1691		
		68	.0345	104.5	.1266	140	.1697		
		69	.0350	105	.1272	140.5	.1703		
		70	.0355	105.5	.1278	141	.1709		
		71	.0360	106	.1285	141.5	.1715		
		72	.0366	106.5	.1291	142	.1721		
		73	.0371	107	.1297	142.5	.1728		
		74	.0376	107.5	.1303	143	.1733		
		75	.0381	108	.1309	143.5	.1739		
				108.5	.1315	144	.1745		
				109	.1321	144.5	.1751		
				109.5	.1327	145	.1757		
				110	.1333	145.5	.1763		
				110.5	.1339	146	.1769		
				111	.1345	146.5	.1775		
				111.5	.1351	147	.1781		
				112	.1357	147.5	.1787		
				112.5	.1363	148	.1794		
				113	.1369	148.5	.1800		
				113.5	.1375	149	.1806		
				114	.1382	149.5	.1812		
						150	.1818		

Waist Minus Wrist Girth Measurement

Body Weight	22	22.5	23	23.5	24	24.5	25	25.5	26	26.5	27	27.5	28	28.5	29	29.5	30	30.5	31	31.5	32	32.5	33	33.5	34	34.5	35	35.5	36	36.5	37	37.5	38	38.5	39	39.5	40	40.5	41	41.5	42	42.5	43	43.5	44	44.5	45	45.5	46	46.5	47	47.5	48	48.5	49	49.5	50
120	4	6	8	10	12	14	16	18	20	21	23	25	27	29	31	33	35	37	39	41	43	45	47	49																																	
125	4	6	7	9	11	13	15	17	19	20	22	24	26	28	30	32	33	35	37	39	41	43	45	46	48	50	52	54	56	58																											
130	3	5	7	9	11	12	14	16	18	20	21	23	25	27	29	31	32	34	36	38	40	41	43	44	46	48	50	52	53	55	57																									
135	3	5	7	8	10	12	14	16	17	19	20	22	24	26	28	29	31	33	34	36	38	40	41	43	44	46	48	50	51	53	54	56																								
140	3	5	6	8	10	11	13	15	16	18	20	21	23	25	27	28	30	31	33	35	36	38	40	41	43	44	46	48	49	51	52	54	56																						
145	3	4	6	8	9	11	13	14	16	17	19	20	22	24	25	27	29	30	32	33	35	37	38	40	41	43	44	46	47	49	51	52	54	55																					
150	2	4	6	7	9	11	12	14	15	17	18	20	21	23	24	26	27	29	30	32	33	35	36	38	40	41	43	44	46	47	49	50	52	53	55																				
155	2	4	6	7	9	10	12	13	15	16	18	19	21	22	24	25	27	28	30	31	32	34	35	37	38	40	41	43	44	46	47	49	50	52	53	55																		
160	2	4	5	7	8	10	11	13	14	16	17	19	20	22	23	24	26	27	29	30	32	33	34	36	37	39	40	42	43	44	46	47	48	50	51	53	54																	
165	2	4	5	6	8	9	11	12	14	15	16	18	19	21	22	24	25	26	28	29	31	32	33	35	36	38	39	40	42	43	44	46	47	48	50	51	52	54															
170	2	3	5	6	8	9	10	12	13	14	16	17	19	20	21	23	24	26	27	28	30	31	32	34	35	36	38	39	40	42	43	44	45	47	48	49	51	52	53													
175	2	3	4	6	7	9	10	11	13	14	15	17	18	19	21	22	23	25	26	27	29	30	31	32	34	35	36	38	39	40	41	43	44	45	47	48	49	50	52	53												
180					3	4	5	7	8	10	11	12	13	15	16	17	19	20	21	22	24	25	26	28	29	30	31	33	34	35	36	38	39	40	41	43	44	45	46	48	49	50	51										
185					3	4	5	6	8	9	10	11	13	14	15	16	18	19	20	21	23	24	25	26	28	29	30	31	33	34	35	36	38	39	40	41	43	44	45	46	48	49	50	51									
190					2	4	5	6	7	8	10	11	12	13	15	16	17	18	20	21	22	23	24	26	27	28	29	31	32	33	34	35	37	38	39	40	41	43	44	45	46	48	49	50	51							
195					2	3	4	5	7	8	9	10	11	13	14	15	16	18	19	20	21	22	24	25	26	27	28	30	31	32	33	34	36	37	38	39	40	41	43	44	45	46	47	49	50	51	52					
200					2	3	4	6	7	8	9	10	12	13	14	15	16	18	19	20	21	22	24	25	26	27	28	29	31	32	33	34	35	36	38	39	40	41	42	44	45	46	47	48	50	51	52					
205					2	3	4	5	6	8	9	10	11	12	14	15	16	17	19	20	21	22	23	25	26	27	28	29	30	32	33	34	35	36	37	39	40	41	42	43	44	46	47	48	49	50	51	52				
210					2	3	4	5	6	7	9	10	11	12	13	15	16	17	18	19	21	22	23	24	25	26	28	29	30	31	32	33	34	36	37	38	39	40	41	42	43	44	46	47	48	49	50	51				
215			2		2	3	4	5	6	7	8	9	11	12	13	14	15	16	18	19	20	21	22	23	24	26	27	28	29	30	31	32	33	35	36	37	38	39	40	41	42	43	44	46	47	48	49	50	51			
220			2		2	3	4	5	6	7	8	9	10	11	13	14	15	16	17	18	19	20	22	23	24	25	26	27	28	29	30	32	33	34	35	36	37	38	39	40	41	42	43	44	45	46	47	48	49	51		
225			2		2	3	4	5	6	7	8	9	10	11	12	13	14	16	17	18	19	20	21	22	23	24	25	26	28	29	30	31	32	33	34	35	36	37	38	39	40	41	42	43	44	45	46	47	48	49	51	
230			2		2	3	4	5	6	7	8	9	10	11	12	13	14	15	16	17	18	20	21	22	23	24	25	26	27	28	29	30	31	32	33	34	35	36	37	38	39	40	41	42	43	44	45	46	47	48	49	50
235			2		2	3	4	5	6	7	8	9	10	11	12	13	14	15	16	17	18	19	20	21	22	23	24	26	27	28	29	30	31	32	33	34	35	36	37	38	39	40	41	42	43	44	45	46	47	48	49	50
240			2		2	3	4	5	6	7	8	9	10	11	12	13	14	15	16	17	18	19	20	21	22	23	24	25	26	27	28	29	30	31	32	34	35	36	37	38	39	40	41	42	43	44	45	46	47	48	49	50
245			2		2	3	4	5	6	7	8	9	9	10	11	12	13	14	15	16	17	18	19	20	21	22	23	24	25	26	27	28	29	30	31	33	34	35	36	37	38	39	40	41	42	43	44	45	46	47	48	49
250			2		2	3	4	5	6	6	7	8	9	10	11	12	13	14	15	16	17	18	19	20	21	22	23	24	25	26	27	28	29	30	31	32	33	34	35	36	37	38	39	40	41	42	43	44	45	46	47	48
255			2		2	3	3	4	5	6	7	8	9	10	11	12	13	14	15	16	17	18	18	19	20	21	22	23	24	25	26	27	28	29	30	31	32	33	34	35	36	37	38	39	40	41	42	43	44	45	46	47
260					2	3	3	4	5	6	7	8	9	10	11	11	12	13	14	15	16	17	18	19	20	21	22	23	24	25	26	27	28	28	29	30	31	32	33	34	35	36	37	38	39	40	41	42	43	44	45	46
265					2	3	3	4	5	6	7	8	9	10	11	11	12	13	14	15	16	17	18	19	20	21	22	23	23	24	25	26	27	28	29	30	31	32	33	34	35	36	37	38	39	40	40	41	42	43	44	45
270					2	3	3	4	5	6	7	8	9	9	10	11	12	13	14	15	16	17	18	18	19	20	21	22	23	24	25	26	27	28	29	30	31	32	33	34	35	36	37	38	39	39	40	41	42	43	43	44
275					2	3	3	4	5	6	7	8	9	9	10	11	12	13	14	15	16	17	17	18	19	20	21	22	23	24	25	26	27	28	29	30	30	31	32	33	34	35	36	37	38	38	39	40	41	42	43	43
280					2	3	3	4	5	6	7	8	8	9	10	11	12	13	14	15	16	16	17	18	19	20	21	22	23	24	25	26	27	28	28	29	30	31	32	33	34	35	36	37	38	38	39	40	41	42	43	43
285					2	3	3	4	5	6	7	7	8	9	10	11	11	12	13	14	15	16	17	18	19	20	21	21	22	23	24	25	26	27	28	29	29	30	31	32	33	34	35	36	37	37	38	39	40	41	42	43
290					2	3	3	4	5	6	6	7	8	9	10	10	11	12	13	14	15	16	17	18	18	19	20	21	22	23	24	25	26	27	28	28	29	30	31	32	33	34	35	36	37	37	38	39	40	41	42	43
295					2	2	3	3	4	5	6	6	7	8	9	10	11	12	12	13	14	15	16	17	18	19	20	21	22	23	23	24	25	26	27	28	29	30	30	31	32	33	34	35	36	36	37	38	39	40	41	42
300					2	2	3	3	4	5	5	6	7	8	9	9	10	11	12	13	14	15	16	17	18	18	19	20	21	22	23	24	25	26	26	27	28	29	30	31	32	33	33	34	35	36	37	38	39	40	41	43

TABLE 9.6 Determination of Body Mass Index

Determine your BMI by looking up the number where your weight and height intersect on the table.
According to your results, look up your disease risk in Table 9.8.

Weight

Height	110	115	120	125	130	135	140	145	150	155	160	165	170	175	180	185	190	195	200	205	210	215	220	225	230	235	240	245	250
5'0"	21	22	23	24	25	26	27	28	29	30	31	32	33	34	35	36	37	38	39	40	41	42	43	44	45	46	47	48	49
5'1"	21	22	23	24	25	26	26	27	28	29	30	31	32	33	34	35	36	37	38	39	40	41	42	43	43	44	45	46	47
5'2"	20	21	22	23	24	25	26	27	27	28	29	30	31	32	33	34	35	36	37	37	38	39	40	41	42	43	44	45	46
5'3"	19	20	21	22	23	24	25	26	27	27	28	29	30	31	32	33	34	35	35	36	37	38	39	40	41	42	43	43	44
5'4"	19	20	21	21	22	23	24	25	26	27	27	28	29	30	31	32	33	33	34	35	36	37	38	39	39	40	41	42	43
5'5"	18	19	20	21	22	22	23	24	25	26	27	27	28	29	30	31	32	32	33	34	35	36	37	37	38	39	40	41	42
5'6"	18	19	19	20	21	22	23	23	24	25	26	27	27	28	29	30	31	31	32	33	34	35	36	36	37	38	39	40	40
5'7"	17	18	19	20	20	21	22	23	23	24	25	26	27	27	28	29	30	31	31	32	33	34	34	35	36	37	38	38	39
5'8"	17	17	18	19	20	21	21	22	23	24	24	25	26	27	27	28	29	30	30	31	32	33	33	34	35	36	36	37	38
5'9"	16	17	18	18	19	20	21	21	22	23	24	24	25	26	27	27	28	29	30	30	31	32	32	33	34	35	35	36	37
5'10"	16	17	17	18	19	19	20	21	22	22	23	24	24	25	26	27	27	28	29	29	30	31	32	32	33	34	34	35	36
5'11"	15	16	17	17	18	19	20	20	21	22	22	23	24	24	25	26	26	27	28	29	29	30	31	31	32	33	33	34	35
6'0"	15	16	16	17	18	18	19	20	20	21	22	22	23	24	24	25	26	26	27	28	28	29	30	31	31	32	33	33	34
6'1"	15	15	16	16	17	18	18	19	20	20	21	22	22	23	24	24	25	26	26	27	28	28	29	30	30	31	32	32	33
6'2"	14	15	15	16	17	17	18	19	19	20	21	21	22	22	23	24	24	25	26	26	27	28	28	29	30	30	31	31	32
6'3"	14	14	15	16	16	17	17	18	19	19	20	21	21	22	22	23	24	24	25	26	26	27	27	28	29	29	30	31	31
6'4"	13	14	15	15	16	16	17	18	18	19	19	20	21	21	22	23	23	24	24	25	26	26	27	27	28	29	29	30	30

(b) multiplying body weight in pounds by 705 and dividing this figure by the square of the height in inches. For example, the BMI for an individual who weighs 172 pounds (78 kg) and is 67 inches (1.7 m) tall would be 27 [$78 \div (1.7)^2$] or [$172 \times 705 \div (67)^2$]. Or you can look up your BMI in Table 9.6 according to your height and weight.

Because of its simplicity and consistency of measurement across populations, BMI is the most widely used measure to determine overweight and obesity. The previously mentioned body composition techniques have various limitations, including cost, availability to the general population, lack of consistency among technicians and laboratories, inconsistent results between techniques, and standard error of measurement of the procedures. Therefore, BMI is used almost exclusively to determine health risks and mortality rates associated with excessive body weight.

Scientific evidence indicates that disease risk starts to increase when BMI exceeds 25.[1] Although a BMI index between 18.5 and 24.99 is considered normal (see Tables 9.7 and 9.9), the lowest risk for chronic disease is in the 22– to-25-year age range.[2] Individuals are classified as overweight if their indexes lie between 25 and 30. BMIs above 30 are classified as obese, and those below 18.5 as **underweight**. Scientific evidence has shown that even though the risk for premature illness and death is greater

TABLE 9.7 Disease Risk According to Body Mass Index (BMI)

BMI	Disease Risk	Classification
<18.5	Increased	Underweight
18.5–21.99	Low	Acceptable
22.0–24.99	Very Low	Acceptable
25.0–29.99	Increased	Overweight
30.0–34.99	High	Obesity I
35.0–39.99	Very High	Obesity II
≥40.00	Extremely High	Obesity III

for those who are overweight, the risk also increases for individuals who are underweight[3] (see Figure 9.4).

Compared to individuals with a BMI between 22 and 25, people with a BMI between 25 and 30 (overweight) exhibit mortality rates up to 25 percent higher; rates for those with a BMI above 30 (obese) are 50 to 100 percent higher.[4] Table 9.7 provides disease risk categories when BMI is used as the sole criteria to identify people at risk. More than one-fifth of the U.S. adult population has a BMI of 30 or more. Overweight and obesity trends starting in 1960 according to BMI are given in Figure 9.5.

Underweight Extremely low body weight.

FIGURE 9.4 Mortality Risk Versus Body Mass Index (BMI)

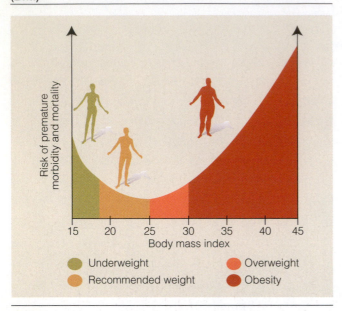

Legend:
- Underweight
- Recommended weight
- Overweight
- Obesity

FIGURE 9.5 Overweight and Obesity Trends in the United States 1960–2000

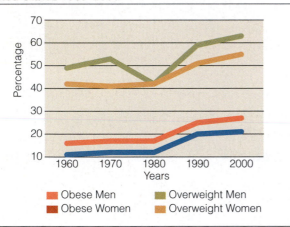

Legend:
- Obese Men
- Obese Women
- Overweight Men
- Overweight Women

Adapted from the National Center for Health Statistics, Centers for Disease Control and Prevention, and the *Journal of the American Medical Association.*

BMI is a useful tool to screen the general population, but its one weakness is that it fails to differentiate fat from lean body mass or note where most of the fat is located (waist circumferences—see discussion that follows). Using BMI, athletes with a large amount of muscle mass (such as body builders and football players) can easily fall in the moderate- or even high-risk categories.

WAIST CIRCUMFERENCE

Scientific evidence suggests that the way people store fat affects their risk for disease. The total amount of body fat by itself is not the best predictor of increased risk for disease but, rather, the location of the fat. **Android obesity** is seen in individuals who tend to store fat in the trunk

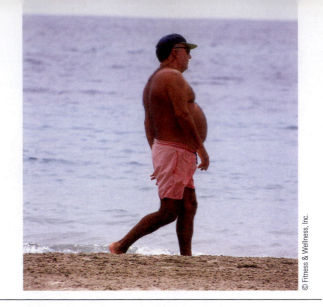

Individuals who accumulate body fat around the midsection have a greater risk for disease than those who accumulate body fat in other areas.

or abdominal area (which produces the "apple" shape). **Gynoid obesity** is seen in people who store fat primarily around the hips and thighs (which creates the "pear" shape).

Obese individuals with abdominal fat are clearly at higher risk for heart disease, hypertension, Type 2 diabetes (non-insulin–dependent diabetes), and stroke than are obese people with similar amounts of body fat stored primarily in the hips and thighs.[5] Evidence also indicates that, among individuals with a lot of abdominal fat, those whose fat deposits are located around internal organs (intra-abdominal or abdominal visceral fat) have an even greater risk for disease than those with fat mainly just beneath the skin (subcutaneous fat).[6]

Because scanning techniques to identify individuals at risk because of high intra-abdominal fatness are costly, a simple **waist circumference (WC)** measure, designed by the National Heart, Lung, and Blood Institute, is used to assess this risk.[7] WC seems to predict abdominal visceral fat as accurately as the DEXA technique.[8] A waist circumference of more than 40 inches in men and 35 inches in women indicates a higher risk for cardiovascular disease, hypertension, and Type 2 diabetes (see Table 9.8). Thus, weight loss is encouraged when individuals exceed these measurements.

One study concluded that WC is a better predictor of the risk for disease than BMI.[9] Thus, BMI in conjunction with WC provides the best combination to identify individuals at higher risk because of excessive body fat. Table 9.9 provides guidelines to identify people at risk according to BMI and WC.

A second procedure that was used for years to identify health risk based on the pattern of fat distribution is the waist-to-hip ratio (WHR) test. In recent years, however, several studies have found that WC is a better indicator than WHR of abdominal visceral obesity.[10] Thus, a combination of BMI and WC, rather than WHR, is now

TABLE 9.8 Disease Risk According to Waist Circumference (WC)

Men	Women	Disease Risk
<35.5	<32.5	Low
35.5–40.0	32.5–35.0	Moderate
>40.0	>35.0	High

TABLE 9.9 Disease Risk According to Body Mass Index (BMI) and Waist Circumference (WC)

		Disease risk relative to normal weight and WC	
Classification	BMI (kg/m²)	Men ≤40" (102 cm) Women ≤35" (88 cm)	Men >40" (102 cm) Women >35" (88 cm)
Underweight	<18.5	Increased	Low
Normal	18.5–24.9	Very low	Increased
Overweight	25.0–29.9	Increased	High
Obesity Class I	30.0–34.9	High	Very high
Obesity Class II	35.0–39.9	Very high	Very high
Obesity Class III	≥40.0	Extremely high	Extremely high

Adapted from Expert Panel, *Executive Summary of the Clinical Guidelines on the Identification, Evaluation, and Treatment of Overweight and Obesity in Adults*, Archives of Internal Medicine 158:1855–1867, 1998.

recommended by health care professionals to assess potential risk for disease.

Determining Recommended Body Weight

After finding out your percent body fat, you can determine your current body composition classification by consulting Table 9.10 which presents percentages of fat according to both the health fitness standard and the high physical fitness standard (see discussion in Chapter 6).

For example, the recommended health fitness fat percentage for a 20-year-old female is 28 percent or less. Although there are no clearly identified percent body fat levels at which the disease risk definitely increases (as is the case with BMI), the health fitness standard in Table 9.10 is currently the best estimate of the point at which there seems to be no harm to health.

According to Table 9.10, the high physical fitness range for this same 20-year-old woman would be between 18 and 23 percent. The high physical fitness standard does not mean that a person cannot be somewhat below this number. Many highly trained male athletes are as low as 3 percent, and some female distance runners have been measured at 6 percent body fat (which may not be healthy).

Although people generally agree that the mortality rate is higher for obese people, some evidence indicates that the same is true for underweight people. "Underweight" and "thin" do not necessarily mean the same thing. The body fat of a healthy thin person is around the high physical fitness standard, whereas an underweight person has extremely low body fat, even to the point of compromising the essential fat.

The 3 percent essential fat for men and 12 percent for women seem to be the lower limits for people to maintain good health. Below these percentages, normal physiological functions can be impaired. Some experts point out that a little storage fat (in addition to the essential fat) is better than none at all. As a result, the health and high fitness standards for percent fat in Table 9.10 are set higher than the minimum essential fat requirements, at a point beneficial to optimal health and well-being. Finally, because lean tissue decreases with age, one extra percentage point is allowed for every additional decade of life.

Critical Thinking

1. Do you think you have a weight problem?
2. Do your body composition results make you feel any different about the way you perceive your current body weight and image?

Your recommended body weight is computed based on the selected health or high fitness fat percentage for your age and sex. Your decision to select a "desired" fat percentage should be based on your current percent body fat and your personal health/fitness objectives. Following are steps to compute your own recommended body weight:

1. Determine the pounds of body weight that are fat (FW) by multiplying your body weight (BW) by the current percent fat (%F) expressed in decimal form (FW = BW × %F).
2. Determine lean body mass (LBM) by subtracting the weight in fat from the total body weight (LBM = BW − FW). (Anything that is not fat must be part of the lean component.)
3. Select a desired body fat percentage (DFP) based on the health or high fitness standards given in Table 9.10.
4. Compute recommended body weight (RBW) according to the formula RBW = LBM ÷ (1.0 × DFP).

Android obesity Obesity pattern in individuals who tend to store fat in the trunk or abdominal area.

Gynoid obesity Obesity pattern in people who store fat primarily around the hips and thighs.

Waist circumference (WC) A waist girth measurement to assess potential risk for disease based on intra-abdominal fat content.

TABLE 9.10 Body Composition Categories According to Percent Body Fat

MEN						
Age	Underweight	Excellent	Good	Moderate	Overweight	Significantly Overweight
≤19	<3	12.0	12.1–17.0	17.1–22.0	22.1–27.0	≥27.1
20–29	<3	13.0	13.1–18.0	18.1–23.0	23.1–28.0	≥28.1
30–39	<3	14.0	14.1–19.0	19.1–24.0	24.1–29.0	≥29.1
40–49	<3	15.0	15.1–20.0	20.1–25.0	25.1–30.0	≥30.1
≥50	<3	16.0	16.1–21.0	21.1–26.0	26.1–31.0	≥31.1
WOMEN						
Age	Underweight	Excellent	Good	Moderate	Overweight	Significantly Overweight
≤19	<12	17.0	17.1–22.0	22.1–27.0	27.1–32.0	≥32.1
20–29	<12	18.0	18.1–23.0	23.1–28.0	28.1–33.0	≥33.1
30–39	<12	19.0	19.1–24.0	24.1–29.0	29.1–34.0	≥34.1
40–49	<12	20.0	20.1–25.0	25.1–30.0	30.1–35.0	≥35.1
≥50	<12	21.0	21.1–26.0	26.1–31.0	31.1–36.0	≥36.1

☐ High physical fitness standard   ☐ Health fitness standard

As an example of these computations, a 19-year-old female who weighs 160 pounds and is 30 percent fat would like to know what her recommended body weight would be at 22 percent:

Sex: female
Age: 19
BW: 160 lbs
%F: 30% (.30 in decimal form)

1. FW = BW × %F
   FW = 160 × .30 = 48 lbs

2. LBM = BW − FW
   LBM = 160 − 48 = 112 lbs

3. DFP: 22% (.22 in decimal form)

4. RBW = LBM ÷ (1.0 − .DFP)
   RBW = 112 ÷ (1.0 − .22)
   RBW = 112 ÷ .78 = 143.6 lbs

In Assessment 9.1 you will have the opportunity to determine your own body composition, recommended body weight, and your risk for disease according to BMI and WC.

Other than hydrostatic weighing and air displacement, skinfold thickness seems to be the most practical and valid technique to estimate body fat. If skinfold calipers are available, use this technique to assess your percent body fat. If none of these techniques is available to you, estimate your percent fat according to girth measurements (or another technique available to you) and use the Profile Plus CD-ROM to obtain your body composition results. You may also wish to use several techniques and compare the results.

Importance of Assessing Body Composition Regularly

Children in the United States do not start with a weight problem. Although a small number struggle with weight throughout life, most are not overweight in the early years of life. Trends indicate that, starting at age 25, the average person in the United States gains 1 to 2 pounds of weight per year. Thus, by age 65, the average American will have gained at least 40 pounds. Because of the typical reduction in physical activity in our society, however, the average person also loses a half a pound of lean tissue each year. Therefore, this span of 40 years has produced an actual fat gain of at least 60 pounds accompanied by a 20-pound loss of lean body mass[11] (see Figure 9.6). These changes cannot be detected unless body composition is assessed periodically.

If you are on a diet/exercise program, you should repeat your percent body fat assessment and recommended weight computations about once a month. This is important because lean body mass is affected by weight reduction and amount of physical activity. As lean body mass

FIGURE 9.6 Typical Body Composition Changes for Adults in the United States

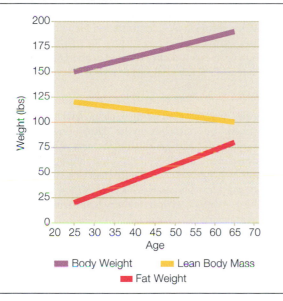

FIGURE 9.7 Effects of a 6-week Aerobics Exercise Program on Body Composition

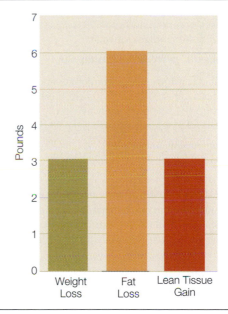

changes, so will your recommended body weight. To make valid comparisons, use the same technique for both pre- and post-program assessments. Knowing your percent body fat also is useful to identify fad diets that promote water loss and lean body mass, especially muscle mass.

Changes in body composition resulting from a weight control/exercise program were illustrated in a co-ed aerobic dance course taught during a 6-week summer term. Students participated in a 60-minute aerobics routine 4 times a week. On the first and last days of class, several physiological parameters, including body composition, were assessed. Students also were given information on diet and nutrition, but they followed their own dietary program.

At the end of the 6 weeks, the average weight loss for the entire class was 3 pounds (see Figure 9.7). But, because body composition was assessed, class members were surprised to find that the average fat loss was actually 6 pounds, accompanied by a 3-pound increase in lean body mass.

When dieting, have your body composition reassessed periodically because of the effects of negative caloric balance on lean body mass. As presented in Chapter 10, dieting does decrease lean body mass. This loss of lean body mass can be offset or eliminated by combining a sensible diet with exercise.

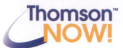

Don't forget to check out the wealth of resources on the ThomsonNOW website at **www.thomsonedu.com/ThomsonNOW** that will:

- Coach you through identifying target goals for behavior change and monitoring your personal change plan throughout the semester
- Help you evaluate your knowledge of the material
- Allow you to take an exam-prep quiz
- Provide a Personalized Learning Plan targeting resources that address areas you should study.

WEB ACTIVITIES

The Exercise and Physical Fitness Laboratory at Georgia State University This university site, from the Department of Kinesiology and Health, describes six methods for measuring body composition and provides information regarding procedure, description, accuracy, and relative cost, as well as a list of advantages and disadvantages for each.

http://www.gsu.edu/~wwwfit/bodycomp.html

Body Fat Lab An informative, interactive, and fun site from Shape Up, America, describing body mass measurements, percent body fat, and the role body fat plays in overall health. You can check your level of knowledge using the Body Fat IQ Test.

http://www.shapeup.org/index.php

InfoTrac®

Additional readings related to wellness via InfoTrac® College Edition are available in an online library of more than 900 journals and publications. Follow the instructions for accessing InfoTrac® that came packaged with your textbook, then search for articles using a key word search.

Suggested Reading Jancin, Bruce. "Maintain young adult weight to limit CV risks," *Family Practice News,* Feb 15, 2005 v35 i4 p10 (1).

1. What can young adults do to prevent the development of cardiovascular disease and metabolic syndromes as they age?
2. Why is weight stabilization a more realistic goal than weight loss?
3. What single step do researchers suggest to hold the line on weight gain?

Web Activity

CyberDiet Tools

http://www.cyberdiet.com

Sponsor Co-founders Cynthia Fink and Timi Gustafson, R.D., created CyberDiet in 1995. The information on CyberDiet is peer-reviewed by licensed registered dietitians as well as other health care providers.

Description Dedicated to the belief that healthy weight management and lifestyle change must come from a combination of balanced nutrition, regular exercise, and behavioral modification, CyberDiet provides a wealth of fun and well-presented

nutritional information. Cyberdiet.com is a comprehensive resource for those seeking a change to a healthier lifestyle. Through articles, meal plans, recipes, interactive tools, nutritional programs, and much more, Cyberdiet.com provides the latest and one of the most comprehensive nutritional and weight management information sites available on the Internet.

Available Activities

1. The "Nutritional Profile" gives specific recommendations for calorie levels and nutritional needs, geared to your specific weight management goals.
2. "Body Mass Index" is a risk predictor that can help determine whether you will be negatively affected by your current weight and/or be at risk for obesity-related diseases, such as heart attacks, strokes, and so on.
3. The "Waist/Hip Ratio Calculator" can pinpoint signs that your weight and weight distribution are becoming health risks.
4. The "CyberDiet Activity Calculator" and "Target Heart Rate Calculator" provide basic information for safe and healthy exercise.
5. Through partnership with Wellmed, CyberDiet provides a complete and confidential health risk assessment.

Web Work

1. From the Cyberdiet.com home page, go to the "Self-Assessment" box and click on the "Nutrition Profile" link.
2. Enter your name, age, gender, height, and weight. Use the pull-down menu to select your preferred units for weight (pounds or kilograms) and height (feet or centimeters).
3. Use the pull-down menu to select your frame size (small, medium, or large) and your activity level (from sedentary to extremely active).
4. Then, click on the "Complete Profile" button at the bottom of the page.
5. You then will receive your calculated BMI reading and helpful tips regarding weight management. You also will be given the opportunity to select your desired weight goals (lose, maintain, or gain) and select a rate of desired weight change (from 1–2 lb. per week to 2 lb. per week). When completed, click on the "Complete Your Profile" button.
6. You then will receive a series of tables describing the appropriate number of calories, as well as amounts of a variety of nutrients (fat, protein, carbohydrates, vitamins, minerals, cholesterol, and fiber) that you should consume daily to help you achieve your weight goal.

Helpful Hints

1. It is most useful to complete all of the assessments because the results of one often are important in the evaluation of another.
2. To obtain the most from your interactive experience at CyberDiet.com, return to the home page and select one of a variety of links, including a daily food planner, eating right, fast-food facts, dining out, diet detective, and smart chef.

For additional Web activities, links, and suggested readings, visit our Health, Fitness, and Wellness Resource Center at http://health.wadsworth.com.

Notes

1. J. Stevens, J. Cai, E. R. Pamuk, D. F. Williamson, M. J. Thun, and J. L. Wood, "The Effect of Age on the Association Between Body Mass Index and Mortality," *New England Journal of Medicine* 338 (1998): 1–7.

2. E. E. Calle, M. J. Thun, J. M. Petrelli, C. Rodriguez, and C. W. Heath, "Body-Mass Index and Mortality in a Prospective Cohort of U.S. Adults," *New England Journal of Medicine* 341 (1999): 1097–1105.

3. American College of Sports Medicine, "Position Stand: Appropriate Intervention Strategies for Weight Loss and Prevention for Weight Regain for Adults," *Medicine and Science in Sports and Exercise* 33 (2001): 2145–2156.

4. K. M. Flegal, M. D. Carrol, R. J. Kuczmarski, and C. L. Johnson, "Overweight and Obesity in the United States: Prevalence and Trends, 1960–1994," *International Journal of Obesity and Related Metabolic Disorders* 22 (1998): 39–47.

5. "Comparing Apples and Pears," *University of California at Berkeley Wellness Letter* (Palm Coast, FL: The Editors, March 2004).

6. C. Bouchard, G. A. Bray, and V. S. Hubbard, "Basic and Clinical Aspects of Regional Fat Distribution," *American Journal of Clinical Nutrition* 52 (1990): 946–950; J. P. Després, I. Lemieux, and D. Prudhomme, "Treatment of Obesity: Need to Focus on High Risk Abdominally Obese Patients," *British Medical Journal* 322 (2001): 716–720; M. C. Pouliot et al., "Waist Circumference and Abdominal Sagittal Diameter: Best Simple Anthropometric Indexes of Abdominal Visceral Adipose Tissue Accumulation and Related Cardiovascular Risk in Men and Women," *American Journal of Cardiology* 73 (1994): 460–468.

7. National Heart, Lung, and Blood Institute, National Institutes of Health, *The Practical Guide: Identification, Evaluation,* *and Treatment of Overweight and Obesity in Adults* (NIH Publication no. 00-4084) (Washington DC: Government Printing Office, 2000).

8. M. B. Snijder, et al., "The Prediction of Visceral Fat by Dual-Energy X-ray Absorptiometry in the Elderly: A Comparison with Computed Tomography and Anthropometry," *International Journal of Obesity* 26 (2002): 984–993.

9. I. Janssen, P. T. Katzmarzyk, and R. Ross, "Waist Circumference and Not Body Mass Index Explains Obesity-Related Health Risk," *American Journal of Clinical Nutrition* 79 (2004): 379–384.

10. P. M. Ribisl, "Toxic 'Waist' Dump: Our Abdominal Visceral Fat," *ACSM's Health & Fitness Journal* 8, no. 4 (2004): 22–25.

11. J. H. Wilmore, "Exercise and Weight Control: Myths, Misconceptions, and Quackery," lecture given at annual meeting of American College of Sports Medicine, Indianapolis, June 1994.

Assess Your Behavior

1. Do you regularly monitor body weight, BMI, and percent body fat for proper weight and disease risk management?

2. As you experience small increases (2 to 3 pounds) in body weight (fat), do you make immediate adjustments in caloric intake and physical activity patterns to decrease the weight gained rather than adapting to the new higher body weight?

Evaluate how well you understand the concepts presented in this chapter by answering the following questions.

1. Body composition incorporates
   a. a fat component.
   b. a non-fat component.
   c. percent body fat.
   d. lean body mass.
   e. all of the four components above.

2. Recommended body weight can be determined through
   a. waist-to-hip ratio.
   b. body composition analysis.
   c. lean body mass assessment.
   d. waist circumference.
   e. all of the above.

3. Essential fat in women is
   a. 3 percent.
   b. 5 percent.
   c. 10 percent.
   d. 12 percent.
   e. 17 percent.

4. Which of the following is not a technique used in the assessment of body fat?
   a. body mass index
   b. skinfold thickness
   c. hydrostatic weighing
   d. circumference measurements
   e. air displacement

5. Which of the following sites is used in the assessment of percent body fat according to skinfold thickness in men?
   a. suprailium
   b. chest
   c. scapular
   d. triceps
   e. All four sites are used.

6. Which variable is not used in the assessment of percent body fat in women according to girth measurements?
   a. age
   b. hip
   c. wrist
   d. upper arm
   e. height

7. Waist circumference can be used to
   a. determine percent body fat.
   b. assess risk for disease.
   c. measure lean body mass.
   d. identify underweight people.
   e. do all of the above.

8. An acceptable BMI is between
   a. 15 and 18.49.
   b. 18.5 and 24.99.
   c. 25 and 29.99.
   d. 30 and 34.99.
   e. 35 and 39.99.

9. The health fitness percent body fat for women of various ages is in the range of
   a. 3 to 7 percent.
   b. 7 to 12 percent.
   c. 12 to 20 percent.
   d. 20 to 27 percent.
   e. 27 to 31 percent.

10. When a previously inactive individual starts an exercise program, the person may
    a. lose weight.
    b. gain weight.
    c. improve body composition.
    d. lose more fat pounds than total weight pounds.
    e. do all of the above.

Correct answers can be found on page 369.

Body Composition Assessment, Recommended Body Weight Determination, and Disease Risk Assessment According to Body Mass Index (BMI) and Waist Circumference (WC)

Name: _____   Date: _____   Grade: _____

Instructor: _____   Course: _____   Section: _____

Necessary Lab Equipment
Skinfold calipers and standard measuring tapes.

Objective
To assess percent body fat using skinfold thickness and/or girth measurements and to determine recommended body weight based on percent body fat.

Instructions
If skinfold calipers are available, use the skinfold thickness technique to assess your percent body fat (see Figure 9.2, page 213). If calipers are unavailable, estimate the percent fat according to the girth measurements technique (see Figure 9.3, page 216). You may wish to use both techniques and compare the results. Compute your recommended body weight according to your current and recommended percent body fat guidelines provided in Table 9.10, page 222).

I. Percent Body Fat According to Skinfold Thickness

Men

Chest (mm):	_____
Abdomen (mm):	_____
Thigh (mm):	_____
Total (mm):	_____
Percent Fat:	_____

Women

Triceps (mm):	_____
Suprailium (mm):	_____
Thigh (mm):	_____
Total (mm):	_____
Percent Fat:	_____

II. Percent Fat According to Girth Measurements

Men

Waist (inches):	_____
Wrist (inches):	_____
Difference:	_____
Body Weight:	_____
Percent Fat:	_____

Women

Upper Arm (cm):	_____	Constant A =	_____
Age:	_____	Constant B =	_____
Hip (cm):	_____	Constant C =	_____
Wrist (cm):	_____	Constant D =	_____

$BD^* = A - B - C + D$

$BD = \underline{\quad} - \underline{\quad} - \underline{\quad} + \underline{\quad} = \underline{\quad}$

$\text{Percent Fat} = (495 \div BD) - 450 = (495 \div \underline{\quad}) - 450 = \underline{\quad}$

*Body density

III. Recommended Body Weight Determination

A. Body Weight (BW): ⬜

B. Current Percent Fat (%F)**: ⬜

C. Fat Weight (FW) = BW × %F

FW = ⬜ × ⬜ = ⬜

D. Lean Body Mass (LBM) = BW − FW = ⬜ − ⬜ = ⬜

E. Age: ⬜

F. Desired Fat Percent (DFP − *see* Table 9.10): ⬜

G. Recommended Body Weight (RBW) = LBM ÷ (1.0 − DFP**)

RBW = ⬜ ÷ (1.0 − ⬜) = ⬜

**Express percentages in decimal form (e.g., 25% = .25)

IV. Body Mass Index

Weight: ⬜ lbs ⬜ kg

Height: ⬜ inches ⬜ meters

BMI = Weight (lbs) × 705 ÷ Height (in) ÷ Height (in)

BMI = ⬜ (lbs) × 705 ÷ ⬜ (in) ÷ ⬜ (in)

BMI = ⬜   Disease Risk: (use Table 9.7, page 219): ⬜

Follow-up   BMI = ⬜   Disease Risk (use Table 9.7, page 219): ⬜

V. Waist Circumference

Follow-up

Waist (inches): ⬜ ⬜

Disease Risk (use Table 9.8, page 221): ⬜ ⬜

VI. Disease Risk According to BMI and WC (use Table 9.9, page 221): ⬜

VII. Briefly state your feelings about your body composition results. Do you need to lose or gain weight? If so, state your body composition, BMI and WC goals, and indicate how you plan to achieve these goals.

_____

_____

_____

_____

_____

_____

_____

_____

_____

_____

_____

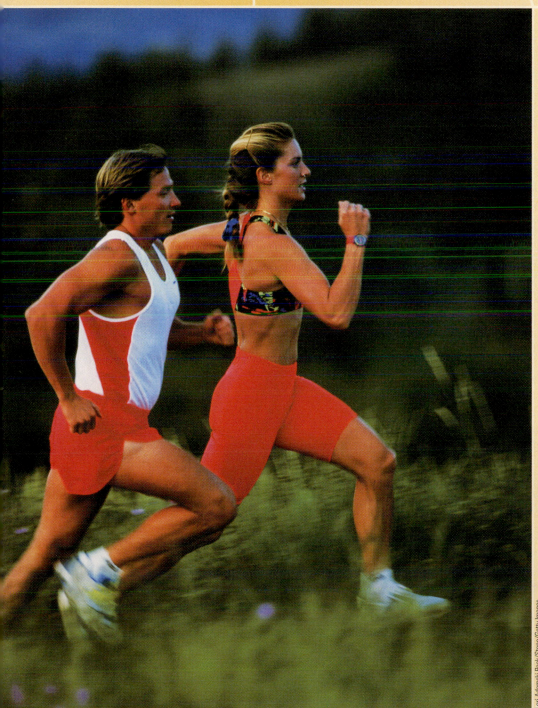

10

CHAPTER

Weight Management

OBJECTIVES

Point out the health consequences of obesity.

Expose some popular fad diets and fallacies regarding weight control.

Identify the eating disorders and describe their behavior patterns and associated medical problems.

Explain the physiology of weight loss, including setpoint theory and the effects of diet on basal metabolic rate.

Explain the role of a lifetime exercise program as the key to a successful weight loss and weight maintenance program.

Learn how to implement a physiologically sound weight reduction and weight maintenance program.

Describe behavior modification techniques that help a person adhere to a lifetime weight maintenance program.

FIGURE 10.1 Percentage of Adult Population That is Obese (BMI ≥ 30) and Overweight (BMI = 25 to 29.9) in the United States

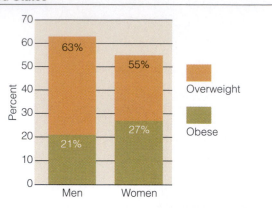

Source: "The Disease Burden Associated with Overweight and Obesity," by A. Must et al., *Journal of the American Medical Association* 282 (1999): 1523–1529.

Two terms commonly used to describe the condition of weighing more than recommended are *overweight* and *obesity*. The obesity level is the point at which excess body fat can lead to serious health problems. Obesity is a health hazard of epidemic proportions in most developed countries around the world. According to the World Health Organization, an estimated 35 percent of the adult population in industrialized nations is obese. **Obesity** has been defined as a body mass index (BMI) of 30 or higher.

In the last several years the number of people who are overweight and obese in the United States has increased dramatically—a direct result of physical inactivity and poor dietary habits. More than 60 percent of adults in the United States do not achieve the recommended amount of physical activity. On the average, American women are consuming 335 more calories daily than they did 20 years ago, and men an additional 170 calories per day.[1]

More than half of American men and women are **overweight** (having a BMI greater than 25), and about a fourth are obese (having a BMI greater than 30) (see Figure 10.1).[2] An estimated 120 million people are overweight and 30 million are obese. Between 1960 and 2000, the overall (men and women combined) prevalence of adult obesity increased from about 13 percent to 24 percent. Most of this increase occurred in the 1990s.

As illustrated in Figure 10.2, the obesity epidemic continues to escalate. Before 1990, not a single state reported an obesity rate above 15 percent of the state's total population (includes both adults and children). By the year 2004, 33 states had an obesity rate between 20 and 24 percent, and nine states had reached a rate above 25 percent.

Most of the blame for the alarming increase in obesity lies in the amount of food that we eat and our lack of physical activity. As the nation continues to evolve into a more mechanized and automated society (relying on escalators, elevators, remote controls, computers, electronic mail, cell phones, and automatic-sensor doors), the amount

FIGURE 10.2 Obesity Trends in the United States 1985–2004, Based on BMI ≥ 30 or 30 Pounds Overweight

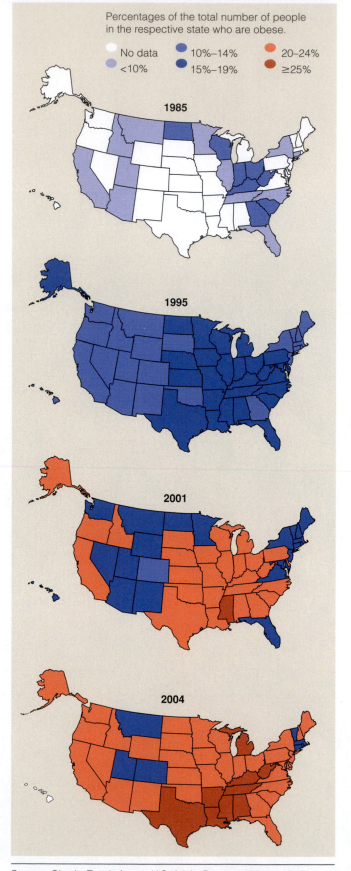

Source: *Obesity Trends Among U.S. Adults Between 1985 and 2004.* (Atlanta: Centers for Disease Control and Prevention, 2004).

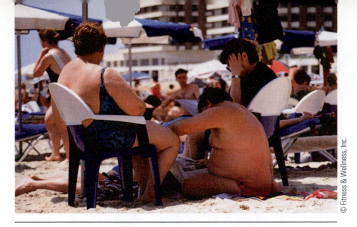

Obesity is a health hazard of epidemic proportions in developed countries.

of required daily physical activity continues to decrease. We are being lulled into a high-risk sedentary lifestyle.

In the last decade alone, the average weight of American adults increased by about 15 pounds. The prevalence of obesity is even higher in ethnic groups, especially African Americans and Hispanic Americans. About 44 percent of all women and 29 percent of all men are on a diet at any given moment.[3] People spend about $40 billion yearly attempting to lose weight. More than $10 billion goes to memberships in weight-reduction centers and another $30 billion to diet food sales. Furthermore, the total cost attributable to treating obesity-related diseases is estimated at $100 billion per year.[4]

As the second leading cause of preventable death in the United States, more than 112,000 deaths each year are caused by excessive body weight and physical inactivity.[5] Obesity is more prevalent than smoking (19 percent), poverty (14 percent), and problem drinking (6 percent).[6] Obesity and unhealthy lifestyle habits are the most critical public health problems that we face in the 21st century.

Excessive body weight and obesity are associated with poor health status and are risk factors for many physical ailments, including cardiovascular disease and cancer. Evidence indicates that health risks associated with increased body weight start at a BMI over 25 and are greatly enhanced at a BMI over 30.

The American Heart Association has identified obesity as one of the six major risk factors for coronary heart disease. Estimates also indicate that 14 percent of all deaths from cancer in men and 20 percent in women are related to overweight and obesity patterns in the United States.[7] Furthermore, excessive body weight is implicated in psychological maladjustment and a higher accidental death rate. Extremely obese people have worse mental health-related quality of life.

Overweight Versus Obesity

Overweight and obesity are not the same thing. Many overweight people (people who weigh about 10 to 20 pounds more than the recommended weight) are not

Health Consequences of Excessive Body Weight

Being overweight or obese increases the risk for

- high blood pressure
- elevated blood lipids (high blood cholesterol and triglycerides
- type 2 (non-insulin–dependent) diabetes
- insulin resistance, glucose intolerance
- coronary heart disease
- angina pectoris
- congestive heart failure
- stroke
- gallbladder disease
- gout
- osteoarthritis
- obstructive sleep apnea and respiratory problems
- some types of cancer (endometrial, breast, prostate, colon)
- complications of pregnancy (gestational diabetes, gestational hypertension, preeclampsia, and complications during C-sections)
- poor female reproductive health (menstrual irregularities, infertility, irregular ovulation)
- bladder-control problems (stress incontinence)
- psychological disorders (depression, eating disorders, distorted body image, discrimination, low self-esteem)
- shortened life expectancy
- decreased quality of life

Source: Centers for Disease Control and Prevention, 2004.

obese. Although a few pounds of excess weight may not be harmful to most people, this is not always the case. People with excessive body fat who have Type 2 diabetes and other cardiovascular risk factors (elevated blood lipids, high blood pressure, physical inactivity, and poor eating habits) benefit from weight loss. People who have a few extra pounds of weight but who are otherwise healthy and physically active, exercise regularly, and eat a healthy diet may not be at greater risk for early death. Such is not the case, however, with obese individuals.

Research indicates that individuals who are 30 or more pounds overweight during middle age (30 to 49 years of age) lose about 7 years of life, whereas being 10 to 30 pounds overweight decreases the lifespan by about three years.[8] These decreases are similar to those seen with tobacco use. Severe obesity (BMI greater than 45) at a young age, nonetheless, may cut up to 20 years off one's life.[9]

Although the loss of years of life is significant, the decreased life expectancy doesn't even begin to address the

Obesity A chronic disease characterized by body mass index (BMI) 30 or higher.

Overweight Excess weight characterized by a body mass index (BMI) greater than 25 but less than 30.

loss in quality of life and increased illness and disability throughout the years. Even a modest reduction of 5 to 10 percent can reduce the risk for chronic diseases including heart disease, high blood pressure, high cholesterol, and diabetes.[10]

A primary objective to achieve overall physical fitness and enhanced quality of life is to attain recommended body composition. Individuals at recommended body weight are able to participate in a wide variety of moderate-to-vigorous activities without functional limitations. These people have the freedom to enjoy most of life's recreational activities to their fullest potential.

Excessive body weight does not afford an individual the fitness level to enjoy many lifetime activities such as basketball, soccer, racquetball, surfing, mountain cycling, or mountain climbing. Maintaining high fitness and recommended body weight gives a person a degree of independence throughout life that most people in developed nations no longer enjoy.

Scientific evidence also recognizes problems with being underweight. Although the social pressure to be thin has declined slightly in recent years, the pressure to attain model-like thinness is still with us and contributes to the gradual increase in the number of people who develop eating disorders (anorexia nervosa and bulimia, discussed under "Eating Disorders," page 235).

Extreme weight loss can lead to medical conditions such as heart damage, gastrointestinal problems, shrinkage of internal organs, immune system abnormalities, disorders of the reproductive system, loss of muscle tissue, damage to the nervous system, and even death. About 14 percent of people in the United States are underweight.

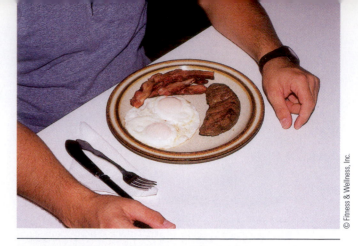

© Fitness & Wellness, Inc.

High-protein/low-carb diets create nutritional deficiencies and contribute to the development of cardiovascular disease, cancer, and osteoporosis.

Failing to attain a "perfect body" may lead to eating disorders in some individuals.

When people set their own target weight, they should be realistic. Attaining the "Excellent" percent of body fat shown in Table 9.10 (page 222) is extremely difficult for some. It is even more difficult to maintain over time, unless the person makes a commitment to a vigorous lifetime exercise program and permanent dietary changes. Few people are willing to do that. The "Moderate" percent body fat category may be more realistic for many people.

The question you should ask yourself is: Am I happy with my weight? Part of enjoying a higher quality of life is being happy with yourself. If you are not, you either need to do something about it or learn to live with it.

If your percent of body fat is higher than those in the "Moderate" category of Table 9.10 (page 222), you should try to reduce it and stay in this category, for health reasons. This is the category that seems to pose no detriment to health. If you are in the "Moderate" category but would like to reduce your percent of body fat further, you need to ask yourself: How badly do I want it? Do I want it badly enough to implement lifetime exercise and dietary changes? If you are not willing to change, you should stop worrying about your weight and deem the "Moderate" category "tolerable" for you.

Critical Thinking

1. Do you consider yourself overweight?
2. If so, how long have you had a weight problem, what attempts have you made to lose weight, and what has worked best for you?

TOLERABLE WEIGHT

Many people want to lose weight so they will look better. That's a noteworthy goal. The problem, however, is that they have a distorted image of what they would really look like if they were to reduce to what they think is their ideal weight. Hereditary factors play a big role, and only few people have the genes for a "perfect body."

The media have a major influence on people's perception of what constitutes ideal body weight. Fashion, fitness, and beauty magazines determine what they should look like. The "ideal" body shapes, physiques, and proportions seen in these magazines are rare and are achieved mainly through airbrushing and medical reconstruction.[11] Many individuals, primarily young women, go to extremes in an attempt to achieve these unrealistic bodies.

THE WEIGHT LOSS DILEMMA

Yo-yo dieting carries as great a health risk as being overweight and remaining overweight in the first place. Epidemiological data show that frequent fluctuations in weight (up or down) markedly increase the risk of dying from cardiovascular diseases. Based on the findings that constant losses and regains can be hazardous to health, quick-fix diets should be replaced by a slow but permanent weight-loss program (as described under "Losing Weight the Sound and Sensible Way," page 245). Individuals reap the benefits of recommended body weight when they get to that weight and stay there throughout life.

Unfortunately, only about 10 percent of all people who begin a traditional weight-loss program without exercise

FIGURE 10.3 Differences Between Self-Reported and Actual Daily Caloric Intake and Exercise in Obese Individuals Attempting to Lose Weight

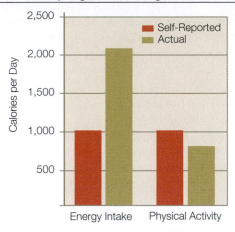

Source: "Discrepancy Between Self-Reported and Actual Caloric Intake and Exercise in Obese Subjects," by S. W. Lichtman et al. *New England Journal of Medicine* 327 (1992): 1893–1898.

are able to lose the desired weight. Worse, only 5 in 100 are able to keep the weight off. The body is highly resistant to permanent weight changes through caloric restrictions alone. Traditional diets have failed because few of them incorporate lifetime changes in food selection and an overall increase in physical activity and exercise as fundamental to successful weight loss and weight maintenance. When the diet stops, weight gain begins. The $40 billion diet industry tries to capitalize on the false idea that weight can be lost quickly without considering the consequences of fast weight loss or the importance of lifetime behavioral changes to ensure proper weight loss and maintenance.

In addition, various studies indicate that most people, especially obese people, underestimate their energy intake. Those who try to lose weight but apparently fail to do so are often described as "diet-resistant." One study found that, while on a "diet," a group of obese individuals with a self-reported history of diet resistance underreported their average daily caloric intake by almost 50 percent (1,028 self-reported versus 2,081 actual calories—see Figure 10.3).[12] These individuals also overestimated their amount of daily physical activity by about 25 percent (1,022 self-reported versus 771 actual calories). These differences represent an additional 1,304 calories of energy per day unaccounted for by the subjects in the study. The findings indicate that failing to lose weight often is related to misreports of actual food intake and level of physical activity.

DIET CRAZES

Capitalizing on hopes that the latest diet to hit the market will really work this time, fad diets continue to appeal to people of all shapes and sizes. These diets may work for awhile, but their success usually is short-lived. Regarding the effectiveness of these diets, Dr. Kelly Brownell, a foremost researcher in the field of weight management, has stated: "When I get the latest diet fad, I imagine a trick birthday cake candle that keeps lighting up and we have to keep blowing it out."

Fad diets deceive people and claim that dieters will lose weight by following all instructions. Most diets are very low in calories and deprive the body of certain nutrients, generating a metabolic imbalance. Under these conditions, a lot of the weight lost is in the form of water and protein, and not fat.

On a crash diet, close to half the weight loss is in lean (protein) tissue. When the body uses protein instead of a combination of fats and carbohydrates as a source of energy, weight is lost as much as 10 times faster. This is because a gram of protein produces half the amount of energy that fat does. In the case of muscle protein, one-fifth of protein is mixed with four-fifths water. Therefore, each pound of muscle yields only one-tenth the amount of energy of a pound of fat. As a result, most of the weight lost is in the form of water, which on the scale, of course, looks good.

Low-Carb Diets Among the most popular diets on the market in recent years are the low-carbohydrate/high-protein (LCHP) diet plans. Although they vary somewhat, in general, "low-carb" diets limit the intake of carbohydrate-rich foods—bread, potatoes, rice, pasta, cereals, crackers, juices, sodas, sweets (candy, cake, cookies), and even fruits and vegetables. Dieters are allowed to eat all the protein-rich foods they desire, including steak, ham, chicken, fish, bacon, eggs, nuts, cheese, tofu, high-fat salad dressings, butter. Typically, these diets are also high in fat content. Examples of these diets are the Atkins Diet, The Zone, Protein Power, the Scarsdale Diet, The Carb Addict's Diet, South Beach Diet, and Sugar Busters.

During digestion, carbohydrates are converted into glucose, a basic fuel used by every cell in the body. As blood glucose rises, the pancreas releases insulin, a hormone that facilitates the entry of glucose into the cells and thereby lowers the glucose level in the bloodstream. If the cells don't soon use the glucose for normal cell functions or to fuel physical activity, glucose is converted to, and stored as, body fat.

Not all carbohydrates cause a similar rise in blood glucose. The rise in glucose is based on the speed of digestion, which depends on a number of factors, including the size of the food particles. Small-particle carbohydrates break down rapidly and cause a quick, sharp rise in blood glucose. Thus, to gauge the effect of a food on blood glucose, carbohydrates are classified by their **glycemic index**.

Yo-yo dieting Constantly losing and gaining weight.

Glycemic index An index that is used to rate the plasma glucose response of carbohydrate-containing foods with the response produced by the same amount of carbohydrate from a standard source, usually glucose or white bread.

TABLE 10.1 Glycemic Index of Selected Foods

Food Item	Index	Food Item	Index
Glucose	100	Muesli	56
Carrots	92	Frosted Flakes	55
Honey	87	Fruit cocktail	55
Baked potatoes	85	Sweet corn	55
Jellybeans	80	Sweet potato	51
White rice	72	Peas	51
White bread	69	White pasta	50
Whole-wheat bread	69	Whole-wheat pasta	42
Pineapple	66	Spaghetti	41
Table sugar	65	Oranges	40
Bananas	62	Apples	39
Boiled potatoes	62	Low-fat yogurt	33
Corn	59	Fructose	20
Oatmeal	59	Peanuts	13

A high glycemic index signifies a food that causes a quick rise in blood glucose. At the top of the 100-point scale is glucose itself. This index is not directly related to simple and complex carbohydrates, and the glycemic values are not always what one might expect. Rather, the index is based on the actual laboratory-measured speed of absorption. Processed foods generally have a high glycemic index, whereas high-fiber foods tend to have a lower index (see Table 10.1).

The body functions best when blood sugar remains at a constant level. Although this is best accomplished with low-glycemic index foods, eliminating all high-glycemic-index foods from the diet is not necessary (foods with a high glycemic index are especially useful to replenish depleted glycogen stores following prolonged or exhaustive exercise). Combining high- and low-glycemic index items or with some fat and protein brings down the average index. Regular consumption of high-glycemic foods, nonetheless, can increase the risk for cardiovascular disease, especially in people at risk for diabetes.

Proponents of LCHP diets say that if a person eats fewer carbohydrates and more protein, the pancreas will produce less insulin, and as insulin drops, the body will turn to its own fat deposits for energy. There is no scientific proof, however, that high levels of insulin lead to weight gain. None of the authors of these diets have published any studies to validate their claims. Yet, these authors base their diets on the faulty premise that high insulin leads to obesity. In fact, we know the opposite to be true: Excessive body fat causes insulin levels to rise, thereby increasing the risk for developing diabetes.

The reason for rapid weight loss during LCHP diets is that a low carbohydrate intake forces the liver to produce glucose. The source for most of this glucose is body proteins—your lean body mass, including muscle. As indicated earlier, protein is mostly water; thus, weight is lost rapidly. When a person terminates the diet, the body rebuilds some of the protein tissue and quickly regains some weight.

A study published in the *New England Journal of Medicine* indicated that individuals on a LCHP (Atkins) diet

Are Low-Carb/High-Protein Diets More Effective?

A few studies suggest that, at least over the short-term, low-carb/high-protein (LCHP) diets are more effective than carbohydrate-based diets in producing weight loss. The results are preliminary and controversial.

- In LCHP diets, much of the weight loss is water and muscle protein, not body fat. Some of this weight is regained quickly upon resuming regular dietary habits.
- In LCHP diets, few people are able to stay with LCHP diets for more than a few weeks at a time. Most stop dieting before completing the targeted program.
- LCHP dieters rarely are found in a national weight-loss registry of people who have lost 30 pounds and kept off the weight for a minimum of 6 years.
- LCHP diets severely restrict food choices. With less variety, individuals tend to eat less (800 to 1,200 calories/day) and thus lose more weight.
- LCHP diets may promote heart disease and cancer and increase the risk for osteoporosis.
- LCHP diets are fundamentally high in fat (about 60 percent fat calories).
- LCHP diets are not recommended for people with diabetes, high blood pressure, heart disease, or kidney disease.
- LCHP diets do not promote long-term healthy eating patterns.

for 12 months lost about twice as much weight as those on a low-fat diet at the mid-point of the study.[13] The effectiveness of the diet, however, seemed to dwindle over time. At 12 months into the diet, participants in the LCHP diet had regained more weight than those on the low-fat diet plan.

Years of research will be required to determine the extent to which long-term adherence to LCHP diets increase the risk for heart disease, cancer, and kidney or bone damage. But low-carb diets are contrary to the nutrition advice of most national leading health organizations (which recommend a diet low in animal fat and saturated fat and high in complex carbohydrates). Without sufficient fruits, vegetables, and whole grains, high-protein diets lack many vitamins, minerals, phytochemicals, and fiber—all dietary factors that protect against an array of ailments and diseases.

The major risk associated with long-term adherence to LCHP diets could be the increased risk for heart disease because high-protein foods also are high in fat content (see Chapter 11). A low-carbohydrate intake also produces a loss of vitamin B, calcium, and potassium. Potential bone loss can accentuate the risk for osteoporosis. Side effects commonly associated with these diets include weakness, nausea, bad breath, constipation, irritability, lightheadedness, and fatigue.

Long-term adherence to an LCHP diet also can increase the risk for cancer. Phytochemicals found in fruits,

How to Recognize Fad Diets

Fad diets have characteristics in common. These diets typically

- are nutritionally unbalanced.
- are based on testimonials.
- were developed according to "confidential research."
- promote rapid and "painless" weight loss.
- promise miraculous results.
- restrict food selection.
- require the use of selected products.
- use liquid formulas instead of foods.
- misrepresent salespeople as individuals qualified to provide nutrition counseling.
- fail to provide information about risks associated with weight loss and use of the diet.
- do not involve physical activity.
- do not encourage healthy behavioral changes.
- are not supported by the scientific community or national health organizations.
- fail to provide information for weight maintenance upon completion of diet phase.

vegetables, and whole grains protect against certain types of cancer. If you choose to go on a LCHP diet for longer than a few weeks, let your physician know so he or she may monitor your blood lipids, bone density, and kidney function.

Combo Diets In addition to the low-carb diets, "combo diets" such as the Schwarzbein and Suzanne Sommers diets are popular. The Schwarzbein diet claims that eating proteins and nonstarchy carbohydrates together will keep the food from being stored as fat. The Suzanne Sommers diet doesn't allow you to eat proteins within 3 hours of carbohydrates, and if you eat fruit, you must wait at least 20 minutes before eating other carbohydrate foods. Both of these diets allow consumption of high-protein/high-fat food items, which can increase the risk for heart disease.

If people only would realize that no magic foods will provide all of the necessary nutrients, that a person has to eat a variety of foods to be well-nourished, the diet industry would not be as successful. Most of these diets create a nutritional deficiency, which at times may be fatal.

The reason many of these diets succeed is that they restrict a large number of foods. Thus, people tend to eat less food overall. With the extraordinary variety of foods available to us, it is unrealistic to think that people will adhere to these diets for very long. People eventually get tired of eating the same thing day in and day out and start eating less, leading to weight loss. If they happen to achieve the lower weight but do not make permanent dietary changes, they regain the weight quickly once they go back to their previous eating habits.

A few diets recommend exercise along with caloric restrictions—the best method to reduce weight, of course. People who adhere to these programs will succeed, so the diet has achieved its purpose. Unfortunately, if the people do not change their food selection and activity level permanently, they gain back the weight once they discontinue dieting and exercise.

Also, let's not forget that we eat for pleasure and for health. Two of the most essential components of a wellness lifestyle are healthy eating and regular physical activity, and they provide the best weight-management program available today.

Eating Disorders

Eating disorders are medical illnesses that involve critical disturbances in eating behaviors thought to stem from some combination of environmental pressures. These disorders are characterized by an intense fear of becoming fat, which does not disappear even when losing extreme amounts of weight. The two most common types of eating disorders are **anorexia nervosa** and bulimia nervosa. A third condition, binge-eating disorder, also known as compulsive overeating, is also recognized as an eating disorder.

Most people who have eating disorders are afflicted by significant family and social problems and may lack fulfillment in many areas of their lives. The eating disorder then becomes the coping mechanism to avoid dealing with these problems. Taking control over their own body weight helps them feel that they are restoring some sense of control over their lives.

Anorexia nervosa and bulimia nervosa are common in industrialized nations where society encourages low-calorie diets and thinness. Although frequently seen in young women, the majority seeking treatment are between the ages of 25 and 50. Surveys indicate that as many as 40 percent of college-age women are struggling with an eating disorder.

Eating disorders are not limited to women. Every one in 10 men has an eating disorder. But because the role of men in society and their body image are viewed differently, these cases often go unreported.

Although genetics may play a role in the development of eating disorders, most cases are environmentally related. Individuals who have clinical depression and obsessive compulsive behavior are more susceptible. About half of all people with eating disorders have some sort of chemical dependency (alcohol and drugs), and a majority of them come from families with alcohol and drug-related problems. Of reported cases of eating disorders, a large

Anorexia nervosa An eating disorder characterized by self-imposed starvation to lose and maintain very low body weight.

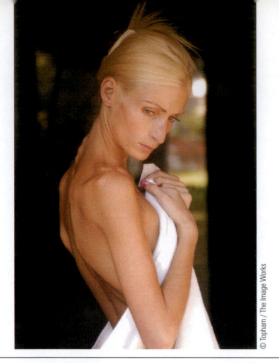

Society's unrealistic view of what constitutes recommended weight and "ideal" body image contributes to the development of eating disorders.

number are individuals who are, or have been, victims of sexual molestation.

Eating disorders develop in stages. Typically, individuals who are already dealing with significant issues in life start a diet. At first they feel in control and are happy about the weight loss even if they are not overweight. Encouraged by the prospect of weight loss and the control they can exert over their own weight, the dieting becomes extreme and often is combined with exhaustive exercise and the overuse of laxatives and diuretics.

Although a genetic predisposition may contribute, the syndrome typically emerges following emotional issues or a stressful life event and the uncertainty about the ability to cope efficiently. Life experiences that can trigger the syndrome might be gaining weight, starting the menstrual period, beginning college, losing a boyfriend, having poor self-esteem, being socially rejected, starting a professional career, or becoming a wife or a mother.

The eating disorder now takes on a life of its own and becomes the primary focus of attention for individuals so afflicted. Self-worth revolves around what the scale reads every day, their relationship with food, and their perception of how they look each day.

ANOREXIA NERVOSA

An estimated 1 percent of the population in the United States is anorexic. Anorexic individuals seem to fear weight gain more than death from starvation. Furthermore, they have a distorted image of their body and think of themselves as being fat even when they are emaciated.

Anorexics commonly develop obsessive and compulsive behaviors and emphatically deny their condition. They are preoccupied with food, meal planning, and grocery shopping, and they have unusual eating habits. As

they lose weight and their health begins to deteriorate, anorexics feel weak and tired. They might realize they have a problem, but they will not stop the starvation and refuse to consider the behavior as abnormal.

Once they have lost a lot of weight and malnutrition sets in, physical changes become more visible. Typical changes are amenorrhea (stopping menstruation), digestive problems, extreme sensitivity to cold, hair and skin problems, fluid and electrolyte abnormalities (which may lead to an irregular heartbeat and sudden stopping of the heart), injuries to nerves and tendons, abnormalities of immune function, anemia, growth of fine body hair, mental confusion, inability to concentrate, lethargy, depression, dry skin, lower skin and body temperature, and osteoporosis.

Diagnostic Criteria and Symptoms Diagnostic criteria for anorexia nervosa are:[14]

- Refusal to maintain body weight over a minimal normal weight for age and height (weight loss leading to maintenance of body weight less than 85 percent of that expected or failure to make expected weight gain during periods of growth, leading to body weight less than 85 percent of that expected).
- Intense fear of gaining weight or becoming fat, even though underweight.
- Disturbance in the way in which one's body weight, size, or shape is perceived, undue influences of body weight or shape on self-evaluation, or denial of the seriousness of the current low body weight.
- In postmenarcheal females, amenorrhea (absence of at least three consecutive menstrual cycles). (A woman is considered to have amenorrhea if her periods occur only following estrogen therapy).

Anorexics strongly deny their condition. They are able to hide it and deceive friends and relatives. Based on their behavior, many of them meet all of the characteristics of anorexia nervosa, but it goes undetected because both thinness and dieting are socially acceptable. Only a well-trained clinician is able to diagnose anorexia nervosa.

Treatment Individuals with anorexia nervosa often turn to bulimia nervosa and some even die as an end result of the disorder. Anorexia nervosa has the highest mortality rate of all psychosomatic illnesses today (approximately 20%). Many of the changes induced by anorexia nervosa, however, can be reversed. This disorder is 100 percent curable, but seldom can anorexics overcome the problem by themselves. Treatment almost always requires professional help.

The sooner treatment is started, the better are the chances for reversibility and cure. Therapy consists of a combination of medical and psychological techniques to restore proper nutrition, prevent medical complications, and modify the environment or events that triggered the syndrome.

BULIMIA NERVOSA

Bulimia nervosa is more prevalent than anorexia nervosa. As many as one in every five women on college campuses may be bulimic, according to some estimates. Bulimia nervosa also is more prevalent than anorexia nervosa in males, although bulimia still is much more prevalent in females.

Bulimics usually are healthy-looking people, well-educated, and near recommended body weight. They seem to enjoy food and often socialize around it. In actuality, they are emotionally insecure, rely on others, and lack self-confidence and self-esteem. Recommended weight and food are important to them.

The binge–purge cycle usually occurs in stages. As a result of stressful life events or the simple compulsion to eat, bulimics engage periodically in binge eating that may last an hour or longer. With some apprehension, bulimics anticipate and plan the cycle. Next they feel an urgency to begin, followed by large and uncontrollable food consumption, during which they may eat several thousand calories (up to 10,000 calories in extreme cases). After a short period of relief and satisfaction, feelings of deep guilt, shame, and intense fear of gaining weight ensue. Purging seems to be an easy answer, as the binging cycle can continue without fear of gaining weight.

Diagnostic Criteria The diagnostic criteria for bulimia nervosa are:[15]

- Recurrent episodes of binge eating. An episode of binge eating is characterized by both of the following:
  - Eating in a discrete period of time (for example, within any 2-hour period), an amount of food that is definitely more than most people would eat during a similar period and under similar circumstances.
  - A sense of lack of control over eating during the episode (a feeling that one cannot stop eating or control what or how much one is eating).
- Recurring inappropriate compensatory behaviors to prevent weight gain, such as self-induced vomiting; misuse of laxatives, diuretics, enemas, or other medications; fasting; or excessive exercise.
- The binge eating and inappropriate compensatory behaviors both occur, on average, at least twice a week for 3 months.
- Self-evaluation is unduly influenced by body shape and weight.

The most typical form of purging is self-induced vomiting. Bulimics, too, frequently ingest strong laxatives and emetics. Near-fasting diets and strenuous bouts of exercise are common. Medical problems associated with bulimia nervosa include cardiac arrhythmias, amenorrhea, kidney and bladder damage, ulcers, colitis, tearing of the esophagus or stomach, tooth erosion, gum damage, and general muscular weakness.

Treatment Unlike anorexics, bulimics realize their behavior is abnormal and feel great shame about it. Fearing social rejection, they pursue the binge–purge cycle in secrecy and at unusual hours of the day.

Bulimia nervosa can be treated successfully when the person realizes that this destructive behavior is not the solution to life's problems. A change in attitude can prevent permanent damage or death.

BINGE-EATING DISORDER

Binge-eating disorder is probably the most common of the three eating disorders. About 2 percent of American adults are afflicted with binge-eating disorder in a 6-month period. Although most people think they overeat from time to time, eating more than a person should now and then does not mean the individual has a binge-eating disorder. The disorder is slightly more common in women than in men; three women for every two men have the disorder.

Binge-eating disorder is characterized by uncontrollable episodes of eating excessive amounts of food within a relatively short time. The causes of binge-eating disorder are unknown, although depression, anger, sadness, boredom, and worry can trigger an episode. Unlike bulimics, binge eaters do not purge; thus, most people with this disorder are either overweight or obese.

Symptoms Typical symptoms of binge-eating disorder include

- eating what most people think is an unusually large amount of food;
- eating until uncomfortably full;
- eating out of control;
- eating much faster than usual during binge episodes;
- eating alone because of embarrassment of how much food is being consumed;
- feeling disgusted, depressed, or guilty after overeating.

Treatment Treatment for eating disorders is available on most school campuses through the school's counseling center or the health center. Local hospitals also offer treatment for these conditions. Many communities have support groups, frequently led by professional personnel and often free of charge. All information and the identity of the individual are kept confidential so the person need not fear embarrassment or repercussion when seeking professional help.

Bulimia nervosa An eating disorder characterized by a pattern of binge eating and purging in an attempt to lose weight and maintain low body weight.

Binge-eating disorder An eating disorder characterized by uncontrollable episodes of eating excessive amounts of food within a relatively short time.

Physiology of Weight Loss

Traditional concepts related to weight control have centered on three assumptions:

1. Balancing food intake against output allows a person to achieve recommended weight.
2. All fat people just eat too much.
3. The human body doesn't care how much (or little) fat it stores.

Although these statements contain some truth, they are open to much debate and research. We now know that the causes of obesity are complex, including a combination of genetics, behavioral, and lifestyle factors.

ENERGY-BALANCING EQUATION

The principle embodied in the **energy-balancing equation** is simple: As long as caloric input equals caloric output, the person will not gain or lose weight. If caloric intake exceeds output, the person gains weight; when output exceeds input, the person loses weight. If daily energy requirements could be determined accurately, caloric intake could be balanced against output. This is not always the case, though, because genetic and lifestyle-related individual differences determine the number of calories required to maintain or lose body weight.

Table 10.3 (page 246) offers general guidelines to determine the **estimated energy requirement (EER)** in calories per day according to lifestyle patterns. This is an estimated figure and (as discussed under "Losing Weight the Sound and Sensible Way," page 245) serves only as a starting point from which individual adjustments have to be made.

The total daily energy requirement has three basic components (see Figure 10.4):

1. resting metabolic rate (RMR)
2. thermic effect of food (TEF)
3. physical activity

The **resting metabolic rate**—the energy requirement to maintain the body's vital processes in the resting state—accounts for approximately 60 to 70 percent of the total daily energy requirement. The thermic effect of food, the energy required to digest, absorb, and store food, accounts for about 5 to 10 percent of the total daily requirement. Physical activity accounts for 15 to 30 percent of the daily total requirement.

One pound of fat is the equivalent of 3,500 calories. If a person's estimated energy requirement is 2,500 calories and that person were to decrease the intake by 500 calories per day, it should result in a loss of 1 pound of fat in 7 days (500 × 7 = 3,500). But research has shown—and many people have experienced—that even when dieters carefully control caloric input and caloric output, weight loss does not always happen as predicted. Furthermore, two people with similar measured caloric intake and output seldom lose weight at the same rate.

FIGURE 10.4 Components of Total Daily Energy Requirement

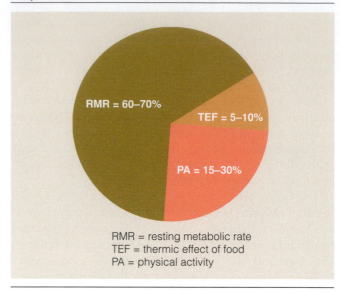

RMR = resting metabolic rate
TEF = thermic effect of food
PA = physical activity

The most common explanation for individual differences in weight loss and weight gain has been the variation in human metabolism from one person to another. We are all familiar with people who seem to eat all day long and not gain an ounce of weight while others say they can't even dream about food without gaining weight. Because experts did not believe that human metabolism alone could account for such extreme differences, they developed several theories that might better explain these individual variations.

SETPOINT THEORY

Results of several research studies point toward a **weight-regulating mechanism (WRM)** that has a **setpoint** for controlling both appetite and the amount of fat stored. Setpoint is hypothesized to work like a thermostat for body fat, maintaining fairly constant body weight, because it "knows" at all times the exact amount of adipose (fat) tissue stored in the fat cells. Some people have high settings, and others have low settings.

If body weight decreases (as in dieting), the setpoint senses this change and triggers the WRM to increase the person's appetite or make the body conserve energy to maintain the "set" weight. The opposite also may be true. Some people have a hard time gaining weight. In this case, the WRM decreases appetite or causes the body to waste energy to maintain the lower weight.

Every person has his or her own certain body fat percentage (as established by the setpoint) that the body attempts to maintain. The genetic instinct to survive tells the body that fat storage is vital, and therefore it sets an acceptable fat level. This level may remain somewhat constant or may climb gradually because of poor lifestyle habits.

For instance, under strict calorie reduction, the body may make extreme metabolic adjustments in an effort to maintain its setpoint for fat. The **basal metabolic rate (BMR)**, the lowest level of caloric intake necessary to sustain life, may drop dramatically when operating under a consistent negative caloric balance, and that person's weight loss may plateau for days or even weeks. A low metabolic rate compounds a person's problems in maintaining recommended body weight.

These findings were substantiated by research conducted at Rockefeller University in New York.[16] The authors showed that the body resists maintaining altered weight. Obese and lifetime non-obese individuals were used in the investigation. Following a 10 percent weight loss, in an attempt to regain the lost weight, the body compensated by burning up to 15 percent fewer calories than expected for the new reduced weight (after accounting for the 10 percent loss). The effects were similar in the obese and non-obese participants. These results imply that after a 10 percent weight loss, a person would have to eat even less or exercise more to compensate for the estimated 15 percent slowdown (a difference of about 200 to 300 calories).

In this same study, when the participants were allowed to increase their weight to 10 percent above their "normal" (pre-weight loss) weight, the body burned 10 to 15 percent *more* calories than expected—attempting to waste energy and maintain the pre-set weight. This is another indication that the body is highly resistant to weight changes unless additional lifestyle changes are incorporated to ensure successful weight management. (These methods are discussed under "Losing Weight the Sound and Sensible Way," page 245.)

Critical Thinking

1. Is there a difference in the amount of food that you are now able to eat compared to the amount you ate in your mid- to late-teen years?
2. If so, to what do you attribute these differences?
3. What actions are you taking to account for the difference?

Dietary restriction alone will not lower the setpoint, even though the person may lose weight and fat. When the dieter goes back to the normal or even below-normal caloric intake (at which the weight may have been stable for a long time), he or she quickly regains the lost fat as the body strives to regain a comfortable fat store.

Effects of a Very Low Calorie Diet Let's use a practical illustration: A person would like to lose some body fat and assumes that his or her current, stable body weight has been reached at an average daily caloric intake of 1,800 calories (no weight gain or loss occurs at this daily intake). In an attempt to lose weight rapidly, this person now goes on a **very low-calorie diet** (defined as under 800 calories per day) or, even worse, a near-fasting diet. This immediately activates the body's survival mechanism

and readjusts the metabolism to a lower caloric balance. After a few weeks of dieting at fewer than 800 calories per day, the body can now maintain its normal functions at 1,300 calories per day. This new figure (1,300) represents a drop of 500 calories per day in the metabolic rate.

Having lost the desired weight, the person terminates the diet but realizes that the original intake of 1,800 calories per day will have to be lower to maintain the new lower weight. To adjust to the new lower body weight, the person restricts the intake to about 1,600 calories per day. The individual is surprised to find that, even at this lower daily intake (200 fewer calories), the weight comes back at a rate of 1 pound every few weeks. After the diet is over, this new, lower metabolic rate may take several months to kick back up to its normal level.

Based on this explanation, individuals clearly should not go on very low-calorie diets. This will slow the resting metabolic rate and also will deprive the body of basic daily nutrients required for normal function. Very low-calorie diets should be used only in conjunction with dietary supplements and under proper medical supervision.[17] Furthermore, people who use very low-calorie diets are not as effective in keeping the weight off once the diet is terminated.

Daily caloric intakes of 1,200 to 1,500 calories provide the necessary nutrients if they are distributed properly over the basic food groups (meeting the daily required servings from each group). Of course, the individual will have to learn which foods meet the requirements and yet are low in fat and sugar.

Under no circumstances should a person go on a diet that calls for under 1,200 calories for women or 1,500 calories for men. Weight (fat) is gained over months and years, not overnight. Likewise, weight loss should be gradual, not abrupt.

Energy-balancing equation A principle holding that as long as caloric input equals caloric output, the person will not gain or lose weight. If caloric intake exceeds output, the person gains weight; when output exceeds input, the person loses weight.

Estimated energy requirement (EER) The average dietary energy (caloric) intake that is predicted to maintain energy balance in a healthy adult of defined age, gender, weight, height, and level of physical activity, consistent with good health.

Resting metabolic rate (RMR) The energy requirement to maintain the body's vital processes in the resting state.

Weight-regulating mechanism (WRM) A feature of the hypothalamus of the brain that controls how much the body should weigh.

Setpoint Weight control theory holding that the body has an established weight and strongly attempts to maintain that weight.

Basal metabolic rate (BMR) The lowest level of oxygen consumption necessary to sustain life.

Very low-calorie diet A diet that allows an energy intake (consumption) of 800 calories or less per day.

The Body "Register" A second way in which the setpoint may work is by keeping track of the nutrients and calories consumed daily. It is thought that the body, like a cash register, records the daily food intake and that the brain will not feel satisfied until the calories and nutrients have been "registered."

This setpoint for calories and nutrients seems to operate even when people participate in moderately intense exercise. Some evidence suggests that people do not become hungrier with moderate physical activity. Therefore, people can choose to lose weight either by going hungry or by combining a sensible calorie-restricted diet with an increase in daily physical activity. Burning more calories through physical activity helps to lower body fat.

Lowering the Setpoint The most common question regarding the setpoint is how it can be lowered so the body will feel comfortable at a reduced fat percentage. These factors seem to affect the setpoint directly by lowering the fat thermostat:

1. Exercise.
2. A diet high in complex carbohydrates.
3. Nicotine.
4. Amphetamines.

Because the last two are more destructive than the extra fat weight, they are not reasonable alternatives (as far as the extra strain on the heart is concerned, smoking one pack of cigarettes per day is said to be the equivalent of carrying 50 to 75 pounds of excess body fat). But a diet high in fats and refined carbohydrates, near-fasting diets, and perhaps even artificial sweeteners seem to raise the setpoint. Therefore, the only practical and sensible way to lower the setpoint and lose fat weight is a combination of exercise and a diet high in complex carbohydrates and only moderate amounts of fat.

Because of the effects of proper food management on the body's setpoint, most of the successful dieters' efforts should be spent in re-forming eating habits, increasing the intake of complex carbohydrates and high-fiber foods, and decreasing the consumption of processed foods that are high in refined carbohydrates (sugars) and fats. This change in eating habits will bring about a decrease in total daily caloric intake. Because 1 gram of carbohydrates provides only 4 calories, compared to 9 calories per gram of fat, you could eat twice the volume of food (by weight) when substituting carbohydrates for fat. Some fat, however, is recommended in the diet—preferably, polyunsaturated and monounsaturated fats. These so-called good fats do more than help protect the heart; they help delay hunger pangs.

A "diet" should not be viewed as a temporary tool to aid in weight loss but, instead, as a permanent change in eating behaviors to ensure weight management and better health. The role of increased physical activity also must be considered, because successful weight loss, maintenance, and recommended body composition seldom are attained without a moderate reduction in caloric intake combined with a regular exercise program.

FIGURE 10.5 Effects of Three Forms of Dieting on Fat Loss

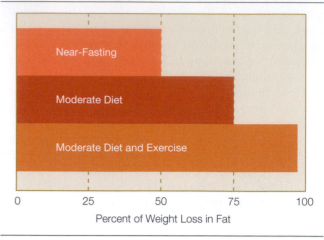

Percent of Weight Loss in Fat

Adapted from *Alive Man: The Physiology of Physical Activity*, by R. J. Shephard (Springfield, IL: Charles C Thomas, 1975): 484–488.

Diet and Metabolism

Fat can be lost by selecting the proper foods, exercising, or restricting calories. When a person tries to lose weight by dietary restrictions alone, lean body mass (muscle protein, along with vital organ protein) always decreases. The amount of lean body mass lost depends entirely on caloric limitation.

When people go on a near-fasting diet, up to half of the weight loss is lean body mass and the other half is actual fat loss (see Figure 10.5).[18] When diet is combined with exercise, close to 100 percent of the weight loss is in the form of fat, and lean tissue actually may increase. Loss of lean body mass is never good because it weakens the organs and muscles and slows metabolism. Large losses in lean tissue can cause disturbances in heart function and also damage other organs. Equally important is not to overindulge (binge) following a very low-calorie diet, as this may cause changes in metabolic rate and electrolyte balance, which could trigger fatal cardiac arrhythmias.

Contrary to some beliefs, aging is not the main reason for the lower metabolic rate. It is not so much that metabolism slows down as that people slow down. As people age, we tend to rely more on the amenities of life (remote controls, cell phones, intercoms, single-level homes, riding lawnmowers) that lull a person into sedentary living.

Basal metabolism is related directly to lean body weight. The more lean tissue, the higher is the metabolic rate. As a consequence of sedentary living and less physical activity, the lean component decreases and fat tissue increases. The human body requires a certain amount of oxygen per pound of lean body mass. Given that fat is considered metabolically inert from the point of view of caloric use, the lean tissue uses most of the oxygen, even at rest. As muscle and organ mass (lean body mass) decrease, so do the energy requirements at rest.

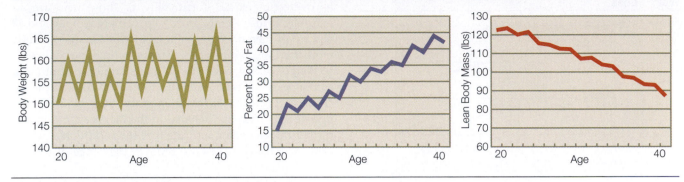

FIGURE 10.6 Effects of Frequent Dieting Without Exercise on Lean Body Mass, Percent Body Fat, and Body Weight

Diets with caloric intakes below 1,200 to 1,500 calories cannot guarantee that lean body mass will be retained. Even at this intake level, some loss is inevitable, unless the diet is combined with exercise. Despite the claims of many diets that they do not alter the lean component, the simple truth is that, regardless of what nutrients may be added to the diet, severe caloric restrictions always prompt the loss of lean tissue. Too many people go on very low-calorie diets as a life pattern, and every time they do, their metabolic rate slows as more lean tissue is lost.

People in their 40s and older who weigh the same as they did when they were 20 tend to think they are at recommended body weight. During this span of 20 years or more, however, they may have dieted many times without participating in an exercise program. After they terminate each diet, they regain the weight, and much of that gain is additional body fat. Maybe at age 20 they weighed 150 pounds, of which only 15 percent was fat. Now at age 40, even though they still weigh 150 pounds, they might be 30 percent fat (see Figure 10.6). At recommended body weight, they wonder why they are eating very little and still having trouble staying at that weight.

Exercise: The Key to Weight Management

A more effective way to tilt the energy-balancing equation in your favor is to burn calories through physical activity. Research shows that the combination of diet and exercise leads to greater weight loss. Further, maintenance of exercise appears to be the best predictor of long-term maintenance of weight loss.[19]

Exercise seems to exert control over how much a person weighs. On the average, starting at age 25, the typical American gains 1 to 2 pounds of weight per year. A 1-pound weight gain represents a simple energy surplus of under 10 calories per day. The additional weight accumulated in middle age comes because people become less physically active and increase their caloric intake. Dr. Jack Wilmore, a leading exercise physiologist and expert weight management researcher, stated:

Physical inactivity is certainly a major, if not the primary, cause of obesity in the United States today. A certain minimal level of activity might be necessary for us to accurately balance our caloric intake to our caloric expenditure. With too little activity, we appear to lose the fine control we normally have to maintain this incredible balance. This fine balance amounts to less than 10 calories per day, or the equivalent of one potato chip.[20]

Exercise enhances the rate of weight loss and is vital in maintaining the weight loss. Exercise will maintain lean tissue, and, in addition, advocates of the setpoint theory say that exercise resets the fat thermostat to a new, lower level. This change may be rapid, or it may take time.

A few individuals lose weight by participating in 30 minutes of exercise per day, but many overweight people need 60 to 90 minutes of daily physical activity to manage their body weight effectively (the 30 minutes of exercise are included as part of the 60 to 90 minutes of physical activity).

Although accumulating 30 minutes of moderate-intensity activity per day provides substantial health benefits from a weight management point of view, the Institute of Medicine of the National Academy of Sciences recommends that people accumulate 60 minutes of moderate-intensity physical activity most days of the week.[21] The evidence shows that people who maintain recommended weight typically accumulate an hour or more of physical activity daily.

As illustrated in Figure 10.7 greater weight loss is achieved by combining a diet with an exercise program. Even more significantly, however, only the individuals who remain physically active for 60 minutes per day are able to keep the weight off (see Figure 10.8).

Further, data from the National Weight Control Registry (http://www.nwcr.ws/) indicates that individuals who have lost at least 30 pounds and kept them off for a minimum of 6 years, typically accumulate 90 minutes of daily activity. Those who are less active gradually regain the lost weight. Individuals who completely stop physical activity regain almost 100 percent of the weight within 18 months of discontinuing the weight loss program (see Figure 10.8). Thus, if weight management is *not* a consideration, 30 minutes of daily activity provides health benefits. To prevent weight gain, 60 minutes of daily activity is the recommendation, and to maintain substantial weight loss, 90 minutes may be required.

FIGURE 10.7 The Roles of Diet and Exercise in Weight Loss

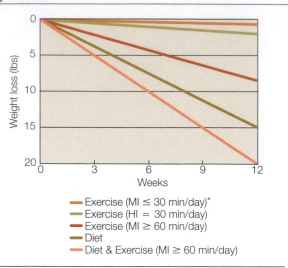

Exercise (MI ≤ 30 min/day)*
Exercise (HI = 30 min/day)
Exercise (MI ≥ 60 min/day)
Diet
Diet & Exercise (MI ≥ 60 min/day)

* Exercise with no change in daily caloric intake
MI = moderate intensity
HI = high intensity
Diet: 1,200–1,500 calories/day

© Fitness & Wellness, Inc.

Based on data from American College of Sports Medicine, "Position Stand: Appropriate Intervention Strategies for Weight Loss and Prevention for Weight Regain for Adults," *Medicine and Science in Sports and Exercise* 33 (2001): 2145–2156.

FIGURE 10.8 Effects of Different Amounts of Daily Energy Expenditure on Weight Maintenance Following a Weight-Reduction Program

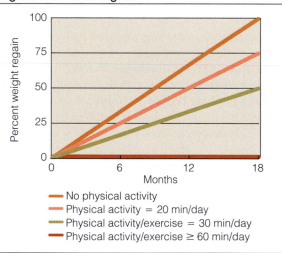

No physical activity
Physical activity = 20 min/day
Physical activity/exercise = 30 min/day
Physical activity/exercise ≥ 60 min/day

Based on data from American College of Sports Medicine, "Position Stand: Appropriate Intervention Strategies for Weight Loss and Prevention for Weight Regain for Adults," *Medicine and Science in Sports and Exercise* 33 (2001): 2145–2156.

COMBINING AEROBIC AND STRENGTH TRAINING

If a person is trying to lose weight, a combination of aerobic and strength-training exercises works best. Aerobic exercise is the best to offset the setpoint, and the continuity and duration of these types of activities cause many calories to be burned in the process. The role of aerobic exercise in successful lifetime weight management cannot be overestimated. Unfortunately, of those who are attempting to lose weight, only 19 percent of women and 22 percent of men decrease their caloric intake and exercise more than an average of 25 or more minutes per day.[22]

Weight loss is likely to be more rapid by combining aerobic exercise with strength training. Although the increase in BMR (basal metabolic rate) through increased muscle mass is being debated in the literature and merits further research, data indicate that each additional pound of muscle tissue raises the BMR in the range of 6 to 35 calories per day.[23]

The number of calories burned during a typical hour-long strength-training session is much lower than during an hour of aerobic exercise. Because of the high intensity of strength training, the exerciser needs frequent rest intervals to recover from each set of exercises. The average person actually lifts weights only 10 to 12 minutes during each hour of exercise. In the long run, however, this person enjoys the benefits of gains in lean tissue. Guidelines for developing aerobic and strength-training programs are given in Chapter 7.

To examine the effects of even a small increase in BMR on long-term body weight, let's use a low estimate of 10 calories per pound of muscle per day. For an individual who adds 3 pounds of muscle tissue as a result of strength training, the increase in BMR would be 30 calories per day (10 × 3). This increase would burn an additional 10,950 calories per year (30 × 365) or the equivalent of 3.1 pounds of fat (10,950 ÷ 3,500). This increase in BMR would more than offset the typical adult weight gain of 1 to 2 pounds per year.

This figure of 10,950 calories per year does not include the actual energy cost of the strength-training workout. If we use an energy expenditure of only 150 calories per strength-training session, done twice per week; over a year's time it would represent 15,600 calories (150 × 2 × 52) or the equivalent of another 4.5 pounds of fat (15,600 ÷ 3,500).

In addition, the previous calculations do not account for the increase in metabolic rate following the strength-training workout (the time it takes the body to return to its pre-workout resting rate—about 2 hours). Depending on the training volume, this recovery energy expenditure ranges from 20 to 100 calories following each strength-training workout.[24] All these "apparently small" changes make a big difference in the long run.

Although size (inches) and percent body fat both decrease when sedentary individuals begin an exercise program, body weight often remains the same or may even increase during the first couple of weeks of the program. Exercise helps to increase muscle tissue, connective tissue, blood volume (as much as 500 ml, or the equivalent of 1 pound, following the first week of aerobic exercise), enzymes and other structures within the cell, and glycogen (which binds water). All of these changes lead to a higher functional capacity of the human body. With exercise, most of the weight loss becomes apparent after a few weeks of training, when the lean component has stabilized.

We know that a negative caloric balance of 3,500 calories does not always result in a loss of exactly 1 pound of fat, and we also know the role of exercise in achieving a negative balance by burning additional calories is significant in weight reduction and maintenance programs. Sadly, some individuals claim that the number of calories burned during exercise is hardly worth the effort. They think that cutting their daily intake by some 300 calories is easier than participating in some sort of exercise that would burn the same amount of calories. The problem is that the willpower to cut those 300 calories lasts only a few weeks, and then the person goes right back to the old eating patterns.

If a person gets into the habit of exercising regularly, say three times a week, jogging 3 miles per exercise session (about 300 calories burned), this represents 900 calories in 1 week, about 3,600 calories in one month, or 46,800 calories per year. This minimal amount of exercise represents as many as 13.5 extra pounds of fat in one year, 27 in two, and so on.

We tend to forget that our weight creeps up gradually over the years, not just overnight. Hardly worth the effort? And we have not even taken into consideration the increase in lean tissue, possible resetting of the setpoint, benefits to the cardiovascular system, and, most important, the improved quality of life. The fundamental reasons for overfatness and obesity, few could argue, are sedentary living and lack of a regular exercise program.

In terms of preventing disease, many of the health benefits that people try to achieve by losing weight are reaped through exercise alone, even without weight loss. Exercise offers protection against premature morbidity and mortality for everyone, including people who already have risk factors for disease.

LOW-INTENSITY VERSUS HIGH-INTENSITY EXERCISE FOR WEIGHT LOSS

Some individuals promote low-intensity exercise over high-intensity for weight loss purposes. Compared with high-intensity exercise, a greater proportion of calories burned during low-intensity exercise is derived from fat. The lower the intensity of exercise, the higher the percentage of fat utilization as an energy source. In theory, if you are trying to lose fat, this principle makes sense, but in reality it is misleading. When trying to lose weight, the bottom line is to burn more calories. When daily caloric expenditure exceeds intake, weight is lost. The more calories burned, the more fat is lost.

During low-intensity exercise, up to 50 percent of the calories burned may be derived from fat (the other 50 percent from glucose [carbohydrates]). With intense exercise, only 30 to 40 percent of the caloric expenditure comes from fat. Overall, however, twice as many calories can be

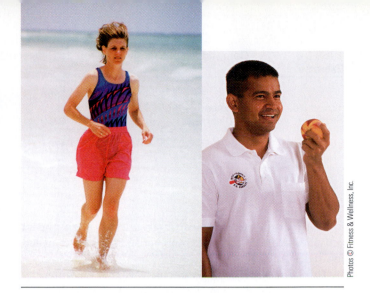

Achieving and maintaining a high physical fitness standard requires a lifetime commitment to regular physical activity and proper nutrition.

burned during high-intensity exercise and, subsequently, more fat as well.

Let's look at a practical illustration (also see Table 10.2). If you exercise for 30–40 minutes at moderate intensity and burn 200 calories, about 100 of those calories (50 percent) would come from fat. If you exercise at high intensity during those same 30–40 minutes, you can burn 400 calories with 120 to 160 of the calories (30–40 percent) coming from fat. Thus, even though the percentage of fat used is greater during low-intensity exercise, the overall amount of fat used is still less during low-intensity exercise. Plus, if you were to exercise at a low intensity, you would have to do so twice as long to burn the same amount of calories. Another benefit is that the metabolic rate remains at a slightly higher level longer after high-intensity exercise, so you continue to burn a few extra calories following exercise.

Moreover, high-intensity exercise by itself appears to trigger greater fat loss than low-intensity exercise. Research conducted at Laval University in Quebec, Canada, showed that subjects who performed a high-intensity intermittent-training program lost more body fat than participants in a low- to moderate-intensity continuous aerobic endurance group.[25] Even more surprisingly, this finding occurred despite the high-intensity group's burning fewer total calories per exercise session. The results support the notion that vigorous exercise is more conducive to weight loss than is low- to moderate-intensity exercise.

Before you start high-intensity exercise sessions, a word of caution is in order: Be sure that it is medically safe for you to participate in these activities and that you build up gradually to that level. If you are cleared to participate in high-intensity exercise, do not attempt to do too much too quickly, because you may incur injuries and become discouraged. You must allow your body a proper conditioning period of 8 to 12 weeks, or even longer for people with a moderate- to-serious weight problem. High

TABLE 10.2 Comparison of Energy Expenditure Between 30–40 Minutes of Low-Intensity Versus High-Intensity Exercise

Exercise Intensity	Total Energy Expenditure (Calories)	Percent Calories From Fat	Total Fat Calories	Percent Calories From CHO*	Total CHO* Calories	Calories Burned per Minute	Calories per Pound per Minute
Low Intensity	200	50%	100	50%	100	6.67	0.045
High Intensity	400	30%	120	70%	280	13.5	0.090

*CHO = Carbohydrates

intensity also does not mean high impact. High-impact activities are the most common cause of exercise-related injuries.

This discussion on high-intensity versus low-intensity exercise does not mean that low intensity is ineffective. Low-intensity exercise provides substantial health benefits, and people who initiate exercise programs are more willing to participate and stay with low-intensity programs. Low-intensity exercise does promote weight loss, but it is not as effective. You will need to exercise longer to obtain the same results.

Healthy Weight Gain

Thin people, too, should realize that the only healthy way to gain weight is through exercise (mainly strength-training exercises) and a slight increase in caloric intake. Attempting to gain weight just by overeating will raise the fat component and not the lean component—which is not the path to better health. Exercise is the best solution to weight (fat) reduction and weight (lean) gain alike.

A strength-training program such as the one outlined in Chapter 7 is the best approach to add body weight. The training program should include at least two exercises of three sets for each major body part. Each set should consist of about 8 to 12 repetitions maximum.

Even though the metabolic cost of synthesizing a pound of muscle tissue is unclear, consuming an estimated 500 additional calories per day is recommended to gain an average of 1 pound of muscle tissue per week. Your diet should include a daily total intake of about 1.5 grams of protein per kilogram of body weight. If your daily protein intake already exceeds 1.5 grams per day, the extra 500 calories should be primarily in the form of complex carbohydrates. The higher caloric intake must be accompanied by a strength-training program. Otherwise, the increase in body weight will be in the form of fat, not muscle tissue (Assessment 10.4 at the end of the chapter can be used to monitor your caloric intake for healthy weight gain).

NUTRITIONAL ACCOMPANIMENTS TO STRENGTH TRAINING

The time of day when carbohydrates and protein are consumed in relation to the strength-training workout plays a role in promoting muscle growth. Studies suggest that consuming a pre-exercise snack consisting of a combination of carbohydrates and protein is beneficial to muscle development. The carbohydrates supply energy for training, and the availability of amino acids (the building blocks of protein) in the blood during training enhances the muscle-building process. Excellent choices for a pre-workout snack are a peanut butter, turkey, or tuna fish sandwich; milk or yogurt and fruit; or nuts and fruit, consumed 30 to 60 minutes before training.

Consuming a carbohydrate/protein snack immediately following strength training, as well as an hour thereafter, further promotes muscle growth and strength development. Post-exercise carbohydrates help restore the muscle glycogen depleted during training, and, in combination with protein, induce an increase in blood insulin and growth hormone levels, which are essential to the muscle-building process.

Muscle fibers also absorb a greater amount of amino acids up to 48 hours following strength-training. The first hour, nonetheless, seems to be the most critical. A higher level of circulating amino acids in the bloodstream immediately after training is believed to increase protein synthesis to a greater extent than amino acids made available later in the day. A ratio of 4-to-1 grams of carbohydrates to protein is recommended for a post-exercise snack.

Weight-Loss Myths

Two common mythical concepts are cellulite and spot reducing. **Cellulite** is nothing but enlarged fat cells that bulge out from accumulated body fat. There is no such thing as **spot reducing**. Doing several sets of daily sit-ups will not get rid of fat in the midsection of the body. When fat comes off, it does so throughout the entire body, not just the exercised area. The greatest proportion of fat may come off the biggest fat deposits, but the caloric output of a few sets of sit-ups has practically no effect on reducing total body fat. A person has to exercise much longer to really see results.

Other touted means toward quick weight loss, such as rubberized sweatsuits, steam baths, and mechanical vibrators, are misleading. When a person wears a sweatsuit or steps into a sauna, the weight lost does not consist of fat, but merely a significant amount of water. Sure, the weight on the scale looks nice when you step on it immediately afterward, but this represents a false loss of weight.

As soon as you replace body fluids, you gain back the weight quickly. Wearing rubberized sweatsuits hastens the rate that body fluid is lost—fluid that is vital during prolonged exercise—and raises core temperature at the same time. This combination puts a person in danger of dehydration, which impairs cellular function and in extreme cases can even cause death.

Similarly, mechanical vibrators are worthless in a weight-control program. Vibrating belts and turning rollers may feel good, but they require no effort whatsoever. Fat cannot be shaken off. It is lost primarily by burning it in muscle tissue.

Losing Weight the Sound and Sensible Way

Dieting never has been fun and never will be. People who are overweight and are serious about losing weight, however, have to include regular exercise in their lives along with proper food management and a sensible reduction in caloric intake.

Because excessive body fat is a risk factor for cardiovascular disease, some precautions are in order. Depending on the extent of the weight problem, a medical examination, and possibly a stress ECG (see Chapter 11, "Resting and Stress Electrocardiograms"), may be a good idea before undertaking the exercise program. A physician should be consulted in this regard.

As another precaution—injuries to joints and muscles are common in excessively overweight individuals who participate in weight-bearing exercises such as walking, jogging, and aerobics. Therefore, significantly overweight individuals may have to choose activities in which they will not have to support their own body weight but that still will be effective in burning calories. If swimming comes to mind, it may not be a good weight loss exercise. More body fat makes a person more buoyant, and many people are not at the skill level required to swim fast enough to get the best training effect, thereby limiting the number of calories burned, as well as the benefits to the cardiorespiratory system.

Better alternatives during the initial stages of exercise include riding a bicycle (either road or stationary), walking in a shallow pool, doing water aerobics, or running in place in deep water (treading water). The latter forms of water exercise are gaining popularity and have proven to be effective in reducing weight without fear of injuries.

How long should each exercise session last? The amount of exercise to promote successful weight loss and weight loss maintenance is different from the amount for improving fitness. For health fitness, accumulating 30 minutes of physical activity on most days of the week is recommended. To develop and maintain cardiorespiratory fitness, 20 to 30 minutes of exercise at the recommended target rate, three to five times per week, is suggested (see Chapter 7). For successful weight loss,

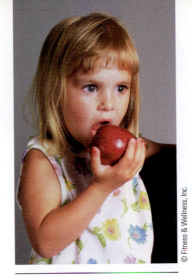

Establishing healthy eating patterns starts at a young age.

60 to 90 minutes of physical activity on most days of the week is recommended.

A person new to exercise should not try to do too much too fast. Unconditioned beginners should start with about 15 minutes of aerobic activity three times a week, and during the next 3 to 4 weeks gradually increase the duration by approximately 5 minutes per week and the frequency by 1 day per week.

One final benefit of long-duration exercise for weight control is that it allows fat to be burned more efficiently. Carbohydrates and fats are both sources of energy. When body glucose levels begin to drop during prolonged exercise, more fat is used as energy substrate. Equally important is that fat-burning enzymes increase with aerobic training. Fat is lost primarily by burning it in muscle. Therefore, as the concentration of the enzymes increases, so does the ability to burn fat.

A SENSIBLE CALORIC INTAKE

In addition to exercise and adequate food management, a sensible reduction in caloric intake and careful monitoring of this intake are recommended. Most research finds that a negative caloric balance is required to lose weight because:

1. Most people underestimate their caloric intake and are eating more than they should be eating.
2. Developing new behaviors takes time, and most people have trouble changing and adjusting to new eating habits.
3. Many individuals are in such poor physical condition that they take a long time to increase their activity level enough to offset the setpoint and burn enough calories to aid in losing body fat.
4. Most successful dieters carefully monitor their daily caloric intake.
5. A few people simply will not alter their food selections. For those who will not (which will still increase their risk for chronic diseases), the only solution to

Cellulite A term frequently used in reference to fat deposits that bulge out; these deposits are nothing but enlarged fat cells from excessive accumulation of body fat.

Spot reducing Fallacious theory holding that exercising a specific body part will result in significant fat reduction in that area.

lose weight successfully is a big increase in physical activity, a negative caloric balance, or a combination of the two.

Perhaps the only exception to a decrease in caloric intake for weight-loss purposes occurs in people who already are eating too few calories. A nutrient analysis often reveals that long-term dieters are not consuming enough calories. These people actually need to increase their daily caloric intake and combine that with an exercise program to get their metabolism to kick back up to a normal level.

You also must learn to make wise food choices. Think in terms of long-term benefits (weight management) rather than instant gratification (unhealthy eating and subsequent weight gain). Making healthful choices allows you to eat more food and more nutritious food and ingest fewer calories. For example, instead of eating a high-fat, 700-calorie scone, you could eat as much as one orange, 1 cup of grapes, a hard-boiled egg, two slices of whole-wheat toast, 2 teaspoons of jam, ½ cup of honey-sweetened oatmeal, and 1 glass of skim milk.

ESTIMATING YOUR DAILY CALORIC REQUIREMENT

You can estimate your daily energy (caloric) requirement by consulting Tables 10.3 and 10.4 and completing Assessment 10.1. Given that this is only an estimated value, individual adjustments related to many of the factors discussed in this chapter may be necessary to establish a more precise value. Nevertheless, the estimated value does offer a beginning guideline for weight control or reduction.

The estimated energy requirement (EER) without additional planned activity and exercise is based on age, total body weight, and gender. Individuals who hold jobs that require a lot of walking or heavy manual labor burn more calories during the day than those who have sedentary jobs such as working behind a desk. To estimate your EER, refer to Table 10.3. For example, the EER computation for a low active 20-year-old man, 71 inches tall, who weighs 160 pounds, would be as follows:

1. Body weight in kilograms = 72.6 kg (160 lbs ÷ 2.2046)
   Height in meters = 1.8 mts (71 × 0.0254)
2. EER = $662 - (9.53 \times Age) + (15.91 \times BW) + (539 \times Ht)$
   EER = $662 - (9.53 \times 20) + (15.91 \times 72.6) + (539 \times 1.8)$
   EER = $662 - 190.6 + 1155 + 970$
   EER = 2,596

Thus, the EER to maintain body weight for this individual would be 2,596 calories per day.

To determine the average number of calories you burn daily as a result of exercise, figure out the total number of minutes you exercise weekly, then figure the daily average exercise time. For instance, if this man exercises "fairly light" five times a week, 60 minutes each time; he exercises 300 minutes per week (5 × 60). The average

TABLE 10.3 Estimated Energy Requirement (EER) Based on Age, Body Weight, and Height

Men	EER = $662 - (9.53 \times Age) + (15.91 \times BW) + (539 \times HT)$
Women	EER = $354 - (6.91 \times Age) + (9.36 \times BW) + (726 \times HT)$

Note: Includes activities of independent living only and no moderate physical activity or exercise.

BW = body weight in kilograms (divide BW in pounds by 2.2046), HT = height in meters (multiply HT in inches by .0254).

TABLE 10.4 Estimated Caloric Expenditure Based on Perceived Exertion of Physical Activity

Perceived Exertion		Caloric Expenditure (Cal/lb/min)
Very, very light	(7)*	0.030
Very light	(9)	0.040
Fairly light	(11)	0.050
Somewhat hard	(13)	0.070
Hard	(15)	0.090
Very hard	(17)	0.100
Very, very hard	(19)	0.110

* Numbers in parentheses indicate the rate of perceived exertion (RPE), see Figure 7.2, Chapter 7.

Adapted from "Caloric Expenditure of Selected Physical Activities," by W. W. K. Hoeger and S. A. Hoeger, *Principles & Labs for Fitness and Wellness* (Wadsworth/Thomson Learning, 2006): 141.

daily exercise time, therefore, is 42 minutes (300 ÷ 7, rounded off to the lowest unit).

Next, from Table 10.4, find the energy expenditure for the activity (or activities) based on the perceived exertion. In the case of "fairly light," the expenditure is .05 calories per pound of body weight per minute of activity (cal/lb/min). With a body weight of 160 pounds, this man would burn 8 calories each minute (body weight × .05, or 160 × .05). In 42 minutes he would burn approximately 336 calories (42 × 8).

Now you can obtain the daily energy requirement, with exercise, needed to maintain body weight. To do this, add the EER obtained from Table 10.3 and the average calories burned through exercise. In our example, it is 2,932 calories (2,596 + 336).

If a negative caloric balance is recommended to lose weight, this person has to consume fewer than 2,932 calories daily to achieve the objective. Because of the many factors that play a role in weight control, this 2,932-calorie value is only an estimated daily requirement. Furthermore, we cannot predict that you will lose exactly 1 pound of fat in 1 week if you cut your daily intake by 500 calories (500 × 7 = 3,500 calories, or the equivalent of 1 pound of fat).

The daily energy requirement figure is only a target guideline for weight control. Periodic readjustments are necessary because individuals differ, and the daily

Calcium and Weight Management

Eating calcium-rich foods—especially from dairy products—may help control or reduce body weight. Individuals with a high calcium intake gain less weight and less body fat than those with a lower intake. Women on low-calcium diets more than double the risk of becoming overweight.

These data indicate that even in the absence of caloric restriction, obese people with high dietary calcium intake (the equivalent of 3 to 4 cups of milk per day) lose body fat and weight. Furthermore, dieters who consume calcium-rich dairy foods lose more fat and less lean body mass than those who consume fewer dairy products. Researchers believe that

- calcium regulates fat storage inside the cell.
- calcium helps the body break down fat or causes fat cells to produce less fat.
- high calcium intake converts more calories into heat rather than fat.
- adequate calcium intake contributes to a decrease in intra-abdominal (visceral) fat.

The data also seem to indicate that calcium from dairy sources is more effective in attenuating weight and fat gain and accelerating fat loss than is calcium obtained from other sources. Most likely, other nutrients found in dairy products may enhance the weight-regulating action of calcium.

Although additional research is needed, the best recommendation at this point is that if you are attempting to lose or maintain weight loss, do not eliminate dairy foods from your diet. Substitute nonfat (skim milk) or low-fat dairy products for other drinks and foods in your diet to help you manage weight and total daily caloric intake.

Sources: "Role of Dietary Calcium and Dairy Products in Modulating Adiposity," by M. B. Zemel, in *Lipids* 38(2): 139–146, 2003; "A Nice Surprise from Calcium" *University of California Berkeley Wellness Letter*, 19, no. 11 (August 2003): 1.

TABLE 10.5 Grams of Fat at 10, 20, and 30 Percent of Total Calories for Selected Energy Intakes

Caloric Intake	Grams of Fat		
	10%	20%	30%
1,200	13	27	40
1,300	14	29	43
1,400	16	31	47
1,500	17	33	50
1,600	18	36	53
1,700	19	38	57
1,800	20	40	60
1,900	21	42	63
2,000	22	44	67
2,100	23	47	70
2,200	24	49	73
2,300	26	51	77
2,400	27	53	80
2,500	28	56	83
2,600	29	58	87
2,700	30	60	90
2,800	31	62	93
2,900	32	64	97
3,000	33	67	100

carbohydrates), less than 30 percent fat, and about 12 percent protein.

REDUCING YOUR FAT INTAKE

Many experts believe that a person can take off weight more efficiently by reducing the amount of daily fat intake to about 20 percent of the total daily caloric intake. Because 1 gram of fat supplies more than twice the amount of calories that carbohydrates and protein do, the general tendency when someone eats less fat is to consume fewer calories. With fat intake at 20 percent of total calories, the individual will have sufficient fat in the diet to feel satisfied and avoid frequent hunger pangs.

Further, it takes only 3 to 5 percent of ingested calories to store fat as fat, whereas it takes approximately 25 percent of ingested calories to convert carbohydrates to fat. Some evidence indicates that if people eat the same number of calories as carbohydrate or as fat, those on the fat diet will store more fat. Long-term successful weight-loss and weight-management programs are low in fat content.

Many people have trouble adhering to a low-fat-calorie diet. During times of weight loss, however, you are strongly encouraged to do so. Refer to Table 10.5 to aid you in determining the grams of fat at 20 percent of the total calories for selected energy intakes. For weight maintenance, data from the National Weight Control Registry show that individuals who have been successful in maintaining an average weight loss of 30 pounds for more than 5 years are consuming about 24 percent of calories from fat, 56 percent from carbohydrates, and 20 percent from protein.[26]

The time of day when food is consumed also may play a part in weight reduction. When a person is attempting

requirement changes as you lose weight and modify your exercise habits.

To determine the target caloric intake to lose weight, multiply your current weight by 5 and subtract this amount from the total daily energy requirement (2,932 in our example) with exercise. For our moderately active male example, this would mean 2,132 calories per day to lose weight ($160 \times 5 = 800$ and $2,932 - 800 = 2,132$ calories).

This final caloric intake to lose weight should never be below 1,200 calories for women and 1,500 for men. If distributed properly over the various food groups, these figures are the lowest caloric intakes that provide the necessary nutrients the body needs. In terms of percentages of total calories, the daily distribution should be approximately 60 percent carbohydrates (mostly complex

1. *Make a commitment to change.* The first necessary ingredient is the desire to modify your behavior. You have to stop pre-contemplating or contemplating change and get going! You must accept that you have a problem and decide by yourself whether you really want to change. Sincere commitment increases your chances for success.

2. *Set realistic goals.* The weight problem developed over several years. Similarly, new lifetime eating and exercise habits take time to develop. A realistic long-term goal also will include short-term objectives that allow for regular evaluation and help maintain motivation and renewed commitment to attain the long-term goal.

3. *Incorporate exercise into the program.* Choosing enjoyable activities, places, times, equipment, and people to work out with will help you adhere to an exercise program.

4. *Differentiate hunger and appetite.* Hunger is the actual physical need for food. Appetite is a desire for food, usually triggered by factors such as stress, habit, boredom, depression, availability of food, or just the thought of food itself. Developing and sticking to a regular meal pattern will help control hunger.

5. *Eat less fat.* Each gram of fat provides 9 calories, and protein and carbohydrates provide only 4. In essence, you can eat more food on a low-fat diet because you consume fewer calories with each meal.

6. *Pay attention to calories.* Just because food is labeled "low-fat" does not mean you can eat as much as you want. When reading food labels—and when eating—don't look at just the fat content. Pay attention to calories as well.

7. *Cut unnecessary items from your diet.* Substituting water for a daily can of soda would cut 51,100 (140 × 365) calories yearly from the diet—the equivalent of 14.6 (51,000 ÷ 3,500) pounds of fat.

8. *Maintain a daily intake of calcium-rich foods,* especially low-fat or nonfat dairy products.

9. *Add foods to your diet that reduce cravings.* Many people have a biological imbalance of insulin. Insulin helps the body use and conserve energy. Some people produce so much insulin that their bodies can't use it all. This imbalance leads to an over-powering craving for carbohydrates. As they eat more carbohydrates, even more insulin is released. Foods that reduce cravings include eggs, red meat, fish, poultry, cheese, tofu, oils, fats, and nonstarchy vegetables such as lettuce, green beans, peppers, asparagus, broccoli, mushrooms, and Brussels sprouts. If you watch your portion sizes, eating foods that reduce cravings at regular meals and for snacks helps to decrease the intense desire for carbohydrates, prevent over-eating, and aid with weight loss.

10. *Avoid automatic eating.* Many people associate certain daily activities with eating—for example, cooking, watching television, reading. Most foods consumed in these situations lack nutritional value or are high in sugar and fat.

11. *Stay busy.* People tend to eat more when they sit around and do nothing. Occupying the mind and body with activities not associated with eating helps take away the desire to eat. Some options are walking; cycling; playing sports; gardening; sewing; or visiting a library, a museum, or a park. You also might develop other skills and interests not associated with food.

12. *Plan meals and shop sensibly.* Always shop on a full stomach, because hungry shoppers tend to buy unhealthy foods impulsively—and then snack on the way home. Always use a shopping list, which should include whole-grain breads and cereals, fruits and vegetables, low-fat milk and dairy products, lean meats, fish, and poultry.

13. *Cook wisely:*

- Use less fat and fewer refined foods in food preparation.
- Trim all visible fat from meats, and remove skin from poultry before cooking.
- Skim the fat off gravies and soups.
- Bake, broil, boil, or steam instead of frying.
- Sparingly use butter, cream, mayonnaise, and salad dressings.
- Avoid coconut oil, palm oil, and cocoa butter.
- Prepare plenty of foods that contain fiber.

---

to lose weight, intake should consist of a minimum of 25 percent of the total daily calories for breakfast, 50 percent for lunch, and 25 percent or lower at dinner. Breakfast, in particular, is a critical meal. Many people skip breakfast because it's the easiest meal to skip. Evidence indicates, however, that people who skip breakfast are hungrier later in the day and end up consuming more total daily calories than those who eat breakfast. Furthermore, regular breakfast eaters have less of a weight problem, lose weight more effectively, and have less difficulty maintaining lost weight.

If most of the daily calories are consumed during one meal (as in the typical evening meal), the body may perceive that something is wrong and will slow the metabolism and store more calories in the form of fat. Also, eating most of the calories during one meal causes a person to go hungry the rest of the day, making it more difficult to adhere to the diet.

Consuming most of the calories earlier in the day seems helpful in losing weight and also in managing atherosclerosis. The time of day when most of the fats and cholesterol are consumed can influence blood lipids and coronary heart disease. Peak digestion time following a heavy meal is about 7 hours after that meal. If most lipids are consumed during the evening meal, digestion peaks while the person is sound asleep, when the metabolism is

- Include whole-grain breads and cereals, vegetables, and legumes in most meals.
- Eat fruits for dessert.
- Stay away from soda pop, fruit juices, and fruit-flavored drinks.
- Use less sugar, and cut down on other refined carbohydrates, such as corn syrup, malt sugar, dextrose, and fructose.
- Drink plenty of water—at least six glasses a day.

14. *Do not serve more food than you should eat.* Measure the food in portions and keep serving dishes away from the table. Do not force yourself or anyone else to "clean the plate" after they are satisfied (including children after they already have had a healthy, nutritious serving).

15. *Try "junior size" instead of "super size."* People who are served larger portions eat more, whether they are hungry or not. Use smaller plates, bowls, cups, and glasses. Try eating half as much food as you commonly eat. Watch for portion sizes at restaurants as well: Supersized foods create supersized people.

16. *Eat out infrequently.* The more often people eat out, the more body fat they have. People who eat out six or more times per week consume an average of about 300 extra calories per day and 30 percent more fat than those who eat out less often.

17. *Eat slowly and at the table only.* Eating on the run promotes overeating because the body doesn't have enough time to "register" consumption and people overeat before the body perceives the fullness signal. Eating at the table encourages people to take time out to eat and deters snacking between meals. After eating, do not sit around the table but, rather, clean up and put away the food to avoid snacking.

18. *Avoid social binges.* Social gatherings tend to entice self-defeating behavior. Use visual imagery to plan ahead. Do not feel pressured to eat or drink and don't rationalize in these situations. Choose low-calorie foods and entertain yourself with other activities, such as dancing and talking.

19. *Do not place unhealthy foods within easy reach.* Ideally, avoid bringing high-calorie, high-sugar, or high-fat foods into the house. If they are there already, store them where they are hard to get to or see—perhaps the garage or basement.

20. *Avoid evening food raids.* Most people do really well during the day but then "lose it" at night. Take control. Stop and think. To avoid excessive nighttime snacking, stay busy after your evening meal. Go for a short walk; floss and brush your teeth, and get to bed earlier.

21. *Practice stress management techniques.* Many people snack and increase their food consumption in stressful situations.

22. *Get support.* People who receive support from friends, relatives, and formal support groups are much more likely to lose and maintain weight loss than those without such support. The more support you receive, the better off you will be.

23. *Monitor changes and reward accomplishments.* Being able to exercise without interruption for 15, 20, 30, or 60 minutes; swimming a certain distance; running a mile—all these accomplishments deserve recognition. Create rewards that are not related to eating: new clothing, a tennis racquet, a bicycle, exercise shoes, or something else that is special and you would not have acquired otherwise.

24. *Prepare for slip-ups.* Most people will slip and occasionally splurge. Do not despair and give up. Reevaluate and continue with your efforts. An occasional slip won't make much difference in the long run.

25. *Think positive.* Avoid negative thoughts about how difficult changing past behaviors might be. Instead, think of the benefits you will reap, such as feeling, looking, and functioning better, plus enjoying better health and improving the quality of life. Avoid negative environments and unsupportive people.

at its lowest rate. Consequently, the body may not metabolize fats and cholesterol as well, leading to a higher blood lipid count and increasing the risk for atherosclerosis and coronary heart disease.

In Assessment 10.2 you will have an opportunity to develop a weight-loss behavior modification program.

Monitoring Your Diet with Daily Food Logs

To help you monitor and adhere to a weight-loss program, use the daily food logs provided in Assessment 10.3.

If the goal is to maintain or increase body weight, use Assessment 10.4.

Evidence indicates that people who monitor their daily caloric intake are more successful at losing weight than those who don't self-monitor. Before using the forms in Assessment 10.3, make a master copy for your files so you can make future copies as needed. Guidelines are provided for 1,200-, 1,500-, 1,800-, and 2,000-calorie diet plans. These plans have been developed based on the MyPyramid food plan and the Dietary Guidelines for Americans to meet the Recommended Dietary Allowances.[27] The objective is to meet (not exceed) the number of servings allowed for each diet plan. Each time you eat a serving of a certain food, record it in the appropriate box.

To lose weight, you should use the diet plan that most closely approximates your target caloric intake. The plan is based on the following caloric allowances for these food groups:

- Grains: 80 calories per serving.
- Fruits: 60 calories per serving.
- Vegetables: 25 calories per serving.
- Milk (use low-fat products): 120 calories per serving.
- Meat and beans: Use low-fat (300 calories per serving) frozen entrees or an equivalent amount if you prepare your own main dish (see the following discussion).

As you start your diet plan, pay particular attention to food serving sizes. Take care with cup and glass sizes. A standard cup is 8 ounces, but most glasses nowadays contain between 12 and 16 ounces. If you drink 12 ounces of fruit juice, in essence you are getting two servings of fruit because a standard serving is ¾ cup of juice.

Read food labels carefully to compare the caloric value of the serving listed on the label with the caloric guidelines provided above. Here are some examples:

- One slice of standard white bread contains about 80 calories. A plain bagel may have 200 to 350 calories. Although it is low in fat, a 350-calorie bagel is equivalent to more than 4 servings in the bread, cereal, rice, and pasta group.
- The standard serving size listed on the food label for most cereals is 1 cup. As you read the nutrition information, however, you will find that for the same cup of cereal, one type of cereal has 120 calories and another cereal has 200 calories. Because a standard serving in the bread, cereal, rice, and pasta group is 80 calories, the first cereal would be 1½ servings and the second one 2½ servings.
- A medium-size fruit usually is considered to be 1 serving. A large fruit could provide as many as 2 or more servings.
- In the milk, yogurt, and cheese groups, 1 serving represents 120 calories. A cup of whole milk has about 160 calories, compared to a cup of skim milk, which contains 88 calories. A cup of whole milk, therefore, would provide 1⅓ servings in this food group.

To be more accurate with caloric intake and to simplify meal preparation, use commercially prepared low-fat frozen entrees as the main dish for lunch and dinner meals (only one entree per meal for the 1,200-calorie diet plan, see Assessment 10.3, page 259). Look for entrees that provide about 300 calories and no more than 6 grams of fat per entree. These two entrees can be used as selections for the meat, poultry, fish, dry beans, eggs, and nuts group and will provide most of your daily protein requirement. Along with each entree, supplement the meal with some of your servings from the other food groups. This diet plan has been used successfully in weight loss research programs.[28] If you choose not to use these low-fat entrees, prepare a similar meal using 3 ounces (cooked) of lean meat, poultry, or fish with additional vegetables, rice, or pasta, which will provide 300 calories with fewer than 6 grams of fat per dish.

In your daily logs, be sure to record the precise amount in each serving. You also may want to run a computerized nutrient analysis to verify your caloric intake and food distribution pattern (percent of total calories from carbohydrate, fat, and protein).

Applying Behavior Modification to a Weight Management Program

Achieving and maintaining recommended body composition requires desire and commitment. If weight management is to become a priority in life, people must realize that they have to transform their behavior to some extent. Modifying old habits and developing new, positive behaviors take time. Individuals who apply behavior management techniques are more successful at changing detrimental behavior and adhering to a positive lifetime weight-control program. In developing a retraining program, people are not expected to incorporate all of the strategies given here but should note the ones that apply to them.

Critical Thinking

1. What behavioral strategies have you used to properly manage your body weight?
2. How do you think those strategies would work for others?

There is no quick and easy way to take off excess body fat and keep it off for good. Weight management is accomplished by making a lifetime commitment to physical activity and proper food selection. When taking part in a weight (fat) reduction program, people also have to decrease their caloric intake moderately, be physically active, and implement strategies to modify unhealthy eating behaviors.

During the process, relapses into past negative behaviors are almost inevitable. The three most common reasons for relapse are:

1. Stress-related factors (such as major life changes, depression, job changes, illness).
2. Social reasons (entertaining, eating out, business travel).
3. Self-enticing behaviors (placing yourself in a situation to see how much you can get away with: "One small taste won't hurt" leads to "I'll eat just one slice"

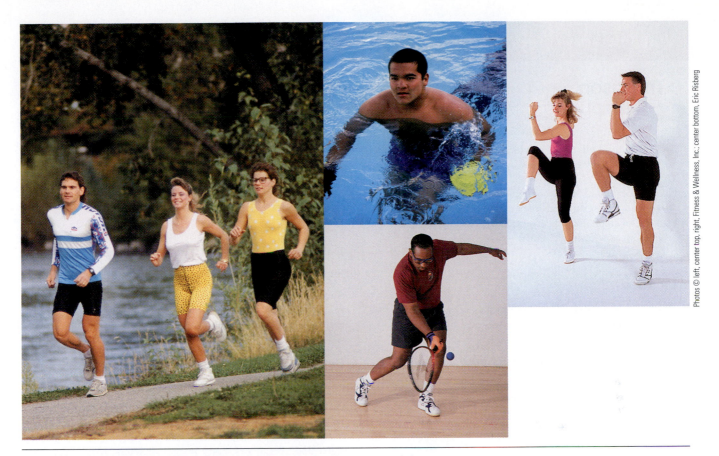

Exercising with other people and in different places helps maintain adherence to exercise.

Photos © left, center top, right, Fitness & Wellness, Inc.; center bottom, Eric Risberg

and finally to "I haven't done well, so I might as well eat some more").

Making mistakes is human and does not necessarily mean failure. Failure comes to those who give up and do not use previous experiences to build upon and, in turn, develop skills that will prevent self-defeating behaviors in the future. Where there's a will, there's a way, and those who persist will reap the rewards.

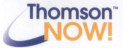 Don't forget to check out the wealth of resources on the ThomsonNOW website at **www.thomsonedu.com/ ThomsonNOW** that will:

- Coach you through identifying target goals for behavior change and monitoring your personal change plan throughout the semester
- Help you evaluate your knowledge of the material
- Allow you to take an exam-prep quiz
- Provide a Personalized Learning Plan targeting resources that address areas you should study.

WEB ACTIVITIES

Weight Management This site describes how to select a safe weight-loss plan combining exercise and healthy diet, including the FDA diet plan.

http://www.wellweb.com/nutri/weight_management.htm

Nutrition Analysis Tool This program was developed at the University of Illinois—Urbana/Champaign, and consists of a free Web-based program that allows you to analyze the foods you eat for a variety of nutrients.

http://www.ag.uiuc.edu/~food-lab/nat

Count Your Calories Because Your Calories Count This interactive site, sponsored by Wake Forest University Baptist Medical Center, features a four-step assessment of your diet, including "How's Your Diet?" "Fit or Not Quiz," "Calorie Counter," and "Drive-Through Diet." There is also an "Eating Disorders Quiz."

http://www1.wfubmc.edu/nutrition

Shape-Up America This excellent fitness and weight management site is endorsed by former U. S. Surgeon General C. Everett Koop, M.D.

http://www.shapeup.org

Eating Disorders This award-winning site, by Mental Health Net, features links describing symptoms, possible causes, consequences, treatment online resources, organizations, online support, and research.

http://eatingdisorders.mentalhelp.net

Mayo Clinic Food and Nutrition Center This site features a wealth of reliable nutrition information including information on different food pyramids and the benefits and dangers of herbs, vitamins, and mineral supplements.

http://www.mayoclinic.com/health/food-and-nutrition/NU99999

InfoTrac®

You can find additional readings related to wellness via InfoTrac® College Edition, an online library of more than 900 journals and publications. Follow the instructions for accessing InfoTrac® that came packaged with your textbook, then search for articles using a key word search.

Suggested Reading Jancin, Bruce. Maintain young adult weight to limit CV risks, *Family Practice News*, Feb. 15, 2005 v35 i4 p10 (1).

1. What can young adults do to prevent the development of cardiovascular disease and metabolic syndromes as they age?
2. Why is weight stabilization a more realistic goal than weight loss?
3. What single step do researchers suggest to hold the line on weight gain?

Web Activity

Eating Disorders Self-Test: Are You in Danger?

http://www.anred.com

Sponsor Anorexia and Related Eating Disorders, Inc., a nonprofit organization that provides information about various food and weight disorders, including warning signs, recovery, and prevention.

Description This excellent Web site features comprehensive descriptions of all types of eating disorders, including anorexia, bulimia, binge eating disorder, anorexia athletica (compulsive exercising), body dysmorphic disorder (bigorexia), and many less-common eating disorders. The site features an overview, definitions and descriptions of each disorder, statistics, warning signs (food behaviors, body image behaviors, social behaviors, and feelings), medical problems, causes, treatment and recovery, and information on how to help someone who has an eating disorder, including tips for parents, partners, and other family members.

Available Activities

1. The Self-Test entitled "Are You in Danger?" consists of 33 Yes/No questions to help you ascertain if you are at risk for developing an eating disorder.

Web Work

1. From the home page, click on "site index."
2. Scroll down the comprehensive table of contents to the "Are You in Danger? A Self-Test" link.
3. Click on this link and print out the list of 33 questions.
4. Circle the number(s) corresponding to the statements that describe you and your eating behaviors.
5. After answering the questions, read the last paragraph on the page to find whether you need to seek medical and/or psychological assistance.

Helpful Hints

1. It is easiest to print out the page and simply circle each statement that applies to you.
2. The self-assessment is not a substitute for appropriate medical and psychological care by qualified licensed professionals. You should show your results of this self-assessment test to your health professional.

For additional Web activities, links, and suggested readings, visit our Health, Fitness, and Wellness Resource Center at http://health.wadsworth.com.

Notes

1. "Wellness Facts," *University of California at Berkeley Wellness Letter* (Palm Coast, FL: The Editors, May 2004).

2. A. Must et al., "The Disease Burden Associated with Overweight and Obesity," *Journal of the American Medical Association* 282 (1999): 1523–1529.

3. M. K. Serdula et al., "Prevalence of Attempting Weight Loss and Strategies for Controlling Weight," *Journal of the American Medical Association* 282 (1999): 1353–1358.

4. A. M. Wolf and G. A. Colditz, "Current Estimates of the Economic Cost of Obesity in the United States," *Obesity Research* 6 (1998): 97–106.

5. A. H. Mokdad, J. S. Marks, D. F. Stroup, and J. L. Gerberding, "Actual Causes of Death in the United States, 2000," *Journal of the American Medical Association* 291 (2004): 1238–1241.

6. R. Sturm and K. B. Wells, "Does Obesity Contribute as Much to Morbidity as Poverty or Smoking?" *Public Health* 115 (2001): 229–235.

7. E. E. Calle et. al., "Overweight, Obesity, and Mortality from Cancer in a Prospectively Studied Cohort of U. S. Adults," *New England Journal of Medicine* 348 (2003): 1625–1638.

8. A. Peeters et al., "Obesity in Adulthood and Its Consequences for Life Expectancy: A Life-Table Analysis," *Annals of Internal Medicine* 138 (2003): 2432.

9. K. R. Fontaine et al., "Years of Life Lost Due to Obesity," *Journal of the American Medical Association* 289 (2003): 187–193.

10. R. R. Wing, E. Venditti, J. M. Jakicic, B. A. Polley, and W. Lang, "Lifestyle Intervention in Overweight Individuals with a Family History of Diabetes," *Diabetes Care* 21 (1998): 350–359.

11. S. Thomsen, "A Steady Diet of Images," *BYU Magazine* 57, no. 3 (2003): 20–21.

12. S. Lichtman et al., "Discrepancy between Self-Reported and Actual Caloric Intake and Exercise in Obese Subjects," *New England Journal of Medicine* 327 (1992): 1893–1898.

13. G. D. Foster et al., "A Randomized Trial of a Low-Carbohydrate Diet for Obesity," *New England Journal of Medicine* 348 (2003): 2082–2090.

14. American Psychiatric Association, *Diagnostic and Statistical Manual of Mental Disorders* (Washington, DC: APA, 2000).

15. See Note 14.

16. R. L. Leibel, M. Rosenbaum, and J. Hirsh, "Changes in Energy Expenditure Resulting from Altered Body Weight," *New England Journal of Medicine* 332 (1995): 621–628.

17. American College of Sports Medicine, "Position Stand: Appropriate Intervention Strategies for Weight Loss and Prevention for Weight Regain for Adults," *Medicine and Science in Sports and Exercise* 33 (2001): 2145–2156.

18. R. J. Shepard, *Alive Man: The Physiology of Physical Activity* (Springfield, IL: Charles C Thomas, 1975): 484–488.

19. W. C. Miller, D. M. Koceja, and E. J. Hamilton, "A Meta-Analysis of the Past 25 Years of Weight Loss Research Using Diet, Exercise, or Diet Plus Exercise Intervention," *International Journal of Obesity* 21 (1997): 941–947.

20. J. H. Wilmore, "Exercise, Obesity, and Weight Control," *Physical Activity and Fitness Research Digest* (Washington DC: President's Council on Physical Fitness & Sports, 1994).

21. National Academy of Sciences, Institute of Medicine, *Dietary Reference Intakes for Energy, Carbohydrates, Fiber, Fat, Protein and Amino Acids (Macronutrients).* Washington, DC: National Academy Press, 2002.

22. See Note 3.

23. E. T. Poehlman et al., "Effects of Endurance and Resistance Training on Total Daily Energy Expenditure in Young Women: A Controlled Randomized Trial," *Journal of Clinical Endocrinology and Metabolism* 87 (2002): 1004–1009; L. M. Van Etten et al., "Effect of an 18-wk Weight-Training Program on Energy Expenditure and Physical Activity," *Journal of Applied Physiology* 82 (1997): 298–304; W. W. Campbell, M. C. Crim, V. R. Young, and W. J. Evans, "Increased Energy Requirements and Changes in Body Composition with Resistance Training in Older Adults," *American Journal of Clinical Nutrition* 60 (1994): 167–175; Z. Wang et al., "Resting Energy Expenditure: Systematic Organization and Critique of Prediction Methods," *Obesity Research* 9 (2001): 331–336.

24. American College of Sports Medicine, *ACSM's Guidelines for Exercise Testing and Prescription* (Baltimore: Williams & Wilkins, 2006).

25. A. Tremblay, J. A. Simoneau, and C. Bouchard, "Impact of Exercise Intensity on Body Fatness and Skeletal Muscle Metabolism," *Metabolism* 43 (1994): 814–818.

26. M. L. Klem, R. R. Wing, M. T. McGuire, H. M. Seagle, and J. O. Hill, "A Descriptive Study of Individuals Successful at Long-Term Maintenance of Substantial Weight Loss," *American Journal of Clinical Nutrition* 66 (1997): 239–246.

27. National Academy of Sciences, Institute of Medicine, *Dietary Reference Intakes for Energy, Carbohydrates, Fiber, Fat, Protein and Amino Acids (Macronutrients)* (Washington, DC: National Academy Press, 2002); U.S. Department of Health and Human Services, Department of Agriculture, *Dietary Guidelines for Americans 2005* (Washington, DC: US DHHS, 2005).

28. W. W. K. Hoeger, C. Harris, E. M. Long, and D. R. Hopkins, "Four-Week Supplementation with a Natural Dietary Compound Produces Favorable Changes in Body Composition," *Advances in Therapy* 15, no. 5 (1998): 305–313; W. W. K. Hoeger, C. Harris, E. M. Long, R. L. Kjorstad, M. Welch, T. L. Hafner, and D. R. Hopkins, "Dietary Supplementation with Chromium Picolinate/L-Carnitine Complex in Combination with Diet and Exercise Enhances Body Composition," *Journal of the American Nutraceutical Association* 2, no. 2 (1999): 40–45.

1. Are physical activity and proper nutrition lifestyle behaviors you use to maintain recommended body weight?

2. Are aerobic exercise and strength training a part of a lifetime weight-management program?

3. Do you employ weight-management strategies when confronted with situations that entice overeating?

Assess Your Knowledge

Evaluate how well you understand the concepts presented in this chapter by answering the following questions.

1. Obesity is defined as a body mass index equal to or above
   a. 10.
   b. 25.
   c. 30.
   d. 45.
   e. 50.

2. The yearly estimated number of deaths attributed to excessive body weight and physical inactivity in the United States is
   a. 28,000.
   b. 55,000.
   c. 93,000.
   d. 112,000.
   e. 350,000.

3. Obesity increases the risk for
   a. high blood pressure.
   b. congestive heart failure.
   c. stroke.
   d. type 2 diabetes.
   e. all of the above.

4. Tolerable weight is a body weight
   a. that is not ideal but one that you can live with.
   b. that will tolerate the increased risk of chronic diseases.
   c. with a BMI range between 25 and 30.
   d. that meets both ideal values for percent body weight and BMI.
   e. All are correct choices.

5. When the body uses protein instead of a combination of fats and carbohydrates as a source of energy,
   a. weight loss is very slow.
   b. a large amount of weight loss is in the form of water.
   c. muscle turns into fat.
   d. fat is lost very rapidly.
   e. fat cannot be lost.

6. One pound of fat represents
   a. 1,200 calories.
   b. 1,500 calories.
   c. 3,500 calories.
   d. 5,000 calories.
   e. None of the above.

7. The mechanism that seems to regulate how much a person weighs is known as
   a. setpoint.
   b. weight factor.
   c. basal metabolic rate.
   d. metabolism.
   e. energy-balancing equation.

8. The key to successful weight management is
   a. frequent dieting.
   b. very low-calorie diets when "normal" dieting doesn't work.
   c. a lifetime exercise program.
   d. regular low carbohydrate/high protein meals.
   e. All are correct choices.

9. The daily amount of physical activity recommended for weight loss maintenance is
   a. 15 to 20 minutes.
   b. 20 to 30 minutes.
   c. 30 to 60 minutes.
   d. 60 to 90 minutes.
   e. Any amount is sufficient as long as it is done daily.

10. A daily energy expenditure of 300 calories through physical activity is the equivalent of approximately _____ pounds of fat per year.
    a. 12
    b. 15
    c. 22
    d. 27
    e. 31

Correct answers can be found on page 369.

Computing Your Daily Caloric Requirement

Name: _____   Date: _____   Grade: _____

Instructor: _____   Course: _____   Section: _____

A. Current body weight (BW) in kilograms (body weight in pounds ÷ 2.2046) . . . . ☐

B. Current height (HT) in meters (HT in inches × .0254) . . . . ☐

C. Estimated energy requirement (EER) (Table 10.3, page 246)

    Men: $EER = 663 - (9.53 \times Age) + (15.91 \times BW) + (539.6 \times HT)$

    Women: $EER = 354 - (6.91 \times Age) + (9.36 \times BW) + (726 \times HT)$

    EER = ☐ − (☐ × ☐) + (☐ × ☐) + (☐ × ☐)

    EER = ☐ − ☐ + ☐ + ☐

    EER = ☐ − ☐ + ☐ = ☐ calories

D. Selected physical activity (e.g., jogging)[a] . . . . ☐

E. Number of exercise sessions per week . . . . ☐

F. Duration of exercise session (in minutes) . . . . ☐

G. Total weekly exercise time in minutes (E × F) . . . . ☐

H. Average daily exercise time in minutes (G ÷ 7) . . . . ☐

I. Caloric expenditure per pound per minute (cal/lb/min) of physical activity (use Table 10.4, page 246) . . . . ☐

J. Total calories burned per minute of physical activity (A × I) . . . . ☐

K. Average daily calories burned as a result of the exercise program (H × J) . . . . ☐

L. Total daily energy requirement with exercise to maintain body weight (C + K) . . . . ☐

Stop here if no weight loss is required, otherwise proceed to items M and N.

M. Number of calories to subtract from daily requirement to achieve a negative caloric

    balance (multiply current body weight by 5) . . . . ☐

N. Target caloric intake to lose weight (L − M)[b] . . . . ☐

---

[a] If more than one physical activity is selected, you will have to estimate the average daily calories burned as a result of each additional activity (steps D through K) and add all of these figures to L above.

[b] This figure should never be below 1,200 calories for women or 1,500 calories for men. See Assessment 10.3 for the 1,200-, 1,500-, 1,800-, and 2,000-calorie diet plans.

Weight-Loss Behavior Modification Plan

Name: _____ Date: _____ Grade: _____

Instructor: _____ Course: _____ Section: _____

1. How much weight do you want to lose? _____ Is it a realistic goal? _____

2. Target caloric intake to lose weight (diet plan—see Assessment 10.1, item N) _____ .

3. How much effort are you willing to put into reaching your weight loss goal?

    _____

    Indicate your feelings about participating in an exercise program.

    _____

4. Will you commit to participate in a combined aerobic and strength-training program?* Yes _____ No _____

    If your answer is "Yes," proceed to the next question; if you answered "No," please review Chapters 8 and 9 again and read Chapters 6 and 7.

5. Select one or two aerobic activities in which you will participate regularly.

    _____   _____

    List facilities available to you where you can carry out the aerobic and strength-training programs.

    _____

    _____

6. Indicate days and times you will set aside for your aerobic and strength-training program (you should devote 5 or 6 days per week to aerobic exercise and 1 to 3 nonconsecutive days per week to strength training).

    Monday: _____

    Tuesday: _____

    Wednesday: _____

    Thursday: _____

    Friday: _____

    Saturday: _____

    Sunday: A complete day of rest once a week is recommended to allow your body to fully recover from exercise.

Behavior Modification

Briefly describe whether you think you can meet the goals of your aerobic and strength-training program. What obstacles will you have to overcome, and how will you overcome them?

_____
_____
_____
_____
_____

* Flexibility programs are necessary for adequate fitness, possible injury prevention, and good health but do not help with weight loss. Stretching exercises can be conducted regularly during the cool-down phase of your aerobic and strength-training programs.

Recording Daily Food Intake:
1,200 Calorie Diet Plan

Name: _____ **Date:** _____ **Grade:** _____

Instructor: _____ **Course:** _____ **Section:** _____

Instructions:

The objective of the diet plan is to meet (not exceed) the number of servings allowed for the food groups listed. Each time you eat a specific food, record it in the space provided for each group along with the amount you ate. Refer to the number of calories below to find out what counts as one serving for each group listed. Instead of the meat and beans group, you are allowed to have a commercially available low-fat frozen entree for your main meal (this entree should provide no more than 300 calories and less than 6 grams of fat). You can make additional copies of this form as needed.

Meat & Beans: 1 low-fat frozen entree
Milk: 2 servings
Fruits: 2 servings
Veggies: 3 servings
Grains: 6 servings

Grains (80 calories/serving): 6 servings

1	
2	
3	
4	
5	
6	

Vegetables (25 calories/serving): 3 servings

1	
2	
3	

Fruits (60 calories/serving): 2 servings

1	
2	

Milk (120 calories/serving, use low-fat milk and milk products): 2 servings

1	
2	

Low-fat Frozen Entree (300 calories and less than 6 grams of fat): 1 serving

1	

Today's physical activity: _____ Intensity: _____ Duration: ____ min Number of steps: _____

ASSESSMENT 10.3

Recording Daily Food Intake:
1,500 Calorie Diet Plan

Instructions

The objective of the diet plan is to meet (not exceed) the number of servings allowed for the food groups listed. Each time you eat a specific food, record it in the space provided for each group along with the amount you ate. Refer to the number of calories below to find out what counts as one serving for each group listed. Instead of the meat and beans group, you are allowed to have 2 commercially available low-fat frozen entrees for your main meal (these entrees should provide no more than 300 calories each and less than 6 grams of fat). You can make additional copies of this form as needed.

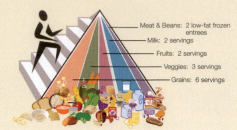

Meat & Beans: 2 low-fat frozen entrees
Milk: 2 servings
Fruits: 2 servings
Veggies: 3 servings
Grains: 6 servings

Grains (80 calories/serving): 6 servings

1
2
3
4
5
6

Vegetables (25 calories/serving): 3 servings

1
2
3

Fruits (60 calories/serving): 2 servings

1
2

Milk (120 calories/serving, use low-fat milk and milk products): 2 servings

1
2

Two Low-fat Frozen Entrees (300 calories and less than 6 grams of fat): 2 servings

1
2

Today's physical activity: _____ Intensity: _____ Duration: ____ min Number of steps: [____]

Wellness: Guidelines for a Healthy Lifestyle

Recording Daily Food Intake: 1,800 Calorie Diet Plan

Instructions

The objective of the diet plan is to meet (not exceed) the number of servings allowed for the food groups listed. Each time you eat a specific food, record it in the space provided for each group along with the amount you ate. Refer to the number of calories below to find out what counts as one serving for each group listed. Instead of the meat and beans group, you are allowed to have 2 commercially available low-fat frozen entrees for your main meal (these entrees should provide no more than 300 calories each and less than 6 grams of fat). You can make additional copies of this form as needed.

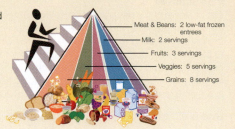

Meat & Beans: 2 low-fat frozen entrees
Milk: 2 servings
Fruits: 3 servings
Veggies: 5 servings
Grains: 8 servings

Grains (80 calories/serving): 8 servings

1
2
3
4
5
6
7
8

Vegetables (25 calories/serving): 5 servings

1
2
3
4
5

Fruits (60 calories/serving): 3 servings

1
2
3

Milk (120 calories/serving, use low-fat milk and milk products): 2 servings

1
2

Two Low-fat Frozen Entrees (300 calories and less than 6 grams of fat): 2 servings

1
2

Today's physical activity: _____   Intensity: _____   Duration: ____ min   Number of steps: _____

Recording Daily Food Intake: 2,000 Calorie Diet Plan

Instructions:

The objective of the diet plan is to meet (not exceed) the number of servings allowed for the food groups listed. Each time you eat a specific food, record it in the space provided for each group along with the amount you ate. Refer to the number of calories below to find out what counts as one serving for each group listed. Instead of the meat and beans group, you are allowed to have 2 commercially available low-fat frozen entrees for your main meal (these entrees should provide no more than 300 calories each and less than 6 grams of fat). You can make additional copies of this form as needed.

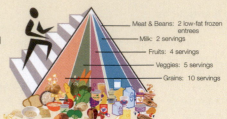

Meat & Beans: 2 low-fat frozen entrees
Milk: 2 servings
Fruits: 4 servings
Veggies: 5 servings
Grains: 10 servings

Grains (80 calories/serving): 10 servings

1.
2.
3.
4.
5.
6.
7.
8.
9.
10.

Vegetables (25 calories/serving): 5 servings

1.
2.
3.
4.
5.

Fruits (60 calories/serving): 4 servings

1.
2.
3.
4.

Milk (120 calories/serving, use low-fat milk and milk products): 2 servings

1.
2.

Two Low-fat Frozen Entrees (300 calories and less than 6 grams of fat): 2 servings

1.
2.

Today's physical activity: _____ Intensity: _____ Duration: ___ min Number of steps: _____ 🚶

Healthy Dietary Plan for Weight Maintenance or Weight Gain

Name: _____ Date: _____ Grade: _____

Instructor: _____ Course: _____ Section: _____

I. Daily Caloric Requirement

A. Current body weight in pounds. . . . . [ ]

B. Current percent body fat . . . . [ ]

C. Current body composition category (Table 9.10, page 222) . . . . [ ]

D. Total daily energy requirement with exercise to maintain body weight (use item L from Assessment 10.1). Use this figure and stop further computations if the goal is to maintain body weight . . . . [ ]

E. Target body weight to increase body weight . . . . [ ]

F. Number of additional daily calories to increase body weight (combine this increased caloric intake with a strength-training program, see Chapter 7) . . . . [500]

G. Total daily energy (caloric) requirement with exercise to increase body weight (D + 500) . . . . [ ]

II. Strength-Training Program

For weight gain purposes, indicate three days during the week and the time when you will engage in a strength-training program.

_____

_____

III. Healthy Diet Plan

Design a sample healthy daily diet plan according to the total daily energy requirement computed in D (maintenance) or G (weight gain) above. Using the Appendix, list all individual food items that you can consume on that day, along with their caloric, carbohydrate, fat, and protein content. Be sure that the diet meets your recommended MyPyramid number of servings from the various food groups.

Breakfast

	Food item	Amount	Calories	Carbohydrates (gr)	Fat (gr)	Protein (gr)
1.						
2.						
3.						
4.						
5.						
6.						
7.						
8.						

Lunch

Food item	Amount	Calories	Carbohydrates (gr)	Fat (gr)	Protein (gr)
1.					
2.					
3.					
4.					
5.					
6.					
7.					
8.					

Snack

1.					

Dinner

1.					
2.					
3.					
4.					
5.					
6.					
7.					
8.					
Totals:					

IV. Percent of Macronutrients

Determine the percent of total calories that are derived from carbohydrates, fat, and protein.

A. Total calories = _____

B. Grams of carbohydrates _____ × 3 ÷ _____ (total calories) = _____ %

C. Grams of fat _____ × 9 ÷ _____ (total calories) = _____ %

D. Grams of protein _____ × 4 ÷ _____ (total calories) = _____ %

E. Body weight (BW) in kilograms (BW in pounds divided by 2.2046) = _____ kg

F. Grams of protein per kilogram of body weight _____ (grams of protein) ÷ _____ (BW in kg) = _____ gr/kg

G. Please summarize your diet and protein intake to either maintain or gain weight.

_____

_____

_____

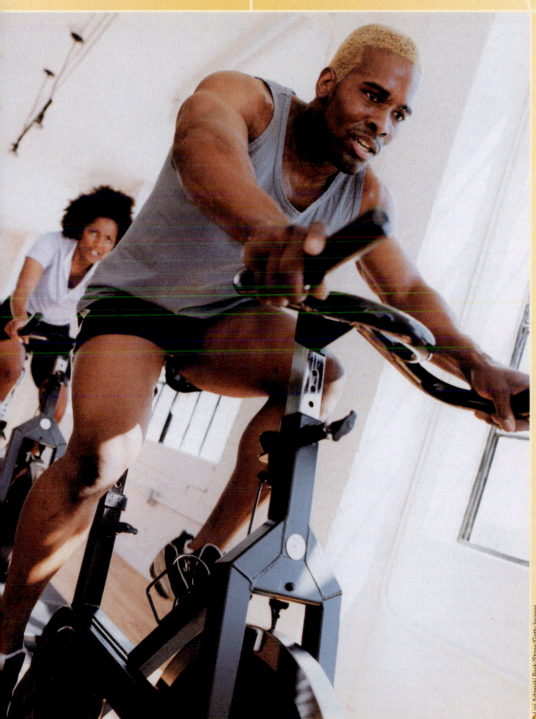

11

CHAPTER

Cardiovascular Wellness

OBJECTIVES

Define cardiovascular diseases and give examples.

Define coronary heart disease and relate its leading risk factors.

Become familiar with the incidence of cardiovascular disease.

Identify and explain the types of cholesterol and how they contribute to CHD.

Define triglycerides, homocysteine, and C-reactive protein (CRP), and explain their relation to CHD.

Define hypertension and know how it is measured.

Identify the major types of diabetes and explain how each is treated.

Describe the role of smoking in CHD.

Explain the "fight or flight" mechanism in relation to heart disease.

Present guidelines for preventing cardiovascular disease.

Estimate your own risk of developing coronary heart disease.

Progress in the field of medicine has largely eliminated the diseases that were most common at the beginning of the 20th century—infectious diseases such as tuberculosis, diphtheria, influenza, kidney disease, polio, and other diseases of infancy. But as the American people started to enjoy the "good life" (sedentary living, excessive consumption of alcohol, fatty foods, and sweets, as well as tobacco, and drugs), a parallel increase was seen in chronic diseases such as cancer, diabetes, emphysema, cirrhosis of the liver, and, in particular, diseases of the cardiovascular system.

Cardiovascular diseases encompass all pathological conditions that affect the heart and the circulatory system (blood vessels). Some examples are coronary heart disease, peripheral vascular disease, congenital heart disease, rheumatic heart disease, atherosclerosis, strokes, high blood pressure, and congestive heart failure.

It has become clear that prevention is the best medicine. People have begun to realize that good health is largely self-controlled and that the leading causes of premature death and illness in the United States can be prevented by adhering to positive lifestyle habits. Consequently, a fitness and wellness trend has emerged.

Incidence of Cardiovascular Disease

At the beginning of the 21st century, cardiovascular diseases continue to be the leading cause of death in the United States, accounting for 37 percent of all yearly deaths. According to estimates by the American Heart Association, about 20 percent of the U.S. population, or one in three adults, has some type of cardiovascular disease.[1] If all deaths from the major cardiovascular diseases were eliminated, life expectancy in the United States would increase by almost seven years.[2]

Although heart and blood vessel disease is still the number-one health problem in the United States, the incidence declined by 26 percent between 1960 and 2000 (see Figure 11.1). The main reasons for this dramatic decrease are health education and better treatment modalities. More people now are aware of the risk factors for cardiovascular disease and are changing their lifestyles to lower their own potential risk for this disease. Further work remains to be done, however, because studies show that the risk of death from cardiovascular disease is greater for the least-educated compared with the most-educated people.

According to the American Heart Association, 71.3 million people in the United States were afflicted with diseases of the cardiovascular system in 2005, including 65 million with hypertension (high blood pressure) and 13.2 million with coronary heart disease. Many of these people have more than one type of cardiovascular disease. The estimated cost of heart and blood vessel disease in 2006 was projected at $403 billion.[3]

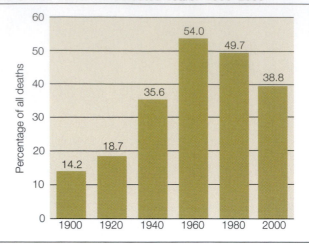

FIGURE 11.1 Incidence of Cardiovascular Disease in the United States for Selected Years: 1900–2000

Source: Centers for Disease Control and Prevention, Atlanta.

Coronary Heart Disease

The major form of cardiovascular disease is **coronary heart disease (CHD)**, a condition in which the arteries that supply the heart muscle with oxygen and nutrients are narrowed by fatty deposits such as cholesterol and triglycerides. Narrowing of the coronary arteries diminishes the blood supply to the heart muscle, which can precipitate a heart attack. Figure 11.2 illustrates this condition.

CHD is the single leading cause of death in the United States, accounting for approximately 20 percent of all deaths and more than half (53 percent) of all cardiovascular deaths.[4] About half of the people who died suddenly from CHD had no previous symptoms of the disease. Further, approximately 80 percent of deaths from CHD in people under age 65 occur during the first heart attack.[5] Almost all of the risk factors for CHD are preventable and reversible, and individuals can reduce their risk. A risk factor analysis to evaluate your personal risk of coronary heart disease is provided in Assessment 11.1 (page 285).

According to the American Heart Association, approximately 7.2 million people have heart attacks each year and more than 479,000 of them die as a result. More than half the time, the first symptom of coronary heart disease is the heart attack itself, and 40 percent of the people who have a first heart attack die within the first 24 hours.

Although genetic inheritance plays a role in CHD, the most important determinant is personal lifestyle. The leading risk factors contributing to CHD are

- physical inactivity
- low HDL cholesterol
- elevated LDL cholesterol
- smoking
- high blood pressure
- diabetes
- excessive body fat
- elevated homocysteine

FIGURE 11.2 Myocardial Infarction (Heart Attack) Resulting from Restricted Blood Flow

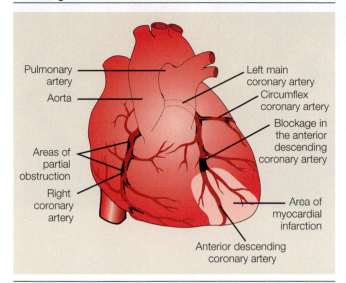

FIGURE 11.3 Interrelationships Among Leading Cardiovascular Risk Factors

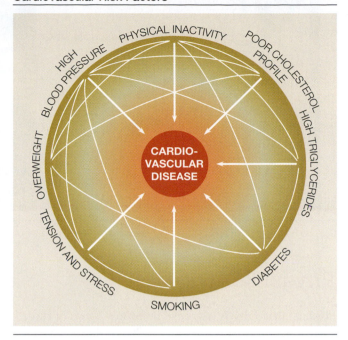

Signs of Heart Attack and Stroke

Any or all of the following signs may occur during a heart attack or a stroke. If you experience any of these symptoms and they last longer than a few minutes, call 911 and seek medical attention immediately. Failure to do so may cause irreparable damage and even result in death.

Warning Signs of a Heart Attack

- Chest pain, discomfort, pressure, or a squeezing sensation that lasts for several minutes. These feelings may go away and return later.
- Pain that radiates to the shoulders, neck, or arms.
- Chest discomfort with shortness of breath, lightheadedness, sweating, nausea, or fainting.

Warning Signs of Stroke

- Sudden weakness or numbness of the face, arm, or leg—particularly on one side of the body.
- Sudden severe headache.
- Sudden confusion, dizziness, or difficulty in speech and understanding.
- Sudden difficulty walking; loss of balance or coordination.
- Sudden difficulty with vision.

- inflammation (elevated C-reactive protein)
- abnormal electrocardiogram (either stress or resting ECG)
- family history of heart disease
- personal history of heart disease
- elevated triglycerides
- tension and stress
- age

With the exception of age, family history of heart disease, and certain electrocardiogram (ECG) abnormalities, the risk factors are preventable and reversible. The leading risk factors for CHD are discussed next, along with general recommendations for reducing the risks.

Studies have documented that risk factors have multiple interrelations. Physical inactivity, for instance, often contributes to an increase in (a) body weight (fat), (b) higher cholesterol, (c) triglycerides, (d) tension and stress, (e) blood pressure, and (f) risk for diabetes. The interrelationships among leading cardiovascular risk factors are depicted in Figure 11.3.

Cardiovascular diseases The array of conditions that affect the heart and the blood vessels.

Coronary heart disease (CHD) Condition in which the arteries that supply the heart muscle with oxygen and nutrients are narrowed by fatty deposits, such as cholesterol and triglycerides.

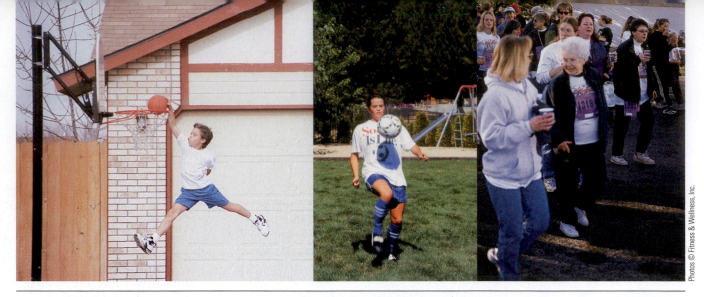

Photos © Fitness & Wellness, Inc.

Lifetime participation in aerobic activities is one of the most important factors in preventing cardiovascular disease.

Physical Inactivity

Physical inactivity is responsible for low levels of cardiorespiratory endurance (defined earlier as the ability of the lungs, heart, and blood vessels to deliver enough oxygen to the cells to meet the demands of prolonged physical activity). Improving cardiorespiratory endurance through aerobic exercise may have the greatest impact in reducing the overall risk for heart disease. Although specific recommendations can be followed to improve each risk factor, a regular aerobic exercise program helps control most of the major risk factors that lead to heart disease. Physical activity and aerobic exercise

- increases cardiorespiratory endurance,
- decreases and controls blood pressure,
- reduces body fat,
- lowers blood lipids (cholesterol and triglycerides),
- improves HDL cholesterol,
- prevents and helps control diabetes,
- decreases low-grade (hidden) inflammation in the body,
- increases and maintains good heart function, sometimes improving certain ECG abnormalities,
- motivates toward smoking cessation,
- alleviates tension and stress,
- counteracts a personal history of heart disease.

The significance of physical inactivity in contributing to cardiovascular risk was clearly shown when the American Heart Association named physical inactivity as one of the six major risk factors for cardiovascular disease (the other five factors are smoking, a poor cholesterol profile, high blood pressure, diabetes, and obesity.)[5] Based on the overwhelming amount of scientific data in this area, evidence of the benefits of aerobic exercise in reducing heart disease is far too impressive to be ignored.

Groundbreaking research at the Institute for Aerobics Research in Dallas, Texas, clearly shows the tie between cardiorespiratory fitness and mortality, regardless of age and other risk factors[6] (see Figure 11.4). A higher level of

FIGURE 11.4 Age-Adjusted Cardiovascular Death Rates by Physical Fitness Groups

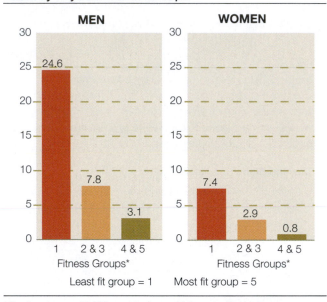

Least fit group = 1   Most fit group = 5

*Death rates per 10,000 person-years of follow-up. One person-year indicates one person that was followed up one year later.

"Physical Fitness and All-Cause Mortality: A Prospective Study of Healthy Men and Women" by S. N. Blair, H. W. Kohl III, R. S. Paffenbarger Jr., D. G. Clark, K. H. Cooper, and L. W. Gibbons, *Journal of the American Medical Association* 262 (1989): 2395–2401.

physical fitness benefits even those who have other risk factors, such as high blood pressure and serum cholesterol, cigarette smoking, and a family history of heart disease. In most cases, unfit people in the study (group 1) without these risk factors had higher death rates than fit people (groups 4 and 5) with these same risk factors.

Although the findings show that the higher the level of cardiorespiratory fitness, the longer the life, the largest drop in premature death is seen between the unfit and the moderately fit groups. Even small improvements in cardiorespiratory endurance greatly decrease the risk for cardiovascular mortality. Most adults who become

FIGURE 11.5 The Atherosclerotic Process

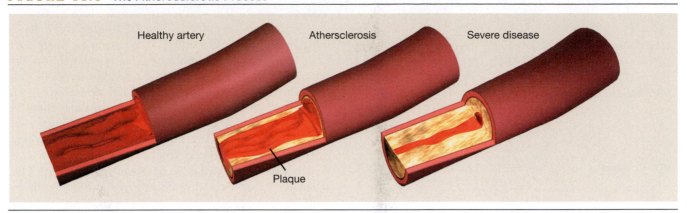

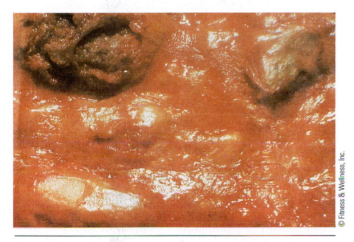

This close-up view shows the build-up of fatty plaque on the inner lining of an artery due to atherosclerosis.

physically active and engage in moderate-intensity activities can attain these fitness levels easily.

Subsequent research substantiated the importance of exercise in preventing CHD.[7] The research indicated that the benefits (to previously inactive adults) of starting a moderate-to-vigorous physical activity program were as important as quitting smoking, managing blood pressure, or controlling cholesterol. The increase in physical activity led to the same decrease as giving up cigarette smoking in relative risk for death from CHD.

Even though physically active individuals have a lower incidence of cardiovascular disease, a regular aerobic exercise program by itself does not guarantee a lifetime free of cardiovascular problems. Poor lifestyle habits—such as smoking, eating too many fatty/salty/sweet foods, being overweight, and having high stress levels—increase cardiovascular risk and will not be eliminated completely through aerobic exercise.

Overall risk factor management is the best guideline to lower the risk for cardiovascular disease. Still, aerobic exercise is one of the most important activities in preventing and reducing cardiovascular problems.

Abnormal Cholesterol Profile

Cholesterol is a waxy substance, technically a steroid alcohol, found only in animal fats and oils. This fatty substance is essential for specific metabolic functions in the body, but an abnormal cholesterol profile contributes to atherosclerotic plaque, a build-up of fatty tissue in the walls of the arteries. As the plaque builds up, it blocks the blood vessels that supply the heart muscle (myocardium) with oxygen and nutrients, and these obstructions can trigger a myocardial infarction or heart attack (see Figure 11.5).

Cholesterol is carried in the bloodstream by molecules of protein known as high-density lipoproteins (HDLs), low-density lipoproteins (LDLs), and very low-density lipoproteins (VLDLs). Although subcategories of these lipoproteins have been identified, the discussion here focuses only on the major categories.

Direct relationships have been established between cholesterol levels (high total cholesterol, high **LDL cholesterol**, and low **HDL cholesterol**) and the rate of CHD in men and women alike. Unfortunately, because the heart disguises its problems quite well, typical symptoms of heart disease, such as angina pectoris and chest pain, do not start until the arteries are about 75 percent blocked. In many cases the first symptom is sudden death.

The general recommendation by the National Cholesterol Education Program (NCEP) is to keep total cholesterol levels below 200 mg/dl. Other health professionals

Cholesterol A waxy substance, technically a steroid alcohol, found only in animal fats and oil; used in making cell membranes, as a building block for some hormones, in the fatty sheath around nerve fibers, and in other necessary substances.

LDL cholesterol Cholesterol-transporting molecules in the blood ("bad cholesterol").

HDL cholesterol Cholesterol-transporting molecules in the blood ("good cholesterol").

TABLE 11.1 Cholesterol Guidelines

	Amount	Rating
Total Cholesterol	<200 mg/dl	Desirable
	200–239 mg/dl	Borderline high
	≥240 mg/dl	High risk
LDL Cholesterol	<100 mg/dl	Optimal
	100–129 mg/dl	Near or above optimal
	130–159 mg/dl	Borderline high
	160–189 mg/dl	High
	≥190 mg/dl	Very high
HDL Cholesterol	<40 mg/dl	Low (high risk)
	≥60 mg/dl	High (low risk)

From National Cholesterol Education Program.

recommend that total cholesterol in individuals age 30 and younger should not be higher than 180 mg/dl, and for children the level should be below 170 mg/dl. Cholesterol levels between 200 and 239 mg/dl are borderline high, and levels of 240 mg/dl and above indicate high risk for disease (see Table 11.1).

Cholesterol is transported primarily in the form of LDL cholesterol and HDL cholesterol. LDL tends to release cholesterol, which then may penetrate the lining or inner membrane of the arteries and speed up the process of atherosclerosis. Thus LDL has been termed the "bad cholesterol. With reference to the NCEP guidelines given in Table 11.1, an LDL cholesterol value below 100 mg/dl is optimal.

HDL cholesterol, the "good cholesterol, tends to attract cholesterol, which then is carried to the liver to be metabolized and excreted. In a process known as **reverse cholesterol transport**, HDLs act as "scavengers," removing cholesterol from the body and preventing plaque from forming in the arteries.

The strength of HDL is in the protein molecules found in the coatings. When HDL comes in contact with cholesterol-filled cells, these protein molecules attach to the cells and take their cholesterol. The more HDL cholesterol, the better, as it offers some protection against heart disease.

Substantial research suggests that a low level of HDL cholesterol has the strongest relationship to CHD at all levels of total cholesterol, including levels below 200 mg/dl.[8] To minimize the risk for CHD, the recommended HDL cholesterol value is at least 40 mg/dl. HDL cholesterol levels above 60 mg/dl help to lower the risk for CHD.

For the most part, HDL cholesterol is determined genetically. Generally, women have higher values than men. This is one of the reasons that heart disease is less common in women. African-American children and adult African-American men have higher values than Caucasians. HDL cholesterol also decreases with age.

Increasing HDL cholesterol improves the cholesterol profile and decreases the risk for CHD. Habitual aerobic exercise, weight loss, and quitting smoking all have been shown to raise HDL cholesterol. Drug therapy can also lead to higher HDL cholesterol levels. Increased HDL cholesterol and a regular aerobic (high-intensity or above 6 METs, for at least 20 minutes three times per week—see Chapter 7) exercise program are clearly related. Individual responses to aerobic exercise differ, but, generally, the more the exercise, the higher is the HDL cholesterol level.

Even when more LDL cholesterol is present than the cells can use, cholesterol seems not to cause a problem until it is oxidized by free radicals. Data suggest that even a single unstable **oxygen free radical** (an oxygen compound produced during metabolism) can damage LDL particles. When oxidation occurs, white blood cells invade the arterial wall, take up the cholesterol, and clog the arteries.

The antioxidant effect of vitamins C and E may provide benefits. Data suggest that a single unstable free radical (an oxygen compound produced during metabolism—see Chapter 8) can damage LDL particles, accelerating the atherosclerotic process. Vitamin C may inactivate free radicals and slow the oxidation of LDL cholesterol. Vitamin E may protect LDL from oxidation, preventing heart disease, but studies suggest that it does not seem to be helpful in reversing damage once it has taken place.[9]

Consumption of saturated fats raises cholesterol levels more than anything else in the diet. Saturated fats produce approximately 1,000 mg of cholesterol per day.[10] Because of individual differences, some people can have a higher-than-normal intake of saturated fats and still maintain normal cholesterol levels. Others who have a lower intake can have abnormally high levels.

Saturated fats are found mostly in meats and dairy products and seldom in foods of plant origin. Poultry and fish contain less saturated fat than beef does but still should be eaten in moderation (about 3 to 6 ounces per day). Unsaturated fats are mainly of plant origin and cannot be converted to cholesterol.

If LDL cholesterol is higher than ideal, it can be lowered by losing body fat, manipulating the diet (through lower intakes of fat, saturated fat and cholesterol, and high in fiber), participating in a regular aerobic exercise program, and possibly taking medication. Exercise is important because dietary manipulation by itself is not as effective in lowering LDL cholesterol as a combination of diet plus aerobic exercise.[11]

Critical Thinking

1. Are you aware of your blood lipid profile?
2. If not, what keeps you from getting a blood chemistry test?
3. What are the benefits of having it done now as opposed to later in life?

Two dietary components—fiber and low-fat foods—merit more detailed discussion.

FIBER

To lower LDL cholesterol significantly, total daily fiber intake must be in the range of 25 to 38 grams per day, total fat consumption must be significantly lower than the current 30 percent of total daily caloric intake guideline, saturated fat consumption has to be under 10 percent of the total daily caloric intake, and the average cholesterol consumption should be much lower than 300 mg per day.

The fiber intake of most people in the United States averages less than 15 grams per day. Fiber, in particular the soluble type, has been shown to lower cholesterol. Soluble fiber dissolves in water and forms a gel-like substance that encloses food particles. This property helps bind and excrete fats from the body. The incidence of heart disease is low in populations where daily fiber intake exceeds 30 grams per day. Further, a 1996 Harvard University Medical School study involving 43,000 middle-aged men who were followed for more than 6 years showed that increasing fiber intake to 30 daily grams was accompanied by a 41 percent reduction in heart attacks.[12]

LOW-FAT DIETS

Research on the effects of a 30-percent-fat diet has shown that it has little or no effect in lowering cholesterol and that CHD actually continues to progress in people who have the disease. The good news came in a study published in the *Archives of Internal Medicine*.[13] Men and women in the study lowered their cholesterol by an average of 23 percent in only 3 weeks following a 10 percent or less fat-calorie diet combined with a regular aerobic exercise program, primarily walking. In this diet, cholesterol intake was less than 25 mg/day. The author of the study concluded that the exact percent-fat guideline (10 or 15 percent) is unknown (it also varies from individual to individual) but that 30 percent total fat calories is definitely too much when attempting to lower blood cholesterol.

A daily 10 percent-total-fat diet requires the person to limit fat intake to an absolute minimum. Some health-care professionals contend that this sort of diet is difficult to follow indefinitely. People with high cholesterol levels, however, may not have to follow that diet indefinitely but should adopt the 10 percent-fat diet while attempting to lower cholesterol. Thereafter, eating a 20- to 30-percent fat diet may be adequate to maintain recommended cholesterol levels.

One drawback of very low-fat diets (less than 25 percent fat) is that they tend to lower HDL cholesterol. If HDL cholesterol is already low, monounsaturated and polyunsaturated fats should be added to the diet. Nuts and olive, canola, corn, and soybean oils are high in monounsaturated fats and polyunsaturated fats. A specialized nutrition book should be consulted to determine other food items that are high in monounsaturated and polyunsaturated fats.

The NCEP guidelines recommend that people consider drug therapy if, after 6 months on a low-cholesterol, low-fat diet, the cholesterol remains unacceptably high. An unacceptable level is an LDL cholesterol above 190 mg/dl for people with fewer than two risk factors and no signs of heart disease. For people with more than two risk factors and with a history of heart disease, LDL cholesterol above 160 mg/dl is unacceptable.

CHOLESTEROL-LOWERING MEDICATIONS

Effective medications are available to treat elevated cholesterol. Most notable among them are the statins group (Lipitor®, Mevacor®, Pravachol®, Lescol®, and Zocor®), which can lower cholesterol by up to 60 percent in 2 to 3 months. Statins slow cholesterol production and increase the liver's ability to remove blood cholesterol. They also decrease triglycerides and produce a small increase in HDL levels.

In general, it is better to lower LDL cholesterol without medication because drugs often cause undesirable side effects. Many people with heart disease, however, must take cholesterol-lowering medication. It is best if medication is combined with lifestyle changes to augment the cholesterol-lowering effect. For example, when Zocor was taken alone over 3 months, LDL cholesterol decreased by 30 percent; but when a Mediterranean diet (a diet focusing on olive oil, grains, legumes, vegetables, fruits, and red wine, and limited amounts of meat, fish, milk, and cheese) was adopted in combination with Zocor therapy, LDL cholesterol decreased by 41 percent.[14]

Other drugs effective in reducing LDL cholesterol are *bile acid sequestrans*, which bind cholesterol found in bile acids. Cholesterol subsequently is excreted in the stools. These drugs are often used in combination with statin drugs.

High doses (1.5 to 3 grams per day) of nicotinic acid or niacin (a B vitamin) also help lower LDL cholesterol and triglycerides and increase HDL cholesterol. A fourth group of drugs, known as *fibrates*, is used primarily to lower triglycerides.

High Triglycerides

Triglycerides, also known as **free fatty acids**, make up most of the fat in our diet and most of the fat that circulates in the blood (called blood lipids). In combination

---

Reverse cholesterol transport A process in which HDL molecules attract cholesterol and carry it to the liver, where it is changed to bile and eventually excreted in the stool.

Oxygen free radicals Substances formed during metabolism that attack and damage proteins and lipids, in particular the cell membrane and DNA, leading to conditions such as heart disease, cancer, and emphysema.

Triglycerides Fats formed by glycerol and three fatty acids. Also known as "free fatty acids."

Free fatty acids (FFA) Fats formed by glycerol and three fatty acids. Also known as triglycerides.

TABLE 11.2 Triglycerides Guidelines

Amount	Rating
≤125 mg/dl	Desirable
126–499 mg/dl	Borderline high
≥500 mg/dl	High risk

with cholesterol, triglycerides speed up formation of plaque in the arteries. Triglycerides are carried in the bloodstream primarily by very low-density lipoproteins (VLDLs) and **chylomicrons**.

Although they are found in poultry skin, lunch meats, and shellfish, these fatty acids are manufactured mainly in the liver from refined sugars, starches, and alcohol. A high intake of alcohol and sugars (honey and fruit juices included) significantly raises triglyceride levels. Triglycerides can be lowered by cutting down on these foods and overall fat consumption, quitting smoking, reducing weight (if overweight), and doing aerobic exercise.

The desirable blood triglyceride level is less than 150 mg/dl (see Table 11.2). For people with cardiovascular problems, this level should be below 100 mg/dl.[15] Levels above 1,000 mg/dl pose an immediate risk for potentially fatal sudden inflammation of the pancreas.

Elevated Homocysteine

Clinical data indicating that many heart attack and stroke victims have normal cholesterol levels have led researchers to look for other risk factors that may contribute to atherosclerosis. Although it is not a blood lipid, a high concentration of the amino acid **homocysteine** in the blood is thought to enhance the formation of plaque and subsequent blockage of the arteries.

The body uses homocysteine to help build proteins and carry out cellular metabolism. It is an intermediate amino acid in the interconversion of two other amino acids—methionine and cysteine. This interconversion requires the B vitamin folate (folic acid) and vitamins B_6 and B_{12}.

Typically, homocysteine is metabolized rapidly, so it does not accumulate in the blood or damage the arteries. Many people, however, have high blood levels of homocysteine. This might result from either a genetic inability to metabolize homocysteine or a deficiency in the vitamins required for its conversion. Homocysteine typically is measured in micromoles per liter (μmol/l). In a 10-year follow-up study of people with high homocysteine levels, the data showed that individuals with a level above 14.25 μmol/l had almost twice the risk of stroke compared to individuals whose level was below 9.25 μmol/l.[16] It is theorized that homocysteine accumulation is toxic because it may

1. damage the inner lining of the arteries (the initial step in atherosclerosis),
2. stimulate the proliferation of cells that contribute to plaque formation, and
3. encourage clotting that may completely obstruct an artery and lead to a heart attack or stroke.

Keeping homocysteine from accumulating in the blood seems to be as simple as eating the recommended daily servings of vegetables, fruits, grains, and some meat and legumes. Five servings of fruits and vegetables daily can provide sufficient levels of folate and vitamin B_6 to remove and clear homocysteine from the blood. Vitamin B_{12} is found primarily in animal flesh and animal products. Vitamin B_{12} deficiency is rarely a problem because 1 cup of milk or an egg provides the daily requirement. The body also recycles most of this vitamin; therefore, a deficiency takes years to develop. People who consume five servings of fruits and vegetables daily are unlikely to derive extra benefits from vitamin-B-complex supplementation.

Increasing evidence that folate can prevent heart attacks has led to the recommendation that people (especially women of childbearing age) consume 400 mcg per day—obtainable from five daily servings of fruits and vegetables. Unfortunately, estimates indicate that more than 80 percent of Americans do not get 400 daily mcg of folate.[17]

Inflammation

Scientists are looking at inflammation as a major risk factor for heart attacks. Low-grade inflammation can occur in a variety of places throughout the body. For years it has been known that inflammation plays a role in CHD and that inflammation hidden deep in the body is a common trigger for heart attacks, even when cholesterol levels are normal or low and arterial plaque is minimal.

FIGURE 11.6 Relationships Among C-reactive Protein, Cholesterol, and Risk of Cardiovascular Disease

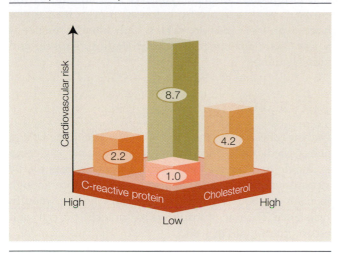

Adapted from "Inflammation and Atherosclerosis" by P. Libby, P. M. Ridker, and A. Maseri, *Circulation* 105 (2002): 1135–1143.

To evaluate ongoing inflammation in the body, physicians have turned to **C-reactive protein (CRP)**, a protein whose levels in the blood increase with inflammation. People with elevated CRP are more prone to cardiovascular events. The evidence shows that CRP blood levels elevate years before a first heart attack or stroke and that individuals with elevated CRP have twice the risk for a heart attack. The risk of a heart attack is even higher in people with both elevated CRP and cholesterol, resulting in an almost ninefold increase in risk (see Figure 11.6).

Because high CRP levels might be a better predictor of future heart attacks than high cholesterol alone, the FDA has approved a test known as high-sensitivity CRP (hs-CRP), which measures inflammation in the blood vessels. The term *high-sensitivity* was derived from the test's capability to detect small amounts of CRP in the blood.

Hs-CRP test results provide a good measure of the probability of plaque rupturing within the arterial wall. Of the two main types of plaque—soft and hard—soft plaque is the most likely to rupture. Ruptured plaque releases clots into the bloodstream that can lead to a heart attack or a stroke. Other evidence has linked high CRP levels to high blood pressure and colon cancer.

Excessive intake of alcohol and high-protein diets increases CRP. Evidence further indicates that high-fat, fast-food meals increase CRP levels for several hours following the meals.[18] And cooking meat and poultry at high temperatures produces damaged proteins (AGEs or advanced glycosylation end products) that trigger inflammation. Further, obesity increases inflammation. With weight loss, CRP levels decrease proportional to the amount of fat lost.

An hs-CRP test is relatively inexpensive, and it is highly recommended for patients at risk for heart attack. Guidelines for hs-CRP levels are given in Table 11.3.

Taking statin drugs results in a decrease in CRP levels, and these drugs also lower cholesterol and reduce

TABLE 11.3 High-Sensitivity CRP Guidelines

Amount	Rating
<1 mg/l	Low risk
1–3 mg/l	Average risk
>3 mg/l	High risk

Source: "Markers of Inflammation and Cardiovascular Disease," by T. A. Pearson, et. al., *Circulation* 107 (2003): 499–511.

inflammation. Also helpful in reducing hs-CRP are exercise, weight loss, proper nutrition, and aspirin. Omega-3 fatty acids (found in salmon, tuna, and mackerel fish) inhibit proteins that cause inflammation. Aspirin therapy also helps control inflammation.

High Blood Pressure (Hypertension)

Blood pressure is a measure of the force exerted against the walls of the blood vessels by the blood flowing through them. Blood pressure is assessed using a sphygmomanometer and a stethoscope.

The **sphygmomanometer** consists of an inflatable bladder contained within a cuff and a mercury gravity manometer or an aneroid manometer from which the pressure is read. The pressure is measured in milliliters of mercury and usually expressed in two numbers. Ideally, blood pressure should be 120/80 or below (see Table 11.4). The first (higher) number reflects the pressure exerted during the forceful contraction of the heart or systole—hence the name **systolic blood pressure**. The second (lower) number, **diastolic blood pressure**, is taken during the heart's relaxation, when no blood is being ejected.

Chylomicrons Triglyceride-transporting molecules in the blood.

Homocysteine An amino acid that, when allowed to accumulate in the blood, may lead to plaque formation and blockage of arteries.

C-reactive protein (CRP) A protein whose blood levels increase with inflammation, at times hidden deep in the body; elevation of this protein is an indicator of potential cardiovascular events.

Blood pressure A measure of the force exerted against the walls of blood vessels by the blood flowing through them.

Sphygmomanometer An inflatable bladder contained within a cuff and a mercury gravity manometer (or an aneroid manometer) from which the blood pressure is read.

Systolic blood pressure Pressure exerted by the blood against the walls of the arteries during the forceful contraction (systole) of the heart.

Diastolic blood pressure Pressure exerted by the blood against the walls of the arteries during the relaxation phase (diastole) of the heart.

TABLE 11.4 Blood Pressure Guidelines (expressed in mm Hg)

Rating	Systolic	Diastolic
Normal	≤120	≤80
Prehypertension	121–139	81–89
Stage 1 hypertension	140–159	90–99
Stage 2 hypertension	≥160	≥100

Source: National High Blood Pressure Education Program.

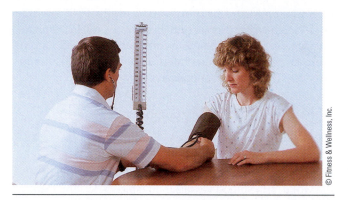

Blood pressure is being assessed using a mercury gravity manometer.

Hypertension is viewed as the point at which the pressure doubles the mortality risk, about 160/96. Statistical evidence clearly indicates, however, that blood pressure readings above 140/90 increase the risk for disease and premature death. Therefore, the American Heart Association considers all blood pressures above 140/90 to be hypertension.

All inner walls of arteries are lined by a layer of smooth endothelial cells. Blood lipids cannot penetrate the healthy lining and start to build up on the walls unless the cells are damaged. High blood pressure is thought to be a leading contributor to destruction of this lining. As blood pressure rises, so does the risk for atherosclerosis. The higher the pressure, the greater is the damage to the arterial wall, making the vessels susceptible to fat deposits, especially if serum cholesterol also is high. Blockage of the coronary vessels decreases blood supply to the heart muscle and can lead to heart attacks. When brain arteries are involved, strokes may follow.

Even though the threshold for hypertension has been set at 140/90, many experts believe that the lower the blood pressure, the better. Even if the pressure is as low as 90/50, as long as individuals do not have any symptoms of low blood pressure, or hypotension, they do not have to be concerned. Typical symptoms of hypotension are dizziness, lightheadedness, and fainting.

Blood pressure may fluctuate during a regular day. Many factors affect blood pressure, and a single reading may not be a true indicator of the real pressure. For example, physical activity and stress increase blood pressure, whereas rest and relaxation decrease it. Consequently, several measurements should be taken before diagnosing elevated pressure.

Hypertension has been called "the silent killer." It does not hurt, it does not make you feel sick, and unless you check it, years may go by before you even realize you have a problem. Besides CHD, high blood pressure is a risk factor for congestive heart failure, strokes, and kidney failure.

Diabetes

Diabetes affects more than 18 million people in the United States. Medically termed **diabetes mellitus**, blood glucose is unable to enter the cells because the pancreas totally stops producing **insulin**, or it does not produce enough to meet the body's needs, or the cells develop **insulin resistance**. The role of insulin is to "unlock" the cells and escort glucose into the cell.

The incidence of cardiovascular disease and death in the diabetic population is quite high. More than 80 percent of people with diabetes mellitus die from cardiovascular disease. People with chronically elevated blood glucose levels may have problems metabolizing fats, which can make them more susceptible to atherosclerosis, coronary heart disease, heart attacks, high blood pressure, and strokes. Diabetics also have lower HDL cholesterol and higher triglyceride levels.

Chronic high blood sugar also can lead to nerve damage, vision loss, kidney damage, and decreased immune function (making the individual more susceptible to infections). Diabetics are four times more likely to become blind and 20 times more likely to develop kidney failure. Because nerve damage in the lower extremities decreases the person's awareness of injury and infection, a small, untreated sore can lead to severe infection, gangrene, and even lead to an amputation.

An 8-hour fasting blood glucose level above 126 mg/dl on two separate tests confirms a diagnosis of diabetes (see Table 11.5). A level of 126 or higher should be brought to the attention of a physician.

Diabetes is of two types: **Type 1 diabetes**, or insulin-dependent diabetes (IDDM), and **Type 2 diabetes**, or non-insulin-dependent diabetes (NIDDM). Type 1 also is called "juvenile diabetes" because it is found mainly in young people. With Type 1, the pancreas produces little or no insulin. With Type 2, the pancreas either does not produce sufficient insulin or it produces adequate amounts but the cells become insulin-resistant, thereby keeping glucose from entering the cells. Type 2 accounts for 90 to 95 percent of all cases of diabetes.

Although diabetes has a genetic predisposition, Type 2, or adult-onset diabetes, is related closely to overeating, obesity, and lack of physical activity. Once limited primarily to overweight adults, Type 2 diabetes now accounts for almost half of the new cases diagnosed in children. More than 80 percent of all Type 2 diabetics are overweight or have a history of excessive weight. In most cases this condition can be corrected through a special diet, a weight-loss program, and a regular exercise program.

TABLE 11.5 Blood Glucose Guidelines

Amount	Rating
≤100 mg/dl	Normal
101–125 mg/dl	Pre-diabetes
≥126 mg/dl	Diabetes*

*Confirmed by two tests on different days.

Aerobic exercise has been shown to prevent diabetes in middle-aged men.[19] The protective effect is even greater in those with risk factors such as obesity, high blood pressure, and family propensity. The preventive effect is attributed to less body fat and better sugar and fat metabolism resulting from the regular exercise program. At 3,500 calories per week, the risk was cut in half, compared to sedentary men. This preventive effect, according to one of the authors of the study, should hold for women, too.

Both moderate-intensity and vigorous physical activity are associated with increased insulin sensitivity and decreased risk for diabetes. The key to increase and maintain proper insulin sensitivity, however, is regularity of the exercise program. Failing to maintain habitual physical activity voids these benefits.

A diet high in complex carbohydrates and water-soluble fibers (found in fruits, vegetables, oats, and beans), low in saturated fat, and low in sugar is helpful in treating diabetes. A simple aerobic exercise program (walking, cycling, or swimming four or five times per week) is often prescribed because it increases the body's sensitivity to insulin. Aggressive weight loss, especially if combined with exercise, often allows diabetic patients to normalize their blood sugar level without medication. Individuals who have high blood glucose levels should consult a physician to decide on the best treatment. (Exercise guidelines for diabetic patients are discussed in detail in Chapter 7 on page 134.)

Although complex carbohydrates are recommended in the diet, diabetics need to pay careful attention to the glycemic index (explained in Chapter 10, page 234). Refined and starchy foods have a high glycemic index (small-particle carbohydrates that are quickly digested); whereas grains, fruits, and vegetables are low-glycemic foods. Foods with a high glycemic index cause a rapid increase in blood sugar. A diet that includes many high-glycemic foods increases the risk for cardiovascular disease in people with high insulin resistance and **glucose intolerance**.[20] Combining a moderate amount of high-glycemic foods with low–glycemic-index foods or with some fat and protein, however, can bring down the average index.

A1c TEST

Individuals who have high blood glucose levels should consult a physician to decide on the best treatment. They also might obtain information about the hemoglobin A1c test (also called HbA1c), which measures the amount of glucose that has been in a person's blood over the last 3 months. Blood glucose can become attached to hemoglobin in the red blood cells. Once attached, it remains there for the life of the red blood cell, about 3 months. The higher the blood glucose, the higher is the concentration of glucose in the red blood cells. Results of this test are given in percentages.

The HbA1c goal for diabetic patients is to keep it at less than 7 percent. At this level, or lower, diabetics have a lower risk for developing diabetic-related problems of the eyes, kidneys, and nerves. Because the test tells a person how well blood glucose has been controlled over the last 3 months, a change in treatment is almost always recommended if the HbA1c results are above 8 percent. All people with Type 2 diabetes should have an HbA1c test twice a year.

METABOLIC SYNDROME

As the cells resist the actions of insulin, the pancreas releases even more insulin in an attempt to keep blood glucose from rising. A chronic rise in insulin seems to trigger a series of abnormalities termed the **metabolic syndrome**. These abnormal conditions include abdominal obesity, elevated blood pressure, high blood glucose, low HDL cholesterol, high triglycerides, and an increased blood-clotting mechanism. All of these conditions increase the risk for CHD and other diabetic-related conditions (blindness, infection, nerve damage, and kidney failure). Approximately 47 million Americans are afflicted with this condition.

Hypertension Chronically elevated blood pressure.

Diabetes mellitus A disease in which the body doesn't produce or utilize insulin properly.

Insulin Hormone secreted by the pancreas; essential for proper metabolism of blood glucose (sugar) and maintenance of blood glucose level.

Insulin resistance Inability of the cells to respond appropriately to insulin.

Type 1 diabetes Insulin-dependent diabetes mellitus (IDDM), a condition in which the pancreas produces little or no insulin; also known as juvenile diabetes because it is seen primarily in young people.

Type 2 diabetes Non-insulin-dependent diabetes mellitus (NIDDM), a condition in which insulin is not processed properly; also known as adult-onset diabetes.

Glucose intolerance A condition characterized by slightly elevated blood glucose levels.

Metabolic syndrome An array of metabolic abnormalities that contribute to development of atherosclerosis triggered by insulin resistance; these conditions include low HDL cholesterol, high triglycerides, high blood pressure, and an increased blood clotting mechanism.

Diagnosis of Metabolic Syndrome

Components	Men	Women
Waist circumference	>40 inches	>35 inches
Blood pressure	>130/85 mm Hg	>130/85 mm Hg
Fasting blood glucose	>110 mg/dl	>110 mg/dl
Fasting HDL cholesterol	<40 mg/dl	<50 mg/dl
Fasting triglycerides	>150 mg/dl	>150 mg/dl

Note: Metabolic syndrome is identified by the presence of at least three of the above components.

People with metabolic syndrome have an abnormal insulin response to carbohydrates, in particular high-glycemic foods. In contrast to the American Heart Association dietary guidelines, researchers on metabolic syndrome indicate that a low-fat, high-carbohydrate diet may not be the best for preventing CHD and actually could increase the risk for disease in people with high insulin resistance and glucose intolerance.[21] These people perhaps should distribute their daily caloric intake so 45 percent of the calories are derived from carbohydrates (primarily low-glycemic), 40 percent from fat, and 15 percent from protein.[22] Of the 40-percent fat calories, most of the fat should come from mono- and polyunsaturated fats and less than 7 percent from saturated fat.

Individuals with metabolic syndrome also benefit from weight loss (if overweight), exercise, and smoking cessation.[23] Insulin resistance drops by about 40 percent in overweight people who lose 20 pounds. Further, 45 minutes of daily aerobic exercise enhances insulin efficiency by 25 percent. Quitting smoking also decreases insulin resistance.

Smoking

More than 48 million adults and 3.5 million adolescents in the United States smoke cigarettes. Cigarette smoking is the single largest preventable cause of illness and premature death in the United States. If we include all related deaths, tobacco is responsible for more than 435,000 unnecessary deaths per year—enough deaths to wipe out the entire population of Miami and Miami Beach in a single year. About 50,000 of those who die are nonsmokers who were exposed to secondhand smoke.

Smoking has been linked to cardiovascular disease, cancer, bronchitis, emphysema, and peptic ulcers. In relation to CHD, smoking speeds up the process of atherosclerosis, and the risk of sudden death following a myocardial infarction increases threefold.

Smoking releases nicotine and another 1,200 toxic compounds or so into the bloodstream. Similar to hypertension, many of these substances destroy the inner membrane that protects artery walls. Once the lining is damaged, cholesterol and triglycerides can be deposited readily in the arterial wall. As the plaque builds up, it obstructs blood flow through the arteries.

Furthermore, smoking encourages the formation of blood clots, which can completely block an artery already narrowed by atherosclerosis. In addition, carbon monoxide, a byproduct of cigarette smoke, decreases the blood's oxygen-carrying capacity. A combination of obstructed arteries, nicotine, and less oxygen in the heart muscle heightens the risk for a serious heart problem.

In addition, smoking increases heart rate, raises blood pressure, and irritates the heart, which can trigger fatal **cardiac arrhythmias** (irregular heart rhythms). Another harmful effect is a decrease in HDL cholesterol, the "good" type that helps control blood lipids. Smoking actually presents a much greater risk of death from heart disease than from lung disease.

Pipe and cigar smoking and chewing tobacco also increase the risk for heart disease. Even if no smoke is inhaled, toxic substances are absorbed through the membranes of the mouth and end up in the bloodstream.

Excessive Body Fat

Body composition, discussed in Chapter 9, is the ratio of lean body weight to fat weight. If the body contains too much fat, the person is considered obese. Although some experts recognize obesity as an independent risk factor for CHD, the risks attributed to obesity actually may be caused by other risk factors that usually accompany excessive body fat. Risk factors such as high blood lipids, hypertension, and diabetes usually improve with increased physical activity. Overweight people who are physically active do not seem to pose increased risk for premature death.

Attaining recommended body composition alleviates some of the CHD risk factors and also improves health and wellness. People with a weight problem who desire to achieve recommended weight must

1. increase daily physical activity up to 90 minutes a day, including aerobic and strength-training programs,
2. follow a diet lower in fat and refined sugars and high in complex carbohydrates and fiber, and
3. reduce total caloric intake moderately while getting the necessary nutrients to sustain normal body functions.

Recommendations for weight management are discussed in Chapter 10.

Personal and Family History

Individuals who have had cardiovascular problems are at higher risk than those who never have had a problem. People with this history should control the other risk factors

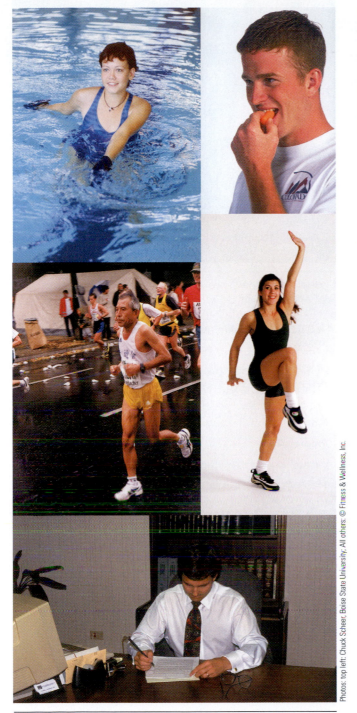

A healthy lifestyle leads to a higher functional capacity throughout life.

In many cases, we have no way of knowing whether a person's genetic predisposition or simply poor lifestyle habits led to a heart problem. A heart attack victim may have been physically inactive, overweight, and a smoker with bad dietary habits. Because we cannot differentiate the effects of these factors reliably, anyone with a family history of cardiovascular problems should watch all other factors closely and maintain the lowest possible risk level. In addition, an annual blood chemistry analysis is strongly recommended to make sure the body is handling blood lipids properly.

Tension and Stress

Tension and stress (discussed in Chapter 3) have become a normal part of life. Everyone has to deal daily with goals, deadlines, responsibilities, pressures. Almost everything in life (whether positive or negative) is a source of stress. The stressor itself is not what creates the health hazard but, rather, the individual's response to it.

The human body responds to stress by producing more catecholamines (hormones) to prepare the body for fight or flight. These hormones elevate the heart rate, blood pressure, and blood glucose levels, enabling the person to take action. If the person "fights or flees"—that is, takes physical action—the higher levels of catecholamines are metabolized and the body returns to a "normal" state. But if a person is under constant stress and unable to take physical action (such as with the death of a close relative or friend, loss of job, trouble at work, or financial insecurity), the catecholamines remain elevated in the bloodstream.

People who are unable to relieve stress put a constant low-level strain on their cardiovascular system that could manifest itself in heart disease. In addition, when a person is in a stressful situation, the coronary arteries that feed the heart muscle constrict, reducing the oxygen supply to the heart. If the blood vessels are significantly blocked by atherosclerosis, abnormal heart rhythms or even a heart attack may follow.

as much as they can. Because most risk factors are reversible, this will greatly decrease their risk for future problems. The more time that has passed since the cardiovascular problem occurred, the lower the risk for recurrence.

Genetic predisposition toward heart disease has been clearly demonstrated and seems to be gaining in importance. All other factors being equal, a person with blood relatives who have or had heart disease before age 60 runs a greater risk than someone who has no such history. The younger the age at which the incident happened to the relative, the greater the risk for the disease.

Cardiac arrhythmias Irregular heart rhythms.

Age

Age is a risk factor because of the greater incidence of heart disease in older people. This tendency may be induced partly by other factors stemming from changes in lifestyle as we get older (less physical activity, poor nutrition, obesity, and so on).

Young people, however, should not think they will escape heart disease. The process begins early in life. This was clearly shown in American soldiers who died during the Korean and Vietnam conflicts. Autopsies conducted on soldiers killed at 22 years of age and younger revealed that approximately 70 percent had early stages of atherosclerosis. Other studies have found elevated blood cholesterol levels in children as young as 10 years old.

Even though the aging process cannot be stopped, it can certainly be slowed down. Physiological versus chronological age is an important concept in preventing disease. Some individuals in their 60s and older have the body of a 20-year-old. And some 20-year-olds are in such poor condition and health that they almost seem to have the body of a 60-year-old. Risk factor management and positive lifestyle habits are the best ways to slow the natural aging process.

Other Factors

Additional evidence points to a few other factors that may be linked to coronary heart disease. Two of these are gum disease and snoring.

GUM DISEASE

A possible factor in CHD is gum disease. The oral bacteria that builds up with dental plaque can enter the bloodstream and contribute to the formation of blood vessel plaque, increase blood clots, and thus increase the risk for heart attack. Daily flossing for 1 to 2 minutes is the best way to prevent gum disease.

SNORING

Loud snoring has been linked to cardiovascular disease. People who snore heavily may suffer from sleep apnea, a sleep disorder in which the throat closes briefly, causing breathing to stop. In one study, individuals who snored heavily tripled their risk for a heart attack and quadrupled the risk for a stroke.[24]

Guidelines for Preventing Cardiovascular Disease

As discussed, most cardiovascular risk factors are preventable and reversible. Overall risk factor management is the best guideline to lower the risk. The key elements in

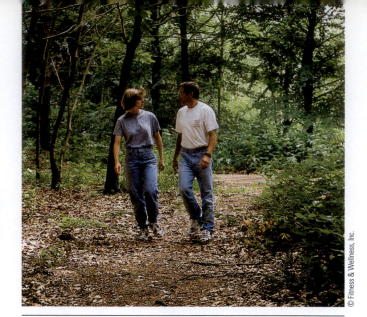

Moderate-intensity activities greatly reduce the risk for premature cardiovascular death.

TABLE 11.6 Minimum Aerobic Exercise for Moderate Fitness

Program 1	Days/ Week	Distance (miles)	Time (min)
Women	≥3	2	≤30
Men	≥3	2	≤27
Program 2			
Women	5–6	2	30–40
Men	6–7	2	30–40

From *Fitness and Mortality*, by S. N. Blair (Dallas: Aerobics Research Center, 1991).

preventing disorders of the cardiovascular system are regular physical activity in combination with proper nutrition, avoidance of tobacco, blood pressure control, stress management, and weight control.

LIFETIME PHYSICAL ACTIVITY

An active lifestyle combined with a systematic aerobic exercise program are two of the most important activities you can do to prevent and reduce the risk for cardiovascular problems. The basic principles for cardiorespiratory exercise are given in Chapter 7.

Although greater benefits are obtained at higher intensity levels, even a moderate-intensity aerobic exercise program can reduce cardiovascular risk considerably[25] (see Figure 11.4, page 268). A simple 40-minute walking (or equivalent) program, six to seven times per week, seems to have a strong inverse relationship with premature cardiovascular mortality. The minimum amount of exercise recommended for adults to achieve moderate fitness is presented in Table 11.6. Program 1 is of higher intensity than Program 2; thus, Program 1 requires a minimum of only three exercise sessions per week (compared to a minimum of five to six for Program 2).

NUTRITION RECOMMENDATIONS

The diet should contain ample amounts of fruits, vegetables, and grains. Because of their antioxidant effect, foods high in vitamins C and E and beta-carotene should be a regular part of the diet. Foods high in sugar and salt should be avoided. Alcohol should be consumed in moderation. (See Chapter 8 for more specific recommendations.)

To lower total and LDL cholesterol levels, the following general dietary guidelines are recommended:

- Consume between 25 and 38 grams of fiber daily, including a minimum of 10 grams of soluble fiber (good sources are oats, fruits, barley, legumes, and psyllium).
- Do not consume more than 200 mg of dietary cholesterol a day.
- Consume 25 grams of soy protein a day.
- Consume red meats (3 ounces per serving) fewer than three times per week, and avoid organ meats (such as liver and kidneys).
- Do not eat commercially baked foods.
- Avoid foods that contain trans fatty acids, hydrogenated fat, or partially hydrogenated vegetable oil.
- Increase intake of omega-3 fatty acids by eating two or three meals per week with fish rich in omega-3 fatty acids.
- Drink low-fat milk (1 percent or less fat, preferably) and use low-fat dairy products.
- Do not use coconut oil, palm oil, or cocoa butter.
- Limit egg consumption to fewer than three eggs per week (this applies only to people with high cholesterol; others may consume eggs in moderation).
- Use margarines and salad dressings that contain stanol ester instead of butter and regular margarine.
- Bake, broil, grill, poach, or steam food instead of frying.
- Refrigerate cooked meat before adding it to other dishes. Remove fat hardened in the refrigerator before mixing the meat with other foods.
- Avoid fatty sauces made with butter, cream, or cheese.
- Maintain recommended body weight.

The combination of a healthy diet, a sound aerobic exercise program, and weight control is the best prescription for controlling blood lipids. If this does not work, a physician can administer a blood test to break down the lipoproteins into their various subcategories.

SMOKING CESSATION

Cigarette smoking is one of the six major risk factors for CHD. Nonetheless, the risk for both cardiovascular disease and cancer starts to decrease the moment you quit smoking. The risk for these two diseases approaches that of a lifetime nonsmoker 10 and 15 years, respectively, after cessation.

Quitting cigarette smoking is no easy task. Only about 20 percent of smokers who try to quit for the first time succeed each year. The addictive properties of nicotine and smoke make quitting difficult. Physical and psychological withdrawal symptoms set in after quitting. Even though giving up smoking can be extremely difficult, it by no means is impossible.

The most crucial factor in quitting cigarette smoking is the person's sincere desire to do so. More than 95 percent of the successful ex-smokers have been able to quit on their own, either by quitting cold turkey or by using self-help kits available from organizations such as the American Cancer Society, the American Heart Association, and the American Lung Association. Only 3 percent of ex-smokers have quit as a result of formal "stop smoking" programs. A plan to help people stop smoking is contained in Chapter 13.

BLOOD PRESSURE CONTROL

Of all hypertension, 90 percent has no definite cause. Referred to as **essential hypertension**, this type is treatable. Aerobic exercise, weight reduction, a low-sodium/high-potassium diet, stress reduction, no smoking, a diet designed to decrease blood lipids, lower caffeine and alcohol intake, and antihypertensive medication—all have been used effectively to treat essential hypertension. The other 10 percent of hypertension is caused by pathological conditions such as narrowing of the kidney arteries, glomerulonephritis (a kidney disease), tumors of the adrenal glands, and narrowing of the aortic artery. With this type of hypertension, the pathological cause has to be treated before the blood pressure problem can be corrected.

A factor contributing to high blood pressure in about half of all hypertensive people is too much sodium in the diet (salt, or sodium chloride, contains approximately 40 percent sodium). With high sodium intake, the body retains more water, which increases the blood volume and, in turn, drives up blood pressure. Although sodium is essential for normal body functions, only 200 mg, or one-tenth of a teaspoon of salt, is required daily. Even under strenuous conditions of job and sports participation that produces heavy perspiration, the amount of sodium required is seldom more than 3,000 mg per day. Yet, sodium intake in the typical American diet ranges between 6,000 and 20,000 mg per day!

When treating high blood pressure (unless it is extremely high), many physicians suggest trying a combination of aerobic exercise, weight loss, smoking cessation (if the person smokes), and reduced sodium before they recommend medication. In most instances, this treatment brings blood pressure under control.

Aerobic exercise is often prescribed for hypertensive patients. Studies have indicated that hypertensive patients who begin a moderate aerobic exercise program can

Essential hypertension Persistent high blood pressure that has no known cause.

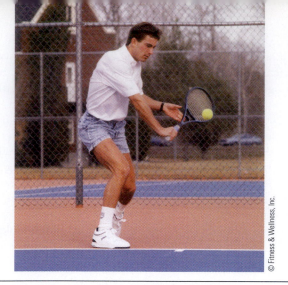

Physical activity is an excellent tool to control stress.

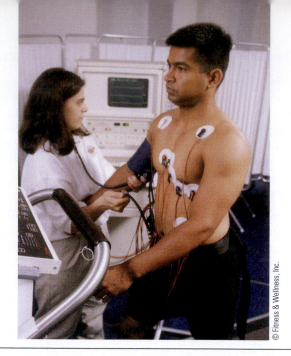

This man is being administered a graded treadmill exercise tolerance test with electrocardiographic monitoring (exercise stress test).

expect a notable decrease in blood pressure after only a few weeks of training. The exercise-related drop in blood pressure may contribute to a 40 percent decrease in the risk for stroke and a 15 percent reduction in the risk for coronary heart disease.[26] Even in the absence of any decrease in resting blood pressure, hypertensive individuals who exercise have a lower risk of all-cause mortality than hypertensive individuals who are sedentary.[27] Research also shows that exercise, not weight loss, is the major contributor to lower blood pressure. If aerobic exercise is discontinued, these changes are not maintained.

The best tip of all is to take a preventive approach. Keeping blood pressure under control is easier than trying to bring it down once it is high. Blood pressure should be checked regularly, regardless of whether it is elevated. Regular physical exercise, weight control, a low-salt diet, no smoking, and stress management are the basic guidelines for blood pressure control.

STRESS MANAGEMENT

Individuals who are under a lot of stress and do not cope well with it need to take measures to counteract the effects of stress in their lives. One of the best suggestions is to identify the sources of stress and learn how to cope with them. People need to take control of themselves, examine and act upon the things that are most important in their lives, and ignore less meaningful details. Relaxation techniques for stress management are presented in Chapter 3.

Physical exercise is one of the best ways to relieve stress. When a person takes part in physical activity, the body metabolizes excess catecholamines and is able to return to a normal state. Exercise also steps up muscular activity, which leads to muscular relaxation after completing the physical activity. Many executives prefer the evening hours for their physical activity programs, stopping after work at a health or fitness club. By doing this, they are able to burn up the excess tension accumulated during the day and enjoy the evening hours.

RESTING AND STRESS ELECTROCARDIOGRAMS

The electrocardiogram (ECG) provides a valuable measure of the heart's function, recording the electrical impulses that stimulate the heart to contract. An ECG shows five general areas of heart function: heart rate, heart rhythm, the heart's axis, enlargement or hypertrophy of the heart, and myocardial infarction or heart attack.

On a standard 12-lead ECG, 10 electrodes are placed on the person's chest. From these 10 electrodes, 12 "pictures" or tracings of electrical impulses are studied from 12 different positions as they travel through the heart muscle (myocardium). By looking at ECG charts, abnormalities in heart functioning can be identified. Based on the findings, the ECG may be interpreted as normal, equivocal, or abnormal. On the one hand, an ECG does not always identify problems, so a normal tracing is not an absolute guarantee. On the other hand, an abnormal tracing does not necessarily signal a serious condition.

ECGs are taken at rest, during stress of exercise, and during recovery. An **exercise ECG** also is known as a "graded exercise stress test" or a "maximal exercise tolerance test." Similar to a high-speed road test on a car, a stress ECG reveals the heart's tolerance to high-intensity exercise. It is a much better test than a resting ECG to discover CHD. Stress ECGs also are used to assess cardiorespiratory fitness levels, screen individuals for preventive and cardiac rehabilitation programs, detect abnormal blood pressure response during exercise, and establish actual or functional maximal heart rate for exercise prescription.

At times, the stress ECG has been questioned as a reliable predictor of CHD. Even so, it remains the most practical, inexpensive, noninvasive procedure available to

Criteria for Stress ECG

Not every adult who wishes to start or continue an exercise program needs a stress ECG. The following criteria can be applied to determine when this type of test should be administered:

- Men over age 45 and women over age 55
- A total cholesterol level above 200 mg/dl or an HDL cholesterol below 35 mg/dl
- Hypertensive and diabetic patients
- Cigarette smokers
- Individuals with a family history of CHD, syncope, or sudden death before age 60
- Hypertensive and diabetic patients
- People with an abnormal resting ECG
- All individuals with symptoms of chest discomfort, dysrhythmias, syncope, or chronotropic incompetence (a heart rate that increases slowly during exercise and never reaches maximum)

diagnose latent (undiagnosed/unknown) CHD. The test is accurate in diagnosing CHD about 65 percent of the time. Part of the problem is that many times those who administer stress ECGs do it without clearly understanding the test's indications and limitations.

The sensitivity of a stress test increases with the severity of the disease. More accurate results also are found for people at high risk for cardiovascular disease, in particular men over age 45 and women over age 55 with a poor cholesterol profile, high blood pressure, or a family history of heart disease. Test protocols, number of leads, electrocardiographic criteria, and the skill of the technicians administering the test also affect its sensitivity. Despite its limitations, a stress ECG test is still a useful tool for identifying people at high risk for exercise-related sudden death.

A Final Word

Most of the risk factors for CHD are reversible and preventable. A person who has a family history of heart disease and possibly some of the other risk factors resulting from a less than healthful lifestyle is not necessarily doomed. A healthier lifestyle—free of cardiovascular problems—is something over which you have much control. You are encouraged to be persistent. Willpower and commitment are necessary to develop patterns that eventually will turn into healthy habits and contribute to your total well-being.

Exercise ECG An exercise test during which workload is increased gradually (until the person reaches maximal fatigue) with blood pressure and 12-lead electrocardiographic monitoring throughout the test.

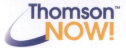

Don't forget to check out the wealth of resources on the ThomsonNOW website at **www.thomsonedu.com/ThomsonNOW** that will:

- Coach you through identifying target goals for behavior change and monitoring your personal change plan throughout the semester
- Help you evaluate your knowledge of the material
- Allow you to take an exam-prep quiz
- Provide a Personalized Learning Plan targeting resources that address areas you should study.

WEB ACTIVITIES

American Heart Association This comprehensive site provides research, cardiac information for health professionals and the general public, as well as advocacy. The site features information on a variety of cardiovascular illnesses, healthy lifestyles, and CPR. It also offers a heart and stroke searchable encyclopedia and a 10-question Healthy Heart Workout quiz.

http://www.americanheart.org

National Cholesterol Education Program This comprehensive site features interactive sessions on planning a low-cholesterol diet and lots more. It provides you with information to prevent heart disease as well as information for people who already have heart disease. You can hear radio messages from the Heart Beat Radio Network. A site highly recommended.

http://rover.nhlbi.nih.gove/chd

The Heart: An Online Exploration This informative and interesting site, developed by the Franklin Institute of Science, provides an interactive multimedia tour of the heart, statistical information, resources, and links. You can learn how to monitor your heart's health by becoming aware of your vital signs, read more about diagnostic tests, and listen to heart sounds via the site's audio and video clips.

http://www.fi.edu/biosci/heart.html

Heart and Vascular Disease Information This comprehensive site sponsored by the National Heart, Lung, and Blood Institute provides a variety of information and interactive sites on topics ranging from a 10-year Risk Calculator, to nutrition, to lowering your blood pressure, and much more.

http://www.nhlbi.nih.gov/health/public/heart/index.htm#other

InfoTrac®

You can find additional readings related to wellness via InfoTrac® College Edition, an online library of more than 900 journals and publications. Follow the instructions for accessing InfoTrac® that came packaged with your textbook, then search for articles using a key word search.

Suggested Reading Studies identify surprising risk factors for heart disease: lower blood sugar, avoiding traffic jams, finishing high school all linked to reduced risk. *Tufts University Health & Nutrition Letter,* Jan. 2005 v22 i11 p6 (1).

1. How might lowering your blood sugar affect your risk of heart disease?
2. How does traffic gridlock threaten the heart?
3. How can education reduce the danger of heart disease?

Web Activity

Texas Heart Institute Risk Factor Assessment

http://hht.texasheartinstitute.org/

Sponsor Texas Heart Institute, St. Luke's Episcopal Hospital, Houston, Texas.

Description Risk factors are your personal characteristics, genetic makeup, and lifestyle behaviors that may increase your chances of incurring a heart attack or stroke. Some factors you can't change or control (age, gender, genetics); some you can, by making a few changes in your daily habits. Are you at risk? Find out by taking this short interactive quiz.

Available Activities

1. The site features 10 simple questions about your personal characteristics and habits designed to determine your personal risk of having a heart attack or stroke.
2. The questions assess your risk based on age, family history, smoking habits, blood cholesterol level, blood pressure, physical activity, weight, diabetes, and past medical history of heart conditions.

Web Work

1. From the home page, answer all 10 questions honestly by clicking on the appropriate radio button or typing in the information requested.
2. Question 4 allows you to calculate your body mass index (BMI) by entering your height and weight. Click on "calculate" button to receive your BMI.
3. When quiz is completed, click the "Submit" button to receive your relative risk and specific information on how to decrease your risks.

Helpful Hints

1. If you check more than three of the 10 risk factors, you should see a health-care provider for a complete assessment of your risks!
2. The evaluation you receive is comprehensive and provides practical guidelines on preventing heart disease by reducing your risk factors.

For additional Web activities, links, and suggested readings, visit our Health, Fitness, and Wellness Resource Center at http://health.wadsworth.com.

Notes

1. American Heart Association, *Heart Disease and Stroke Statistics—2006 Update* (Dallas: AHA, 2006).
2. See Note 1.
3. See Note 1.
4. See Note 1.
5. American Heart Association, *1999 Heart and Stroke Facts Statistical Update* (Dallas: AHA, 1998).
6. S. N. Blair, H. W. Kohl III, R. S. Paffenbarger Jr., D. G. Clark, K. H. Cooper, and L. W. Gibbons, "Physical Fitness and All-Cause Mortality: A Prospective Study of Healthy Men and Women," *Journal of the American Medical Association* 262 (1989): 2395–2401.
7. R. S. Paffenbarger Jr., R. T. Hyde, A. L. Wing, I. Lee, D. L. Jung, and J. B. Kampert, "The Association of Changes in Physical-Activity Level and Other Lifestyle Characteristics with Mortality Among Men," *New England Journal of Medicine* 328 (1993): 538–545.
8. P. A. Romm, M. K. Hong, and C. E. Rackley, "High-Density-Lipoprotein Cholesterol and Risk of Coronary Heart Disease," *Practical Cardiology* 16 (1990): 28–40.
9. "From Starring Role to Bit Part: Has the Curtain Come Down on Vitamin E?" *Environmental Nutrition* 25 no. 5 (May 2002): 1, 4.
10. American Heart Association, *2000 Heart and Stroke Facts Statistical Update* (Dallas: AHA, 1999).
11. M. L. Stefanick et al., "Effects of Diet in Men and Postmenopausal Women with Low Levels of HDL Cholesterol and High Levels of LDL Cholesterol," *New England Journal of Medicine* 339 (1998): 12–20.

12. E. B. Rimm, A. Ascherio, E. Giovannucci, D. Spiegelman, M. J. Stampfer, and W. C. Willett, "Vegetable, Fruit, and Cereal Fiber Intake and Risk of Coronary Heart Disease Among Men," *Journal of the American Medical Association* 275 (1996): 447–451.
13. R. J. Barnard, "Effects of Lifestyle Modification on Serum Lipids," *Archives of Internal Medicine* 151 (1991): 1389–1394.
14. Jula et al., "Effects of Diet and Simvastatin on Serum Lipids, Insulin, and Antioxidants in Hypercholesterolemic Men," *Journal of the American Medical Association* 287 (2002): 598–605.
15. W. Castelli, "Smart Heart Strategies: Best Ways to Beat Heart Disease," *Bottom Line/Health* 19, no. 4 (1998): 1–3.
16. "The Homocysteine-CVD Connection," *HealthNews* (October 25, 1999).
17. C. J. Boushey, S. A. A. Beresford, G. S. Omenn, and A. G. Motulsky, "A Quantitative Assessment of Plasma Homocysteine as a Risk Factor for Vascular Disease," *Journal of the American Medical Association* 274 (1995): 1049–1057.
18. "Inflammation May Be Key Cause of Heart Disease and More: Diet's Role" *Environmental Nutrition* 27 no. 7 (July 2004): 1, 4.
19. S. P. Helmrich, D. R. Ragland, R. W. Leung, and R. S. Paffenbarger, "Physical Activity and Reduced Occurrences of Non-Insulin-Dependent Diabetes Mellitus," *New England Journal of Medicine* 325 (1991): 147–152.

20. S. Liu et al., "A Prospective Study of Dietary Glycemic Load, Carbohydrate Intake, and Risk of Coronary Heart Disease in U. S. Women," *American Journal of Clinical Nutrition* 71 (2000): 1455–1461.
21. E. J. Mayer et al., "Intensity and Amount of Physical Activity in Relation to Insulin Sensitivity," *Journal of the American Medical Association* 279 (1998): 669–674.
22. G. M. Reaven, T. K. Strom, and B. Fox, *Syndrome X: Overcoming the Silent Killer That Can Give You a Heart Attack* (Englewood Cliffs, NJ: Simon & Schuster, 2000).
23. G. M. Reaven, "Syndrome X: The Little Known Cause of Many Heart Attacks," *Bottom Line/Health* 14 (June 2000).
24. "Checkup for the New Millennium," *Consumer Reports on Health* (December, 1999).
25. See Note 6.
26. R. Collins et al., "Blood Pressure, Stroke, and Coronary Heart Disease: Part 2. Short-Term Reductions in Blood Pressure: Overview of Randomized Drug Trials in Their Epidemiological Context," *Lancet* 335 (1990): 827–838.
27. S. N. Blair et al., "Influences of Cardiorespiratory Fitness and Other Precursors on Cardiovascular Disease and All-Cause Mortality in Men and Women," *Journal of the American Medical Association* 276 (1996): 205–210.

Assess Your Behavior

1. Are you accumulating a minimum of 30 minutes of physical activity on most days of the week?
2. Do you know your current BMI, blood pressure, and blood lipid profile?
3. Do you avoid all forms of tobacco use?
4. Is your current diet low in saturated fat and high in fiber intake?

Evaluate how well you understand the concepts presented in this chapter by answering the following questions.

1. The incidence of cardiovascular disease during the past 40 years in the United States has
   a. increased.
   b. decreased.
   c. remained constant.
   d. increased in some years and decreased in others.
   e. fluctuated according to medical technology.

2. Coronary heart disease
   a. is the single leading cause of death in the United States.
   b. is the leading cause of sudden cardiac deaths.
   c. is a condition in which the arteries that supply the heart muscle with oxygen and nutrients are narrowed by fatty deposits.
   d. accounts for approximately 20 percent of all cardio-vascular deaths.
   e. All of the above.

3. Regular aerobic activity helps
   a. lower LDL cholesterol.
   b. lower HDL cholesterol.
   c. increase triglycerides.
   d. decrease insulin sensitivity.
   e. All of the above.

4. The risk of heart disease increases with
   a. high LDL cholesterol.
   b. low HDL cholesterol.
   c. high concentration of homocysteine.
   d. high levels of hs-CRP.
   e. All of the above factors.

5. An optimal level of LDL cholesterol is
   a. between 200 and 239 mg/dl.
   b. at about 200 mg/dl.
   c. between 150 and 200 mg/dl.
   d. between 100 and 150 mg/dl.
   e. below 100 mg/dl.

6. To keep homocysteine from accumulating in the blood a person needs to
   a. decrease the intake of saturated fat.
   b. lower consumption of foods high in triglycerides.
   c. eat at five daily servings of fruits and vegetables.
   d. increase aerobic exercise.
   e. All of the above.

7. Statin drugs
   a. increase the liver's ability to remove blood cholesterol.
   b. decrease cholesterol.
   c. slow cholesterol production.
   d. decrease triglycerides.
   e. All of the above.

8. Type 2 diabetes is related closely to
   a. overeating.
   b. obesity.
   c. lack of physical activity.
   d. insulin resistance.
   e. All of the above factors.

9. Metabolic syndrome is related to
   a. low HDL cholesterol.
   b. high triglycerides.
   c. increased blood-clotting mechanism.
   d. an abnormal insulin response to carbohydrates.
   e. All of the above.

10. Which of the following factors may be linked to coronary heart disease?
    a. inflammation
    b. low HDL cholesterol
    c. gum disease
    d. smoking
    e. All factors may be linked to coronary heart disease.

Correct answers can be found on page 369.

Cardiovascular Disease Risk Analysis

Name: _____   Date: _____   Grade: _____

Instructor: _____   Course: _____   Section: _____

Necessary Lab Equipment
None required.

Objective
Evaluate family and lifestyle factors that may affect your risk for cardiovascular disease and cancer.

I. Cardiovascular Disease

	Yes	No
1. I accumulate between 30 and 60 minutes of physical activity on most days of the week.	☐	☐
2. I exercise aerobically a minimum of three times a week in the appropriate target zone for at least 20 minutes per session.	☐	☐
3. I am at or slightly below the health fitness recommended percent body fat (see Table 9.10, page 222, or a BMI below 25).	☐	☐
4. My blood lipids are within normal range.	☐	☐
5. I get 25 (women) to 38 (men) grams of fiber in my daily diet.	☐	☐
6. I eat more than five servings of fruits and vegetables every day.	☐	☐
7. I limit saturated fat, and cholesterol in my daily diet.	☐	☐
8. I am not a diabetic.	☐	☐
9. My blood pressure is normal.	☐	☐
10. I do not smoke cigarettes or use tobacco in any other form.	☐	☐
11. I manage stress adequately in daily life.	☐	☐
12. I do not have a personal or family history of heart disease.	☐	☐

Evaluation

Risk Category	Number of "no" Answers
Very Low Risk	0
Low Risk	1 or less
Moderate Risk	2
High Risk	3
Very High Risk	4 or more

II. In a few sentences, discuss your family and personal risk for cardiovascular disease:

_____

_____

_____

_____

_____

_____

_____

_____

_____

_____

_____

_____

III. Discuss lifestyle changes that you have already implemented in this course, as well as additional changes that you can make to decrease your own risk of developing cardiovascular disease in the future.

_____

_____

_____

_____

_____

_____

_____

_____

_____

_____

_____

_____

IV. Physical Activity Rating

Current number of daily steps: [   ]

Activity category (use Table 1.2, page 15): [   ]

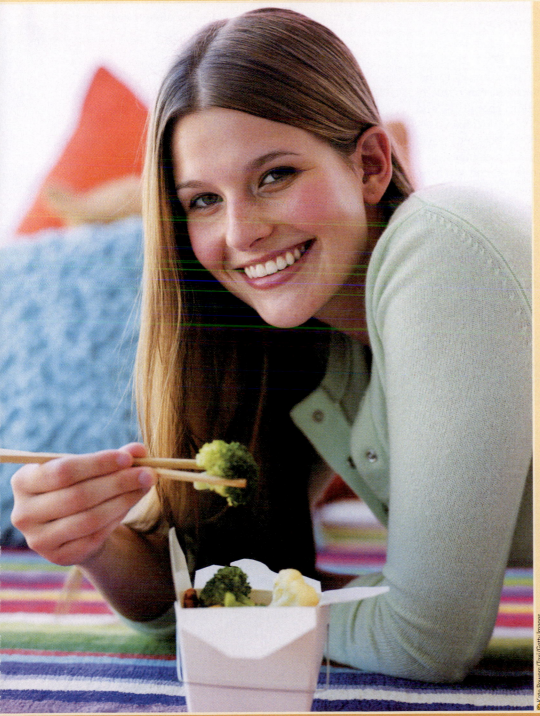

12

Cancer Prevention and Wellness

OBJECTIVES

Know the differences in characteristics of benign and malignant tumors.

Differentiate the major types of cancer.

Recognize precancerous conditions and warning signs of cancer.

Identify the three basic kinds of skin cancers.

Learn about the gender-specific cancers, their incidence, and their risk factors.

List guidelines for preventing cancer, including dietary guidelines.

Understand the role of self-examinations (and how to conduct them) and examinations by physicians.

© Kate Powers/Taxi/Getty Images

Cancer is second only to heart disease as the leading killer in the United States, accounting for about 23 percent of all deaths yearly. For the first time since statistics for cancer were initiated in the 1930s, the cancer rate declined slightly in 1996 and has stabilized since then. This decline is attributed to improved prevention and treatment, most markedly a reduction in cigarette smoking. Although the decline in mortality is certainly good news, cancer remains the number-one health fear of the American people. The American Cancer Society urges us to redouble our efforts to get people to stop smoking and to eat a healthier diet as the best preventive measures.

Development of Cancer

Cancer starts when an "initiator" alters DNA, the cell's basic genetic material, in a way that allows the cell to dictate its own rate of growth. The alteration can occur in minutes, or days, initiated by radiation, chemicals, and viruses. Having a cell with altered DNA, however, does not guarantee cancer. Fortunately, special enzymes travel up and down the DNA to repair breaks and changes.

Anything that accelerates the rate of cell division lessens the chance that repair enzymes will find the altered part of the DNA in time. Once a cell multiplies and incorporates its newly altered DNA into its genetic instructions, the cell no longer realizes that its DNA has been changed.

Compounds that increase cell division are called "promoters." They are thought to promote cancer either by reducing the time available for repair enzymes to act or by encouraging cells with altered DNA to develop and grow. Development and growth of these altered cells may take up to 20 years. Some common promoters are thought to be estrogen, alcohol, and dietary fat in excess.

Even after an altered cell has multiplied, cancer does not necessarily result. First, a cell mass must grow large enough to affect body metabolism. During this initial stage of growth, the immune system may find the altered cells and destroy them. Or the cancer cells themselves may be so defective that their own DNA limits their ability to grow, and they die anyway.

Actually, most of us probably have cancerous or **precancerous** cells in our bodies at some time. Many of these cells die because of mutation. Many more are destroyed by a healthy immune system. Occasionally, though, the immune system is unable to dominate, and cancer develops.

Benign and **malignant** tumors differ in the following ways:

1. Benign tumors resemble the normal tissues that surround them; malignant tumors do not.
2. The cells of benign tumors do not break off and metastasize; the cells of malignant tumors do.
3. Benign tumors do not invade surrounding tissues; malignant tumors do.
4. Benign tumors can be controlled by normal methods used to control any tissue growth; malignant tumors cannot.
5. Almost all benign tumors are encased (contained) in a fibrous capsule; very few malignant tumors are.
6. Benign tumors are not dangerous unless they interfere with blood flow; malignant tumors are fatal if untreated.

Survival depends on how early the cancer is diagnosed, what tissues are involved, the strength of the immune system, and potential treatment options. Cures have been discovered for some kinds of cancer. Equally important is that more than 9.8 million Americans with a history of cancer were alive in 2005. Currently, six in 10 people diagnosed with cancer are expected to be alive 5 years from the initial diagnosis.[1]

Incidence of Cancer

Someone in the United States dies of cancer every minute. It strikes people of all ages and is the leading killer of children between ages 3 and 14. More than half a million people in the United States die from cancer each year, and more than a million are diagnosed with cancer each year. One in every five deaths from any cause in the United States is from cancer.[2]

The incidence of cancer varies slightly between men and women. The most common cancers in men are prostate, lung, colon/rectal, and urinary/bladder, in that order. The most common cancers in women are lung, breast, colon/rectal, and uterine. Leading sites and deaths from cancer in men and women are shown in Figure 12.1.

Risk Factors for Cancer

In more than half of all diagnosed cases, the cancer has **metastasized**, making treatment more difficult. The American Cancer Society estimates that two in every five people who die from cancer could have been saved if they had been diagnosed sooner. In addition, we can go a long way toward preventing cancer by changing our behaviors.

The probable causes of cancer are many. We know that cancer is caused by certain substances in the environment. We also know that cigarette smoking and dietary factors play a role. So do heredity (the inherited tendency for certain kinds of cancers) and race. Some cancers can be caused by viruses. Viruses that increase the risk for cancer include Epstein-Barr, human papilloma, Hepatitis B, and T-cell leukemia/lymphoma. Although some controversy still surrounds the notion, increasing evidence suggests that attitudes and emotions might increase susceptibility to cancer and could cause physiological changes in the body that can lead to the development of cancer.

FIGURE 12.1 Estimated Cancer Incidence and Deaths by Site and Sex, 2005

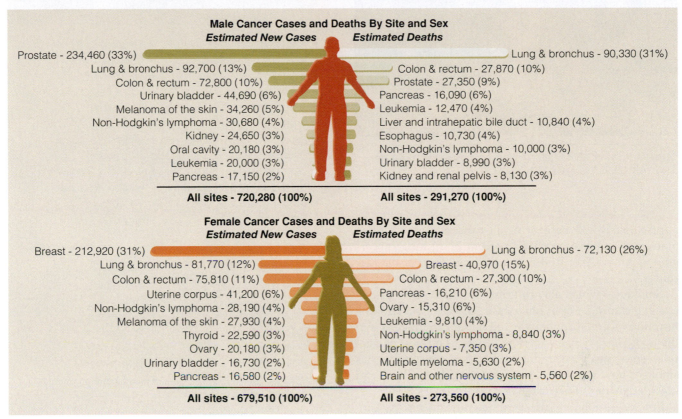

Male Cancer Cases and Deaths By Site and Sex
Estimated New Cases   *Estimated Deaths*

Prostate - 234,460 (33%)
Lung & bronchus - 92,700 (13%)
Colon & rectum - 72,800 (10%)
Urinary bladder - 44,690 (6%)
Melanoma of the skin - 34,260 (5%)
Non-Hodgkin's lymphoma - 30,680 (4%)
Kidney - 24,650 (3%)
Oral cavity - 20,180 (3%)
Leukemia - 20,000 (3%)
Pancreas - 17,150 (2%)

Lung & bronchus - 90,330 (31%)
Colon & rectum - 27,870 (10%)
Prostate - 27,350 (9%)
Pancreas - 16,090 (6%)
Leukemia - 12,470 (4%)
Liver and intrahepatic bile duct - 10,840 (4%)
Esophagus - 10,730 (4%)
Non-Hodgkin's lymphoma - 10,000 (3%)
Urinary bladder - 8,990 (3%)
Kidney and renal pelvis - 8,130 (3%)

All sites - 720,280 (100%)   **All sites - 291,270 (100%)**

Female Cancer Cases and Deaths By Site and Sex
Estimated New Cases   *Estimated Deaths*

Breast - 212,920 (31%)
Lung & bronchus - 81,770 (12%)
Colon & rectum - 75,810 (11%)
Uterine corpus - 41,200 (6%)
Non-Hodgkin's lymphoma - 28,190 (4%)
Melanoma of the skin - 27,930 (4%)
Thyroid - 22,590 (3%)
Ovary - 20,180 (3%)
Urinary bladder - 16,730 (2%)
Pancreas - 16,580 (2%)

Lung & bronchus - 72,130 (26%)
Breast - 40,970 (15%)
Colon & rectum - 27,300 (10%)
Pancreas - 16,210 (6%)
Ovary - 15,310 (6%)
Leukemia - 9,810 (4%)
Non-Hodgkin's lymphoma - 8,840 (3%)
Uterine corpus - 7,350 (3%)
Multiple myeloma - 5,630 (2%)
Brain and other nervous system - 5,560 (2%)

All sites - 679,510 (100%)   **All sites - 273,560 (100%)**

Note: These statistics exclude basal and squamous cell skin cancers and in situ carcinoma except cancer of the urinary bladder. Percentages may not total 100% because of rounding.

Source: From American Cancer Society, *Cancer Facts & Figures.* © 2004, American Cancer Society.

TABLE 12.1 Chances of Developing Invasive Cancers

Site	Sex	Birth to 39 Years	40 to 59 Years	60 to 79 Years	Ever (Birth to Death)
All sites	Male	1 in 58	1 in 13	1 in 3	1 in 2
	Female	1 in 52	1 in 11	1 in 4	1 in 3
Breast	Female	1 in 217	1 in 26	1 in 15	1 in 8
Colon and Rectum	Male	1 in 1,667	1 in 108	1 in 23	1 in 16
	Female	1 in 2,000	1 in 137	1 in 30	1 in 17
Prostate	Male	<1 in 10,000	1 in 103	1 in 8	1 in 6

Source: *CA—A Cancer Journal for Clinicians*, 45, no. 1.

FIGURE 12.2 Estimate of the Relative Roles of the Major Cancer-Causing Factors

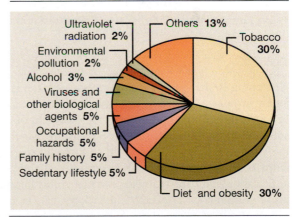

Ultraviolet radiation 2%
Environmental pollution 2%
Alcohol 3%
Viruses and other biological agents 5%
Occupational hazards 5%
Family history 5%
Sedentary lifestyle 5%
Others 13%
Tobacco 30%
Diet and obesity 30%

Table 12.1 shows the probability of developing invasive cancers. You can't control some causes of cancer—heredity and race, for instance—but you can actively reduce many identified risk factors and help beat the odds of developing cancer (see Figure 12.2). Proven, general risk factors are discussed next.

TOBACCO

Cigarette smoking has been called the number one preventable cause of death in the United States. It is estimated to directly cause

Cancer A group of more than a hundred diseases in which cells grow at an uncontrolled rate, mature in an abnormal way, and invade nearby tissues.

Precancerous Describes any of the conditions in which a benign (noncancerous) condition has the potential to become cancerous.

Benign Noncancerous.

Malignant Cancerous.

Metastasis The process that occurs when cancer cells from one growth break off, enter the bloodstream or lymph system, and are carried to a distant part of the body, where they cause another cancerous growth to begin.

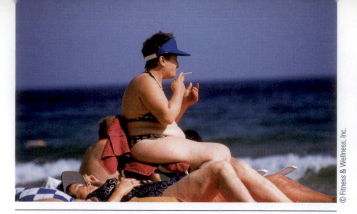

Cigarette smoking, obesity, and excessive exposure to the sun are major risk factors for cancer.

© Fitness & Wellness, Inc.

approximately 30 percent of all cancers in the United States and approximately 87 percent of all lung cancers among Americans. It also is a leading cause of bladder cancer.[3]

Smoking—which also contributes to other serious diseases, including emphysema, heart disease, and stroke—introduces carbon monoxide and lethal **carcinogens** into the body. The chance of getting cancer as a result of cigarette smoking is related to how long the person has smoked, how many packs a day he or she smokes, and how deeply the smoke is inhaled.

Smokeless tobacco also poses significant risk for cancer, despite the persistent myth that it's okay to "chew" as long as you don't smoke. Smokeless or chewing tobacco is a leading cause of cancer of the mouth, throat, esophagus, and larynx.

Also of concern is **secondhand smoke**. Children are at particular risk for lung diseases such as bronchitis. Nonsmokers who live with smokers have been found to develop lung cancer at a higher rate than other nonsmokers.

DIET

According to the American Cancer Society, diet is a major factor in nearly a third of all cancers. Some scientists believe the role of diet may be equivalent to that of cigarette smoking in boosting the risk for developing cancer. A diet high in saturated fats increases the risk for cancer. Specific culprits are tropical oils (such as coconut oil and palm oil) and animal fats (fatty meats, whole milk, cheese, and other animal-source foods). The risk for cancer increases substantially if more than 30 percent of daily calories comes from fat and more than 10 percent comes from saturated fats.

Also, if the diet doesn't contain enough fiber, the risk of certain kinds of cancers, especially cancer of the colon, may increase significantly. Other dietary factors that increase the risk for cancer include

- foods cured or pickled with salt or nitrites, such as lunch meats,
- smoked foods,
- charcoal-broiled foods,
- foods containing cyclamates (a type of artificial sweetener),
- vitamin and mineral deficiency, and
- excessive alcohol consumption.

ENVIRONMENTAL CARCINOGENS

Carcinogens include atmospheric agents ranging from electromagnetic radiation and radon gas to chemicals such as vinyl chloride and arsenic. In most cases of environmental carcinogens, the risk of cancer is related to the dose. A one-time massive exposure to a carcinogen may cause cancer, as can prolonged, long-term exposure to small amounts.

As carcinogens are identified, policies are instituted to protect the public from exposure. For example, strict building codes now ban the use of asbestos. Accidental exposure still occurs, however, when old buildings are demolished or remodeled. Schools, in particular, have to take extreme measures to prevent children from being exposed to the asbestos, which formerly was used for fireproofing.

The chemicals in the water we drink, the hydrocarbons emitted in automobile exhaust, and the agents in some insecticides and pesticides have been shown to cause cancer at certain levels. Few people are exposed to high levels of these pollutants, but the effects of chronic, low-level exposure are being studied.

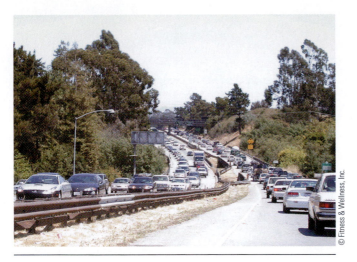

Automobile exhaust was a leading source of environmental carcinogens before the advent of catalytic converters.

MEDICAL SUBSTANCES

Cancer can follow exposure to certain medical substances such as drugs, agents used in chemotherapy, medications used to suppress the immune system, hormones, and X-rays. For example, the drug diethylstilbestrol (DES)—used to treat complications and prevent miscarriages until the mid-1960s—was found to cause cancer of the female reproductive organs in the daughters of women who took the drug.

Although cancer caused by X-rays is rare, it can happen from exposure to large doses of radiation. In most cases, precise calibration of X-ray equipment has helped prevent accidental exposure to large doses. The effects of radiation are cumulative, so repeated small doses over a long time may be a cause for concern. Lead shields are used to protect parts of the body that are not being X-rayed from accidental exposure.

VIRUSES

The first virus known to cause cancer was identified in 1911 by a scientist who injected it into chickens and cancerous tumors resulted. Since that time, exhaustive research has been conducted in the attempt to identify viruses that may cause cancers in humans.

One group of viruses—three variants of the human papilloma virus (HPV), which causes genital warts—is suspected of causing cervical cancer and other genital malignancies. These cancer-causing viruses can be transmitted sexually.

Approximately 2 percent of all cancers in the United States may be related to viruses. In some cases the virus may be responsible for causing or initiating the cancer, and once the disease takes hold, the virus no longer is in the picture. In other situations the viruses may not actually cause the cancer but may increase the risk of developing cancer in the first place.

Scientists also have identified a particular kind of virus called **retroviruses**. The human immunodeficiency virus (HIV), which causes AIDS, is a retrovirus.

Controversy still surrounds the notion of cancer-causing viruses. Most scientists conclude that certain viruses may cause cancer only under certain circumstances. For example, Epstein-Barr virus (EBV), which causes mononucleosis in the United States, causes a cancer called Burkitt's lymphoma among children in Africa. Scientists now are researching the possibility that EBV, or similar viruses responsible for herpes, may sharply increase the risk of Hodgkin's disease, cervical cancer, and some forms of leukemia.

HEREDITY

Heredity is a factor in an estimated 10 percent of all cancers in the United States. Approximately 14 million Americans are at risk because they inherited the tendency for certain malignancies.[4] Cancers caused by hereditary factors often begin in childhood. Such factors can increase the likelihood of developing the cancer by as much as 30 times normal odds.

Critical Thinking

1. Have you ever had, or do you now have, any family members with cancer?
2. Can you identify lifestyle or environmental factors as possible contributors to the disease?
3. If not, are you concerned about your genetic predisposition, and, if so, are you making lifestyle changes to decrease your risk?

In some cases, genetic markers called **oncogenes** can be used to predict cancer. Cancer also can be predicted if **suppressor genes**, which protect against cancer, are missing from certain genetic material.

In a few cases, the cancer itself is inherited. One example is retinoblastoma, a cancer of the eye that occurs in infants and young children. More often, what is inherited is not the actual cancer but, rather, the predisposition for

Carcinogens Cancer-causing substances.

Secondhand smoke A mixture of smoke exhaled by smokers and smoke from the burning portion of a cigarette, pipe, or cigar.

Retroviruses Viruses that invade a cell's genetic structure and are passed on to each succeeding generation of cells as the cells divide.

Oncogenes Pieces of genetic material that serve as markers to predict later mutation and development of certain cancers, probably by encouraging mutation of related cells.

Suppressor genes Pieces of genetic material that are part of a cell's normal protective mechanism against development of cancer.

(or the tendency to develop) that cancer. Exciting research has identified, for example, a gene that predisposes its carriers to cancer of the colon. Once the gene is identified, a person carrying the gene can take certain precautions and undergo aggressive early screening to improve the odds of preventing or successfully treating the disease.

The risk for certain leukemias can be genetically passed from parent to child. Also, the tendency for lung, colon, breast, uterine, prostate, bone, brain, stomach, and adrenal gland cancers can be inherited.

STRESS

An individual's response to stress has been linked to the risk for developing cancer, as well as certain other diseases such as heart disease. Chronic stress and the hormones it unleashes on the body interfere with the ability of the immune system to recognize cancerous cells and destroy them.

Although controversy surrounds the idea, researchers have identified a "cancer-prone" personality, a collection of traits that seem to occur in people who later develop cancer. Called the "Type C" personality, it is characterized by unusual compliance and the tendency to internalize conflict. It also is marked by the individual's inability to deal with stress in a healthy way (see Chapter 2).

CHRONIC IRRITATION

Evidence indicates that chronic irritation of cells or tissues can lead to the development of cancer. Linked to certain kinds of cancers and increased risk for cancer are

- chronic low-grade infections;
- repeated bladder infections;
- repeated ulceration of tissues;
- chronic infection of scar tissue;
- constant irritation of a mole or other benign growth;
- certain kinds of injuries; and
- long-term irritation of gallstones against the gallbladder.

ESTROGEN-REPLACEMENT THERAPY

When the level of estrogen, normally produced by the ovaries, tapers off as a woman reaches menopause, physicians traditionally prescribed estrogen-replacement therapy to ease or delay the troublesome symptoms of menopause. Evidence shows that estrogen-replacement therapy also helps prevent osteoporosis, a loss of bone tissue that affects mostly older women. Estrogen-replacement therapy, however, increases the risk of breast cancer and endometrial cancer (a cancer of the lining of the uterus).

Types of Cancer

In addition to being familiar with general risk factors, if you know the specific risk factors for various kinds of cancers, you will be able to reduce the odds of developing one or more of the types of cancer. Cancers have been classified according to six general types:

1. *Carcinomas*. Spread through the bloodstream and lymph system, carcinomas—the most common kind of cancers—affect the tissues that line most body cavities and cover body surfaces. Examples are lung cancer, breast cancer, skin cancer, colon cancer, and uterine cancer. (If the cancer occurs in a gland, it is called an *adenocarcinoma*.)
2. *Sarcomas*. Spread through the bloodstream, sarcomas affect the connective tissues of the body, such as the muscles, bones, and cartilage. Although sarcomas are not as common as carcinomas, they grow and spread more rapidly and form more solid tumors.
3. *Lymphomas*. Spread through the lymph system, lymphomas are cancers of the lymphatic, or infection-fighting, cells. Lymph nodes in the groin, armpits, and neck can be affected. An example of lymphoma is Hodgkin's disease.
4. *Melanomas*. Spread through the bloodstream, melanomas affect the skin. Generally beginning as a mole that later becomes cancerous, they grow and spread rapidly.

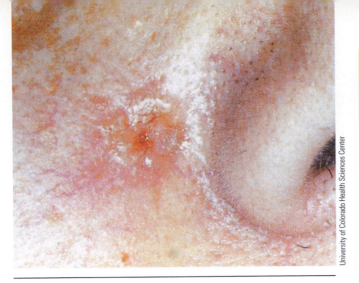

Basal cell carcinoma.

5. *Leukemias.* Spread through the bloodstream, leukemias affect the tissues that manufacture blood, especially the spleen and the bone marrow.

6. *Neuroblastomas.* Spread through the bloodstream, neuroblastomas affect the nervous system or the adrenal glands. Relatively uncommon, they occur most often in children under age 10.

Cancer Sites

Following are some common cancer sites and risk factors that contribute to these cancers. Table 12.2 summarizes pertinent data on these cancers.

SKIN CANCER

More than a million Americans were diagnosed with some form of skin cancer in the year 2005. Skin cancer is probably the most underrated type of cancer. It accounts for approximately 40 percent of all cancers and is the fastest-growing type of cancer in men over 50. The sharp increase in the incidence of skin cancer is alarming. Over the past decade, it has increased about 90 percent. As many as 1 in every 90 Americans has some type of skin cancer.

The three basic kinds of skin cancers are:

1. *Basal cell carcinoma.* This is the most common, and least serious, of the skin cancers. It grows slowly and usually does not spread. Most basal cell carcinomas occur on the face, neck, and hands—areas of frequent exposure to the sun.

2. *Squamous cell carcinoma.* This type of cancer grows faster than the basal cell type and involves deeper layers of skin, but it rarely spreads to other parts of the body.

3. *Malignant melanoma.* This rapidly growing cancer is the most dangerous of the skin cancers and almost always spreads to other organs. According to the American Cancer Society, of the 9,600 people who die

Skin Types

A fair-skinned person (Type 1) in the sun at noon and at an elevation of about 5,000 feet stands a good chance of beginning to burn within 10 minutes. The times are determined by multiplying the sun-protection factor (SPF) number by 10 minutes. For example, SPF 15 × 10 min = 150 min = 2 hrs 30 min. To determine how long a given SPF will protect your skin, this six-point standard scale used by dermatologists gives guidelines for your exposure limits.

Type 1—Fair skin with blue or green eyes and light blond or red hair; typical time for skin to burn: 10–20 minutes.

Type 2—Fair skin with deep blue, hazel, or brown eyes and ash blond, deep red, or light brown hair; typical burn time: 15–30 minutes.

Type 3—Medium skin with brown eyes and brown hair; typical burn time: 20–40 minutes.

Type 4—Light to medium brown skin with dark brown eyes and hair; typical burn time: 25–50 minutes.

Type 5—Light to golden brown skin with dark brown eyes and black hair; typical burn time: 30–60 minutes.

Type 6—Brown to deepest brown skin with dark brown eyes and black hair; typical burn time: 40–75 minutes.

from skin cancer each year, approximately 7,700 succumb to malignant melanoma. It is the number-one cancer killer of American women ages 25 to 29 and number two for women ages 30 to 34.

Basal and squamous cell carcinomas are detected and treated quite easily. Malignant melanoma can be treated successfully if it is diagnosed and treated early. If not treated early, metastasis makes treatment extremely difficult.

The risk factors for skin cancer include

- sun exposure (most dangerous are ultraviolet B rays, at their strongest between 10 AM and 4 PM),
- fair skin that burns easily and rarely tans,
- blonde and red hair,
- artificial sources of ultraviolet rays, such as tanning booths and sunlamps,
- a history of one or more severe sunburns,
- a dark brown or black wart,
- birthmarks and congenital moles (although these do not always become cancerous, they should be watched closely and removed if they begin to grow or change in appearance),
- moles that are irritated chronically (moles at the waistline, bra line, or other areas where clothing rubs them constantly), and
- occupational exposure to creosote, coal tar, pitch, arsenic, or radium.

Danger signs of skin cancer are given in Figure 12.3.

TABLE 12.2 Common Cancers

	Risk Factors	Warning Signals	Early Detection	Treatment	5-Year Survival with Treatment
Lung cancer	Cigarette smoking for 20 or more years; exposure to certain industrial substances, particularly asbestos; secondhand smoke; radiation; radon.	Persistent cough, sputum streaked with blood, chest pain, recurring bronchitis or pneumonia.	Difficult to detect early. Diagnosis based on chest x-ray, sputum testing, fiberoptic bronchoscopy (direct examination of the lungs by means of a specially lighted tube).	Surgery, radiation therapy, chemotherapy.	The leading cause of cancer death among both men and women.
Breast cancer	Over age 50, personal or family history of breast cancer, no children or first child after age 30, dense breast tissue, obesity, high fat intake, alcohol, estrogen replacement therapy after menopause.	Breast changes: lumps, thickening, swelling, puckering, dimpling, skin irritation, nipple distortion, scaliness, discharge, pain, tenderness.	Monthly breast self-examination. Professional breast exam every 3 years for women ages 20–40 and every year over age 40. Yearly mammography for all women over 50, every 1 or 2 years for women 40–49; baseline mammogram for those 35–39. Tissue biopsy confirms diagnosis.	Surgery, from lumpectomy (local removal of tumor) to a modified radical mastectomy (removal of breast and lymph glands, leaving underlying muscle intact); radiation; chemotherapy; or all three. For metastatic breast cancer, autologous bone marrow transplantation.	Until recently, the leading cause of cancer death in women; now surpassed by lung cancer.
Uterine and cervical cancer	For cervical cancer: early age of first intercourse, multiple sex partners, genital herpes, human papilloma virus infection, significant exposure to secondhand smoke. For uterine cancer: infertility, failure to ovulate, prolonged estrogen therapy, obesity.	Unusual vaginal bleeding or discharge.	Pap smear every 3 years after two initial negative tests 1 year apart.	Surgery, radiation, or a combination of the two. In precancerous stages, cervical cells may be destroyed by extreme cold or intense heat. Precancerous endometrial changes are treated with the hormone progesterone.	Cervical cancer mortality has declined 70% during the last 40 years with wider application of the Pap smear. Postmenopausal women with abnormal bleeding should be checked.
Ovarian cancer	Family history of ovarian cancer; personal history of breast cancer; obesity; infertility (because the abnormality that interferes with conception may also play a role in cancer development); low levels of transferase, an enzyme involved in metabolism of dairy foods.	Often no obvious symptoms until advanced stages. Painless swelling of abdomen; irregular bleeding; lower abdominal pain; digestive and urinary abnormalities; fatigue; backache; bloating; weight gain.	Women with family history: annual pelvic and abdominal exams; blood test for a tumor marker called CA125 every 6 months; annual pelvic ultrasound. (In cases of very high risk, some oncologists recommend prophylactic removal of ovaries no later than age 35.)	Surgery, sometimes in combination with chemotherapy or radiation.	85% if detected and treated early; 23% in advanced cases.

Cancer type	Risk factors	Detection	Treatment	Notes
Colon and rectum cancer	Personal or family history of colon and rectal cancer or polyps (growths) in the colon or rectum; inflammatory bowel disease; high-fat, low-fiber diet.	Unusual bleeding from rectum, blood in stool, a change in bowel habits.	Digital rectal exam (once a year after age 40); stool-blood slide test that detects blood in feces (every year after age 50); proctosigmoidoscopy, a rectal exam using a hollow, lighted tube (every 3–5 years after age 50, following 2 consecutive normal annual exams). Diagnosis may require a colonoscopy (viewing the entire colon) or a barium enema.	Surgery, sometimes in combination with chemotherapy or radiation.	Considered a highly curable disease when digital and proctoscopy examinations are included in routine checkups.
Skin cancer (melanoma)	Excessive exposure to sun, fair complexion, occupational exposure to carcinogens. (Inherited skin disorders, such as xeroderma pigmentosum and familial atypical multiple mole melanoma, account for 10% of cases.)	Unusual skin condition, especially a change in size or color of a mole; appearance of darkly pigmented growth or spot; oozing, scaliness, bleeding; appearance of a bump; change in sensation, itchiness, tenderness, or pain.	Examine moles on your skin once a month.	Surgery, radiation, electrodesiccation (tissue destruction by heat), cryosurgery (tissue destruction by cold), or a combination of therapies.	Melanoma is readily detected by observation and diagnosed by simple biopsy.
Oral cancer	Heavy smoking of cigarettes, cigars, pipes; excessive drinking; use of chewing tobacco.	A sore that bleeds easily and doesn't heal; a lump or thickening; a reddish or whitish patch; difficulty chewing, swallowing, or moving the tongue or jaws.	Regular exams by your dentist or primary-care physician.	Surgery and radiation.	Many more lives should be saved because the mouth is easily accessible to visual examination by physicians and dentists.
Leukemia	Down syndrome and other inherited abnormalities; excessive exposure to radiation and to certain chemicals, such as benzene.	Difficult to detect early because its symptoms are often similar to those of less serious conditions, such as flu. Diagnosis is based on blood tests and bone-marrow biopsy.	Chemotherapy, drugs, blood transfusions, and antibiotics; bone-marrow transplants.	Leukemias are cancers of blood-forming tissues and are characterized by the abnormal production of immature white blood cells. Acute leukemia strikes mainly children and is treated by drugs that have extended life from a few months to as much as 10 years. Chronic leukemia strikes usually after age 25 and progresses less rapidly.
Testicular cancer	Young men under age 35.	Testicular self-examinations.	Surgical removal of the diseased testis, radiation therapy, chemotherapy, removal of nearby lymph nodes.	96% if the cancer is localized; 89% overall.
Prostate cancer	Risk increases with age, African-American men more susceptible than whites. Suspected risk factors: family history, high-fat diet, exposure to heavy metal cadmium, high number of sexual partners, history of frequent STDs.	Frequent urination, difficulty urinating, blood in the urine, lower back pain.	Rectal exam; PSA blood test available.	Surgical removal of prostate, conventional radiation, or implanting "seeds" of radioactive iodine in the prostate; hormone therapy.	Occurs mainly in men over 60; can be detected by digital rectal exam at annual checkup.

Adapted from the American Cancer Society, *Cancer Facts and Figures* (2000).

FIGURE 12.3 Danger Signs of Skin Cancer

The American Academy of Dermatology advises: Know your spots and do a spot check. Also, have your skin checked by a doctor for any changes once a year. If you notice one of the following changes in your skin, you should see your family doctor or dermatologist immediately:

- Basal-cell or squamous-cell carcinomas: any lesion that is new, starts growing, starts changing, bleeds, is scabby, or doesn't heal.
- Melanoma:

    A. *Asymmetry:* One half of a mole or lesion doesn't look like the other half.

    B. *Border:* A mole has an irregular, scalloped, or not clearly defined border.

    C. *Color:* The color varies or is not uniform from one area of a mole or lesion to another, whether the color is tan, brown, black, white, red, or blue.

    D. *Diameter:* The lesion is larger than 6 millimeters (one-quarter inch) or larger than a pencil eraser.

- Actinic keratosis: a precancerous skin lesion that is dry, scaly, reddish, and slightly raised.

Melanoma Warnings

Asymmetrical

Border irregular

Color varied

Diameter larger than ¼"

Adapted from *FDA Consumer*, May 1991.

Precancerous Skin Conditions

Precancerous conditions are those in which a benign, or non-cancerous, condition becomes cancerous for one reason or another. Generally, physicians recommend that the following precancerous skin conditions be surgically removed or repaired to prevent their becoming cancerous, regardless of how low the risk may be:

- Benign tumors
- Chronic scaly patches on the skin
- Brown or black warts
- Moles subject to chronic irritation (such as those on the waist that are constantly rubbed by a waistband or belt)
- A lump on the lip, tongue, or inside the cheek
- A scaly patch on the inside of the cheek

The UV Index

The Ultraviolet Index is a measure of the sun's damaging ultraviolet rays during the hottest part of the day. This chart can help you interpret the UV Index the next time you see one:

Solar-hazard Rating	Health Risk	Time to Burn*
0–2	Very low	More than 30 minutes
3–4	Low	15 to 90 minutes
5–6	Moderate	10 to 60 minutes
7–9	High	7 to 35 minutes
10 & over	Very high	5 to 30 minutes

* The "time to burn" ranges are based on the amount of time it takes for a person to sunburn and varies widely by skin type.

Critical Thinking

1. What significance does a "healthy tan" have in your social life?
2. Are you a "sun worshiper," or are you concerned about skin damage, premature aging, and potential skin cancer in your future?

LUNG CANCER

The leading cancer killer among both men and women, lung cancer caused an estimated 163,510 deaths in 2005. Lung cancer occurs almost exclusively among cigarette smokers, although a few cases do develop in individuals who have never smoked. According to the U.S. Department of Health and Human Services, the cellular changes and tissue damage that lead to lung cancer have been observed in 93 percent of active smokers and 6 percent of former smokers but in only 1 percent of those who have never smoked. Researchers estimate that close to 90 percent of all lung cancers could be eliminated if people did not smoke.

Once a disease affecting men predominantly, lung cancer in women has risen along with higher smoking rates among women. Today, lung cancer is decreasing steadily in men while increasing steadily in African Americans, teenagers, and women. Lung cancer now surpasses breast cancer as the leading cause of cancer deaths in women.

Lung cancer spreads rapidly, and it is rarely detected early, because it usually does not cause symptoms or show up on an X-ray until it is quite advanced. By that time, the damage usually is too extensive to treat successfully. The 5-year survival rate of lung cancer patients is only about 15 percent.

When symptoms do arise, they might be manifested by persistent hoarseness, a nagging cough, repeated bouts of pneumonia or bronchitis, or spitting up blood. Treatment

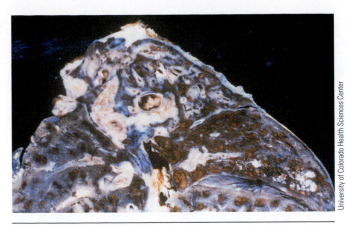

University of Colorado Health Sciences Center

Lung cancer is the frequent result of smoking.

consists of surgery for localized cancers combined with radiation and chemotherapy if the cancer has spread.

The number-one risk factor for lung cancer is cigarette smoking. Most at risk are those who have smoked more than 20 years. Secondhand smoke inhaled by nonsmokers who live or work with smokers also increases the risk for lung cancer significantly. The Centers for Disease Control and Prevention estimate that 3,000 nonsmokers die each year from lung cancer caused by secondhand tobacco smoke. Other risk factors for lung cancer include

- exposure to asbestos,
- high-level air pollution,
- exposure to carcinogenic chemicals,
- exposure to certain metals (cadmium, cobalt, chromium, silver, nickel, steel),
- exposure to arsenic or radioactive ores, and
- exposure to radon gas.

All other risk factors for lung cancer are much more marked if the individual also smokes.

COLON AND RECTAL CANCER

Cancer of the colon and rectum—also called colorectal cancer—is the third leading cancer killer in the United States among both men and women. According to the American Cancer Society, about 145,000 new cases are diagnosed each year, and almost 56,000 Americans die of colorectal cancer annually. If detected early, colorectal cancer usually can be treated successfully because it grows and spreads quite slowly. Treatment usually consists of radiation or surgery.

The most common signs of colorectal cancer are changes in bowel habits and bleeding from the rectum not attributable to hemorrhoids. Another sign is bright red blood in the stools that is not attributable to hemorrhoids. Risk factors include

- a personal or family history of polyps (benign growths) in the colon or rectum,
- a family history of colorectal cancer,
- a diet high in fats and low in fiber, and
- inflammatory bowel problems, such as colitis.

Age also is a risk factor, which increases sharply after age 40. Researchers believe that at least half, and possibly all, cases of colorectal cancer can be attributed to a genetic tendency for polyps in the colon or rectum combined with a high-fat, low-fiber diet.

The American Cancer Society recommends a colon exam called a flexible sigmoidoscopy every 5 years for men and women alike beginning at age 50. Those with a family history of colorectal cancer or ulcerative colitis should be tested beginning at age 40.

BREAST CANCER

The second leading cancer killer of women (lung cancer is number one), breast cancer kills more than 40,000 American women each year (and 400 men). Approximately 211,000 women in the United States were diagnosed with breast cancer in 2005. American Cancer Society projects that one in eight American women will develop breast cancer at some time in her life.

Early detection is the key. With early detection and treatment, the 5-year survival rate for breast cancer can be over 90 percent. Heightened awareness of the disease, together with breast self-examination and regular mammograms beginning at a younger age, have improved survival rates because cancers are being diagnosed earlier.

General symptoms of breast cancer include a thickening or lump in the breast; distortion or dimpling of a breast; swollen lymph nodes under the arm; or retraction, pain, discharge, or scaliness of the nipple. General risk factors for breast cancer include

- a grandmother, mother, or sister who has had breast cancer,
- early onset of menstruation (before age 12),
- delayed onset of menopause (after age 55),
- first pregnancy after age 30,
- obesity,
- a woman who has never been pregnant,
- a woman who has never breastfed, and
- age (dramatic increase after age 50).

A report from the Utah Population Database suggests that 17 to 19 percent of breast cancer cases may be attributable to a family history of the disease. Also, women with a first-degree relative with colon cancer had a 30-percent increase in risk for breast cancer. A family history of breast cancer, however, does not necessarily affect the prognosis or outcome adversely.

Hormone replacement therapy (HRT) may be associated with a higher risk. Some researchers believe the progestin component of HRT may have a greater impact on risk than the estrogen component. Because of the increased risk, some gynecologists advise against long-term use of oral contraceptives in young women who have not borne children.

Despite earlier findings that a high-fat diet raises the risk, more recent studies have found little support for a role of dietary fat in the onset of breast cancer. Evidence is mounting that daily alcohol consumption does increase the risk, however. Daily consumption of vitamin A—as little as one carrot—may reduce the risk.

Exercise also may reduce the risk for breast cancer. Some researchers think exercise may change the proportions of estrogen and progesterone produced during the menstrual cycle, which may affect the risk. Other studies reveal interesting findings. According to one of these, the longer a woman breastfeeds and the more babies she nurses, the less is her risk for breast cancer. Environmental factors—specifically, pesticide residues in food—also have been implicated, but this is difficult to study systematically.

Many factors probably contribute to a woman's risk for developing breast cancer, and the known risk factors account for only a small percentage. The majority of patients (60 to 70 percent) have no known risk factors for the disease except older age. Thus, age is the most influential known risk factor for breast cancer.

CERVICAL CANCER

More than half of all uterine cancers start in the cervix, the neck of the uterus that protrudes into the top end of the vagina. The death rate from cancer of the cervix has decreased more than 70 percent during the past four decades because of early detection, mainly in the form of Pap smears (especially among younger women) and regular gynecological examinations.

With early diagnosis, treatment of cervical cancer usually is successful because the cancer has not spread. Unusual vaginal bleeding or discharge is often an early symptom. Risk factors for cervical cancer include

- early age at first intercourse,
- multiple sex partners,
- a history of viral genital infections, especially herpes and the human papilloma virus, and
- cigarette smoking.

UTERINE CANCER

Uterine cancer, which involves the endometrium, or lining, of the uterus, strikes approximately 41,000 women in the United States each year. Because of improved early detection, the death rate from uterine cancer has fallen dramatically, and only about 7,300 deaths a year in the United States were attributed to uterine cancer. With early detection, treatment generally is successful. Symptoms of uterine cancer might be unusual vaginal discharge, unusual vaginal bleeding, or bleeding between menstrual periods. Risk factors for uterine cancer include

- late onset of menopause,
- history of infertility/failure to ovulate,
- prolonged estrogen replacement therapy,
- obesity, and
- diabetes.

OVARIAN CANCER

Although ovarian cancer claims a relatively few 16,000 American women each year, it is a particularly difficult cancer because it typically reveals no symptoms and can be difficult to diagnose until it is in its latest stages. Late symptoms include abdominal swelling or bloating (the most common sign), persistent abdominal gas, and unexplained stomachaches or indigestion.

Age is a factor. The risk increases with age and is highest for women in their 60s. For unknown reasons, the rates are higher in Jewish women. This form of cancer also strikes Americans, Scandinavians, and Scots at three times the rate it is found in Japanese women. Other risk factors include

- a grandmother, mother, or sister who has had ovarian cancer,
- never having children (doubles the risk),
- use of oral contraceptives,
- occurrence of colorectal, breast, or uterine cancer (doubles the risk), and
- early onset of ovulation.

A diet high in fat may be a risk factor for ovarian cancer, though more research is needed.

PROSTATE CANCER

The leading cancer in American men and the second leading cause of cancer death in men (after lung cancer), prostate cancer strikes more than 232,000 men in the United States every year and about 30,000 die from it. Prostate cancer often is detected early because it generally provokes an array of symptoms fairly early in its development. The symptoms, however, can be mistaken for signs of other, more common ailments, such as an enlarged prostate or bladder infection.

If detected early, prostate cancer has been treated successfully in more than 80 percent of the cases. A blood test that measures the amount of prostate-specific antigen (PSA) in the blood can be used to help diagnose prostate cancer. This test is recommended for men beginning at age 50.

Signs and symptoms of prostate cancer include pain in the pelvis, lower back, or upper thighs; blood in the urine or semen; pain or burning during urination; frequent urination; and weak or interrupted urine, difficulty starting or stopping the flow of urine, or inability to urinate.

The risk for prostate cancer increases with age. For that reason, the American Cancer Society recommends an annual prostate exam beginning at age 50. At highest risk are men over age 65, in whom more than 80 percent of all prostate cancers are diagnosed. Another substantial risk factor is race: African-American men have the highest rate of prostate cancer in the world (30 percent higher than for Caucasians). Oddly enough, the cancer is relatively rare in Africa; and is much more common in North America and northwest Europe than it is in Central and South America and the Near East.

Other risk factors include

- a family history of prostate cancer,
- occupational exposure to cadmium, and
- a high-fat diet.

TESTICULAR CANCER

Although testicular cancer is not one of the most common types of cancer in the United States, it is the most common cancer in young men between ages 17 and 34. Of all deaths from cancer in that age group, 12 percent are from testicular cancer. For unknown reasons, the incidence of testicular cancer in this age group has been increasing steadily.

If this cancer is found in its early stages, the chances for cure are nearly 100 percent. Early detection is the key to successful treatment. Many men discover the cancer themselves, through self-examination. The major warning sign is an often-painless thickening or hard lump in the testicle. Other signs include pain or a sensation of heaviness in the affected testicle, an accumulation of fluid or blood in the scrotum, and a dull ache in the groin that may involve the lower abdomen. Although the exact cause of testicular cancer is not known, identified risk factors for testicular cancer include

- a testicle that did not descend until after age 6 (the risk can be 40 times as high), and
- a grandfather, father, or brother who has had testicular cancer.

BLADDER CANCER

Approximately 53,000 new cases of bladder cancer are diagnosed each year in the United States, and more than 13,000 Americans die from this form of cancer each year. If the cancer is detected while it is still confined to the bladder—before it has metastasized to involve other organs—almost nine in 10 cases can be cured. A new test called "flow cytometry" currently is being evaluated as an early detection tool for bladder cancer.

The most common signs of bladder cancer are more frequent urination, and blood in the urine. The cancer is four times more common in men than in women. Other risk factors are

- cigarette smoking (smoking is believed to cause almost half the bladder cancers in men and approximately 40 percent of the bladder cancers in women),
- occupational exposure to leather and rubber,
- occupational exposure to dyes, and
- living in an urban area.

PANCREATIC CANCER

Although pancreatic cancer is not one of the most common cancers, its incidence has more than doubled in the past two decades, making it the fourth most common cancer killer in U.S. men and the fifth most common cancer killer among U.S. women.

About 32,180 new cases are diagnosed in the United States each year, and 31,800 Americans die of pancreatic cancer yearly. The survival rate from pancreatic cancer is low because the disease spreads rapidly. Few patients with pancreatic cancer survive more than 3 years. In addition, pancreatic cancer is a "silent" disease, usually progressing without symptoms until it is in extremely advanced stages.

The risk for pancreatic cancer increases with age. The highest risk is between ages 65 and 79. Although more men die of pancreatic cancer each year, more women are diagnosed with pancreatic cancer. African Americans are at higher risk than people of other races. Other risk factors include

- smoking cigarettes,
- consuming alcohol,
- eating a high-fat diet, and
- being exposed to gasoline or some chemical cleaners on the job.

ORAL CANCER

The incidence of oral cancer has increased substantially over the past two decades, and this correlates with the popularity of smokeless tobacco, or chewing tobacco. Twice as many men as women get oral cancer. More than 29,000 Americans are diagnosed with oral cancer each year, and approximately 7,300 die.

Oral cancer can develop anywhere in the oral cavity. Most often it develops on the lining of the cheeks, the lips, the gums, and the floor of the mouth. Signs of oral cancer typically include a sore that fails to heal or that bleeds easily; a whitish patch that does not go away (called leukoplakia); a lump or thickening in the cheek, tongue, or lips; and difficulty chewing or swallowing.

The most common risk factor is the use of smokeless tobacco. Other risk factors are smoking cigarettes, cigars, or a pipe; and excessive alcohol consumption.

LEUKEMIA

Leukemia, a cancer of the blood-forming tissues (such as the spleen and the bone marrow), can strike people of any age. Though most people believe it is more common among children, leukemia actually strikes 12 times more adults than children. Approximately 34,810 people are diagnosed with leukemia each year in the United States. With advances in treatment, survival rates have improved dramatically over the past three decades.

Leukemia can be chronic or acute, and it has a number of varieties. Two of the known risk factors for leukemia are excessive exposure to radiation and exposure to benzenes and other hydrocarbons.

Many forms of leukemia develop slowly and cause few, if any, symptoms. As the immature white blood cells

TABLE 12.3 Preventing Cancer

Stop smoking	Cigarette smoking is responsible for 85% of lung cancer cases among men and 75% among women—about 83% overall. Smoking accounts for about 30% of all cancer deaths. Those who smoke two or more packs of cigarettes a day have lung cancer mortality rates 15 to 25 times greater than nonsmokers.
Limit sunlight exposure	Almost all of the more than 600,000 cases of nonmelanoma skin cancer diagnosed each year in the United States are considered to be sun-related. Sun exposure is a major factor in the development of melanoma, and the incidence increases for those living near the equator and at high altitudes.
Limit alcohol intake	Oral cancer and cancers of the larynx, throat, esophagus, and liver occur more frequently among heavy drinkers of alcohol.
Avoid smokeless tobacco	Use of chewing tobacco or snuff increases risk of cancer of the mouth, larynx, throat, and esophagus and is highly habit-forming.
Monitor estrogen intake	For mature women, estrogen treatment to control menopausal symptoms increases risk of endometrial cancer. Estrogen use by menopausal women calls for careful discussion between the woman and her physician.
Monitor radiation exposure	Excessive exposure to ionizing radiation can increase cancer risk. Most medical and dental X-rays are adjusted to deliver the lowest dose possible without sacrificing image quality. Excessive radon exposure in homes may increase risk of lung cancer, especially in cigarette smokers. If levels are found to be too high, remedial actions should be taken.
Avoid occupational hazards	Exposure to several different industrial agents (nickel, chromate, asbestos, vinyl chloride, etc.) increases risk of various cancers. Risk from asbestos is greatly increased when combined with cigarette smoking.
Improve nutrition	Risk for colon, breast, and uterine cancers increases in obese people. High-fat diets may contribute to the development of cancers of the colon and prostate. High-fiber foods may help reduce risk of colon cancer. A varied diet containing plenty of vegetables and fruits rich in vitamins A and C may reduce risk for a wide range of cancers. Salt-cured, smoked, and nitrite-cured foods have been linked to esophageal and stomach cancer. Heavy use of alcohol, especially when accompanied by cigarette smoking or chewing tobacco, increases risk of cancers of the mouth, larynx, throat, esophagus, and liver.
Increase physical activity	Accumulate at least 30 minutes of moderate intensity physical activity on most days of the week.
Monitor body weight	Stay within your recommended (healthy) body weight range.

Adapted from the American Cancer Society.

progressively crowd out the red blood cells, normal white blood cells, and platelets, symptoms begin to develop. Leukemia often is misdiagnosed in adults because the most common initial symptom is fatigue, which is a symptom of a number of conditions. Leukemia usually is diagnosed much more quickly in children because additional symptoms—such as weight loss, paleness, frequent nosebleeds, easy bruising, and repeated infections—tend to develop suddenly and rapidly in children.

Guidelines for Preventing Cancer

As much as 80 percent of all cancer is related to lifestyle and environmental factors over which we have control. Assessment 12.1 can help you determine how well you are taking control of your personal lifestyle habits to prevent cancer. Table 12.3 summarizes major preventive measures. By changing your lifestyle and taking control over your environment, you have a good chance to avoid cancer. Your general risk for cancer can be cut dramatically if you

- avoid substances known to cause cancer, such as tobacco and overuse of alcohol,
- avoid overexposure to sunlight,
- avoid overeating and eat an anti-cancer diet,
- do appropriate self-examinations, and
- get regular checkups to boost your chances of early detection.

QUIT SMOKING

The single best thing that a person can do to lower the risk for cancer is to stop smoking if you smoke and to avoid exposure to cigarette smoke if you are a non-smoker. Smoking causes about 87 percent of all lung cancers and 30 percent of all cancers. If you don't smoke, don't start. If you're smoking now, stop. That holds true for any tobacco in any form, not just cigarette smoking.

As soon as you stop smoking, your lungs will start to heal. Your risk will be slightly higher than if you never smoked, but eventually the risk can be the same as non-smokers. A smoking cessation program is presented in Chapter 13.

Even if you don't smoke, you should limit the amount of cigarette smoke you are exposed to. Nonsmokers who are forced to breathe the cigarette smoke of others run an increased risk of developing cancer.

LIMIT SUN EXPOSURE

The major cause of skin cancer is too much sun, so if you want to lower your risk for developing skin cancer, you should limit your exposure to the sun. Sunscreens protect against the sun's ultraviolet rays. The sun protection factor (SPF) indicates the protection you're getting. An SPF of 10, for example, lets you stay in the sun 10 times as long as you normally would without burning. If your skin normally starts to redden after 20 minutes, a sunscreen with an SPF of 10 lets you stay in the sun 200 minutes before you start to burn. After that time, you'll begin to burn.

If you're going outside for longer than 15 minutes, use a sunscreen even if you think you won't be getting that much sun exposure. Choose a sunscreen that provides adequate protection for your skin type. Choose a broad-spectrum sunscreen that protects against both UVA and UVB radiation. Apply it at least 30–45 minutes before exposure to the sun. If you're in and out of the water, apply the sunscreen frequently (look for a waterproof or water-resistant sunscreen).

Sunscreen should be applied heavily to areas where your skin is thin, such as your nose, face, neck, and hands. Use sunscreen even on cloudy days (clouds don't block the ultraviolet rays) and during the winter when you're outside. Sunscreen is increasingly important the closer you are to the equator and the higher the altitude where you live or visit, as both of these situations afford less atmospheric protection from UV rays.

To further cut your risk for overexposure to the sun, do the following:

- Even when using a sunscreen, avoid being in the sun between 10 AM and 3 PM, when UV rays are at their most intense. If your shadow is shorter than your height, the sun is strong enough to burn your skin quickly. You can burn even if you're sitting in the shade. Plan outdoor activities during the early morning or early evening hours, when sun is less intense and temperatures are cooler.
- Even if you are using a sunscreen, avoid lengthy exposure to the sun whenever possible.
- If you have to stay outside for long periods, wear protective clothing—long pants, a long-sleeved shirt, a hat with a brim or visor. Wear tightly woven cottons, and avoid white and thin fabrics. Don't sit in the sun in wet clothing.
- Don't assume that because your skin isn't red, it isn't getting burned. A sunburn becomes most evident 6 to 24 hours after being in the sun.

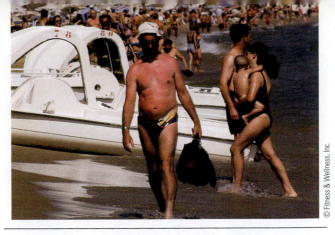

© Fitness & Wellness, Inc.

Sunburns pose a risk for skin cancer from overexposure to the sun's ultraviolet rays.

- Avoid surfaces that reflect the sun's rays more intensely—concrete, snow, expanses of metal, expanses of sand.
- Stay out of the sun or take extra precautions if you are taking antibiotics (especially penicillin or tetracycline), birth control pills, insulin (especially oral insulin), diuretics, and some medications used to lower blood pressure. These increase the damage from ultraviolet rays.
- Don't drink alcohol if you will be exposed to sunlight. Alcohol increases the damage from ultraviolet rays.
- Don't patronize tanning salons or booths, and don't use a sunlamp. Tanned skin is damaged skin. There is no such thing as a "safe" tan.

Most important, do whatever you can to avoid a sunburn. The risk of skin cancer from exposure to sunlight is cumulative. Each time you are unprotected and exposed to sunlight, some amount of damage accrues. With increasing damage, you also increase your risk for developing skin cancer. Sunburns are especially dangerous. Experts say that even one bad sunburn during childhood can double your risk for acquiring skin cancer later on.

FOLLOW AN ANTI-CANCER DIET

The first specific recommendations relating to an "anti-cancer diet" were published almost 30 years ago, when the National Academy of Sciences issued a report stating that certain changes in diet could reduce the risk of cancer. Since then, the National Institutes of Health, the U.S. Surgeon General, the U.S. Department of Agriculture, and the U.S. Department of Health and Human Services have joined the National Academy of Sciences in continuing research on the link between diet and cancer. They conclude that at least 30 percent of cancer deaths are caused by what people eat.

Food affects the risk of cancer in at least three ways:

1. Foods that contain certain chemicals (phytochemicals) and other compounds actually can stop or reverse the development of cancer. These substances also boost the body's natural defenses against various carcinogens.

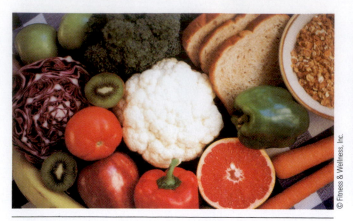

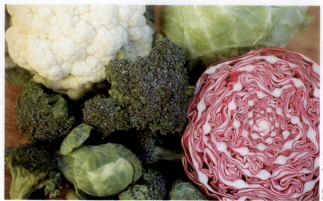

A diet high in fruits, vegetables, and grains decreases the risk for cancer.

Cruciferous vegetables are recommended for a cancer-prevention diet.

2. Some foods (such as smoked foods) contain carcinogens. Others contain chemicals (such as nitrite) that are converted into carcinogens during digestion.

3. If eaten regularly for long periods, certain foods, especially those high in fat, provide an environment in which cancer cells can grow more readily.

Based on research by the U. S. Surgeon General and a variety of scientific agencies, the American Institute for Cancer Research issued a four-part dietary guideline to reduce the risk of cancer:

1. Reduce total dietary fat to no more than 30 percent of total calories. In particular, reduce saturated fat (fat that is solid at room temperature) to less than 10 percent of total calories.
2. Eat more fruits, vegetables, and whole grains.
3. Eat salt-cured, salt-pickled, and smoked foods rarely.
4. Drink alcoholic beverages in moderation or not at all.

The American Cancer Society and the National Academy of Science jointly released the following detailed dietary guidelines for reducing the risk for cancer:

- *Maintain normal weight.* A 12-year study involving almost a million Americans showed that those who were overweight—especially those who were 40 percent or more overweight—ran substantially higher risks for cancer. According to the study, those who are obese run a one-and-a-half times greater risk for cancer of the breast and colon, two times higher risk for cancer of the prostate, three times greater risk for cancer of the gallbladder, and five times greater risk for uterine cancer. The American Cancer Society recommends limiting calories and increasing exercise to maintain recommended weight.

- *Reduce the amount of fat in the diet.* Major sources of fat in the American diet are visible fats (the fats we add to foods, such as butter, mayonnaise, and salad dressings) as well as the less visible fats that are found in eggs, dairy foods, meats, and baked and processed foods.

  You need to make a conscientious effort to cut down on foods high in fats, such as red meats, whole milk and whole milk products, cheeses, butter, pastries, candies, and oils. Trim all visible fat from your meat before cooking it, and remove skin and fat from chicken before cooking. Instead of frying foods, use low-fat methods of cooking such as broiling, steaming, and baking. Use less cooking oil than a recipe calls for. Skim all visible fats from soups, stews, and gravies; preferably, refrigerate them overnight, then remove the hardened fat that rises to the surface. Cut back on the use of cream, butter, margarine, shortening, mayonnaise, and salad dressing. Substitute foods naturally low in fat, such as whole grains, legumes, fruits, and vegetables.

- *Eat a wide variety of more high-fiber foods,* such as whole-grain cereals, whole-grain breads, bran cereals, legumes (including kidney beans), lima beans, pinto beans, rice, popcorn, and brown rice. Leave well-scrubbed skins on fruits and vegetables. Eat foods with visible hulls, seeds, and textured skins, such as strawberries, raspberries, and peaches.

- *Eat food rich in vitamins A and C every day.* Good sources of vitamin A are fresh foods that are dark green or deep yellow in color: spinach, broccoli, carrots, sweet potatoes, squash, apricots, and peaches. Good sources of vitamin C are citrus fruits (such as oranges, grapefruit, and tangerines), strawberries, cantaloupes, tomatoes, and green peppers. Many of these foods also are rich in beta-carotene.

- *Eat cruciferous vegetables* such as cabbage, broccoli, cauliflower, Brussels sprouts, and kohlrabi.

- *Cut down on salt-cured, smoked, and nitrite-cured foods.* Nitrites in salt-cured and salt-pickled foods become carcinogenic during the digestive process. Limit your intake of bacon, ham, hot dogs, beef jerky, smoked fish, smoked meats, and salt-cured fish. If you barbecue often, cook food at lower temperatures or farther from the flame so the food doesn't get charred.

- *If you drink, use alcohol moderately.* Alcohol significantly increases your risk for a number of cancers, especially if you also smoke cigarettes. Besides the harmful effects of the alcohol itself, alcohol can interfere with eating a healthy, balanced diet.

TABLE 12.4 Anti-Cancer Dietary Measures

Substance	Associated Cancers	Comments	Steps to Take
Fiber	May *decrease* risk of colorectal cancer.	Different types of fiber may affect cancer risk differently. Benefits also may be due to lower fat intakes usually associated with high-fiber diets.	Eat 4 to 5 servings a day of a variety of vegetables, fruits, whole-grain cereals, and legumes. Maximize fiber in vegetables and fruits by eating them unpeeled.
Fruits and vegetables	May *decrease* risk of colorectal and breast cancers.	Eat good sources of fiber (see above). Cruciferous vegetables, such as broccoli, cabbage, and Brussels sprouts, also contain indoles—nitrogen compounds that, in some studies, have knocked out carcinogens that can lead to breast cancer.	To maximize indole intake, eat vegetables raw, steamed, or microwaved; boiling leaches up to half the indoles.
Fat	May *increase* risk of breast, colon, and prostate cancers.	Lowering fat intake will almost automatically lower caloric intake and boost fiber intake—steps that will also lower cancer risk.	Decrease calories from fat to 25% to 30% of total daily calories. (Current average intake is 40% of total calories.)
Alcohol	Heavy use *increases* risk of cancers of the oral cavity, larynx, and esophagus; moderate use may *increase* breast cancer risk.	Cigarette smoking in conjunction with alcohol drinking greatly increases cancer risk. Alcohol use also can cause liver cirrhosis, which may lead to liver cancer.	Drink only occasionally and sparingly.
Salt-cured, smoked, barbecued, and nitrite-preserved foods	May *increase* risk of stomach, esophageal, and lung cancers.	Smoking and charcoal-grilling foods produces tars that are similar to those in cigarette smoke and are absorbed by the food. Manufacturers have substantially decreased nitrites used in meat preservation.	Opt for other cooking methods; limit intake of salt-cured and nitrite-preserved foods.
Beta-carotene and antioxidant vitamins (A, C, and E)	Inconclusive	Vitamin E and beta-carotene have been associated with lower rates of cancer in humans; a lesser effect has been noted with the other antioxidant nutrients. More research is needed.	Eat a balanced and varied diet to ensure that you get the RDA for all vitamins; do not take megadose vitamin supplements.
Selenium	Inconclusive	Limited evidence shows this trace element may protect against breast and colon cancers; however, it is highly toxic in high doses.	Taking selenium supplements can be dangerous; you get all the selenium you need from a varied diet.
Artificial sweeteners	Inconclusive	High levels of saccharin cause bladder cancer in rats, but no evidence of this in humans. Long-term effects of aspartame are unknown.	Moderate use poses no risk.
Coffee and caffeine	None	Both coffee and caffeine have received a clean bill of health.	Moderate use of coffee and caffeine does not appear to be a risk.
Food additives	None	Chemical additives found to be carcinogenic in animals have been banned; insufficient evidence that additives currently in use have any cancer risk or benefit.	None

Reprinted with permission of the *Johns Hopkins Medical Letter Health After 50,* © MedLetter Associates, 1992.

In addition to these guidelines, the following dietary suggestions can further reduce your risk of cancer:

- Get adequate amounts of calcium. It seems to help neutralize carcinogenic substances in the digestive tract. Early studies indicate calcium may help prevent colon cancer. Low-fat milk and nonfat milk and dairy products are good sources, as are dark-green vegetables, and foods that have been fortified with calcium.
- Avoid foods that have been treated heavily with chemicals or pesticides or processed with large amounts of

additives. Wash fruits and vegetables well before you eat them.

- Refrigerate foods that need it, especially fruits and vegetables. Fruits and vegetables naturally produce nitrites, a process that refrigeration slows down.

Table 12.4 summarizes the dietary measures that may lower your risk for cancer. The key seems to be variety and moderation.

Appropriate Self-Exams

One of the keys to successful treatment for cancer is early detection. You should examine yourself regularly for skin and breast or testicular cancer.

SKIN SELF-EXAMS

One of the easiest and quickest self-exams is a brief survey to detect possible skin cancers (see Figure 12.4). A simple skin self-exam can reduce deaths from melanoma by as much as 63 percent, saving as many as 4,500 lives in the United States each year.

- Make a drawing of yourself. Include a full front view, a full back view, and close-up views of your head (both sides), the soles of your feet, the tops of your feet, and the backs of your hands.
- After you get out of the bath or shower, examine yourself closely in a full-length mirror. On your sketch

make note of any moles, warts, or other skin marks you find anywhere on your body. Pay particular attention to areas that are exposed to the sun constantly, such as your face, the tops of your ears, and your hands.

- Briefly describe each mark on your sketch: its size, color, texture, and so on.
- Repeat the exam about once a month. Watch for changes in the size, texture, or color of a mole, wart, or other skin mark. If you notice any difference, contact your physician. You also should contact a doctor if you have a sore that does not heal.

BREAST SELF-EXAMS

Early detection of breast cancer is vital to successful treatment, and a woman who does regular monthly self-exams has a much better chance of detecting changes that could indicate problems. When you're doing self-exams regularly, you can detect a growth when it's about the size of a pea. A physician doing a breast exam probably wouldn't detect it until it's two to three times that size.

Perform the exam on both breasts regularly, once a month. A week after your menstrual period is the best time, as your breasts won't be subject to the swelling that sometimes precedes menstruation, and it will be a regular reminder. If you don't have periods, pick a day you can remember easily (such as the first day of the month). Figure 12.5 illustrates the breast self-exam.

FIGURE 12.4 Self-Exam for Skin Cancer

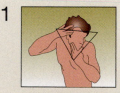

1 Examine your face, especially the nose, lips, mouth, and ears—front and back. Use one or more mirrors to get a clear view.

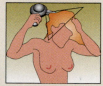

2 Thoroughly inspect your scalp, using a blow dryer and mirror to expose each section to view. Get a friend or family member to help, if you can.

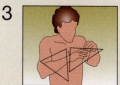

3 Check your hands carefully: palms and backs, between the fingers, and under the fingernails. Continue up the wrists to examine both front and back of your forearms.

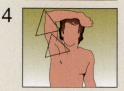

4 Standing in front of a full-length mirror, begin at the elbows and scan all sides of your upper arms. Don't forget the underarms.

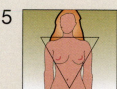

5 Next focus on the neck, chest, and torso. Women should lift breasts to view the underside.

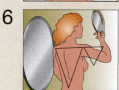

6 With your back to the full-length mirror, use the hand mirror to inspect the back of your neck, shoulders, upper back, and any part of the back of your upper arms you could not view in step 4.

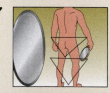

7 Still using both mirrors, scan your lower back, buttocks, and backs of both legs.

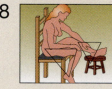

8 Sit down; prop each leg in turn on another stool or chair. Use the hand mirror to examine the genitals. Check front and sides of both legs, thigh to shin; ankles, tops of feet, between toes, and under toenails. Examine soles of feet and heels.

Reprinted with permission from *Family Practice Recertification*, 14, no. 3, (March, 1992).

FIGURE 12.5 Breast Self-Exam

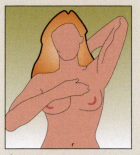
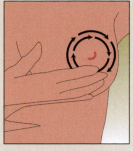

1 Raising one arm at a time over your head, use the fingertips of the opposite hand to check for any changes, lumps, or thickening.

2 Start near the nipple and work outward in widening circles.

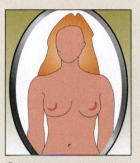
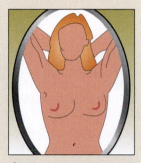

3 Visually examine your breasts in a mirror with your arms at your sides.

4 Visually examine your breasts in a mirror with your arms raised above your head.

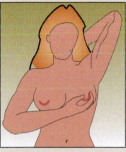
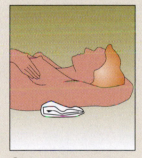

5 Check your nipples by squeezing them gently. Unless you have recently had a baby, any discharge is abnormal.

6 Place a pillow under your shoulder and your arm under your head. With your other hand, feel your breast and armpit for lumps, thickening, or other changes.

Adapted from *Family Practice Recertification* 14(3), March 1992. Used by permission.

The key to breast self-examination is to do the exam regularly. Cancer is detected soonest when you notice a change from one month to the next. If you notice a change or anything unusual, immediately report this your doctor. And don't forego your yearly medical exam.

TESTICULAR SELF-EXAM

Testicular cancer detected early can be treated successfully a good deal of the time. The key to early detection is

FIGURE 12.6 Testicular Self-Exam

Checking yourself for testicular cancer

Cancer of the testicle is a disease that usually strikes men between ages 15 and 34, although it can start at any age. All men are at risk, but if you have a testicle that did not come down into the scrotum normally or if you have a brother or father with the disease, your risk is higher. Fortunately, this is among the most curable of cancers —if it is caught early. Many doctors recommend that all men examine their testicles on a regular basis.

How do I do the examination?
- Set aside a few minutes to do the examination while you're in the shower.
- Roll each testicle between your thumb and fingers several times (see the illustration).

What should I feel?
- A normal testicle is most often compared to a hard-boiled egg. It should be egg-shaped and have a smooth surface.
- In back of each testicle lies the epididymis. This is a small cord that has the same shape as a small candy cane or comma.

What is abnormal?
Promptly make an appointment with your doctor if you have any of the following:
- A usually pain-less lump on one testicle.
- Swelling in a testicle.
- A persistent ache or dragging feeling in the groin.

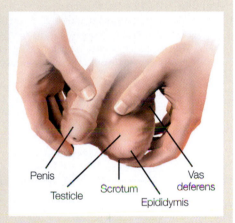

Penis — Testicle — Scrotum — Epididymis — Vas deferens

What if it's cancer?
No man wants to face the possibility of testicular cancer. Remember, not all lumps in scrotum are cancerous—but only your doctor can help you find out. Other possibilities include infections and cysts.

If it turns out that you do have testicular cancer, you should know that it is highly curable. Most men are cured even if the cancer has started to spread. In addition, most men who want to have children now are able to do so after treatment.

Reprinted with permission from *Patient Care* (May 30, 2000), Medical Economics, and Tim Phelps.

a simple, 3-minute self-exam done once a month. Choose a day each month that is easy to remember (such as the first of the month) and do the exam while you take a warm bath or shower, because the testicles and scrotal skin are most relaxed then. You need to examine both testicles one at a time as demonstrated in Figure 12.6.

1. Using both hands, roll the testicle gently between your thumbs and fingers. You'll feel a rope-like structure toward the back of the testicle. That's the epididymis, and it's normal. Most cancers occur toward the front of the testicle, and they will feel like a pea-sized lump or hard knot.

Site	Recommendation
Breast	• Yearly mammograms are recommended starting at age 40. The age at which screening should be stopped should be individualized by considering the potential risks and benefits of screening in the context of overall health status and longevity. • Clinical breast exam should be part of a periodic health exam, about every three years for women in their 20s and 30s, and every year for women 40 and older. • Women should know how their breasts normally feel and report any breast change promptly to their health care providers. Breast self-exam is an option for women starting in their 20s. • Women at increased risk (e.g., family history, genetic tendency, past breast cancer) should talk with their doctors about the benefits and limitations of starting mammography screening earlier, having additional tests (i.e., breast ultrasound and MRI), or having more frequent exams.
Colon & Rectum	Beginning at age 50, men and women should begin screening with 1 of the examination schedules below: • A fecal occult blood test (FOBT) or fecal immunochemical test (FIT) every year • A flexible sigmoidoscopy (FSIG) every five years • Annual FOBT or FIT and flexible sigmoidoscopy every five years* • A double-contrast barium enema every five years • A colonoscopy every 10 years * Combined testing is preferred over either annual FOBT or FIT, or FSIG every five years, alone. People who are at moderate or high risk for colorectal cancer should talk with a doctor about a different testing schedule.
Prostate	The PSA test and the digital rectal exam should be offered annually, beginning at age 50, to men who have a life expectancy of at least 10 years. Men at high risk (African-American men and men with a strong family history of one or more first-degree relatives diagnosed with prostate cancer at an early age) should begin testing at age 45. For both men at average risk and high risk, information should be provided about what is known and what is uncertain about the benefits and limitations of early detection and treatment of prostate cancer so that they can make an informed decision about testing.
Uterus	**Cervix:** Screening should begin approximately three years after a woman begins having vaginal intercourse, but no later than 21 years of age. Screening should be done every year with regular Pap tests or every two years using liquid-based tests. At or after age 30, women who have had three normal test results in a row may get screened every two to three years. Alternatively, cervical cancer screening with HPV DNA testing and conventional or liquid-based cytology could be performed every three years. However, doctors may suggest a woman get screened more often if she has certain risk factors, such as HIV infection or a weak immune system. Women 70 years and older who have had three or more consecutive normal Pap tests in the last 10 years may choose to stop cervical cancer screening. Screening after total hysterectomy (with removal of the cervix) is not necessary unless the surgery was done as a treatment for cervical cancer. **Endometrium:** The American Cancer Society recommends that at the time of menopause all women should be informed about the risks and symptoms of endometrial cancer, and strongly encouraged to report any unexpected bleeding or spotting to their physicians. Annual screening for endometrial cancer with endometrial biopsy beginning at age 35 should be offered to women with or at risk for hereditary nonpolyposis colon cancer (HNPCC).
Cancer-related Checkup	For individuals undergoing periodic health examinations, a cancer-related checkup should include health counseling and, depending on a person's age and gender, might include examinations for cancers of the thyroid, oral cavity, skin, lymph nodes, testes, and ovaries, as well as for some nonmalignant diseases.

From *Cancer Facts and Figures.* © 2006, American Cancer Society, Inc.

2. Repeat the exam on the other testicle.
3. Immediately report to your doctor any nodules or lumps.

AGE-APPROPRIATE CHECKUPS

In addition to self-exams you do at home, your physician can do examinations and tests to enable early detection of cancer. The exams suggested in Table 12.5 are the final weapons in your arsenal against cancer.

If you are at high risk for a certain type of cancer, you should have screening tests more often. Check with your physician. Sexually active women should have annual Pap smears and pelvic exams as soon as sexual activity begins. Women also should have a mammogram beginning while a woman is in her 40s. One of the advantages of earlier mammograms is that almost half the breast cancers in women under age 50 are noninvasive forms that are virtually 100 percent curable if detected early. Left undetected and untreated, these cancers progress into invasive cancers that are more difficult to cure.

To get the best reading from your mammogram, make sure the X-ray technician is certified by the American Registry of Radiological Technologists or a state licensing board; that the technician has mammogram training; and that the facility is accredited by the American College of Radiology (ACR).

In addition to monthly breast self-exams, the American Cancer Society recommends a breast exam by a physician every 3 years for women ages 20 to 40 and annual exams by a physician every year beginning at age 40.

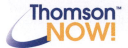

Don't forget to check out the wealth of resources on the ThomsonNOW website at **www.thomsonedu.com/ ThomsonNOW** that will:

- Coach you through identifying target goals for behavior change and monitoring your personal change plan throughout the semester
- Help you evaluate your knowledge of the material
- Allow you to take an exam-prep quiz
- Provide a Personalized Learning Plan targeting resources that address areas you should study.

WEB ACTIVITIES

American Cancer Society This site features current topics, research, statistics and information concerning prevention and early detection. It offers links to community American Cancer Society organizations, a calendar of local events, and extensive resources.

http://www.cancer.org

National Cancer Institute This comprehensive site features information on various types of cancers, treatments, clinical trials, statistics, publications, and health risk factors.

http://www.nci.nih.gov

Types of Cancers This searchable database, which covers all major types of cancers, sponsored by the National Cancer Institute. Information concerning known causes, prevention, detection, and treatment is available.

http://cancernet.nci.nih.gov/cancertopics

Susan G. Komen Breast Cancer Foundation This site provides a wealth of breast cancer information including a video showing the correct way to perform a breast self-exam, and the Komen NetQuiz, which allows you to test your knowledge of breast cancer.

http://www.komen.org/bci/

National Center for Chronic Disease Prevention and Health Promotion, Cancer Prevention and Control This site, sponsored by the Centers for Disease Control and Prevention (CDC), features current information on cancers of the breast, cervix, prostate, skin, and colon. The site also provides monthly spotlights on specific cancers, as well as links to the National Comprehensive Cancer Control Program and the National Program of Cancer Registries.

http://www.cdc.gov/cancer/index.htm

InfoTrac®

You can find additional readings related to wellness via InfoTrac® College Edition, an online library of more than 900 journals and publications. Follow the instructions for accessing InfoTrac® that came packaged with your textbook, then search for articles using a key word search.

Suggested Reading Liebman, Bonnie. "Antioxidants: still hazy after all these years," *Nutrition Action Healthletter,* Nov 2005 v32 i9 p1 (6).

1. How has scientific opinion of the value of antioxidants in preventing major diseases such as cancer changed in recent years?
2. Should you believe the health claims of products, such as teas and dietary supplements, that contain antioxidants?
3. What is the best advice for consumers until scientists sort out the possible benefits of antioxidants?

Web Activity

Cancer Prevention and Detection

http://www.cancer.org/docroot/PED/ped_0.asp

Sponsor The American Cancer Society (ACS) is a nationwide, community-based voluntary health organization.

Description Can you prevent cancer or reduce your cancer risk? How can you detect cancer early? What are the risk factors for different types of cancer? Concerned about cancer because it runs in your family? Frequently exposed to tobacco or environmental hazards? Just want to stay healthy? You can find answers to these questions and more with the ACS website on prevention and detection.

Available Activities

1. Tobacco risk assessment.
2. UV rays and cancer.
3. Learn how food and fitness affect cancer risk.
4. Learn about the cancer risk posed by your surroundings.
5. How early detection works, and how to get tested.
6. What men and women each need to know about cancer.

Web Work

1. From the home page, click on Men's and Women's Health.
2. Navigate to the appropriate Cancer Prevention and Early Detection Worksheet for your gender.
3. Complete the worksheet, identifying factors or behaviors that contribute to your cancer risk.
4. Choose an Action Plan for both prevention and detection.

Helpful Hints

1. Check out the Cancer Facts for Men and Women just below the Worksheet links for more information on the prevalent cancers for each gender.
2. Explore the Prevention and Detection sections on the home page to gather more specific information as you craft your personalized Action Plan.

For additional Web activities, links, and suggested readings, visit our Health, Fitness, and Wellness Resource Center at http://health.wadsworth.com.

1. American Cancer Society, *Cancer Facts & Figures, 2005* (Atlanta: American Cancer Society, 2005).

2. See Note 1.
3. See Note 1.

4. American Cancer Society, *Cancer Facts & Figures, 1994* (Atlanta: American Cancer Society, 1994).

Assess Your Behavior

1. In your daily diet do you include ample amounts of fruits, vegetables, whole grains, and limit overall fat intake?

2. Are you physically active most days of the week?

3. Do you avoid all forms of tobacco products and exposure to second hand smoke?

Assess Your Knowledge

Evaluate how well you understand the concepts presented in this chapter by answering the following questions.

1. Cancer can be defined as
   a. a process whereby some cells invade and destroy the immune system.
   b. an uncontrolled growth and spread of abnormal cells.
   c. the spread of benign tumors throughout the body.
   d. interference of normal body functions through blood-flow disruption caused by angiogenesis.
   e. All are correct choices.

2. Benign tumors
   a. resemble normal tissues that surround them.
   b. do not metastasize.
   c. do not invade surrounding tissues.
   d. are almost always encased in a fibrous capsule.
   e. All are correct choices.

3. Which of the following factors is not a risk factor for cancer?
   a. tobacco use
   b. viruses
   c. hereditary
   d. stress
   e. All of the above are risk factors for cancer.

4. The following foods protect against cancer.
   a. cruciferous vegetables
   b. salt-cured foods
   c. cyclamate-containing foods
   d. charcoal-broiled foods
   e. All of the above protect against cancer.

5. Cancer
   a. is primarily a preventable disease.
   b. is often related to tobacco use.
   c. has been linked to dietary habits.
   d. risk increases with obesity.
   e. All are correct choices.

6. The most common kind of cancers are
   a. melanomas.
   b. carcinomas.
   c. sarcomas.
   d. lymphomas.
   e. neuroblastomas.

7. The leading cancer killer in women is
   a. cervical cancer.
   b. breast cancer.
   c. uterine cancer.
   d. lung cancer.
   d. skin cancer.

8. The most common risk factor for oral cancer is
   a. smokeless tobacco.
   b. inadequate fruits and vegetables in the diet.
   c. lack of dental hygiene.
   d. a high fat diet.
   e. excessive intake of smoked foods.

9. The risk of breast cancer is higher in women
   a. under age 50.
   b. with a family history of breast cancer.
   c. who started menstruating after the age of 15.
   d. who became pregnant prior to age 30.
   e. with an early onset of menopause (prior to age 50).

10. A cancer prevention diet includes
    a. high fiber foods.
    b. cruciferous vegetables.
    c. proper weight management.
    d. lower fat intake.
    e. All of the above.

Correct answers can be found on page 370.

Cancer Prevention Questionnaire

Name: _____   Date: _____   Grade: _____

Instructor: _____   Course: _____   Section: _____

Today, scientists think most cancers may be related to lifestyle and environment—what you eat and drink, whether you smoke, and where you work and play. The good news, then, is that you can help reduce your own cancer risk by taking control of things in your daily life.

I. 10 Steps to a Healthier Life and Reduced Cancer Risk   Yes   No

1. Are you eating more cabbage-family vegetables?
   They include broccoli, cauliflower, Brussels sprouts, all cabbages, and kale.   ☐   ☐

2. Does your diet include high-fiber foods?
   Fiber is found in whole grains, fruits, and vegetables including peaches, strawberries, potatoes, spinach, tomatoes, wheat and bran cereals, rice, popcorn, and whole-wheat bread.   ☐   ☐

3. Do you choose foods with vitamin A?
   Fresh foods with beta-carotene, including carrots, peaches, apricots, squash, and broccoli are the best source—not vitamin pills.   ☐   ☐

4. Is vitamin C included in your diet?
   You'll find it naturally in lots of fresh fruits and vegetables including grapefruit, cantaloupe, oranges, strawberries, red and green peppers, broccoli, and tomatoes.   ☐   ☐

5. Are you physically active and do you monitor calorie intake to avoid weight gain?   ☐   ☐

   Total number of daily steps: [_____] 🚶 Total minutes of daily physical activity: [_____]

6. Are you cutting overall fat intake?
   Do this by eating lean meat, fish, skinned poultry, and low-fat dairy products.   ☐   ☐

7. Do you limit salt-cured, smoked, nitrite-cured foods?
   Choose bacon, ham, hot dogs, or salt-cured fish only occasionally if you like them a lot.   ☐   ☐

8. If you smoke, have you tried to quit?   ☐   ☐

9. If you drink alcohol, is your intake moderate?   ☐   ☐

10. Do you respect the sun's rays?
    Protect yourself with sunscreen (at least SPE 15) and wear long sleeves and a hat, especially during midday hours—10 AM to 3 PM   ☐   ☐

11. Do you have a family history of any type of cancer? If so, have you brought this to the attention of your personal physician?   ☐   ☐

12. Are you familiar with the seven warning signals for cancer?

If you answered "yes" to most of these questions, congratulations. You are taking control of simple lifestyle factors that will help you feel better and reduce your risk for cancer.

Adapted from the American Cancer Society, Texas Division.

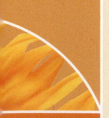

II. In the space below, discuss your risk for the various cancer sites. State your feelings about cancer and comment on any experiences that you may have had with cancer patients.

_____
_____
_____
_____
_____
_____
_____
_____
_____
_____
_____
_____

III. Discuss lifestyle changes that you need to implement to reduce your own risk of cancer. Indicate how you can best comply with these changes.

_____
_____
_____
_____
_____
_____
_____
_____
_____
_____
_____

13 CHAPTER

Addictive Behavior and Wellness

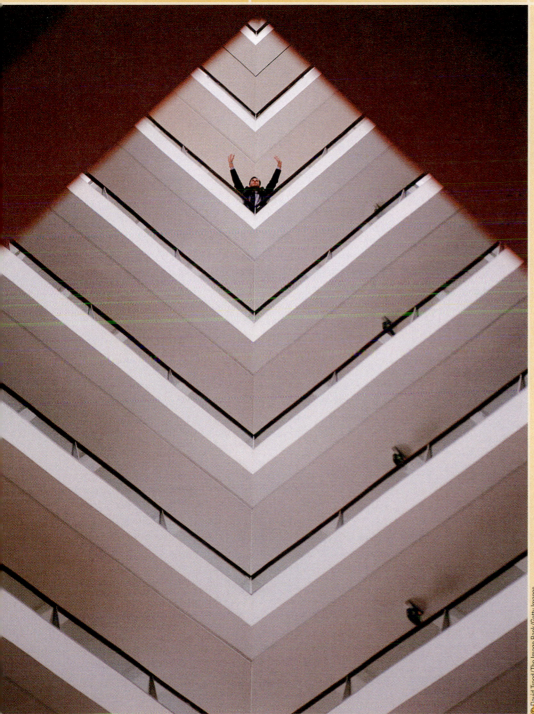

© David Trood/The Image Bank/Getty Images

OBJECTIVES

Define addiction and differentiate it from habit.

Delineate the difference between physiological addiction and psychological addiction.

Cite the threats of addiction to each of the dimensions of wellness.

Define the addictive personality and discuss addictive personality traits.

List the major risk factors for addiction.

Describe the health risks of tobacco, alcohol, and other drug use and abuse.

Cite some guidelines for managing and changing addictive behavior.

All of us have habits. You might have the habit of flopping down in front of the TV as soon as you get home every day, or you might have a habit of biting your nails when you are bored. Most habits are harmless, but when a habit escalates into an addiction, it threatens wellness. Broadly defined, an **addiction** is an abnormal or disordered relationship with an object (such as tobacco or alcohol) or an event or behavior (such as shoplifting or gambling). Continued involvement with the object or activity may have harmful consequences.

Addiction evolves over time. It almost always begins as a pleasurable, voluntary activity, but it eventually causes continuous disruption in an addict's life. Typical characteristics of addictive behavior are

- a compulsive need to do a particular thing,
- loss of control of actions, and
- repeating the action even though the results are harmful.

Most people with addictions deny they have a problem. **Denial**, is a common component of addiction. The addicted person refuses to admit, or fails to see, that he or she has a problem. Addicts cannot see it even though people around them see it clearly. Denial prevents people from seeking treatment long after their problems have become unmanageable.

Physiological Versus Psychological Addiction

Addiction can be either physiological or psychological. **Physiological addiction** denotes a change in the body's biochemistry so it demands a substance (a drug) not for pleasure but to function normally. As the body begins to clear the substance from its system, the altered body chemistry disrupts normal functioning, and the symptoms of withdrawal ensue. Withdrawal is extremely unpleasant and creates an urgent need for another dose of the drug. By this stage in the addictive process, the drug may be producing little or no euphoria. Figure 13.1 illustrates the downward negative spiral of drug addiction. In some instances, the withdrawal is so miserable that it can precipitate suicidal behavior.[1]

A drug is a substance that modifies one or more of the body's functions. Drugs that produce euphoria (an enhanced feeling of well-being) are more likely to be abused. To be addictive, a substance must be able to produce a change in mood. It is physiologically addictive when its use results in tolerance—when ever-larger doses are needed to achieve the effect. When a person is addicted to a substance and the substance is withheld, brainwave patterns change, mood alters, and drug-seeking behavior follows.

Physiological addiction also has a psychological component—a strong craving for the addictive substance. **Psychological addiction** can occur without physiological

FIGURE 13.1 The Downward Spiral of Physiological Addiction

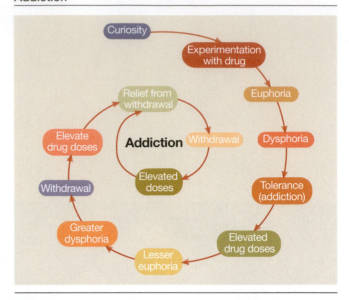

Signs of Addictive Behavior

- No matter how much you get, it's never enough. You constantly need to do more or get more.
- You derive no pleasure from the behavior, or it doesn't contribute to an overall sense of well-being.
- The behavior becomes predictable. You know you'll do a certain thing a certain way.
- You become inflexible about the behavior.
- Your self-worth or self-esteem is lower because of the behavior, but you can't seem to stop.
- You don't enjoy the behavior, but you feel driven to it. Even though your behavior makes you feel disgusted with yourself, or physically ill, you can't seem to stop.
- The behavior dulls your senses, provides escape, or otherwise helps you get away from stress, unhappiness, boredom, or frustration. Whenever you get a chance for challenge or reward, you resort to the addictive behavior instead of taking a chance on some other behavior.

addiction, though. People can become addicted to gambling, computers, exercise, television, work, sex, cleanliness, or over-the-counter medications. College students are at risk for developing addictions to the Internet.[2] Too, a person may switch addictions from one object or behavior to another.

People who have a psychological addiction have not learned healthy ways to cope with emotional pain. They crave relief from emotional hurt and use a substance or behavior to distract themselves. Regardless of the behavior used to relieve the emotional pain, the underlying motive is the same: People who are addicted can achieve temporary numbness and short-term relief, but if the behavior is destructive, or if involvement in the behavior keeps people

FIGURE 13.2 The Cycle of Psychological Addiction

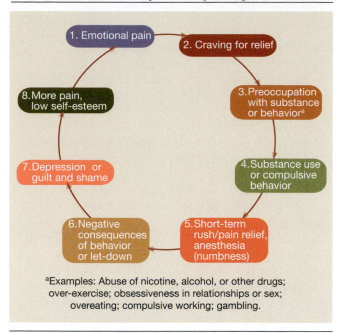

1. Emotional pain
2. Craving for relief
3. Preoccupation with substance or behavior[a]
4. Substance use or compulsive behavior
5. Short-term rush/pain relief, anesthesia (numbness)
6. Negative consequences of behavior or let-down
7. Depression or guilt and shame
8. More pain, low self-esteem

[a]Examples: Abuse of nicotine, alcohol, or other drugs; over-exercise; obsessiveness in relationships or sex; overeating; compulsive working; gambling.

from taking care of themselves, they experience negative consequences. If the person turns to the behavior or substance repeatedly, he or she is caught up in the cycle of psychological addiction depicted in Figure 13.2.

Addiction Related to Wellness Dimensions

Addiction is a staggering problem in the United States.[3] Drug addiction is alarmingly widespread. Addiction threatens all of the dimensions of wellness—physical, emotional, social, intellectual, spiritual, occupational, and environmental—as follows:

1. *Physical wellness.* People who are addicted to an object or an event typically fail to take good care of themselves because they are preoccupied with the addictive behavior. They might not get enough sleep, may skip meals, and could even put themselves in dangerous situations. Certain addictive behaviors damage the body itself. As examples, bulimia damages the throat and alcoholism damages the liver. The stress accompanying some addictions can injure virtually every organ and system in the body. In the extreme, addictions can result in death either from intentional or unintentional drug overdose.

2. *Emotional wellness.* Physiological and psychological addiction lowers self-esteem. The addict usually feels guilty, anxious, angry, depressed, and ashamed. Many addicts have unexplained mood swings or episodes of rage and violence.

3. *Social wellness.* Other than the interaction the addiction requires, the addict often becomes a loner who gradually cuts off relationships with family members, friends, colleagues, and classmates. Addiction brings with it a powerful preoccupation that takes priority over people, places, and events outside of the addictive behavior.

4. *Mental wellness.* Addiction impairs reasoning, judgment, and logic. Things that formerly provided intellectual challenge or stimulation to a student—coursework in a stimulating class, exploration of nearby geological sites, debates over a current topic—no longer matter.

5. *Spiritual wellness.* Because of the time and energy demands of an addiction, addicts have difficulty maintaining the same priorities and values they once had. Addicts gradually lose a sense of self and a feeling of being connected to the people and the world around them. They can't focus on something beyond themselves, nor can they appreciate themselves in a meaningful way.

6. *Occupational wellness.* A person with an addiction is involved in the addictive behavior to the extent that it leaves little time for school or work. Absenteeism increases; work quality suffers; relationships with professors, other students, colleagues, and supervisors are impaired.

7. *Environmental wellness.* People with addictions are distracted by their dependence and unable to be concerned about protecting themselves and others against hazards in the environment or in protecting the environment.

Personality and Addiction

The notion of an addictive personality is controversial. One school of thought flatly believes there is no such thing as an addictive personality. Another believes no set of personality traits leads to addiction but has identified a constellation of traits that disposes someone to addiction. The more of these characteristics a person has, and the stronger each trait or condition is, the more vulnerable that person is to addiction.

THE NONADDICTIVE PERSONALITY

Some traits of people who are less likely to show addictive behavior include the ability to face problems head-on

Addiction An abnormal or disordered relationship with an object, event, or behavior.

Denial Refusal or inability to acknowledge that a problem exists.

Physiological addiction A change in the body's biochemistry so that the substance is required for functioning.

Psychological addiction A strong craving for a substance or behavior.

with optimism and realism. These people work to overcome their problems. They recognize their own limitations and pace themselves accordingly to maximize their ability to cope.

People who are less prone to addictions are able to look at their circumstances realistically. They set reasonable goals and work toward achieving their goals in a structured way. They are not too hard on themselves when they don't achieve a goal. They recognize their limitations and weaknesses and also appreciate their strengths and good qualities.

The person who is less likely to become addicted has a keen interest in other people, allows others the freedom to pursue their own interests, and has at least a few deep relationships with other people. People with a nonaddictive personality have the ability to love and be loved and consider others' feelings, desires, and needs. They are not controlled by others but at the same time are sensitive to others.

THE ADDICTIVE PERSONALITY

The objects, events, or behaviors involved in some addictions may not be harmful, but an addict has an unhealthy or abnormal relationship with those objects, events, or behaviors. For example, food provides us with nutrition and energy, but food addicts eat compulsively and endanger their health. Sex provides intimacy, but a sex addict becomes preoccupied with pornography or an ever-expanding cadre of sexual partners. Drugs can treat disease, but drug addicts harm themselves by abusing the substance.

People who are emotionally unhealthy are at greater risk for addiction (see Chapter 2 for more details about traits of emotionally unhealthy people). Two traits often observed in addicts are low self-esteem and a strong need for immediate gratification. The addictive personality is one who has learned not to trust people, does not have healthy relationships, and has not learned to connect with other people, his or her own emotions, or the surrounding world.[4] People who have an external locus of control (discussed in Chapter 5) may be more prone to developing certain types of addictions.

Risk Factors for Addiction

Addictive behavior covers a wide spectrum—use of the Internet, sexual addiction, eating disorders, compulsive gambling, shoplifting, compulsive spending, and alcoholism, to name a few. Factors leading to addiction include the following:

- The behavior is reinforced.
- The addiction is an attempt to meet basic human needs, such as physical needs, the need to feel safe, the need to belong, or the need to feel important.
- The addiction seems to temporarily relieve stress.

Is Caffeine Harmful?

Many Americans consume caffeine regularly, and almost half of all Americans drink coffee every day. Caffeine is found in coffee, tea, cocoa, chocolate, colas, a variety of soft drinks, and a number of prescription and over-the-counter drugs. It is a common ingredient in nonprescription drugs for cold and allergy relief, pain relief, weight control, alleviation of fluid retention, and alertness. Caffeine occurs naturally in coffee, tea, and chocolate, and it is added to other products during manufacturing.

Caffeine is a stimulant that, if consumed in excess, elicits a number of physiological and psychological effects in the body including stomach upset, nervousness, irritability, headaches, and diarrhea. Caffeine should be used in moderation (1–2 cups per day). Drinking the equivalent of five cups of coffee may increase the risk of heart attack. Caffeine-containing beverages should not be regularly substituted for dairy, juice, and water. If this happens, the person will not only experience the negative effects of excessive caffeine but also will be less likely to obtain adequate intake of needed nutrients.

- The addiction can be compatible with the person's value system (a person whose values wouldn't let him or her shoot heroin may be able to rationalize compulsive eating or obsessive television watching, for example).
- If the person has a serious illness, the addiction can provide escape from pain or fear of disfigurement.
- There is pressure to perform or succeed.
- The person is afflicted by self-hate.
- Society allows addiction. Advertising even encourages it, for some harmful addictions.

Most people with addictions deny their problem. Even when the addiction is clear to people around them, they continue to deny that they are addicted. Instead, they tend to get angry when someone tries to talk about the behavior and are likely to make excuses. Many addicts also blame others for the problem. In some cases, an addict admits the problem but fails to take any steps to change.

Probably no one who starts out using a substance intends to get hooked, but it happens nevertheless. A person tries it for one reason but continues the behavior because addiction has set in. People who experiment with harmful substances often want to believe that they will not become addicted. It will happen only to others who are not able to handle it. The truth is that no one is exempt. The only way to escape addiction is to refrain from experimenting with the substance that produces it.

The same general characteristics and behaviors are involved in all kinds of addictions, whether they involve food, sex, gambling, shopping, alcohol, tobacco, or other drugs. The following discussion covers addictions to tobacco, alcohol, marijuana, and cocaine.

Tobacco Addiction

Tobacco products—cigarettes, cigars, pipes, smokeless tobacco—all contain the addictive drug **nicotine**. The dysphoria (unpleasant mood that occurs when the drug wears off) associated with nicotine withdrawal is so intense that quitting tobacco use is extremely difficult. For this reason, it is wise to never start smoking.

The percentage of the U.S. population that smokes has declined over the last three decades, although the percentage of young people who smoke remains high.[5] Adults with less than a 12th-grade education are more than twice as likely to smoke as are those with a college degree. About 28 percent of students in grades 9–12 smoke cigarettes, compared to 22.5 percent of adults.

HEALTH RISKS

People who engage in any form of tobacco use put themselves at tremendous risk. They contract an assortment of diseases and suffering, and they die at earlier ages. The most commonly known of tobacco-related diseases is lung cancer. The particulates in tobacco smoke are 500,000 times greater than the most heavily polluted air in the world. Lung cancer is the leading cause of deaths from cancer in the United States, killing more than 153,000 Americans every year.

Another risk to health is exposure to carbon monoxide, which reduces the ability of red blood cells to carry oxygen. The concentration of carbon monoxide in tobacco smoke is 800 times higher than the level considered safe by the U.S. Environmental Protection Agency.

Other cancers observed in tobacco users are oral cancer (cancer of the mouth, palate, larynx, pharynx, and esophagus) and, in pipe smokers, cancers of the lip, tongue, and jaw. Seventy percent of all oral cancer cases are caused by cigarettes or chewing tobacco. Cancer of the pancreas, bladder, and cervix also are associated with smoking.

Chronic obstructive pulmonary diseases, including emphysema, asthma, and chronic bronchitis, are 25 times more prevalent in smokers. Smoking also damages the respiratory system, increasing the risk for pneumonia, influenza, and colds. Smoke destroys the air sacs in the lungs, reducing their ability to absorb oxygen and eliminate carbon dioxide. Smokers are 18 times more likely than nonsmokers to die from these lung diseases.

Smokers have a greater frequency of heart attacks, strokes, and coronary artery disease, including damage to the inner surface of coronary arteries. Smoking reduces the amount of oxygen that gets to the heart, weakening it. Smokers are twice as likely as nonsmokers to have a stroke. Smoking also adds an estimated 10 years of aging

Facts About Secondhand Tobacco Smoke

Every year in America, an estimated 3,000 nonsmokers die from lung cancer caused by secondhand tobacco smoke, also known as environmental tobacco smoke. If you breathe it regularly, you're probably at risk.

- Exposure to secondhand smoke causes 30 times as many deaths from lung cancer as all regulated air pollutants combined.
- Secondhand smoke leads to coughing, phlegm, chest discomfort, reduced lung function, and reddening, itching, and watering of the eyes.
- Of the more than 4,000 chemical compounds that have been identified in tobacco smoke, at least 43 are known to cause cancer in humans or animals.
- Women who are exposed to secondhand smoke have a 15% greater risk of dying from coronary heart disease.
- Exposure to secondhand smoke contributes to up to 300,000 infections annually in children younger than 18 months. Infections include potentially serious conditions, such as pneumonia and bronchitis. Between 7,500 and 15,000 children are hospitalized each year as a result of these infections.
- Annually, secondhand smoke triggers 8,000 to 26,000 new cases of asthma in children and worsens symptoms in 400,000 to 1 million asthmatic children.
- Infants are three times more likely to die from sudden infant death syndrome (SIDS) if their mothers smoke during and after pregnancy.
- There is no safe level of exposure to secondhand cigarette smoke.

Sources: Centers for Disease Control and Prevention, Atlanta, and U.S. Environmental Protection Agency.

to the arteries. More than a quarter of a million deaths from heart disease each year (half of those who die from heart disease) are attributed directly to cigarette smoking. Smokers have a 70 percent higher death rate from heart disease; heavy smokers, a 200 percent higher death rate than moderate smokers.

Further, smoking increases the risk for peptic ulcers, miscarriage, stillbirths, death during infancy, low-birthweight babies, sudden infant death syndrome (SIDS) among babies born to mothers who smoke, and higher rates of asthma and middle-ear infections in children of smoking parents.

Even though smoking is considered the leading preventable cause of death and disability in the United States,

Nicotine A poisonous, addictive component of tobacco, inhaled by smokers or absorbed through the lining of the mouth by people who use smokeless tobacco.

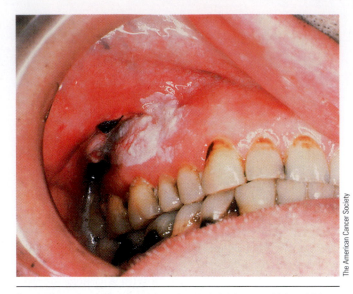

The American Cancer Society

Smokeless tobacco can lead to oral cancer (white growth) in addition to gum and teeth damage.

many college students are unaware of the magnitude of this problem. College students are surprisingly uninformed regarding the devastating and harmful outcomes related to smoking.[6] Smoking drastically shortens life and reduces the years of healthy life. Many smokers experience years of pain and suffering from smoking-related illnesses. And many of the harmful effects begin to take effect in people by age 30.[7]

Years ago, smoking was socially acceptable, but currently, as more people become informed about the vast negative health effects, society as a whole views smoking negatively. Smoking can limit social opportunities because, to the majority of nonsmokers, smoking is offensive. Smoking discolors the teeth and leaves unpleasant odors in clothes, mouth, hair, furniture, and dwellings. Nonsmokers are concerned about their own health risks of being around a smoker.

Another health concern regarding smoking is that nicotine is considered a gateway drug. Most cocaine or heroin addicts, for example, do not begin their drug use with those drugs. When past patterns of heavy drug abusers are studied, a trend is obvious: These abusers first used tobacco. Tobacco use creates a gateway or path to other drug use and abuse. People who use tobacco often experiment with other, more dangerous drugs. Researchers attribute the gateway effect to social and pharmacologic factors related to nicotine.[8]

Smoking is associated with additional unhealthy behaviors. People who smoke are more likely to abuse alcohol, eat poorly, and be physically inactive. Adolescents who use tobacco also are more likely to be involved in reckless and aggressive behaviors, and more likely to have more sex partners and take other sexual risks. Smoking seems to be associated with a risk-taking personality.[9] Assessments 13.2 and 13.3 provide insights into tobacco behavior.

SMOKELESS TOBACCO

The use of smokeless tobacco (chew and snuff) has increased dramatically over the past few decades. Almost 16 percent of high school males use smokeless tobacco.

Chewing tobacco is made by treating tobacco leaves with molasses and other flavorings. A plug of the tobacco is placed between the lower lip and the gums, where it is sucked to release the nicotine. A dip of chewing tobacco contains two to three times more nicotine than a cigarette. An average-sized dip held in the mouth for 30 minutes provides the same nicotine response as smoking four cigarettes. Someone who uses two cans of chewing tobacco a week gets as much nicotine as someone who smokes a pack and a half of cigarettes every day. Smokeless tobacco also contains cancer-causing nitrosamines at levels higher than foods may legally contain. Snuff is even more dangerous, because powdered tobacco releases more of its chemicals in the mouth.

Smokeless tobacco causes oral cancer as well as a variety of mouth and gum diseases and conditions, including loss of taste, bad breath, gingivitis, pyorrhea, tooth loss, unusual wear on tooth surfaces, tooth decay, receding gums, damage to the jawbone, and leukoplakia (precancerous thick, rough, leathery, white patches on the tongue, gums, or inner cheek). One in five people who develop leukoplakia is eventually diagnosed with oral cancer. Smokeless tobacco has also been shown to increase blood pressure and to interfere with the body's ability to use the nutrients in food effectively.

Alcohol Addiction

The term *alcohol*, as it is commonly used, refers to the active ingredient of alcoholic beverages—ethanol or ethyl alcohol. The percentage of alcohol in distilled liquor is stated as "proof." "100-proof" liquor is 50 percent alcohol. A drink is considered to be a dose of any alcoholic beverage that delivers 1/2 ounce of pure ethanol, such as 3 to 4 ounces of wine, a 10 oz standard wine cooler, a 12 oz standard beer, or 1 oz of hard liquor (whiskey, gin, rum, or vodka).

Alcohol is a drug that modifies one or more of the body's functions. Pure alcohol is toxic and, taken in large doses, can be poisonous. If sufficiently diluted and taken in small enough doses, however, alcohol produces euphoria, or a sense of well-being and pleasure, but this effect does not occur without risk. Like other substances that produce euphoria, alcohol carries with it the risk of abuse and addiction. The cycle of addiction, both physiological and psychological, entraps about one in 10 users of alcohol. The effects of alcohol overuse go beyond harming the individual users to disrupting the lives of those who surround them in the family and on the job. Alcohol use becomes abuse when it interferes with family, work, school, or social life or when it involves any violation of the law (including drunk driving).

One-third of students report **binge drinking**—the quick consumption of several alcoholic drinks in a short time for the purpose of becoming intoxicated. Binge drinking and participating in drinking games are popular on college campuses. The drinking games designed to ensure overconsumption of alcohol are life-threatening.

REASONS FOR DRINKING

People drink for many reasons, among them: to celebrate, to unwind, to get high, or because they like the taste of alcoholic beverages. Many people drink because peer pressure demands it, and young people may drink because they think drinking shows their maturity. Still-younger people use it as a way of rebelling against authority. Some people use alcohol as an escape from the pressures of life.

A typical reason that college students give for drinking alcohol is to overcome shyness. Many people long to have the courage to meet new friends, particularly members of the other sex, but have not developed the social skills or confidence to do so with ease. They claim that drinking alcohol makes them feel more confident, and they are able to be outgoing, carefree, and bold under its influence. They do admit, however, that their drinking can lead to problems. They often become intoxicated, embarrass themselves, and suffer bruised egos the next day. People who use "liquid courage" to help with socialization learn that they still do not have the skills necessary to engage in successful social interaction.

The deceptive appeals of the alcohol industry encourage people, particularly young people, to drink. Billboards, magazines, ads, TV dramas, and movies project an image of the alcohol drinker in a variety of appealing ways to encourage drinking and increase alcohol sales. These appeals suggest that consuming alcohol can help people achieve the qualities they most desire, such as being sophisticated or more social, having sex appeal, or being athletic.

Looked at with a rational eye, alcohol use hinders the attainment of the qualities used to promote it. People striving for sophistication and for rewarding social and sexual interactions do not have to lose control of themselves and their behaviors and would find the control they seek by practicing social skills. A person seeking success in sports will not find it by drinking beer but, instead, by faithfully practicing the sport. The ads deceive people by not mentioning that alcohol abuse causes accidents, impotence, and various health problems and can destroy relationships. These advertisements conceal the facts and strengthen the emotional impulse to consume alcohol.

Another reason cited for drinking, especially heavy drinking or problem drinking, is the inability to cope with negative moods and distress. People who have learned how to handle or cope with unpleasant mood states are much less likely than people with poor self-regulating skills to engage in problem drinking. Weak emotional health contributes to alcohol abuse. People are more likely to abuse alcohol if they are depressed, lonely, or have inadequate social support systems.

HEALTH RISKS

Alcohol is involved in more than half of all fatal automobile accidents in the United States. Someone is injured every minute, and someone dies every 23 minutes from an alcohol-related accident. One in every two of us is projected to be involved in an alcohol-related accident at some time in our lives. Our entire society suffers the consequences of alcohol abuse in terms of crimes, medical expenses, and emotional health.

Binge drinking is a particular concern because it has many serious health consequences, including death. Students who participate in binge drinking and drinking games experience more alcohol-related ill effects than other students.[10] Female students who are involved in drinking games also are more likely than others to be involved in sexual victimization.

Alcohol abuse impairs health status both in the short-term and the long-term. Short-term risks include, in addition to those mentioned above, the danger of acute alcohol poisoning, which can result in death. Another effect is fatty liver, the accumulation of fat in the liver cells, which interferes with the distribution of nutrients and oxygen to the liver cells. If drinking episodes are so close together that the liver cannot recover between drinking bouts, liver disease develops. This is a common problem among people who drink excessively on the weekends.

Binge drinking Imbibing at least five alcoholic beverages in one sitting for men, and four for women.

FIGURE 13.3 Long-Term Risks Associated with Chronic Alcohol Use

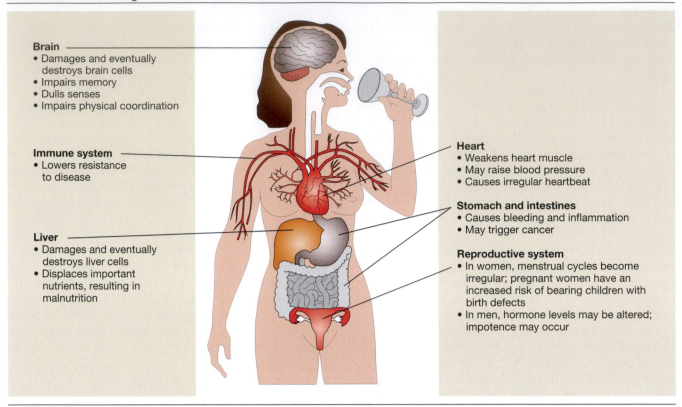

Brain
- Damages and eventually destroys brain cells
- Impairs memory
- Dulls senses
- Impairs physical coordination

Immune system
- Lowers resistance to disease

Liver
- Damages and eventually destroys liver cells
- Displaces important nutrients, resulting in malnutrition

Heart
- Weakens heart muscle
- May raise blood pressure
- Causes irregular heartbeat

Stomach and intestines
- Causes bleeding and inflammation
- May trigger cancer

Reproductive system
- In women, menstrual cycles become irregular; pregnant women have an increased risk of bearing children with birth defects
- In men, hormone levels may be altered; impotence may occur

The hangover—the awful feeling of headache and nausea on the "morning after" is a mild form of drug withdrawal. The hangover is caused by dehydration of brain cells. When brain cells begin to rehydrate, nerve pain accompanies their swelling back to normal size. Another contributor to the hangover is the accumulation of formaldehyde, a byproduct of alcohol metabolism.

The only cure for a hangover is time (to metabolize the alcohol). Simple-minded remedies clearly will not work (for example, taking vitamins, drinking more alcohol, drinking coffee). Taking Tylenol (or acetaminophen) when drinking can cause dangerous liver damage. Some people decide to drink less next time!

Like tobacco, alcohol is considered a **gateway drug** to the use of other, more dangerous drugs. In addition, alcohol abuse is linked to involvement in harmful health behaviors. For example, adolescent girls who abuse alcohol are more likely to take sexual risks, putting them at risk for pregnancy and for STDs including AIDS.

Long-term risks associated with alcohol are many and are depicted in Figure 13.3. The most commonly observed effects include liver disease, nutritional deficiencies, and impotence.[11] In addition to the devastating physical harm alcohol abuse causes, it also results in considerable emotional and social damage.[12] Problem drinkers affect family, friends, fellow employees, and the community. Assessment 13.4 can help you determine if you may have a problem with alcohol.

FETAL ALCOHOL SYNDROME

Women who use alcohol when pregnant run the risk of giving birth to a baby with **fetal alcohol syndrome** (FAS), the second leading cause of mental retardation in the United States and the third most common birth defect. Another, more common condition is fetal alcohol effects (FAE), which occurs when babies are exposed to alcohol in the womb but do not have the classic signs of fetal alcohol syndrome.

Even a few drinks during the entire term of a pregnancy or one episode of heavy drinking can be harmful to the fetus. Women who are, or think they may be, pregnant should not consume alcohol. Tests show that blood alcohol content is much higher in the fetus than in the mother who drank the alcohol. The greatest harm probably is done during the first 3 months of pregnancy, when the fetus is most susceptible, but alcohol at any time during fetal development can cause damage. Generally, drinking during the first trimester damages organ development; during the last trimester, it damages development of the central nervous system.

FAS is characterized by low birthweight, small head size, mental retardation, poor motor development, long-term developmental disabilities, and a distinctive set of facial malformations (short eye openings, low nasal bridge, thin upper lip, and absence of a groove above the upper lip).

Marijuana Addiction

Made from the dried, crushed leaves and flowers of the *Cannabis sativa* plant, marijuana—which looks a lot like tobacco—most often is rolled into papers and smoked like cigarettes. Some users pack it firmly into a pipe or smoke it through a water pipe. Less often, it is brewed into tea or baked in brownies. Although marijuana is a chemically complex plant with more than 400 identified substances, the one that has made marijuana popular is its chief psychoactive agent, **THC** (delta-9-tetrahydro-cannabinol).

The marijuana that today's college students smoke is much more potent than that used by earlier generations. Plants cultivated today have as much as three times the amount of THC as those cultivated just 10 years ago.

Marijuana is fat-soluble, stored in the fatty tissues of the brain, body, and reproductive organs. The user feels the effects of marijuana intoxication within 10 to 30 minutes, the "high" usually last several hours, and marijuana actually stays in the system as long as a month. The body has difficulty completely eliminating the THC, and the effects are cumulative, building up over time. What this means is that if someone smokes a joint every weekend—which may not seem all that bad—the body is permeated with the drug constantly. The immediate effects of use are bloodshot eyes, dry mouth and throat, coughing, and mild muscular weakness.

HEALTH EFFECTS

Though marijuana may be considered less toxic than some other illegal drugs, it has harmful effects on short-term memory and other cognitive functions. Marijuana distorts perceptions of the passage of time and impairs depth perception. It alters perceptions and delays reaction time. For this reason, it is dangerous to drive under its influence. In addition, marijuana use presents the following risks and long-term effects:

- Inhibited brain and motor functions.
- Changes in cell membranes, especially those in the brain and reproductive tracts, interfering with cells' ability to absorb energy.
- Interference with immunity, compromising the ability to fight infection.
- Faster heart rate and heightened blood pressure, leading to long-term cardiac damage (this is a problem particularly for people who already have arteriosclerosis, angina, or some other heart disease).
- Lung damage as much as four times that caused by inhaling the same amount of tobacco smoke. Marijuana is higher in tars and contains more carcinogens.
- Impaired oxygen and carbon dioxide exchange in the lungs.
- Depressed sex drive and impotence.
- Impaired male fertility because of lowered sperm count, reducing sperm motility (movement) and damaging sperm (causing irregularly shaped sperm).

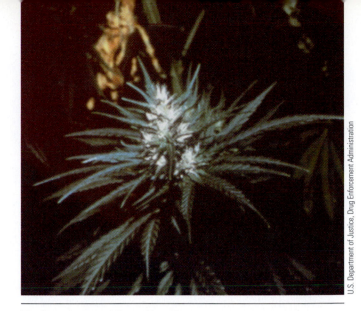

The flowering top of *Cannabis sativa*.

- Reduced female fertility by inhibiting ovulation.
- Birth defects in babies born to mothers who smoke it during pregnancy (especially low birth weight, premature birth, and congenital deformities similar to those of fetal alcohol syndrome). Marijuana may cause breaks in both the ova and the sperm, resulting in birth defects.

Some people respond to long-term use by developing amotivational syndrome, losing ambition and drive. Some people develop a psychological addiction to marijuana and require therapy to overcome dependence.

Perhaps one of the most serious risks from marijuana use is its status as a gateway drug to other drug use and abuse. Those who use marijuana regularly are much more likely to experiment with other, more dangerous drugs, such as cocaine, LSD, and even heroin.

Cocaine Addiction

Commonly known as "coke" and "snow," cocaine is a crystalline powder extracted from the leaves of the coca plant grown in Central and South America. It can be injected, smoked—called **freebasing**—or inhaled through the nose. It acts as both a powerful local anesthetic and a central nervous system stimulant. In fact, mixtures of novocaine and caffeine have been sold on the street as cocaine.

Gateway drugs Drugs (such as tobacco and alcohol) that were followed by use of other, more dangerous drugs.

Fetal alcohol syndrome A set of mental and physical characteristics in a newborn caused by moderate-to-heavy alcohol drinking during pregnancy.

THC (delta-9-tetrahydrocannabinol) The psychoactive ingredient in marijuana.

Freebasing Smoking cocaine that has been separated from its hydrochloric salt by mixing it with a volatile chemical.

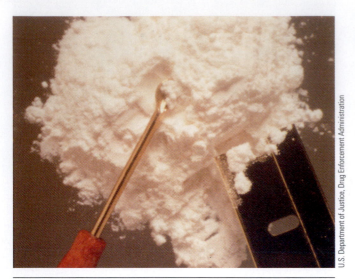

Powdered cocaine.

The effects of cocaine can be immediate and devastating. Cocaine that is snorted reaches the brain within 3 minutes; when smoked or injected, it reaches the brain within seconds. Powdered cocaine that is snorted can destroy the sense of smell, damage the mucous membranes, destroy the septum of the nose, and cause sinusitis. Smoking cocaine causes lung and liver damage, weight loss, and an increase in blood pressure and heart rate. Injecting cocaine can damage the linings of the arteries, damage the heart, and cause skin infections. Cocaine has been known to cause sudden death.

A particularly dangerous and addictive form of cocaine is **crack**, which derives its name from a popping or crackling sound that happens when it is smoked. Crack cocaine reaches the brain within 4 to 6 seconds, creating intense euphoria. Addiction to crack is so powerful that it has been defined as one of the most serious drug problems in the United States.

HEALTH EFFECTS

Health effects of cocaine and crack include the following:

- Rapid increase in heart rate and blood pressure (can cause strokes or bleeding in the brain, even in young, healthy people).
- Increased breathing rate.
- Heart and respiratory failure, including fluid buildup in the lungs.
- Raised body temperature.
- Lowered immune system response.
- Damaged upper respiratory system (if inhaled).
- Reduced appetite (can lead to malnutrition).
- Liver damage.
- Impotence.
- "Cocaine psychosis," characterized by paranoia, delusions, and violence.

Babies born to cocaine users incur significant developmental problems before birth. Cocaine crosses the placenta,

exposing the fetus to the drug. In addition, fluctuations in the mother's blood pressure cause blood vessels in the baby's brain to deteriorate, eventually resulting in strokes. Babies who are born cocaine-addicted are jittery, unable to sleep, irritable, and have long-lasting emotional and social problems, brain damage, heart defects, kidney damage, possible malformed head, arms, and fingers, and increased risk for sudden infant death syndrome (SIDS).

To determine if you have an addiction, Assessment 13.1 provides a self-questionnaire.

Other Addictive Drugs and Cautions

Other drugs, legal and illegal, carry risk factors as well. Table 13.1 presents types of drugs and their short-term and long-term effects. Two important issues concerning illegal drug use are, first, the user risks problems with the law; and second, illegal drugs are not standardized. No watchdog agency, such as the Food and Drug Administration, screens illegal drugs for safety, purity, or concentration.

Therefore, substances provided by an illicit source are of unpredictable composition, and they vary from batch to batch. Illegal drug sales provide a profit at each level of sale, so sellers tend to mix them liberally with extenders. For example, "consumer quality" cocaine is expected to contain some quantity of white powder other than pure cocaine, usually talcum powder or sugar lactose. Some sellers of cocaine maximize their profits by adding sugar, then masking the weakened effect with cheaper drugs such as amphetamines, caffeine, or anesthetics that mimic some of the effects of cocaine. In addition, many illegal drugs are manufactured under unsanitary conditions and may contain rodent droppings and other unknown substances, increasing the danger to users. As great a danger as the drugs themselves may pose to the users, greater still may be the dangers from unknown substances they contain.

Another important issue related to drug use is the **synergistic effect**. If you are taking any kind of medication—even over-the-counter drugs such as a cold medicine—you could get into serious trouble if you drink at the same time. Alcohol blocks the actions of some drugs and vastly increases the effects of many others, resulting in something similar to a severe overdose. We cannot list all the drugs here, but be especially cautious if you are taking any of the following:

- pain pills, both narcotic (e.g., Darvon) and non-narcotic (e.g., aspirin),
- over-the-counter cold medication,
- antihistamines for colds or allergies,
- antibiotics,
- sleeping pills,
- diet pills,
- tranquilizers, or
- medication for depression.

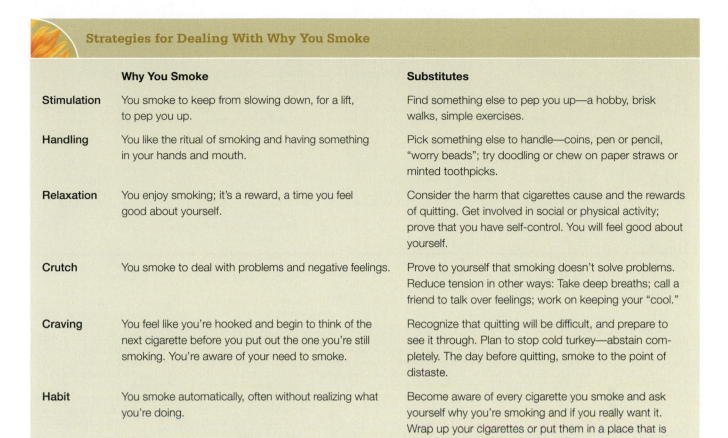

Strategies for Dealing With Why You Smoke

	Why You Smoke	Substitutes
Stimulation	You smoke to keep from slowing down, for a lift, to pep you up.	Find something else to pep you up—a hobby, brisk walks, simple exercises.
Handling	You like the ritual of smoking and having something in your hands and mouth.	Pick something else to handle—coins, pen or pencil, "worry beads"; try doodling or chew on paper straws or minted toothpicks.
Relaxation	You enjoy smoking; it's a reward, a time you feel good about yourself.	Consider the harm that cigarettes cause and the rewards of quitting. Get involved in social or physical activity; prove that you have self-control. You will feel good about yourself.
Crutch	You smoke to deal with problems and negative feelings.	Prove to yourself that smoking doesn't solve problems. Reduce tension in other ways: Take deep breaths; call a friend to talk over feelings; work on keeping your "cool."
Craving	You feel like you're hooked and begin to think of the next cigarette before you put out the one you're still smoking. You're aware of your need to smoke.	Recognize that quitting will be difficult, and prepare to see it through. Plan to stop cold turkey—abstain completely. The day before quitting, smoke to the point of distaste.
Habit	You smoke automatically, often without realizing what you're doing.	Become aware of every cigarette you smoke and ask yourself why you're smoking and if you really want it. Wrap up your cigarettes or put them in a place that is difficult to access.

Alcohol also can have serious, even fatal, consequences if you drink while you are taking the medications commonly prescribed for high blood pressure, water retention, epilepsy, diabetes, hemophilia, or heart disease. To be safe, abstain from alcohol completely when you are taking medications, or at least talk to your doctor or pharmacist about possible drug-alcohol interactions before you have a drink.

Overcoming Tobacco Addiction

If a person quits using tobacco, the benefits start almost immediately, and 15 years after quitting smoking the risk of death and disease will be no higher than if the person had never smoked at all (assuming the person is not already ill at the time of quitting). The risk of dying of heart attack is cut in half after only 1 year of not smoking. Some think that nothing else a person can do for health can have such immediate, far-reaching dividends as quitting smoking.

Quitting smoking is extremely difficult. A smoker not only must overcome the addiction to nicotine but also must break the habit of reaching for a cigarette at certain times associated with smoking. Further, nicotine withdrawal can be unpleasant, causing nausea, vomiting, restlessness, and irritability, in addition to the intense craving for tobacco.

No one method of quitting works for everyone. Your reasons for smoking and your habits are unique to you, as your life circumstances. Some suggest that if you are severely depressed, going through a major life crisis, or having severe emotional problems, you should reduce the number of cigarettes you smoke instead of quitting completely until the problem is resolved. If you smoke two or more packs of cigarettes a day, you might do better by first trying to cut down the number of cigarettes you smoke, then gradually stopping completely.

Some of the following suggestions may help in quitting smoking:

- There are no safe cigarettes and there is no safe way to smoke. While you are quitting, though, choose a brand lower in tar and nicotine than the brand you use now, smoke fewer cigarettes each day, inhale less deeply, and put out the cigarette after you've smoked only half of it.
- Set a goal. Determine a date when you want to quit smoking. Start now to quit, and tell those around you about it.

Crack A particularly dangerous and addictive form of cocaine.

Synergistic effect A phenomenon in which the effects of using more than one drug simultaneously are different and greater than using any of the drugs alone.

TABLE 13.1 Drugs and Their Effects on the Body

	Alcohol	Amphetamines ("speed," "bennies," "black beauties," "uppers")	Cocaine ("crack")	LSD (and other hallucinogens)
Type of Drug (Chemical)	• ethyl alcohol (ethanol), a clear liquid (in beer, wine, spirits) • made synthetically or from gain, fruit, or vegetables • favored for its relaxing, intoxicating properties • beers contain about 5% alcohol, wines to 12%, and spirits about 40% (about 13.6 g per drink) • a sedative-hypnotic and central nervous system (CNS) depressant	• synthetically produced: amphetamine (speed), dextroamphetamine (dexedrine), methylamphetamine or "ice," methylphenidate (Ritalin), and so on. • used as pills, inhaled or injected (speed) • CNS stimulants that resemble action of adrenaline (natural body hormone)	• derived from South American coca bush (still chewed in Andes to offset fatigue) • crack is mixture of cocaine and baking soda • cocaine hydrochloride is white powder ("coke," "C," "flake," "snow") • formerly used in many medicines (until 1920) • stimulant action—like amphetamine, but now legally classed as a narcotic	• derived from mushrooms (psilocybin) or cactus (mescaline) or synthetically—e.g., lysergic acid (LSD or "acid") and phencyclidine (PCP or "hog," "angel dust") • structures resemble catecholamines—normal brain neurotransmitters • hallucinogens can distort reality and produce severe delusions
Short-Term Effects (after a single dose)	• Effects vary with user's size, sex, and amount of food in stomach • initial relaxation and loss of inhibitions • increased sociability • impaired coordination • slowing down of reflexes and mental processes • attitude changes, increased risk-taking, and bad judgment/danger in driving car, operating machinery • sleepiness	• nervous system briefly stimulated • reduced appetite • increased energy, offsetting fatigue • talkative, restless, more alert • faster breathing • rise in heart rate and blood pressure (with risk of burst blood vessels and heart failure) • raised temperature, dry mouth, sweaty skin • dilated pupils • alleviated nose stuffiness (original medicinal use)	• short-acting, powerful CNS stimulant, also a local anesthetic • effects vary depending whether drug is "snorted" (inhaled); injected; put in mouth, rectum, or vagina; or smoked (as crack) • transient euphoria and increased energy • loss of appetite • rise in heart rate and breathing • dilated pupils • agitated, restless talkativeness • brief rise in sex drive	• unpredictable effects—at first, like amphetamine • excitation, arousal • raised temperature • altered sense of smell, shape, size, color, distance • exhilaration, perceived "mind expansion" or anxiety—depending on user • rapid pulse, dilated pupils, blank stare • exaggerated sense of power with possibly violent behavior • later, dramatic perceptual distortions • occasionally, convulsions
With Larger Doses and Longer Use	• blackouts (memory loss) • facial flushing, slurred speech • staggering gait, stupor • rise in blood pressure • pancreatitis, hepatitis, stomach ulcers, injuries (broken bones) • effects magnified by other depressants (e.g., opiates, barbiturates, tranquilizers, antihistamines, sleep aids, cold remedies) • alone or combined with other drugs can increase accident rates • overdose may be fatal, from respiratory distress	• bizarre behavior, talkativeness, restlessness, tremors, excitability • sense of power, superiority, aggression • illusions and hallucinations • some users become paranoid, suspicious, panicky, violent • raised blood pressure • insomnia	• permanently stuffy nose (if snorted) and risk of perforated nasal septum • brief euphoria followed by "crash" (depression) • anesthetic effect can depress brain function • bizarre, erratic, perhaps violent actions • paranoid "psychosis" (disappears if drug is discontinued) • sensation of "crawling under the skin" • convulsions, disturbed heart action, even death	• anxiety, panic attacks, paranoid delusions, occasionally psychosis (like schizophrenia) • injury or accidents because of drug-induced delusions or distance misjudgment • increased risk of fetal abnormalities • tolerance develops rapidly but also disappears fast with renewed drug sensitivity • with PCP, high fever, muscle spasm, erratic behavior, psychosis lasting weeks or more
Long-Term Effects (prolonged repeated use)	• harms many body organs—pancreas, heart, liver, kidney, brain—and gastrointestinal tract, blood circulation • may produce liver cirrhosis, ulcers, memory loss, impotence • increased risk of cancers (mouth, larynx, throat, maybe breast) • depletes vitamins • damages offspring • dependence	• malnutrition, emaciation (owing to appetite loss) • anxiety states • "amphetamine-psychosis" (with schizophrenia-like hallucinations) • kidney damage • susceptibility to infection • sleep disorders • psychological dependence	• weight loss, malnutrition • destroyed nose tissues (if sniffed) • restlessness, mood swings, insomnia, extreme excitability, suspiciousness/paranoia, delusions ("psychosis") • depression • impotence • risk of heart attacks • strong psychological dependence	• long-term medical effects not known • may include muscle tenseness or flashbacks—brief, spontaneous recurrence of prior LSD (hallucinogenic) experiences • prolonged, profound depression • panic attacks • psychological dependence
Withdrawal Symptoms	• insomnia, headache • nausea • shakiness, tremors • sweating, seizures	• long sleep, chills • ravenous hunger • depression	• little or no withdrawal sickness; sleepiness • extreme exhaustion • possibly "cocaine blues" (depression)	• few withdrawal effects, possible "flashbacks," anxiety

Adapted from Health News (May 1990).

Nicotine	Caffeine	Cannabis (marijuana, "pot," "grass," hashish)	Narcotic (opioid) Analgesics (painkillers)	Solvents (Inhalants)
• derived from tobacco • used medicinally in South America • Tobacco smoke contains 4,000 chemicals, but nicotine is the most addictive • A typical Canadian cigarette contains one mg nicotine, but amount absorbed varies with smoker • CNS stimulant	• derived from tea, coffee beans, kola nuts, chocolate • used in many medicines (e.g., with painkillers, cold/cough, pain remedies, antihistamines) • average cup of coffee contains 60–75 mg caffeine, colas about 35 mg (per 250 ml) • CNS stimulant	• derived from cannabis sativa, or hemp plant; preparations vary in potency; hash is most potent, marijuana least potent • smoked in "joints" or chewed (sometimes with food) • medicinally used for epilepsy, glaucoma, against nausea • classed as hallucinogen	• poppy derivatives (opium, codeine, morphine, heroin) and synthetics (Demerol, Methadone, Dilaudid, Percodan) • smoked, eaten, or injected • ancient painkillers used medicinally • deaden pain, produce euphoria and drowsiness	• volatile organic hydro-carbons from petroleum and natural gas (e.g., gasoline, toluene, hexane, chloroform, carbon tetrachloride, nail polish remover or acetone, lighter fluid, paint thinners, clean-ing fluid, airplane cement, plastic glue) • hallucinogenic effects
• faster pulse • increased, then reduced brain and nervous system activity • increased blood pressure • sense of relaxation • reduced urine output • impaired cleansing action of lung's cilia (hairs)	• stimulates brain, speeds nerve-cell transmission • elevated mood and alertness • stimulated mental activity • enhanced mental performance • reduced fatigue • shortened sleep • more urine output • increased stomach acidity • decreased appetite	• dreamlike euphoria, laugh-ter, relaxation • altered sense of space, time • increased heart rate • reddened eyes • dreamy, "stoned" look • at later stages, users are quiet, reflective, sleepy • combined with alcohol, increased effects, distorted behavior • impaired short-term memory, thinking, and abil-ity to drive car or perform complex tasks	• briefly stimulated, then depressed higher brain centers • quick surge of pleasure (for few minutes) then stupor (which mutes hunger, pain, sex drive) • pupils tiny, body warm, limbs heavy • dry mouth, itchy skin • users may "nod" off, alter-nately awake or asleep, oblivious to surroundings • taken by mouth, effects slower, no initial pleasure surge	• exhilaration, lightheaded-ness, excitability, disorientation • confusion, slurred speech, dizziness • distorted perception • visual and auditory hallucinations • impaired muscular control • possible nausea, increased saliva, sneezing • dampened reflexes • recklessness, feelings of power, invincibility
• lung damage • damaged blood circulation • slower wound-healing • vitamin C depletion • shortness of breath • more upper respiratory infections • cancer-formation risks	• nervousness, hand tremors • delayed sleep onset, reduces "depth" of sleep, insomnia • abnormally rapid heartbeat • jitteriness • mild delirium possible • convulsions (rare)	• slowed digestive (gastrointestinal) activity • misjudgment of time • sharpened or distorted sense of color, sound • slow and confused thinking • apathy, loss of motivation/drive • large doses can produce severe confusion, panic attacks • hallucinations (even psychosis)	• feeling of heaviness in extremities • permanent drowsiness • pinpoint pupils • cold, moist, bluish skin • progressively slower and depressed breathing • dangers increase with alcohol intake	• drowsiness and possible unconsciousness • severe disorientation • risks increase with fume concentration • irregular heartbeat, dis-turbed heart action • large doses may cause heart failure (e.g., "sudden sniffing death" especially with spot removers or air-plane cement)
• narrowed blood vessels, risk of heart attack, stroke • bronchitis, emphysema • raised risk of cancers of mouth, lung, larynx, throat, bladder, pancreas, possibly cervix • stomach ulcers • impairs fetal growth • strong dependence	• risk of stomach ulcers • possible damage to unborn baby • regular coffee use (more than 5 cups daily) can lead to dependence	• loss of drive, energy • regular use increases risk of — bronchitis, lung cancer — reduced sex hormones — impaired learning — memory loss • decrease in immunity • psychological dependence	• constipation • moodiness • risk of endocarditis (heart infection) and other infections (AIDS) from needle sharing • hormone upsets (menstrual irregularities) • liver damage • damaged offspring • strong dependence	• pallor; thirst; nose, eye, or mouth sores • irritability, hostility, forgetful-ness • may damage liver, kidney, and brain • nosebleeds, impaired blood-cell formation • depression, weight loss • other drugs compound damage • dependence possible
• anxiety, jitteriness • inability to concentrate • increased appetite	• severe headache • irritability • tiredness	• possible nausea, insomnia, anxiety, irritability	• striking withdrawal effects (4–5 hours after last dose): sweating, anxiety, diarrhea, "gooseflesh," shivering, tremors	• restlessness, anxiety, irritability, headaches • stomach upsets • delirium (rare)

The following six-step plan has been developed as a guide to help you quit smoking. The total program should be completed in 4 weeks or less. Steps 1 through 4 should take no longer than 2 weeks. A maximum of 2 additional weeks is allowed for the rest of the program.

Step One Decide positively that you want to quit. Prepare a list of the reasons you smoke and why you want to quit.

Step Two Initiate a personal diet and exercise program. Exercise and reduced body weight create more awareness of healthy living and increase motivation for giving up cigarettes.

Step Three Decide what approach you will use to stop smoking. You may quit cold turkey or gradually decrease the number of cigarettes you smoke daily. Many people have found that quitting cold turkey is the easiest way to do it. Although it may not work the first time, after several attempts, all of a sudden smokers are able to overcome the habit without too much difficulty. Tapering off cigarettes can be done in several ways. You may start by eliminating cigarettes you do not necessarily need, switch to a brand lower in nicotine or tar every couple of days, smoke less of each cigarette, or simply cut down the total number of cigarettes you smoke each day.

Step Four Set a target date for quitting. In choosing the target date, a special date may add a little extra incentive—an upcoming birthday, anniversary, vacation, graduation, family reunion.

Step Five Stock up on low-calorie foods—carrots, broccoli, cauliflower, celery, popcorn (butter- and salt-free), fruits, sunflower seeds (in the shell), sugarless gum, and plenty of water. Keep these handy on the day you stop and the first few days afterward. Replace cigarettes with these foods when you want one.

Step Six This is the day you will quit smoking. On this day and the first few days thereafter, don't keep cigarettes handy. Stay away from friends and events that trigger your desire to smoke. Drink large amounts of water and fruit juices, and eat low-calorie foods. Replace smoking time with new, positive substitutes that will make smoking difficult or impossible. When you desire a cigarette, take a few deep breaths and then occupy yourself by talking to someone else, washing your hands, brushing your teeth, eating a healthy snack, chewing on a straw, doing dishes, playing sports, going for a walk or bike ride, going swimming, and so on.

If you have been successful and stopped smoking, a lot of events can still trigger your urge to smoke. When confronted with such events, people rationalize and think, "One won't hurt." This rationalization won't work! Before you know it, you'll be back to the regular nasty habit. Therefore, be prepared to take action in those situations. Find adequate substitutes for smoking. Remind yourself how difficult it has been and how long it has taken you to get to this point. Keep in mind that it will only get easier rather than worse as time goes on.

From *Fitness & Wellness*, 5th ed., by Werner W. K. Hoeger and Sharon A. Hoeger (Belmont, CA: Thomson Learning, 2002).

- Use an aid such as nicotine gum or a nicotine patch, which is applied to the skin and delivers a continuous flow of nicotine to the body 24 hours a day. The patch is used in decreasing strengths for 8 to 12 weeks, gradually weaning the user from nicotine. One in four people who use nicotine replacement therapy eventually quits smoking.[13]
- Use relaxation techniques to help overcome the urge to smoke and also to counteract the physical withdrawal symptoms and inability to sleep.
- Switch progressively to brands of cigarettes that have progressively less nicotine. As your body's demand for nicotine diminishes, it will be easier to stop smoking without difficult withdrawal symptoms.
- Change your brand of cigarettes to one that doesn't taste good to you.
- Each time you resist smoking, put aside the money you would have spent on that pack of cigarettes. Keep it in a separate account. When you've succeeded in quitting, use the money to buy something you've always wanted.
- As you quit, you'll struggle with common withdrawal symptoms, such as irritability, headaches, dry mouth, hunger, constipation, and trouble going to sleep. Anticipate these symptoms and compensate for them. Soak in a hot bath when you're feeling irritable or get a headache. Chew gum or sip fruit juice to moisten a dry mouth. To ease hunger, keep on hand plenty of low-fat, low-calorie snacks (such as raw fruits and vegetables or air-popped popcorn). Include plenty of fiber (such as whole-grain breads and cereals) in your diet.
- Have substitutes on hand for times when you want a cigarette. Chew sugarless gum, eat raw carrot sticks, suck on hard candy, or nibble on sunflower seeds.
- Avoid situations, people, and routines that have made it easy for you to smoke. If you always smoke after you eat a meal, for example, finish with a piece of fresh fruit instead, then swish out your mouth with a great-tasting mouthwash.
- Set aside a regular time to walk briskly once a day.
- Know that most people who quit have attempted quitting several times. Be persistent. If it does not work, keep trying until you are successful.
- Many communities have smoking cessation programs and support groups. Consider joining a local group to get the support you need. Look in the yellow pages

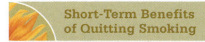

- For former smokers, the decline in risk of death begins shortly after quitting.
- Smoking cessation halves the risks for cancers of the oral cavity and the esophagus, compared with continued smoking, as soon as 5 years after cessation, with further reduction over a longer period of abstinence.
- The risk of cervical cancer is substantially lower among former smokers in comparison with continuing smokers, even in the first few years after cessation.
- The excess risk of coronary heart disease (CHD) caused by smoking is reduced by about half after a year of abstaining from smoking and then declines gradually.
- After smoking cessation, the risk of stroke returns to the level of lifetime nonsmokers; in some studies this has occurred within 5 years, and in others as long as 15 years.
- For those without overt chronic obstructive pulmonary disease (COPD), smoking cessation improves pulmonary function about 5 percent within a few months after quitting.
- Pregnant smokers who stop smoking at any time up to the 30th week of gestation have infants with higher birthweight than women who smoke throughout pregnancy. Quitting in the first 3 to 4 months of pregnancy and abstaining throughout the remainder of pregnancy protects the fetus from the adverse effects of smoking on birth weight.

under "Smokers' Treatment," ask your physician to recommend a group, or call the local chapter of the American Cancer Society.

Overcoming Alcohol Addiction

Alcoholism has been designated as a disease of addiction to alcohol. The addicting sequence is well defined. It typically progresses from the first drink, through increasing involvement with alcohol to a point where alcohol dominates the person's life, damaging family and relationships, work life, and physical health. Full-blown alcoholism typically takes from 3 to 10 years to develop after heavy drinking has begun. Assessment 13.4 explores issues related to problem drinking

SOME DANGER SIGNS

A key feature of alcoholism is denial. The person refuses to acknowledge that he or she is addicted. As a result, a diagnosis made by someone else usually cannot lead to effective treatment because the person with alcoholism will not cooperate. The best diagnosis for alcoholism, therefore, is self-diagnosis—which is why experts encourage the widespread use of self-tests, and why they emphasize certain symptoms that only the drinker can recognize. Here are some danger signs:

- You're preoccupied with drinking alcohol. You think about it or plan it even when you're not drinking.
- You drink to escape your problems or relieve stress.
- You need a drink to help you go to sleep.
- You need a drink to help you get going in the morning.
- You get drunk often or stay drunk several days at a time.
- You sneak drinks or drink alone.
- You make excuses for why you drink.
- You hide the amount you drink from your mate, children, friends.
- You gulp your drinks.
- You have had blackouts (periods during which you can't remember what happened).
- You've had frequent accidents because of drinking.
- You've been ill a lot because of drinking.
- You've missed work or school because of drinking.
- You've had financial or legal problems because of drinking.
- Your personality or behavior changes when you drink.
- Once you sober up, you regret the things you did while you were drinking.
- Other people tell you that you drink too much.
- You feel guilty about your drinking.
- You've tried to stop drinking but can't.
- You don't want to talk about the negative effects of drinking.

CAUSES AND CHARACTERISTICS

The causes of alcoholism are varied and not completely understood. Alcoholism seems to have a genetic component and also may be related to the surrounding environment. Why some people can drink socially for years without becoming addicted and others follow the downward spiral of alcoholism is not understood. Figure 13.4 illustrates the different fates of two drinkers.

Alcoholism is characterized by memory blackouts—episodes of temporary amnesia that occur after (not during) times when a person is drinking. During an event a person may function normally—not appear drunk and not pass out (a memory blackout is different from passing out). Often people will not be able to tell that anything is wrong or even whether the drinker is drinking at the time. But afterward (typically the morning after), the drinker will remember nothing about the event. Blackouts are so striking that some people, upon experiencing a blackout for the first time, have quit drinking for life.

Alcoholism is not the addict's fault, but recovery is the addict's responsibility. If a person with alcoholism chooses to continue the addictive behavior, he or she alone should accept the negative consequences of that choice. Family members and friends should not cover up or fix problems the addict has caused. This response is called enabling—

Typical 12-Step Program

1. We admitted we were powerless over the obsession or compulsion (such as drinking alcohol, using other drugs, gambling, overworking, overexercising, overeating, or excessively depending on other people)—that our lives had become unmanageable.
2. We came to believe that a power greater than ourselves could restore us to sanity.
3. We made a decision to turn our will and our lives over to the care of God as we understood Him.
4. We made a searching and fearless moral inventory of ourselves.
5. We admitted to God, to ourselves, and to another human being the exact nature of our wrongs.
6. We were entirely ready to have God remove all these defects of character.
7. We humbly asked Him to remove our shortcomings.
8. We made a list of all the persons we had harmed and became willing to make amends to them all.
9. We made direct amends to such people wherever possible, except when doing so would hurt them or others.
10. We continued to take personal inventory, and when we were wrong, promptly admitted it.
11. We sought through prayer and meditation to improve our conscious contact with God as we understood Him, praying only for knowledge of His will for us and the power to carry that out.
12. Having had a spiritual awakening as the result of these steps, we tried to carry this message to other people who suffer from the same compulsions and to practice these principles in all our affairs.

misguided helping that actually delays or hinders the alcohol addict from getting better.

Alcoholism is a complex problem that requires treatment. The first step is to break the denial. The person has to admit to having a problem, take responsibility, and be willing to abstain from alcohol. Some people need to go to a treatment center; others are able to recover with the help of specific support groups such as Alcoholics Anonymous (AA).

AA groups meet frequently in most communities. Their programs are based on a 12-step program that begins with the attendee's admitting the problem and, after healing and recovery, helping others with the disease. The 12-step program is very spiritual in nature and the most effective system for recovery.

Recovery from alcoholism is similar to recovery from any addiction. It involves, first, learning to abstain from the substance, and second, overcoming the problems that contributed to the addiction as well as the problems the addiction caused.

FIGURE 13.4 The Fates of Two Drinkers

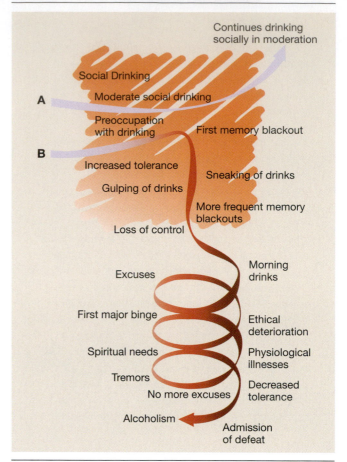

HOW TO DRINK AND HOW TO REFUSE

Those who choose to drink need to learn to handle drinking responsibly. Those who choose to abstain may need to learn to do so gracefully. Those who succeed in drinking moderately drink at appropriate times and in appropriate settings only. They limit their intake, and they remain in control. They acknowledge their responsibility not to damage themselves or society, and they know that being intoxicated is irresponsible drinking behavior.[14] Among the skills they report to be useful are the following:

"I get together with my friends, and we decide ahead of time who will drive us home. The designated driver agrees not to drink at all at the party."

"I decide in advance how much I'm going to drink. I decide on two drinks and then I drink non-alcohol beverages."

"If they're serving beer by the pitcher, I still order it by the glass." (Ordering beer by the pitcher tends to double a drinker's intake.)

"I eat before and during a party, and then I drink slowly."

"I allow time to metabolize the alcohol I've drunk before I drive home."

Finding Drug-Free Highs

Pleasure is there for the taking, for those who know where to look. To get high, try any of the following:

1. Run, walk, or skip across an open field, through a park, or along a beach.
2. Ask one of your grandparents what life is about.
3. Play with a baby.
4. Give a friend a gift that you made with your own hands.
5. Get involved in worthwhile activities with groups in which you feel you are contributing and are needed.
6. Work hard at something and see it through to completion.
7. Have a good cry about that thing you have been hiding from for too long.
8. Learn to meditate.
9. Eat nourishing food.
10. Write some poetry for yourself (it doesn't have to rhyme).
11. Climb a mountain.
12. Visit a river.
13. Say "thank you" more often.
14. Beat the feathers out of a pillow next time you are very angry.
15. Stop biting your nails (or shed another bad habit).
16. Read a good book.
17. Give someone a long hug.
18. Call your parents and say, "I love you."

Source: Inspired in part by S. J. Levy, *Managing the Drugs in Your Life* (New York: McGraw-Hill, 1983), p. 104.

Strategies: Refusing a Drink

To refuse an unwanted drink gracefully:

1. **Don't apologize.** It may take nerve to say, "No, thanks." Say it calmly, casually, firmly. Keep it brief; don't give excuses, explanations, or arguments. A discussion period is a good time for explanations; a party is not.
2. **Expect others to respect your choice.** When you're confident of your choice, your firm manner will make your confidence clear to others, and you'll get respect. If you're hesitant, you'll pave the way for others to tease or argue.
3. **Respect the drinker's choice to drink.** Give the person who drinks the same acceptance you want to receive. If you don't, you're backing the person into a corner, and people who are cornered have to fight their way out. The person probably will try to embarrass you for your decision not to drink.
4. **Consider another group of friends.** If you continue to be pressured to drink from those who are drinking, even after trying the above suggestions, consider developing other friendships. Those who push alcohol on nondrinkers are often problem drinkers themselves and are uncomfortable if those around them are not drinking. If they base the friendship on your drinking, you may be better off looking elsewhere for quality friendships.

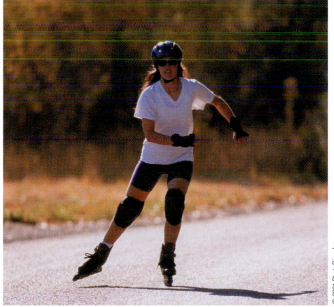
Life without the substance may be better.

"I sip my drinks; I add ice cubes or water; and if I'm thirsty, I drink water."

"I use fruit juices for mixers. They meet my calorie need and keep my blood sugar up."

"When I want dessert, I eat ice cream. A piña colada has too many calories!"

"I don't accept drinks I don't want."

"I go slowly with unfamiliar drinks."

"I know my capacity and I don't exceed it."

Many people choose to not drink at all. They have the ability to socialize without alcohol, and they don't want to risk becoming addicted or experiencing any other negative effects of alcohol use. Sometimes drinkers pressure others to drink alcohol, and refusing can be a challenge. People who abstain successfully have mastered many social skills to resist social pressure to drink.

The only two healthy alternatives are to abstain from alcohol or to use it responsibly in moderation. Excessive alcohol consumption results in short-term and long-term risks to health, family life, and society. Few addicts who attempt recovery make it all the way. This is why health professionals recommend not starting to use drugs, including alcohol. Most people with addictions get caught in something like a revolving door—undergoing treatment, giving up the drug, getting out of treatment, taking the drug again, going back into treatment, and so on indefinitely. Consider drug-free alternatives. Being able to enjoy life without artificial highs is truly satisfying.

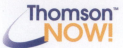

Don't forget to check out the wealth of resources on the ThomsonNOW website at **www.thomsonedu.com/ ThomsonNOW** that will:

- Coach you through identifying target goals for behavior change and monitoring your personal change plan throughout the semester
- Help you evaluate your knowledge of the material
- Allow you to take an exam-prep quiz
- Provide a Personalized Learning Plan targeting resources that address areas you should study.

WEB ACTIVITIES

National Institute of Drug Abuse This site, sponsored by the National Institutes of Health, provides information on a variety of abused drugs, research, and current events. The site features research on addictions and a link to additional information on club drugs and steroids.

http://www.nida.nih.gov

Web of Addictions This site features comprehensive and factual information on a variety of addictions, including alcohol and other drug abuse.

http://www.well.com/user/woa

Truth: The Facts About Tobacco This is a fun, creative site on tobacco education, designed for teens and young adults.

http://www.thetruth.com/

The College Alcohol Study: Harvard University School of Public Health This site describes the ongoing survey (1993, 1997, 1999, 2000, 2001) of more than 15,000 students at 140 four-year colleges in 40 states. The CAS examines high-risk behaviors among college students, such as binge drinking, smoking, illicit drug use, violence, and other behavioral, social, and health problems. The principal investigator is Henry Wechsler, Ph.D.

http://www.hsph.harvard.edu/cas

Club Drugs Information from the National Institute of Drug Abuse features factual information concerning these drugs: alcohol, LSD (acid), MDMA (ecstasy), GHB, GBL, ketamine (Special-K), Fentanyl, Rohypnol, amphetamines, and methamphetamine.

http://www.nida.nih.gov/drugpages/clubdrugs.html

InfoTrac®

You can find additional readings related to wellness via InfoTrac® College Edition, an online library of more than 900 journals and publications. Follow the instructions for accessing InfoTrac® that came packaged with your textbook, then search for articles using a key word search.

Suggested Reading Sheffield, Felicia et al. Binge drinking and alcohol-related problems among community college students: implications for prevention policy. *Journal of American College Health,* Nov–Dec 2005 v54 i3 p137 (5).

1. What are some of the consequences of binge-drinking by college students?

2. Describe the most common patterns of drinking among the community college students in this study.
3. What are some reasons why binge-drinking rates may be lower at community colleges than at four-year universities?

Web Activity

Facts On Tap: Alcohol and Student Life

http://www.factsontap.org

Sponsor The Children of Alcoholics Foundation and the American Council for Drug Education, two of the nation's leaders in substance abuse prevention education. The major funding sponsor is the Metropolitan Life Foundation.

Description This colorful and interactive Web site features a variety of activities and straightforward information written specifically for college students. Some of the topics include alcohol and the college experience, the effects of alcohol on the nondrinker, alcohol and the family, and a true/false quiz to test your knowledge about alcohol and its effects.

Available Activities Among the many informative links are three interactive activities to explore.

1. Under the "Alcohol and Student Life" link is a quiz to reveal whether you have a problem with alcohol.
2. Another quiz to help you figure out if your relationship depends too heavily on alcohol is located under the "Alcohol and Sex" link.
3. A true/false quiz designed to test your alcohol knowledge is located under the "Alcohol and Your Body" link.

Web Work

1. From the home page, first click on "Facts on Tap," choose "College Students," then click on "Alcohol and Student Life" to learn sobering statistics about the use of alcohol among college students, tips to help you cut down on or stop using alcohol, common misconceptions and the real truth, resources to go to for help, as well as a test to reveal if you have a problem with alcohol. Return to the home page.
2. Click on the link to take the short quiz to help you figure out if your relationship depends too heavily on alcohol.
3. From the home page, click on "Alcohol and Your Body" link to go to a site that features a true/false quiz designed to test your alcohol knowledge. The site also includes information on how to determine your blood alcohol level and how your behavior changes as your blood alcohol level increases.
4. The "Someone Else's Drinking" link features stories from students who were affected by someone else's drinking, as well as information on how to help a friend whose drinking is out of control.

Helpful Hint

Resources are included for college students and college staff, as well as links to college health centers that sponsor model alcohol education programs.

For additional Web activities, links, and suggested readings, visit our Health, Fitness, and Wellness Resource Center at http://health.wadsworth.com.

Notes

1. J. R. Cornelius et al., "Cocaine Use Associated with Increased Suicidal Behavior in Depressed Alcoholics," *Addictive Behaviors* 23 (1998): 119–121.
2. K. Clark, L. Leung, "Shyness and Locus of Control as Predictors for Internet Addiction and Internet Use," *Cyberpsychology and Behavior* 7 (2003): 559–570.
3. J. D. Kassel, "Generalized Expectancies for Negative Mood Regulation and Problem Drinking Among College Students," *Journal of Studies on Alcohol* 61 (2000): 332–337.
4. B. Johnson, "Psychological Addiction, Physical Addiction, Addictive Character, and Addictive Personality Disorder: A Nosology of Addictive Disorders," *Canadian Journal of Psychoanalysis* 11 (2002): 135–160.
5. U. S. Centers for Disease Control and Prevention, "Tobacco Use, Access, and Exposure to Tobacco in Media Among Middle and High School Students—United States," *Morbidity and Mortality Weekly* 54 (2005): 5412.
6. R. Murphy-Hoefer, S. Alder, C. Higbee, "Perceptions About Cigarette Smoking and Risks Among College Students," *Nicotine and Tobacco Research*, 6 (2004): S371–S374.
7. J. S. Brook, D. W. Brook, and C. Zhand, "Tobacco Use and Health in Young Adulthood," *Journal of Genetic Psychology* 165 (2004): 310–323.
8. G. B. Lindsay et al., "Psychosocial and Pharmacologic Explanations of Nicotine's Gateway Drug Function," *Journal of School Health* 67 (1997): 123–127.
9. F. J. Kelley, S. A. Thomas, E. Friedmann, "Health Risk Behaviors in Smoking and Nonsmoking Young Women," *Journal of the American Academy of Nurse Practitioners* 15 (2003): 179–184.
10. T. J. Johnson, J. Wendel, and S. Hamilton, "Social Anxiety, Alcohol Expectancies, and Drinking-Game Participation," *Addictive Behaviors* 23 (1998): 65–79.
11. R. H. Moos, P. L. Brennan, K. K. Schutte, and B. S. Moos, High-Risk Alcohol Consumption and Late-Life Alcohol Use Problems," *American Journal of Public Health* 94 (2004): 1985–1991.
12. M. A. Ichiyama, "The Social Context of Binge Drinking among Private University Freshmen," *Journal of Alcohol and Drug Education* 44 (1998): 18–33.
13. L. Lamberg, "Patients Need More Help to Quit Smoking," *Journal of the American Medical Association*, 292 (2004): 1286–1290.
14. R. C. Engs, "Responsibility and Alcohol: Teaching Responsible Decisions about Alcohol and Its Use for Those Who Choose to Drink," *Health Education* (January/February 1989): 20–22.

Assess Your Behavior

1. Think about the risk factors for addiction. Are you at risk for addiction? If so, what can you do to reduce your risk?

2. Is your alcohol, tobacco, or other drug behavior causing you problems in the areas of health, work, school, or relationships? If so, what are some resources that you can use to help?

Evaluate how well you understand the concepts presented in this chapter by answering the following questions.

1. An abnormal or disordered relationship with a substance or behavior is called:
   a. denial.
   b. addiction.
   c. habit.
   d. depression.
   e. All of the above.

2. This denotes a change in the body's biochemistry so that it demands a substance to function.
   a. psychological addition
   b. physiological addiction
   c. obsessive compulsion
   d. euphoria

3. Risk factors for addiction include:
   a. the addiction seems to temporarily reduce stress.
   b. society discourages the addictive behavior.
   c. the addition can provide escape from pain.
   d. a and b.
   e. a and c.

4. Reasons for quitting smoking include:
   a. it increases risk for heart attacks and strokes.
   b. it increases risk of ulcers, miscarriages, low birthweight.
   c. it is socially unacceptable.
   d. it limits social opportunities.
   e. All of the above.

5. A product that is 120 proof is what percent alcohol?
   a. 50
   b. 60
   c. 70
   d. 80

6. Reasons to avoid binge drinking include:
   a. it can cause death.
   b. it can increase your risk of sexual victimization.
   c. it can make you more popular.
   d. a and b.
   e. b and c.

7. Causes of the hangover include:
   a. rehydration of nerve cells.
   b. accumulation of formaldehyde.
   c. fatty liver.
   d. a and b.

8. Health effects of marijuana include:
   a. lung damage.
   b. reduced sex drive.
   c. reduced short term memory.
   d. interference with immunity.
   e. All of the above.

Correct answers can be found on page 370.

Am I an Addict?

The following questions were written by recovering addicts in Narcotics Anonymous.

	Yes	No
1. Do you ever use alone?	☐	☐
2. Have you ever substituted one drug for another, thinking that one particular drug was the problem?	☐	☐
3. Have you ever manipulated or lied to a doctor to obtain prescription drugs?	☐	☐
4. Have you ever stolen drugs or stolen to obtain drugs?	☐	☐
5. Do you regularly use a drug when you wake up or when you go to bed?	☐	☐
6. Have you ever taken one drug to overcome the effects of another drug?	☐	☐
7. Do you avoid people or places that do not approve of you using drugs?	☐	☐
8. Have you ever used a drug without knowing what it was or what it would do to you?	☐	☐
9. Has your job or school performance ever suffered from the effects of your drug use?	☐	☐
10. Have you ever been arrested as a result of using drugs?	☐	☐
11. Have you ever lied about what or how much you use?	☐	☐
12. Do you put the purchase of drugs ahead of your financial responsibilities?	☐	☐
13. Have you ever tried to stop or control your using?	☐	☐
14. Have you ever been in a jail, hospital, or drug rehabilitation center because of your using?	☐	☐
15. Does using interfere with your sleeping or eating?	☐	☐
16. Does the thought of running out of drugs terrify you?	☐	☐
17. Do you feel it is impossible for you to live without drugs?	☐	☐
18. Do you ever question your own sanity?	☐	☐
19. Is your drug use making life at home unhappy?	☐	☐
20. Have you ever thought you couldn't fit in or have a good time without using drugs?	☐	☐
21. Have you ever felt defensive, guilty, or ashamed about your using?	☐	☐
22. Do you think a lot about drugs?	☐	☐
23. Have you had irrational or indefinable fears?	☐	☐
24. Has using affected your sexual relationship?	☐	☐

	Yes	No
25. Have you ever taken drugs you didn't prefer?	☐	☐
26. Have you ever used drugs because of emotional pain or stress?	☐	☐
27. Have you ever overdosed on any drugs?	☐	☐
28. Do you continue to use despite negative consequences?	☐	☐
29. Do you think you might have a drug problem?	☐	☐

"Am I an addict?" This is a question only you can answer. Members of Narcotics Anonymous found that they all answered different numbers of these questions "yes." The actual number of *yes* responses isn't as important as how you feel inside and how addiction has affected your life. If you are an addict, you must first admit that you have a problem with drugs before any progress can be made toward recovery.

Nicotine Dependence: Are You Hooked?

Answer each question in the list below, giving yourself the appropriate points.

		0 points	1 point	2 points
☐	**1.** How soon after you wake up do you smoke your first cigarette?	After 30 minutes	Within 30 minutes	—
☐	**2.** Do you find it difficult to refrain from smoking in places where it is forbidden, such as the library, theater, doctor's office?	No	Yes	—
☐	**3.** Which of all the cigarettes you smoke in a day is the most satisfying?	Any other than the first one in the morning	The first one in the morning	—
☐	**4.** How many cigarettes a day do you smoke?	1–15	16–25	26+
☐	**5.** Do you smoke more during the morning than during the rest of the day?	No	Yes	—
☐	**6.** Do you smoke when you are so ill that you are in bed most of the day?	No	Yes	—
☐	**7.** Does the brand you smoke have a low, medium, or high nicotine content?	Low	Medium	High
☐	**8.** How often do you inhale the smoke?	Never	Sometimes	Always

☐ **Total**

Scoring

- More than 6 points—very dependent
- Less than 6 points—low-to-moderate dependence

Why Do You Smoke?

		Always	Fre-quently	Occa-sionally	Seldom	Never
A.	I smoke cigarettes in order to keep myself from slowing down.	5	4	3	2	1
B.	Handling a cigarette is part of the enjoyment of smoking it.	5	4	3	2	1
C.	Smoking cigarettes is pleasant and relaxing.	5	4	3	2	1
D.	I light up a cigarette when I feel angry about something.	5	4	3	2	1
E.	When I have run out of cigarettes, I find it almost unbearable until I can get them.	5	4	3	2	1
F.	I smoke cigarettes automatically without even being aware of it.	5	4	3	2	1
G.	I smoke cigarettes to stimulate me, to perk myself up.	5	4	3	2	1
H.	Part of the enjoyment of smoking a cigarette comes from the steps I take to light up.	5	4	3	2	1
I.	I find cigarettes pleasurable.	5	4	3	2	1
J.	When I feel uncomfortable or upset about something, I light up a cigarette.	5	4	3	2	1
K.	I am very much aware of the fact when I am not smoking a cigarette.	5	4	3	2	1
L.	I light up a cigarette without realizing I still have one burning in the ashtray.	5	4	3	2	1
M.	I smoke cigarettes to give me a "lift."	5	4	3	2	1
N.	When I smoke a cigarette, part of the enjoyment is watching the smoke as I exhale it.	5	4	3	2	1
O.	I want a cigarette most when I am comfortable and relaxed.	5	4	3	2	1
P.	When I feel "blue" or want to take my mind off cares and worries, I smoke cigarettes.	5	4	3	2	1
Q.	I get a real gnawing hunger for a cigarette when I haven't smoked for a while.	5	4	3	2	1
R.	I've found a cigarette in my mouth and didn't remember putting it there.	5	4	3	2	1

From *A Self-Test for Smokers* (U.S. Department of Health and Human Services, 1983).

Scoring Your Test:

Enter the numbers you have circled on the test questions in the spaces provided below, putting the number you have circled to question A on line A, to question B on line B, and so on. Add the three scores on each line to get a total for each factor. For example, the sum of your scores on lines A, G, and M gives you your score on "Stimulation,"; lines B, H, and N give the score on "Handling"; and so on. Scores can vary from 3 to 15. Any score 11 and above is high; any score 7 and below is low.

A   _____ + G _____ + M _____ = _____   Stimulation

B   _____ + H _____ + N _____ = _____   Handling

C   _____ + I _____ + O _____ = _____   Pleasure / Relaxation

D   _____ + J _____ + P _____ = _____   Crutch: Tension Reduction

E   _____ + K _____ + Q _____ = _____   Craving: Psychological Addiction

F   _____ + L _____ + R _____ = _____   Habit

A score of 11 or above on any factor indicates that smoking is an important source of satisfaction for you. The higher you score (15 is the highest), the more important a given factor is in your smoking. See page 324 for strategies for dealing with why you smoke.

Do You Have a Problem With Alcohol?

Instructions

To determine if you have a problem with alcohol, answer yes (Y) or no (N) to the following questions about your drinking. Refer to the scale at the end of the quiz for evaluation of your answers.

1. Do you occasionally drink heavily after a disappointment or a quarrel or when your parents or boss gives you a hard time?

2. When you have trouble or feel pressured at school or at work, do you drink more heavily than usual?

3. Have you noticed that you are able to handle more liquor than you did when you were first drinking?

4. Did you ever wake up the "morning after" and discover that you couldn't remember part of the evening before, even though your friends tell you that you didn't pass out?

5. When drinking with other people, do you try to have a few extra drinks that others don't notice?

6. Are there certain occasions when you feel uncomfortable if alcohol is not available?

7. Have you recently noticed that when you begin drinking, you are in more of a hurry to get the first drink than you used to be?

8. Do you sometimes feel a little guilty about your drinking?

9. Are you secretly irritated when your family or friends discuss your drinking?

10. Have you recently noticed an increase in the frequency of your memory blackouts?

11. Do you often find that you wish to continue drinking after your friends say they have had enough?

12. Do you usually have a reason for the occasions when you drink heavily?

13. When you are sober, do you often regret things you did or said while drinking?

14. Have you tried switching brands or following different plans for controlling your drinking?

15. Have you often failed to keep the promises you've made to yourself about controlling or cutting down on your drinking?

16. Have you ever tried to control your drinking by changing jobs or moving to a new location?

17. Do you try to avoid family or close friends while you are drinking?

18. Are you having more financial and academic problems than you used to?

19. Do more people seem to treat you unfairly without good reason?

20. Do you eat very little or irregularly when you are drinking?

21. Do you sometimes have the shakes in the morning and find that it helps to have a drink?

22. Have you recently noticed that you cannot drink as much as you once did?

23. Do you sometimes stay drunk for several days at a time?

24. Do you sometimes feel very depressed and wonder whether life is worth living?

25. Sometimes after a period of drinking, do you see or hear things that aren't there?

26. Do you get terribly frightened after you have been drinking heavily?

If you answer "*yes*" to two or three of these questions, you may wish to evaluate your drinking in these areas. Yes answers to several of these questions may indicate one of the following stages of alcoholism:

- **Questions 1–8 (early stage):** Drinking is a regular part of your life.

- **Questions 9–21 (middle stage):** You are having trouble controlling when, where, and how much you drink.

- **Questions 22–26 (beginning of the final stage):** You no longer can control your desire to drink.

14

CHAPTER

Sexually Transmitted Infections

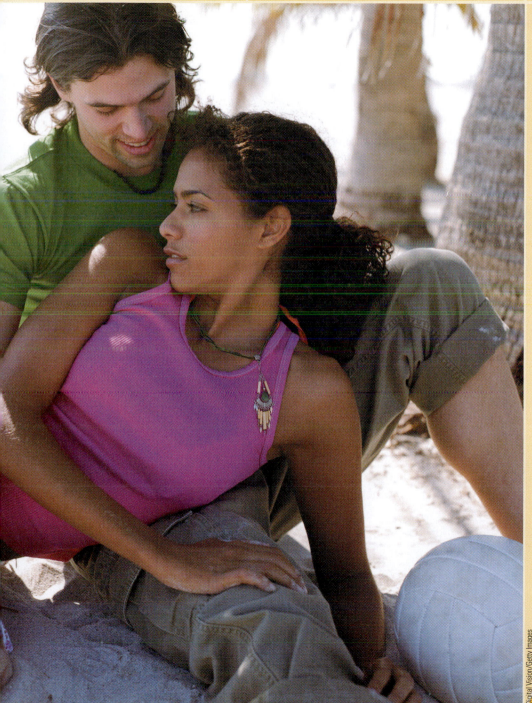

© Digital Vision/Getty Images

OBJECTIVES

Describe how sexually transmitted infections are passed from one person to another.

Discuss the reasons for the prevalence of STIs.

List the symptoms, risks, and treatment for various STIs: chlamydia, gonorrhea, genital warts, herpes, viral hepatitis, pelvic inflammatory disease, pubic lice and scabies, syphilis, and AIDS.

Describe guidelines for preventing and treating STIs.

Sexually transmitted diseases (STDs) or **sexually transmitted infections (STIs)**, as their name implies, are transmitted from one person to another through sexual contact. Several STIs also can be passed to another person through infected blood. Typically, the organisms that cause these infections are fragile and cannot exist outside the protective environment of the human reproductive tract. Therefore, in most cases they cannot be transmitted by toilet seats, soap dishes, towels, or door knobs. Some sexually transmitted infections can be cured, and others can be treated but not cured. These infections can be life-threatening and life-changing. Fortunately, most STIs can be prevented.

More than 25 identified STIs are among the most prevalent infectious infections in the United States. Of the more than 19 million new cases reported to the Centers for Disease Control and Prevention (CDC) every year, half occur among people 15 to 24 years of age.[1] More than 68 million Americans have incurable STIs. Only the common cold and flu are more prevalent than these infections. Figure 14.1 shows the estimated annual cases of common STIs.

Many STIs have reached epidemic proportions, even though some of them can be cured with proper medication. These diseases are rampant for a number of reasons:

- Some STIs have no symptoms, so victims are unaware that they are infected. Others have only mild symptoms that can be easily confused with other ailments.
- When birth control pills became widely available, many people stopped using condoms as a form of birth control, and even though condoms offer some protection against STIs, birth control pills do not.
- As a trend, some people are becoming sexually active at earlier ages and are having more than one sexual partner.
- Some STIs cannot be treated, and others have developed strains that resist antibiotics.
- Fear of social stigma, disapproval, and condemnation stop some people from seeking treatment, even when they suspect they might be infected.[2] Others become complacent because of the past successes of penicillin and other antibiotics.
- Many victims deny the possibility that they are infected, believing that "it can never happen to me," or they believe that STIs affect only high-risk groups.
- Some people erroneously believe that STIs are only minor irritations and are unaware of the serious complications that can result if these infections go untreated.

Causes

STIs are caused by pathogens (disease-causing microorganisms) including bacteria, viruses, parasites, and fungi. STI infections can recur with every new exposure. The body generally does not build up a resistance to the

FIGURE 14.1 Estimated Annual U.S. Cases of Common Sexually Transmitted Infections

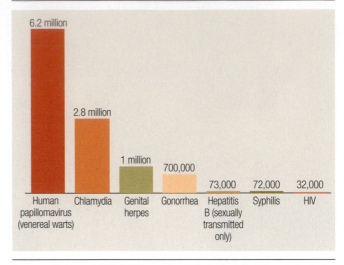

Source: Division of STD/HIV Prevention U.S. Centers for Disease Control and Prevention.

organisms that cause these infections, most of which initially affect the genitals, anus, mouth, and throat. Left untreated, many have serious complications that affect the entire body. The STI of greatest concern, **acquired immune deficiency syndrome (AIDS)**, is caused by the **human immunodeficiency virus (HIV)**, which disables the immune system, leaving the body open to various opportunistic infections and, eventually, to death.

Strictly speaking, anyone who engages in sexual activity is at risk for STIs. People who have more than one sexual partner or who have sex with someone who has or had more than one sexual partner is at risk. The risk also increases substantially if condoms are not used. Sexual behavior that tears or damages the vagina, anus, or penis increases the risk, and anal intercourse is especially dangerous. Women are at greater risk than men because they have a greater area of mucous membranes in their genital tissues. At highest risk are men who have sex with men, their sexual partners, intravenous drug users, and their partners. An infected mother can pass the disease to her child during gestation and birth.

Signs and Symptoms

Because signs and symptoms are often slower to develop and more difficult to detect in women than in men, women may not have as early an indication of infection. General signs and symptoms of STIs include

- sores on or near the genitals, anus, or mouth;
- pain in the genitals, anus, or mouth;
- a burning sensation in the genitals, anus, or mouth;
- discharge from the vagina or penis;
- itching around the genitals, in the vagina, in the rectum, around the anus, or in and around the mou;
- abdominal pain; and

- growths or warts in the genital area, anus, or mouth; these may be skin-colored or dark, flat or raised.

Sores, warts, itching, rashes, and burning in areas of the body other than the genitals, vagina, rectum, and mouth usually do not indicate STIs. If you develop these symptoms and think you may have been exposed to an STI, however, you should see a physician.

Common STIs

Understanding the incidence, signs and symptoms, and risks for specific STIs may help you reduce your risk of becoming infected.

CHLAMYDIA

About 2.8 million new cases of **chlamydia** are reported each year. An estimated 15 percent of all college students in the United States are infected. As many as half a million cases in women progress to pelvic inflammatory disease (PID), which can cause sterility and death. An estimated 4 percent of all pregnant women are infected. If left untreated, chlamydia will worsen.

Caused by the *Chlamydia trachomatis* bacteria, chlamydia often occurs simultaneously with other STIs, most commonly gonorrhea and herpes. If unidentified for many years, the bacteria also can cause non-gonococcal urethritis (NGU).

About 90 percent of all men who are infected with chlamydia have symptoms. Only about 20 percent of all women who are infected have symptoms unless the infection progresses to pelvic inflammatory disease. Even when women do have symptoms, these often are mild and can disappear on their own even though the woman is still infected. When symptoms occur, they usually appear 1 to 3 weeks after infection.

Chlamydia infects the mucous membranes that line the genitals, rectum, anus, mouth, and eyes. It is transmitted by contact with infected mucous membranes and occurs most commonly between heterosexuals. The most

common complications for newborns are pneumonia and conjunctivitis (an infection of the membranes in the eyes), found in more than 30,000 newborn babies each year in the United States.

In men, the most common symptoms of chlamydia are

- whitish or pus-like discharge from the penis;
- pain during urination; and a watery, clear discharge after urination;
- frequent urination;
- urethral itching;
- a painful, swollen scrotum; and
- abdominal discomfort.

Women who experience symptoms may have any of the following:

- a whitish vaginal discharge;
- itching or burning of the genitals;
- mild pain during urination;
- abdominal discomfort;
- bleeding between menstrual periods; and
- symptoms of pelvic inflammatory disease (fever, painful intercourse, pelvic pain, vaginal discharge).

Complications of chlamydia in men include infections of the urinary tract and sterility. In women, chlamydia is the leading cause of pelvic inflammatory disease, which also can cause ectopic pregnancy and sterility. Chlamydia that is untreated can damage the arteries, heart valves, and heart muscle in men and women alike. At particular risk for chlamydia are people with more than one sexual partner and people who do not use some kind of barrier (such as condoms) during intercourse.

Treatment for chlamydia consists of a full course of antibiotics, usually tetracycline or erythromycin. Infected and diagnosed individuals should

1. take all the antibiotics the doctor prescribes,
2. have a follow-up culture 2 weeks after finishing the antibiotics to make sure the bacteria have been destroyed completely,
3. avoid all sexual activity until the infection is gone, at least until the follow-up culture is clean, and

Sexually transmitted disease (STD) A disease that is passed from one person to another through sexual contact.

Sexually transmitted infection (STI) An infection that is passed from one person to another through sexual contact.

Acquired immunodeficiency syndrome (AIDS) The final stage of HIV infection, characterized by opportunistic infections that are rare or harmless in people with normal immune function.

Human immunodeficiency virus (HIV) The virus that weakens and destroys the immune system and gradually leads to AIDS.

Chlamydia An STI caused by bacteria that infects the mucous membranes that line the genitals, rectum, anus, mouth, and eyes.

4. tell sexual partners so they can get tested and treated for chlamydia; if you have sex again with an infected partner during or after your treatment, you could be reinfected.

GONORRHEA

Known most commonly as "the clap," about 700,000 new cases of **gonorrhea** are reported each year. The actual number of infected people in the United States may be as many as five times that high, because it is believed that only about 20 percent of all cases are reported. Gonorrhea is most common among people aged 20 to 24, and its incidence is increasing most rapidly among non-white adolescents and young adults.

Gonorrhea is caused by bacteria that infect the cervix, rectum, urethra, or mouth. The bacteria die rapidly when removed from the warmth and moisture of the mucous membranes, so it cannot be transmitted by inanimate objects. It is transmitted by vaginal intercourse, anal–genital sex, and oral–genital sex. Because the environment of the vagina is so conducive to growth of the bacteria that causes gonorrhea, women who are exposed to these bacteria through intercourse have an 80 percent chance of developing gonorrhea. The most common site of infection is the cervix. If left untreated, gonorrhea is chronic and progressive. People infected with gonorrhea do not become immune to it, so they can become reinfected many times.

The symptoms of gonorrhea generally develop within 2 days to 2 weeks after infection but may not appear for as long as 30 days. As with chlamydia, it may have no symptoms at all or only mild symptoms, especially in women.

Men generally tend to have more noticeable signs and symptoms, which include

- a profuse, yellowish or milky, foul-smelling discharge from the penis;

- burning, frequent urination;
- fever;
- abdominal pain;
- swollen lymph glands in the groin; and
- swelling of the testicles, sometimes accompanied by testicular pain.

An estimated 80 percent of women infected with gonorrhea do not have immediate symptoms. If women develop symptoms, they are usually mild and include

- slight burning or pain in the genital area;
- slight foul-smelling vaginal discharge that has a different color or odor than a woman's usual discharg;
- possible pain during urination; and
- abnormally heavy menstrual bleeding or bleeding between periods.

Gonorrhea transmitted during oral sex can cause a mild sore throat (often no more severe than the sore throat that accompanies the common cold). If gonorrhea was transmitted during anal intercourse, it can cause pain, burning, and discharge from the anus or the presence of mucous, pus, or blood in the stools.

Babies born to infected mothers may become blind. Because gonorrhea is so prevalent, the eyes of newborns are treated routinely with silver nitrate. Other complications include pneumonia and infections of the anus or rectum.

If left untreated, gonorrhea can cause epididymitis, a painful condition of the testicles that can lead to permanent sterility. Other complications include heart damage, brain damage, liver damage, arthritis, skin lesions, and meningitis. The bacteria responsible for gonorrhea can survive in the reproductive tract for years, enabling a man or a woman without symptoms to infect multiple partners unknowingly.

Gonorrhea most often is treated with antibiotics. Gonorrhea can be stubborn to treat especially among men who have sex with men: As many as 40 percent of gonorrhea infections are resistant to standard antibiotics and must be treated with newer drugs and administered by injection, rather than orally.

Anyone who is infected and diagnosed with this STI should

1. take the full course of antibiotics prescribed by a doctor, even though the symptoms will probably ease up within 12 hours and disappear within 3 days;
2. return for a follow-up culture a week after finishing the antibiotics;
3. avoid sexual intercourse or other sexual contact that could spread the infection until the doctor verifies that the infection is completely gone; and
4. contact your sex partner(s) who could be infected; if they are not treated and you have sex with them during or after your treatment, you could get reinfected.

Gonorrhea is so common that some health officials recommend regular screening (usually once every 6 months) for all sexually active people.

PELVIC INFLAMMATORY DISEASE

Pelvic inflammatory disease (PID) usually is caused by other sexually transmitted infections, most commonly chlamydia and gonorrhea. It is a severe infection of the lining of the abdominal cavity in women. One of the factors that makes PID so dangerous is that it is difficult to diagnose and, unless treated immediately, it can cause infection to progress and scar tissue to form in the fallopian tubes.

Signs and symptoms of PID include

- menstrual irregularities, including irregular cycles, profuse bleeding during menstruation, and vaginal bleeding between cycles;
- severe menstrual cramps;
- unusual vaginal discharge;
- pain or tenderness in the abdomen or lower back;
- fever and chills;
- nausea and vomiting;
- loss of appetite; and
- a burning sensation during urination.

Some women who develop PID become sterile. Of those who do get pregnant, the risks for ectopic pregnancy (a fetus that attaches to the fallopian tube instead of the uterus), miscarriage, and stillbirth increase dramatically. If an ectopic pregnancy is undiagnosed, the fetus continues to grow until it ruptures the fallopian tube. This can cause severe bleeding and result in death. Clearly, PID can be life-threatening.

Antibiotics are used to treat PID. Early treatment is essential. Later treatment can kill the bacteria but cannot repair the damage already done from the infection. A person who is diagnosed and treated should

1. follow the complete course of antibiotics prescribed by a doctor, even if the symptoms disappear;
2. not use an intrauterine device for birth control;
3. avoid sexual activity until the infection has cleared up;
4. ask that any sexual partners be treated; if they are not and you have sex with them during or after treatment, you can become reinfected;
5. not douche, because it can spread the infection.

GENITAL WARTS

Genital warts are wart-like growths caused by the **human papilloma virus (HPV)**. Genital warts are the most common STI, epidemic on America's college campuses and infecting an estimated 6.2 million Americans each year. More than 65 different strains of HPV cause genital warts, and a person can be infected by more than one strain at the same time.

The most common symptom—warts on the penis, scrotum, anus, cervix, vagina, or around the urethra—may develop as soon as 1 to 3 months following infection or as long as 8 months after infection. Outbreaks of warts are more common during pregnancy and in people who

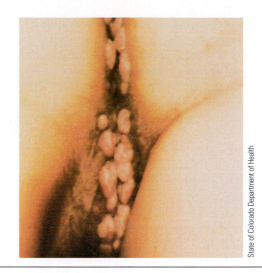

Genital warts on the male.

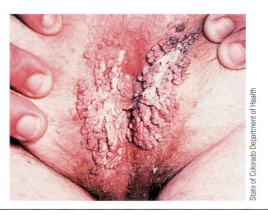

An advanced case of genital warts on the female.

have weak immune systems. Genital warts can be transmitted by skin-to-skin contact during vaginal or anal intercourse or by oral-genital contact during oral sex.

Genital warts usually start with localized irritation and itching, followed by the presence of painless warts, which may be soft or hard, flat, small, yellowish, and dry. They usually are shaped irregularly and may be white, pink, or gray. Often warts are inside the vagina or rectum or on the cervix, so they may not be noticed unless a physician discovers them during an examination. Flat warts are so small that they may not be visible to the human eye.

Gonorrhea An STI caused by bacteria that infects the cervix, rectum, urethra, or mouth.

Pelvic inflammatory disease (PID) A severe infection of the lining of the abdominal cavity in women, usually caused by bacterial STIs.

Genital warts An STI caused by the human papilloma virus (HPV) and characterized by warts around the genitals or mouth.

Human papilloma virus (HPV) The virus that causes genital warts; some strains of the virus also have been linked to cervical cancer.

In advanced stages, genital warts often clump together, interfering with urination and sexual intercourse. If the infection was passed via oral sex, the warts may grow in and around the mouth.

Even though many people who have HPV do not develop obvious symptoms, everyone who carries the virus is at risk for the complications. HPV presents life-threatening risks in people who have symptoms as well as those who do not. The complications of genital warts are potentially deadly. HPV is associated with more than 90 percent of all cervical cancers, and it is associated with other genital cancers as well, including cancer of the penis and anus.

Newborns infected by their mothers can develop warts in the mouth and bronchial passages. This can interfere with breathing.

Although treatment can remove the warts, it cannot completely kill the virus that causes the warts. Recurrence is extremely common. The typical treatment for genital warts is the drug podophyllin, which causes the wart to slough off. A physician normally applies it once a week for 5 or 6 weeks until the wart has disappeared completely. Podophyllin cannot be used by pregnant women or to treat warts in the cervical area.

Warts that resist treatment with podophyllin sometimes can be removed by surgery, electrocautery (burning), or cryotherapy (freezing). All of these options result in scarring.

A person diagnosed and treated for genital warts should

1. follow the physician's instructions carefully; repeated treatment usually is necessary to remove the warts;
2. use any antibiotic ointments the physician prescribes;
3. avoid sexual contact during an outbreak of warts; use condoms when warts are not visible;
4. for women—have a pelvic exam, including a Pap smear, every year to monitor the risk for cervical cancer; and
5. never use over-the-counter wart removers; they are useless against genital warts and can cause tissue damage if applied to the genital area.

Treatment does not kill the virus that causes genital warts. Once infected, the person always carries the virus, even though it may be dormant for months or years at a time.

HERPES

Of the different strains of herpes simplex virus, the most common is herpes simplex-1, the culprit behind the common cold sore or fever blister. Other viruses in the herpes family cause chicken pox, shingles, and infectious mononucleosis. The herpes simplex-2 virus causes the herpes STI, also known as **herpes genitalis**.

Once a person gets genital herpes, it remains forever. It has no cure, but the symptoms can be treated with limited success. The virus always will reside in the body, even

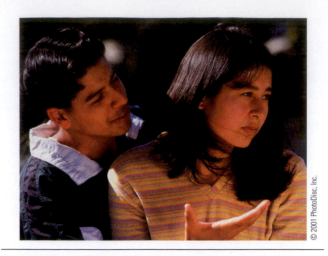

If you care enough to hesitate, you care enough to tell your partner.

when the blistering sores characteristic of a herpes outbreak are not present. Some people have only one or two outbreaks a year; others may have outbreaks more often. The virus can be spread even when no lesions are visible. Herpes is transmitted by contact with an active sore or with the virus-containing secretions from the vagina or penis, even when an outbreak is not occurring.

Approximately one million new cases of herpes are reported to the CDC each year. More than 37 million Americans have the virus. It is most common among those aged 18 to 25 years. Usually within 10 days of infection, flu-like symptoms arise that may include

- fever;
- swollen glands, especially in the groin;
- muscle aches and pains;
- fatigue; and
- occasionally, shooting or stabbing pains in the abdomen and legs.

During this initial period, the infected person may feel pain during intercourse or urination. The characteristic blisters that appear on the genitals or mouth follow the flu-like symptoms. These sores shed the herpes virus and are highly contagious. Herpes sores progress through four stages:

1. At the site where the virus entered the body, the skin starts to itch or tingle, turns red, and becomes extremely sensitive. This stage of infection, called the **prodrome**, typically precedes all outbreaks. During this stage the virus is present and the person is contagious.
2. One or more small, painful blisters or sores erupt on the glans and shaft of the penis, around the anus, at the opening of the vagina, on the clitoris, on the cervix, or on the labia. If oral–genital contact occurred, the sores may be in or around the mouth. The blisters rupture and the resulting painful, itching, open sores may weep a yellowish secretion or pus. During this stage, the risk of transmission is high.

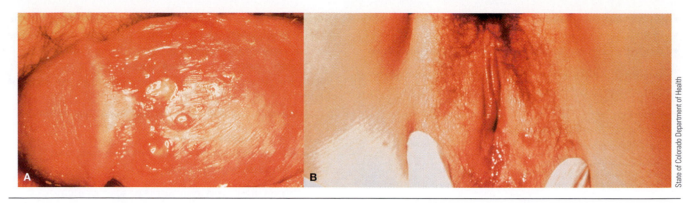

Genital herpes on the penis (A) and labia (B).

3. Without treatment, the sores diminish; scabs form and fall off within 1 to 2 weeks. Pain, fever, and other symptoms subside.

4. The virus lies dormant in the nerve endings until the next outbreak. The recurrence of blisters is usually less severe and of shorter duration. Recurrence can be caused by unrelated illness, fever, emotional stress, lack of sleep, exposure to cold or heat, sunburn, poor nutrition, and menstruation.

One complication of herpes is **autoinoculation**, in which the mouth, eyes, or other part of the body can become infected. If people experiencing an outbreak touch the blisters, then rub their eyes, the eyes can become infected. Women are at higher risk for cervical cancer if they are infected with herpes.

Possibly the most serious complications involve babies born to mothers with herpes. If a woman with an active herpes lesion delivers a baby vaginally, the baby has a one-in-four chance of being infected and can become blind, have mental retardation, have damage to internal organs, and may even die. During a herpes outbreak or presence of the virus in the vagina, a pregnant woman should have a cesarean section delivery to lessen the risk of infecting the baby.

Herpes is caused by a virus, and it has no known cure. Drug treatments using antiviral drugs have helped relieve symptoms. A person diagnosed with herpes should

1. wash the hands thoroughly after touching infected areas to avoid spreading the disease to other areas of the body;

2. keep the infected lesions clean and dry;

3. wear loose clothing to avoid irritating the infected areas; avoid scratching, rubbing, touching, or picking at sores;

4. avoid sexual contact of any kind during the prodrome and when lesions are active;

5. use a latex condom to help prevent spread of the infection when blisters are not present;

6. practice good health habits to avoid getting fatigued or stressed, which can lead to recurrences; and

7. for women—have a pelvic exam including a Pap smear every 6 to 12 months to monitor the risk for cervical cancer. If pregnant, discuss the history of the infection with the doctor. Physicians usually recommend that the baby of an infected mother be delivered by cesarean section.

HEPATITIS

Hepatitis, an infection that causes inflammation of the liver, is caused by one or more viruses. Of the four identified types of hepatitis, the most common is hepatitis A, more often called "infectious hepatitis." Hepatitis A is spread through unsanitary conditions, poor hygiene, direct exposure to the virus, or infected food and water. An estimated half of all adults in the United States have developed antibodies to hepatitis A, and it can be prevented with gamma globulin injections within 10 days of exposure.

Hepatitis B is spread through exposure to the contaminated blood or body fluids of an infected person. Besides being spread through semen and vagina secretions, it can be transmitted through breast milk, saliva, and perspiration. Hepatitis B is a resilient pathogen; it can be spread through less-direct contact.

The first signs and symptoms of hepatitis B, which develop within 6 months of infection, include

- mild fever;
- loss of appetite;
- nausea and vomiting;
- diarrhea;
- severe fatigue;

Herpes genitalis An infection caused by the herpes simplex-2 virus and characterized by blistering sores on the genitals.

Prodrome The stage of infection when early symptoms erupt; in the case of herpes, a sensation in which the skin starts to itch or tingle; precedes onset of the blisters and sores.

Autoinoculation Spreading an infection to other parts of one's own body.

Hepatitis B A form of hepatitis spread through exposure to the contaminated blood or body fluids of an infected person; can cause long-term liver damage.

- pain in the muscles and joints;
- headache; and
- tenderness in the upper right section of the abdomen.

Within 2 weeks after symptoms first appear, signs of liver damage may become apparent, including

- **jaundice**;
- light gray or whitish stools;
- dark urine; and
- tender, enlarged liver.

Because the symptoms of hepatitis B are so much like those of the flu or infectious mononucleosis, a blood test is needed for proper diagnosis. Long-term complications from hepatitis B, which can be devastating, include chronic progressive hepatitis, liver cancer, liver failure, cirrhosis of the liver, and death.

Although hepatitis B has no cure, an effective vaccine is available to make uninfected people immune and prevent infection. Anyone in the high-risk group should ask for the vaccine. High-risk individuals include

- sexually active people and their partners;
- sexual partners of an infected person or a person living in the house with an infected person, even if not sexually involved;
- intravenous drug users and their partners;
- people in health-care professions; and
- natives of or travelers to Africa, Asia, Alaska, and the Pacific Islands.

People diagnosed with hepatitis B should do the following:

1. Get plenty of rest. Follow the physician's guidelines for limiting activity during the acute stage of infection.
2. Avoid using drugs, including alcohol, that are metabolized by the liver, because these substances can put an excess burden on the liver.
3. Avoid sexual contact.
4. If pregnant, discuss the disease with a physician. Do not breastfeed your baby.
5. Have regular follow-up checkups to determine the risk for liver disease.

PUBIC LICE AND SCABIES

Commonly called "crabs," **pubic lice** are tiny parasites that move from partner to partner during sexual activity. Pubic lice actually are one of three different kinds of lice that attach to various parts of the body. Pubic lice grip the pubic hair and feed on the small blood vessels of the underlying skin, and other forms of lice attach to skin or the hair of the head.

With a life cycle of approximately 2 months, pubic lice attach to the pubic hair, where females can lay as many as 10 eggs (nits) a day. The nits adhere to the pubic hair with a thick, sticky substance. Body warmth incubates the eggs

until they hatch, and the new lice start feeding on the blood vessels as the old lice drop off. As they drop off, the lice are visible to the naked eye in bedding and clothing.

The tiny mite that causes **scabies** has a similar life cycle, but the female mite burrows under the skin at night.

Common signs and symptoms of pubic lice include

- intense itching in the pubic area;
- visible lice or whitish nits in the pubic hair; and
- swollen glands in the groin.

Common signs and symptoms of scabies include

- characteristic patterns of burrowing, most commonly on the buttocks, under the breasts, between the fingers, and on the wrists;
- a discharge of pus from the burrowed areas; and
- intense itching.

Treatment options for pubic lice include shampoos and lotions available by prescription and over the counter. Both are applied to the pubic hair, and a fine-tooth comb is then used to remove nits. Pregnant women should check with a doctor before using any of these products.

Individuals diagnosed with scabies should follow the doctor's directions, because scabies can be transmitted by close nonsexual contact. If diagnosed with pubic lice or scabies, the infected person should follow these steps:

1. Follow treatment directions carefully.
2. Dip the comb in vinegar, then water, to dissolve the sticky substance holding nits to the pubic hair.
3. Wash all clothing, bedding, and linens that were contacted prior to treatment. Towels or sheets can infect a person who does not have sexual contact.
4. Clean all upholstery and furniture that were contacted prior to treatment.
5. Avoid sexual contact and inform all sexual partners to seek treatment. If they are not treated, and you have sex with them during or after treatment, you could become reinfected.

SYPHILIS

Approximately 72,000 new cases of **syphilis** are reported each year. Caused by a spirochete (corkscrew-shaped type of bacteria), syphilis is transmitted through direct contact with infectious sores, skin rashes, or mucous patches caused by the disease.

Syphilis is transmitted most often through penile–vaginal intercourse, anal–genital contact, and oral–genital contact, though kissing a person who has a sore or mucous patches on the mouth also can transmit the infection. And syphilis can be transmitted from a pregnant woman to her baby after the fourth month of pregnancy. (For the first 4 months, a special temporary membrane in the placenta protects the fetus from infectious agents in the mother's bloodstream.) After the fourth month, the bacterium that causes syphilis is passed easily across the placenta from the mother's bloodstream to the baby's circulatory system.

Syphilis has four identifiable stages:

1. *Primary stage.* Occurring 2 to 3 weeks after the bacteria enter the body, a **chancre** (sore) develops at the site where the bacteria entered, usually on the genitals. The chancre may look like a blister or pimple but is often an open sore. It may be as large as a dime but commonly is as small as a pinhead and may go unnoticed, especially if it is in the vagina, rectum, anus, or mouth. The sore looks like it would be painful but actually is painless and may be accompanied by painless swollen lymph nodes in the groin.

   Within 3 to 6 weeks, the chancre clears up without treatment; so many infected people assume it was something else. Even though the chancre has healed, infectious bacteria remain in the system.

2. *Secondary stage.* Any time from 6 weeks to a year after the chancre heals, the symptoms of secondary syphilis appear. These symptoms, which may be mild to severe and can last anywhere from a few days to a few months, include

   - low-grade fever;
   - nausea and loss of appetite;
   - whitish patches on the mouth and throat (infectious patches);
   - sore throat;
   - painless rash anywhere on the skin, especially on the soles of the feet and palms of the hands; though the rash does not itch, it spreads infection;
   - headache;
   - swollen glands;
   - hair loss, usually patchy;
   - arthritic-type joint pain; and
   - large sores on the genitals or around the mouth.

   Even if untreated, these symptoms usually run their course, then disappear. This does not mean the infection is gone. The infection remains dormant, and symptoms can reappear at any time. The person remains infectious during this stage, even though symptoms have cleared up.

3. *Latent stage.* No outward symptoms are present during the latent stage, which usually lasts as long as 30 years. During the latent stage, the person is no longer contagious unless moist lesions erupt. One exception is a pregnant woman, who can pass syphilis to her fetus during the latent stage. Even though nothing seems to be happening on the outside during the latent stage, the spirochetes attack the body's organs, causing substantial damage to the brain, heart, and central nervous system. Maladies characteristic of the latent stage include heart disease, senility, blindness, deterioration of the central nervous system, and sometimes death.

4. *Late (tertiary) stage.* The late stage of syphilis usually begins 5 to 20 years after the initial infection.

Two-thirds of people with untreated infections have no further symptoms. About one-third of people with untreated infections develop blindness, deafness, central nervous system destruction, damage to the heart, paralysis, psychosis, and, finally, death during the late stage of syphilis.

A fetus infected by the mother's blood may develop mild to severe organ damage as a result. Syphilis also can result in stillbirth.

Penicillin is the drug of choice in treating syphilis. With treatment, syphilis can be cured at any stage. Early detection and treatment is best, because treatment is effective at killing the bacteria and stopping the infection, but it cannot repair the damage that the infection already caused.

A person diagnosed and treated for syphilis should do the following:

1. Follow the complete course of antibiotics as prescribed by a doctor, even if symptoms are not apparent.
2. Discuss with the doctor the possibility of simultaneous STI infections, such as gonorrhea or chlamydia. If additional infections are present, higher doses of various antibiotics are necessary.
3. Avoid sexual activity until cured.
4. Have follow-up blood tests for a year after finishing antibiotic treatment.

HIV AND AIDS

In the United States, approximately 580,000 people are infected with HIV, the virus that causes AIDS. Each year about 32,000 new cases are reported, and more than 400,000 Americans have died of the consistently fatal disorder. The number of women infected with HIV is increasing faster than any other population. Currently no vaccine is available, and no cure.

Differentiating HIV and AIDS At first, people who become infected with HIV may not know they are infected. An incubation period of weeks, months, or years may go by during which no symptoms appear. HIV may live in the body 10 years or longer before symptoms develop. The

Jaundice Liver condition in which the skin and whites of the eyes appear yellow.

Pubic lice Commonly called "crabs," tiny parasites that feed on the small blood vessels of the skin beneath the pubic hair.

Scabies Tiny mites that burrow under the skin; may be spread by sexual or nonsexual contact.

Syphilis An STI caused by bacteria, occurring in four stages; untreated, it is fatal.

Chancre A painless, red-rimmed sore that develops at the site where syphilis bacteria enter the body.

person can spread HIV to others even though no symptoms have appeared during the early stages of infection.

As the infection progresses to the point at which certain diseases develop, the person is said to have AIDS. HIV itself does not kill people, nor do people die of AIDS. AIDS is the term used to define the final stage of HIV infection, when death results from a weakened immune system that is unable to fight off the opportunistic diseases that develop. To test your knowledge of AIDS, see Assessment 14.1.

Earliest symptoms of the disease include unexplained weight loss, constant fatigue, mild fever, swollen lymph glands, diarrhea, and sore throat. Among the symptoms in the more advanced stages are loss of appetite, skin diseases, night sweats, and deterioration of mucous membranes. Though fatal to AIDS victims, most of the illnesses that AIDS patients develop are harmless and rare in the general population. The two most common fatal conditions in AIDS patients are pneumocystis carinii pneumonia (a parasitic infection of the lungs) and Kaposi's sarcoma (a type of skin cancer). The AIDS virus also may attack the nervous system, causing damage to the brain and spinal cord.

Upon HIV infection, the immune system's line of defense against the virus is to form antibodies that bind to the virus. On average, the body takes 3 months to manufacture enough antibodies to show up positive in an HIV antibody test. Sometimes this may take 6 months or even longer. If HIV infection is suspected, a prudent waiting period of 3 to 6 months is suggested prior to testing. During this time, and from there on, individuals should refrain from further endangering themselves and others through risky behaviors such as sexual activity or IV drug use.

HIV Transmission Two basic conditions have to be present for HIV to be transmitted:

1. One person has to be infected.
2. The virus has to be transmitted to an area in the body where body fluids can be exchanged.

HIV is transmitted by the exchange of body fluids including blood, semen, vaginal secretions, and maternal milk. These fluids may be exchanged during sexual intercourse, by using hypodermic needles used previously by infected individuals, between a pregnant woman and her developing fetus, by infection of babies from the mother during childbirth, less frequently during breast-feeding, and rarely from a blood transfusion or organ transplant.

The risk of being infected with HIV from a blood transfusion today is slight. Prior to 1985, several cases of HIV infection came from blood transfusions because HIV-infected individuals donated the blood. Today, all donated blood is tested for HIV.

A myth regarding HIV is that donating blood can transmit it. People cannot get HIV from giving blood. Health professionals use a new needle every time they withdraw blood from a person. These needles are used only once and are thrown away immediately after each person has donated blood.

HIV and AIDS can threaten anyone, anywhere, regardless of gender, race, income, or education. It is considered an equal-opportunity destroyer. HIV can be transmitted between males, between females, from male to female, or from female to male. The good news is that HIV and AIDS are preventable. Almost everyone who contracts HIV does so because they choose to engage in risky behaviors.

Risky Behaviors You cannot tell if people are infected with HIV or have AIDS by simply looking at them or taking their word. Although many people who have been infected with HIV look normal and healthy for years, they are capable of passing the virus to others. Therefore, every time you engage in a risky behavior, you run the risk of contracting HIV. The two most basic risky behaviors are unprotected sex and needle-sharing.

1. *Having unprotected vaginal, anal, or oral sex with an HIV-infected person.* Unprotected sex means having sex without the proper use of a condom. A person should select only latex (rubber or prophylactic) condoms that include "disease prevention" on the package. Although you might have unprotected sex with an infected person and not get the virus, you also can get it by having unprotected sex only once with that infected person.

Rubbing during sexual intercourse often damages mucous membranes and causes unseen bleeding (even in the mouth). During vaginal, anal, or oral sexual contact, the infected blood, semen, or vaginal fluids can penetrate the mucous membranes that line the vagina, the penis, the rectum, the mouth, or the throat. From the membrane, HIV then can travel into the blood of the previously uninfected person.

Health experts believe that unprotected anal sex is the riskiest type of sex. Even though bleeding is not visible in some cases, anal sex almost always causes tiny tears and bleeding in the rectum. This happens because the rectum does not stretch easily, the mucous membrane is quite thin, and small blood vessels lie directly beneath the membrane. Condoms also are more likely to break during anal intercourse because more friction takes place in a smaller cavity. All of these factors greatly enhance the risk of transmitting HIV.

Although latex condoms reduce risk if they are used correctly, they are not 100 percent foolproof. Abstaining from sex is the only way to completely protect yourself from HIV infection and other STIs.

2. *Sharing hypodermic needles or other drug paraphernalia with someone who is infected.* Following an injection, a small amount of blood remains in the needle and sometimes in the syringe itself. If the person who used the syringe is infected with HIV and someone else uses that same syringe, regardless of the drug used (legal or illegal), that small amount of blood is sufficient to spread

- **Do** use condoms during every sexual encounter.
- **Do** use condoms for vaginal intercourse, anal intercourse, and oral sex.
- **Do** use only latex condoms. Natural membranes have pores through which the virus can travel.
- **Do** use caution when opening a condom. Teeth, fingernails, or other sharp objects could tear the condom.
- **Do** put on the condom as the penis is erect, roll it all the way to the base of the penis, and be sure it stays on until the penis is fully withdrawn. Also make sure there is no air in the tip of the condom.

- **Do** use plenty of water-based lubricant, not oil- or alcohol-based lubricants such as Vaseline or baby oil, as these weaken latex and make condoms break more easily.
- **Do** look for a date within 2½ years from this date (all condoms are stamped with a date of manufacture)
- **Don't** use a condom more than once.
- **Don't** continue using a condom if it breaks during sex. Stop and put on a new condom.
- **Don't** expose condoms to extreme light or temperature.
- **Don't** carry condoms in wallets, as these conditions may cause a condom to dry out and break.
- **Don't** stretch or inflate a condom before use.

the virus. All used syringes should be destroyed and disposed of immediately after they are used.

In addition, a person must be cautious when receiving acupuncture, getting a tattoo, or having the ears pierced. If the needle was used previously on someone who is HIV-infected and was not disinfected properly, the person risks contracting HIV as well.

Infrequent use of drugs, including alcohol, also heightens the risk of spreading HIV. Otherwise-prudent people often act irrationally and engage in risky behaviors when they are under the influence of alcohol and other drugs. Getting high can result in your willingness to have sex when you didn't plan to, and thereby run the risk of contracting HIV infection.

How HIV Is Not Transmitted No evidence suggests that HIV transmission can be airborne. HIV cannot be passed by coughing or sneezing. Small concentrations of the virus have been found in saliva, so if the person has cuts in the lips, mouth, or gums or engages in passionate open-mouthed kissing, HIV potentially could be transmitted through open-mouthed kissing, (though such a case has not been documented).

The virus cannot be transmitted through perspiration either. Sporting activities with no physical contact pose no risk to uninfected individuals unless they have open wounds through which blood from an infected person can come in direct contact with the open wound of the uninfected person. The skin is an excellent line of defense against HIV. Blood from an infected person cannot penetrate the skin except through an opening in the skin. As a precaution, a person should use vinyl or latex gloves when performing work that requires direct contact with someone else's blood or open wounds.

Some people fear getting HIV from health-care professionals. The chances of getting infected during physical or medical procedures are extremely low. Health-care workers take extra care to protect themselves and their patients from HIV.

HIV is not transmitted through normal social contact. HIV cannot be caught by spending time with, shaking hands with, or hugging an infected person; by using a public telephone, toilet seat, drinking fountain, swimming pool, dishes, or silverware used by an HIV patient; or by sharing a drink, food, a towel, or clothes with a person who has HIV.

A person cannot catch HIV from insects or animals, because they do not get infected with HIV. A mosquito that picks up the virus may carry the virus in its stomach, but the virus cannot reproduce in the mosquito or travel to the mosquito's saliva.

HIV Testing HIV testing usually is free of charge, and the results are kept confidential. Many states also conduct anonymous testing, which means the name is never recorded. Instead, a number is assigned as a link to the test.

Two types of tests are used to detect HIV:

1. *The EIA or ELISA*. This simple, inexpensive screening test measures whether the person has developed antibodies to the virus. If the test is negative and the person has not been exposed to HIV within the previous 3 months, he or she can be relatively certain of not being infected. Generally, no further testing is required. If the test is positive, the person usually is asked to take a second screening test to reduce the chance of a false-positive result.
2. *The Western Blot Test*. If the second EIA/ELISA test is positive, this more sophisticated, expensive test is given to confirm the positive results. If the Western Blot is positive, HIV infection is certain. If the test is negative, the person can be reasonably certain of not being infected, because false negative results are rare.

Neither of these tests can tell if a person has AIDS. The tests can determine only if he or she has been infected with HIV. A diagnosis of AIDS is given only if the person is infected with HIV and

- the T-lymphocyte count is low, or
- the person has one of the opportunistic infections listed by the Centers for Disease Control and Prevention. These

infections are rare or harmless in people with normal immunity.

As with any other serious illness, people with AIDS deserve respect, understanding, and support. Rejection and discrimination are traits of immature, hateful, and ignorant people. Education, knowledge, and responsible behaviors are the best ways to minimize fear and discrimination.

HIV / AIDS Treatment Even though several drugs are being tested to treat and slow the disease process, AIDS has no known cure. At least 30 different approaches to an AIDS vaccine are being explored. The best advice at this point is to take a preventive approach. Although HIV has no cure, medications are available that allow HIV-infected patients to live longer. The sooner treatment is initiated following infection, the better the chances for delaying the onset of AIDS.

Developing a vaccine to prevent HIV infection or AIDS seems highly unlikely in the next few years. People should not expect a medical breakthrough. Treatment modalities, however, should continue to improve and allow HIV-infected persons and AIDS patients to live longer and more productive lives.

Table 14.1 summarizes and compares the information about STIs presented so far in this chapter. This includes symptoms, outlook, complications, diagnosis, and treatment.

Preventing Sexually Transmitted Infections

Knowing that STIs are life-threatening and life-changing in their consequences, you will want to avoid risk and take precautions to keep yourself from becoming a victim. The one strategy that is 100 percent effective is abstinence. More and more young people are taking this approach to secure a high quality of life. The next-best prevention technique is a mutually monogamous sexual relationship—two uninfected people having a sexual relationship only with each other. A mutually monogamous relationship is effective in preventing STIs, but first you need to know that you and your partner are uninfected and, second, you need to know if your partner is being monogamous or sexually faithful.

In today's society, people often have difficulty knowing when to trust a person. In sharing information about past and present sexual behavior, most people are dishonest.[3] You may be led to believe that you are in a monogamous relationship when your partner actually (a) may be cheating on you and gets infected, (b) ends up having a one-night stand with someone who is infected, (c) got the virus several years before the present relationship and still doesn't know of the infection, (d) may not be honest with you and chooses not to tell you about the infection,

or (e) is shooting up drugs and becomes infected. In any of these cases, an STI can be passed on to you.

In addition to the medical consequences of acquiring an STI, negative emotional outcomes result from these infections. When people develop diseases that cannot be cured, their self-esteem and self-respect plummet. They often report a loss of dignity and hope. Depression results as they realize the betrayal of a partner who cheated and lied and they anticipate having a infection for the rest of their life and having to tell a future life partner about it.

Because your future and your life are at stake, and because you cannot be completely sure if your partner is infected, you should give serious and careful consideration to postponing sex until you believe you have found a lifetime monogamous relationship. In doing so, you will not have to live with the fear of contracting STIs or deal with an unplanned pregnancy. Many people postpone sexual activity until they are married. Married life will provide plenty of time for a fulfilling and rewarding sexual relationship.

Some people would have you believe you are not a "real" man or woman if you don't have sex early in your life. Manhood and womanhood are not proven during sexual intercourse but, instead, through mature, responsible, and healthy choices. Other people may lead you to believe that love cannot exist without sex. Sex in the early stages of a relationship is not the product of love but is simply the fulfillment of a physical, and often selfish, drive. Then there are those who enjoy bragging about their sexual conquests and mock people who choose to wait. In essence, many of these "conquests" are only fantasies or attempts to gain popularity with peers.

Sexual promiscuity never leads to a trusting, loving, and lasting relationship. Mature people respect others' choices. If someone does not respect your choice to wait, he or she certainly does not deserve your friendship. Sexual intercourse lasts only a few minutes. The consequences of irresponsible sex, however, may last a lifetime. In some cases, these consequences are fatal.

A loving relationship develops over a long time with mutual respect for each other. There is no better sex relationship than that between two loving and responsible individuals who mutually trust and admire each other.

TABLE 14.1 Comparing Selected Sexually Transmitted Infections

Infection	Symptoms	Outlook	Complications	Diagnosis and Treatment
Syphilis	Spirochete infection. Curable in early stages. Transmitted by oral, genital, anal contact. After a decline, case numbers rising again in North America, mainly related to drug use or exchange of sex for drugs.	Painless sore (chancre) appears 3–6 weeks after infection on genitals, mouth, or rectal area; most obvious in men, hardly noticed if vaginal. Heals without scarring. About 4–10 weeks later, second stage: fever, rash, which disappears but may reappear.	If untreated, chronic, occasionally fatal. Third stage appears up to 30 years later with brain and spinal cord damage, blindness, insanity. Untreated, can cause miscarriage and birth defects; infants of infected mother may be born with syphilis (congenital syphilis).	Even if no symptoms, can diagnose by simple blood test; test results usually positive by time chancre (ulcer) appears. Antibiotics, taken as prescribed, a dependable cure in early stages.
Gonorrhea ("clap")	Bacterial infection, transmitted by oral, vaginal, or anal sex. Prevalent in young women, teens. Untreated, can result in pelvic inflammatory disease (PID) and infertility. Up to half of infected people have no symptoms.	Symptoms (if any) within 7 days of contact: painful urination, thick vaginal or penile discharge, bleeding between periods, sore throat (if contracted via oral sex), rectal pain or discharge (if through anal sex).	May lead to tubal scarring, PID, ectopic pregnancy (outside womb; dangerous for mother). Can cause permanent sterility in both sexes. Eye infection and possible blindness in infected newborns.	Diagnosed by smear and lab culture. Antibiotics a reliable cure, but some strains now resistant to standard antibiotics (e.g., penicillin) and require cefixime, ceftriaxone, or other new drugs.
Herpes	Viral infection due to Herpes virus types I or II. Spreads via oral, vaginal, or anal sex or kissing. Can spread silently, via asymptomatic people. Most easily transmitted by direct contact with active sores or genital secretions.	Symptoms within 10 days: slight fever, tingling, shooting pains, swollen lymph glands, then painful blisters, anywhere on genitals—mainly penis, vulva, or anal areas. Subsides without treatment, but can recur. First outbreak usually worst, but sometimes unnoticed.	Virus remains permanently in nerves, stays dormant for months or years. Newborns may get herpes during birth, resulting in central nervous system damage or death. Cesarean delivery may be advised for babies of infected mothers.	Diagnosis from blisters (scraping or culture). Medicine, not a cure, eases symptoms and reduces length of attack and its severity. Herpes support groups helpful in combating psychological problems.
Chlamydia	Bacterial infection, very common, in teens, 60–80 percent without symptoms. Spreads via anal, vaginal, or oral sex with infected partners. Often occurs together with gonorrhea.	Like gonorrhea: painful urination, vaginal or penile discharge, abdominal pain, genital itching. But often mild, unnoticed in carriers, can disappear without treatment.	In women, leading cause of PID, ectopic pregnancy, infertility. In men, can produce urinary tract diseases and prostatitis. Babies of infected mothers prone to eye infections, pneumonia.	Diagnosed by culture or other tests. Antibiotic treatment a reliable cure (if caught early).
Genital Warts	Caused by human papilloma virus (HPV). Highly contagious, spread by intimate bodily contact, especially sexual activity, often accompanies other STIs.	Warts—tiny growths on and around genitals—usually itchy, pinkish, flat, irregularly surfaced, may increase in size. Often undetectable in women in vagina or on cervix, except by physician.	Certain HPV strains linked to cervical cancer in women (and possibly penile cancer in men). Infants born to mothers with HPV may develop warts.	Removal advised—chemically, by freezing, or with lasers. Women should have regular Pap smears to detect HPV infection and early cervical cancer changes.
Hepatitis B	Virus passed on via blood, semen, vaginal secretions, saliva, needles, razors, toothbrushes. Can go from mother to infant at birth. Groups most at risk: those practicing anal sex, those with many partners, injection drug users, babies of infected mothers.	Usually subclinical with few or no symptoms. Possibly flu-like malaise, fever, fatigue typically lasting 6 weeks, perhaps jaundice/skin and eye-white yellowing. May linger in body unnoticed.	60–90 percent of infected children and 10 percent infected as adults become lifelong carriers, at risk of cirrhosis and liver cancer. Unsuspecting carriers can infect others. Fulminant is a rapidly fatal form occurring in 1 per 100 cases.	Detected by blood tests for viral markers. No cure. Effective safe vaccine recommended for all at risk—especially health care workers and those living with or close to known hepatitis B carriers.

Adapted from *Health News,* a bimonthly publication of the University of Toronto Faculty of Medicine. Subscriptions and back issues can be obtained by writing to *Health News,* 109 Vanderhoof Ave., Suite 205, Toronto, Ontario M4G 2H7 or by calling (416) 696-8818.

Contrary to many beliefs, these relationships are possible. They are built upon unselfish attitudes and behaviors.

As you look around, you will find that many of your peers believe the same way you do. Seek them out and build your friendships and future around people who respect you for who you are and what you believe. You do not have to compromise your choices or values. In the end, you will reap the greater rewards of a fulfilling and lasting relationship, free of STIs. You will enjoy self-respect and enhanced self-esteem.

In addition, be prepared for social situations, and avoid placing yourself in sexually intimate situations. Look for common interests and become involved in social settings and activities that do not involve time alone in places where sexual involvement is tempting. Communication is important, too,[4] with an honest, open expression of your feelings: "I'm not ready for sex; I just want to have fun, and kissing is fine with me."[5] If your friend doesn't accept your answer and is not willing to stop the advances, be prepared with a strong response. Statements such as, "Please stop" and "Don't!" are ineffective for the most part. Use a firm statement such as: "No, I'm not willing to do it," or "I've already thought about this and I'm not going to have sex." If the person continues the sexual advance, you have every right to say, "This is rape, and I'm going to call the police."

The following precautions will reduce your risk for contracting STIs:

1. Postpone sex until you and your uninfected partner are prepared to enter into a lifetime monogamous relationship. The famous basketball player Magic Johnson stated, in his revelation that he had HIV:

   > If I had known what I do now when I was younger, I would have postponed sex as long as I could, and I would have tried to have it the first time with somebody that I knew I wanted to spend the rest of my life with. I certainly want my children to postpone sex. Now the rest of my life may be a lot shorter than I thought it was going to be.[6]

2. Unless you are in a monogamous relationship and you know your partner is not infected (which you may never know for sure), practice safer sex every time you have sex. This means you should use a latex condom from start to finish (before any sexual contact until after the penis is withdrawn) for each sexual act, including oral sex. Put on the condom as soon as the penis is erect; pinch the condom to allow a little extra space at the tip, but do not let any air get trapped in the condom. Roll it all the way to the base of the penis, and keep it all the way on until the penis is fully withdrawn. When withdrawing the penis from the vagina, hold the condom tight at the base of the penis to prevent leakage. Inspect the condom for tears.

   If you ask your partner to use a condom but he or she refuses to do so, say no to sex with that person.

   Many experts believe greater protection can be obtained by placing a small amount of the spermicide

Safety Measures to Prevent STIs

To reduce your risk of contracting STIs:

- Plan before you get into a sexual situation. Determine the conditions under which you will allow sex to take place. If you decide to have sex, practice safer sex.
- Discuss STIs with the person you are contemplating having sex with before you do so. Talking about STIs might be awkward, but the short-lived embarrassment of addressing intimate questions can keep you from contracting or spreading infection. If you don't know the person well enough to address this issue, or you are uncertain about the answers, don't have sex with this individual.
- Eliminate your risk of getting an STI by not having sexual contact with anyone or by having contact only with a noninfected partner who has contact only with you. Limit the number of sexual partners you have. Having one partner lowers your chance of infection.
- Unless you're sure your partner is free of an STI, protect yourself by using a latex condom every time you have sexual intercourse. For extra protection, use a spermicide with the condom, as spermicide can kill the bacteria and viruses that cause some STIs.
- Avoid mixing alcohol or other drugs with sexual activities. This could cloud your judgment and lead you to engage in unsafe sexual practices.
- Thoroughly wash immediately after sexual activity. Washing with hot, soapy water will not guarantee safety against STIs, but it can prevent you from spreading certain germs on your fingers and may wash away bacteria and viruses that have not entered the body yet.
- If you suspect that your partner is infected with a STI, ask. Also, look for signs of infection, such as sores, redness, inflammations, a rash, growths, warts, or discharge. If you're unsure, abstain.
- Consider abstaining from sexual relations if you have any kind of an illness or disease, even a common cold. Any kind of illness lowers immunity and can make you extra-vulnerable to STIs.
- If you think you might have a STI, go to your doctor right away. Ask your partner to get tested, too, so you won't pass STIs back and forth.

nonoxynol–9 inside the condom at its tip and then lubricating the outside with additional spermicide. Nonoxynol–9 is used to kill the sperm for birth-control purposes. In test tubes, it has been shown to kill some STI pathogens including HIV. This spermicide, however, should not be used in place of a condom, because it will not offer the same protection as the condom does by itself.

3. Avoid having multiple and anonymous sexual partners. Anyone you have sex with could be infected with a STI.

4. Don't have sexual contact with anyone who does not practice safer sex.

5. Avoid sexual contact with anyone who has had sex with people at risk for STIs, even if they are now practicing safer sex.

6. Be cautious when communicating on the Internet. People who seek sex using the Internet have a greater chance of having STIs.[7]

7. Do not have sex with prostitutes.

8. If you do have sex with someone who might be infected with a STI or whose history is unknown to you, avoid exchange of body fluids.

9. Don't share toothbrushes, razors, or other implements that could become contaminated with blood with anyone who is, or who might be, infected with a STI.

10. Be cautious regarding procedures such as acupuncture, tattooing, and ear piercing, in which needles or other nonsterile instruments may be reused to pierce the skin or mucous membranes. These procedures are safe only if proper sterilization methods or disposable needles are used. Before undergoing any such procedure, ask about the precautions.

11. If you are planning to undergo artificial insemination, insist on frozen sperm obtained from a laboratory that tests all donors for infection with STIs. Donors should be tested twice before the lab accepts the sperm—once at the time of donation and again a few months later.

Avoiding risky behaviors that destroy quality of life and life itself are critical components in a healthy lifestyle. Preventing sexually transmitted infections is a key to averting both physical and psychological damage. Learning the facts so you can make responsible choices can protect you and those around you from life-changing and life-threatening diseases.

WEB Interactive

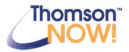

Don't forget to check out the wealth of resources on the ThomsonNOW website at **www.thomsonedu.com/ThomsonNOW** that will:

- Coach you through identifying target goals for behavior change and monitoring your personal change plan throughout the semester
- Help you evaluate your knowledge of the material
- Allow you to take an exam-prep quiz
- Provide a Personalized Learning Plan targeting resources that address areas you should study.

WEB ACTIVITIES

Planned Parenthood This excellent site features information on sexual health, including family planning, emergency contraception, and sexually transmitted infections. It also features a clinic locator to help you find places where you can receive confidential diagnosis and treatment.

http://www.plannedparenthood.org

Assess Your Risk for HIV and Other Sexually Transmitted Infections By completing this simple 24-question multiple-choice questionnaire, you will obtain an accurate portrayal of your personal risk for acquiring HIV and other types of sexually transmitted infections.

http://www.thebody.com/surveys/sexsurvey.html

CDC National Center for HIV, STI, and TB Prevention This comprehensive site features a variety of links to information regarding HIV/AIDS presentation, including the latest statistics.

http://www.cdc.gov/hiv/dhap.htm

InfoTrac®

You can find additional readings related to wellness via InfoTrac® College Edition, an online library of more than 900 journals and publications. Follow the instructions for accessing InfoTrac® that came packaged with your textbook, then search for articles using a key word search.

Suggested Reading Grosby, Richard et al. Condom discomfort and association with their use among university sudents. *Journal of American College Health,* Nov–Dec 2005 v54 i3 p143 (5).

1. In this study, what percentage of students reported discomfort when using a condom?
2. What can condom users do to avoid discomfort?
3. Is there an association between discomfort and condom breakage? What can be done to prevent this problem?

Web Activity

http://www.thebody.com/index.html

Sponsor The Body—the complete HIV/AIDS resource.

Description The Body's mission is to use the Web to lower barriers between patients and clinicians, demystify HIV/AIDS and its treatment, improve patients' quality of life, and foster community through human connection.

Available Activities

1. Risk assessment for HIV and other STDs.
2. Test your knowledge about HIV.
3. Take a quiz to measure your stress.
4. Explore HIV myth versus reality.
5. Learn how HIV medications function.

Web Work

1. From the home page, click on the tools tab.
2. In the Tools for HIV Awareness box, click on the "Assess your risk" link.
3. Complete the survey to the best of your knowledge.
4. Be sure to take advantage of the "look up a word" function and the link to the basics of safe sex and STD prevention.

5. Identify your risky behavior, if any, and follow the recommended links to implement effective behavior change!

Helpful Hints

1. Navigate to the Ask the Experts tab, and then the Safe Sex and HIV Prevention Forum.

2. Browse the forum by topic and read Q&A between the public and a M.D. specialist on HIV and other STDs.

For additional Web activities, links, and suggested readings, visit our Health, Fitness, and Wellness Resource Center at http://health.wadsworth.com.

Notes

1. Unless otherwise noted, all the statistics regarding STIs are from the Centers for Disease Control and Prevention, Atlanta.

2. J. Fortenberry, M. McFarlane, A. Bleakley, M. Fishbein, et al., "Relationships of Stigma and Shame to Gonorrhea and HIV Screening," *American Journal of Public Health* 92 (2002): 378–381.

3. J. M. Ellen et al., "Individuals' Perceptions About Their Sex Partners' Risk Behavior," *Journal of Sex Research* 35 (1998): 328–331.

4. R. Luquis, E. Garcia, and D. Ashford, "A Qualitative Assessment of College Students' Perceptions of Health Behaviors," *American Journal of Health Studies* 18 (2003): 156–164.

5. "Sexual Risk," *Dermatology Nursing* 10 (1998): 436.

6. J. Mason, *What You Can Do to Avoid AIDS* (New York: Random House, 1991).

7. M. McFarlane et al., "The Internet as Newly Emerging Risk Environment for Sexually Transmitted Diseases," *Journal of the American Medical Association* 284 (2000): 443–446.

Assess Your Behavior

1. Are you at risk for contracting a sexually transmitted infection? If so, what can you do to reduce your risk?

2. Do you know the signs and symptoms of STIs? If you were to develop a STI, what should you do to take care of it?

Assess Your Knowledge

Evaluate how well you understand the concepts presented in this chapter by answering the following questions.

1. Which of the following statements is true about STIs?
   a. All STIs have outward symptoms.
   b. Birth control pills help in the prevention of STIs.
   c. STIs affect only high-risk groups.
   d. STIs are life-changing and life-threatening.

2. General signs and symptoms of STIs include:
   a. sores on or near the genitals, mouth, or anus.
   b. pain in the genitals, mouth, or anus.
   c. discharge from the vagina or penis.
   d. itching around the genitals.
   e. All of the above.

3. This STI is bacterial and usually causes pelvic inflammatory disease in women.
   a. chlamydia
   b. gonorrhea
   c. genital warts
   d. genital herpes

4. This condition is caused by other infections and can cause ectopic pregnancy.
   a. chlamydia
   b. pelvic inflammatory disease
   c. gonorrhea
   d. syphilis

5. This pathogen causes genital warts.
   a. genital herpes
   b. acquired immune deficiency syndrome
   c. human immunodeficiency virus
   d. human papilloma virus

6. This STI causes fever and outbreaks of blistering sores on the genitals.
   a. genital warts
   b. genital herpes
   c. autoinoculation
   d. hepatitis

7. This infection is caused by a corkscrew-shaped type of bacteria.
   a. genital warts
   b. genital herpes
   c. syphilis
   d. HIV

8. To completely reduce risk of STIs
   a. postpone sex until you and your uninfected partner are prepared to enter into a lifetime monogamous relationship.
   b. use a condom every time you have sex.
   c. avoid multiple partners.
   d. do not have sex with a prostitute.

Correct answers can be found on page 370.

How Much Do You Know About AIDS?

Name: _____   Date: _____   Grade: _____

Instructor: _____   Course: _____   Section: _____

	Yes	No
1. AIDS is the end stage of infection caused by HIV.	☐	☐
2. HIV is a chronic infectious disease that spreads among individuals who engage in risky behaviors, such as unprotected sex or the sharing of hypodermic needles.	☐	☐
3. AIDS now has a cure.	☐	☐
4. Condoms are 100 percent effective in protection against HIV infection.	☐	☐
5. If you're sexually active, latex condoms provide the best protection against HIV infection.	☐	☐
6. Each year more and more teens are getting infected with HIV.	☐	☐
7. You can become HIV-infected by donating blood.	☐	☐
8. You can tell by looking at someone if he or she is HIV-infected.	☐	☐
9. The only means to determine whether someone has HIV is through an HIV antibody test.	☐	☐
10. HIV can completely destroy the immune system.	☐	☐
11. The HIV virus may live in the body 10 years or longer before AIDS symptoms develop.	☐	☐
12. People infected with HIV have AIDS.	☐	☐
13. Once infected with HIV, a person never becomes uninfected.	☐	☐
14. HIV infection is preventable.	☐	☐

Adapted from *Test Your Survival Smarts: Self-Quiz on Drugs and AIDS,* National Institute on Drug Abuse, U. S. Department of Health & Human Services; and *Principles and Labs for Physical Fitness and Wellness,* 3d edition, by Werner W. K. Hoeger and Sharon A. Hoeger (Englewood, CO: Morton Publishing, 1994), pp. 375–376.

Answers:

1. Yes. "AIDS" is the term used to define the manifestation of opportunistic diseases and cancers that occur as a result of HIV infection.

2. Yes. People do not get HIV because of who they are but, rather, because of what they do. Almost all of the people who get HIV do so because they choose to engage in risky behaviors.

3. No. AIDS has no cure, and none seems likely soon.

4. No. Only abstaining from sex gives you 100 percent protection, but latex condoms are somewhat effective in protecting against HIV infection if they're used correctly.

5. Yes. Proper use, however, is necessary to minimize the risk of infection.

6. Yes. In the early 1990s, the number of infected teens increased by 96 percent over a short span of 2 years. Probably about 20 percent of the AIDS patients today were infected as teenagers.

7. No. A myth regarding HIV is that donating blood can transmit it. People cannot get HIV from giving blood. Health professionals use a new needle every time they draw blood. These needles are used only once and are thrown away and destroyed immediately after each individual has donated blood.

8. No. The symptoms of AIDS often are not noticeable until several years after a person has been infected with HIV.

9. Yes. Nobody can tell if an HIV infection is present unless an HIV antibody test is done. Upon HIV infection, the immune system's line of defense against the virus is to form antibodies that bind to the virus. On the average, the body takes 3 months to manufacture enough antibodies to show up positive in an HIV antibody test. Sometimes it may take 6 months or longer.

10. Yes. The virus multiplies, attacks, and destroys white blood cells. These cells are part of the immune system, and their function is to fight off infections and diseases in the body. As the number of white blood cells killed increases, the body's immune system gradually breaks down and may be completely destroyed.

11. Yes. Up to 10 years or more may go by before the person develops AIDS.

12. No. Being HIV-positive does not necessarily mean the person has AIDS. On the average, it takes 7 to 8 years following infection before the individual develops the symptoms that fit the case definition of AIDS. From that point on, the person may live another 2 to 3 years. In essence, from the point of infection, the individual may have the chronic disease 8 to 10 years.

13. Yes. There is no second chance.

14. Yes. The best prevention technique is to abstain from sex until the time comes for a mutually monogamous sexual relationship. In the absence of sharing needles, this will almost completely remove the risk of contracting HIV or developing any other sexually transmitted infection.

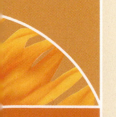

Nutritive Value of Selected Foods

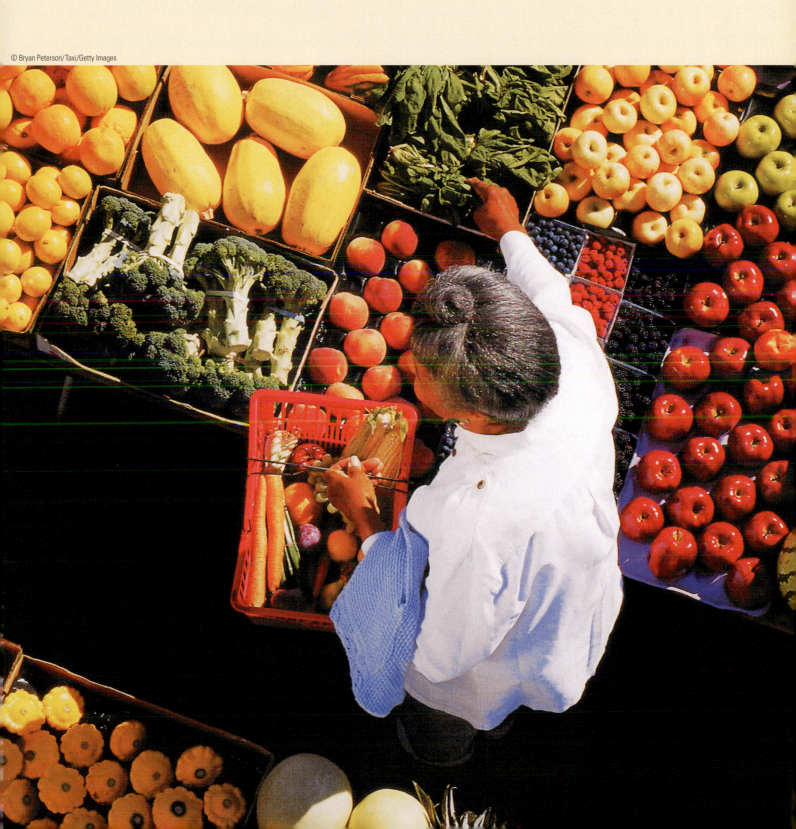

Food	Amount	Weight (g)	Calories	Protein (g)	Fat (g)	Sat. Fat (g)	Cholesterol (g)	Carbohydrate (g)	Fiber (g)	Calcium (mg)	Iron (mg)	Sodium (mg)	Vit A (IU)	Thiamin (Vit B₁) (mg)	Riboflavin (Vit B₂) (mg)	Niacin (mg)	Vit C (mg)	Folate (mcg)
Apples, fresh, w/peel, lrg	1 ea	150	88	0.3	1	0.1	0	23	4.1	10	0.3	0	80	0.03	0.02	0.1	9	4.2
Applesauce, swtnd, w/o salt, cnd	1 cup	255	194	0.5	0	0.1	0	51	3.1	10	0.9	8	28	0.03	0.07	0.5	4	1.53
Apricots, pitted, fresh, whole	3 ea	114	55	1.6	0	0	0	13	2.7	16	0.6	1	2978	0.03	0.05	0.7	11	9.8
Apricots, w/skin, in heavy syrup, cnd, whole	½ cup	120	100	0.6	0	0	0	26	1.9	11	0.4	5	1476	0.02	0.03	0.5	4	2.04
Asparagus, spears, ckd w/o salt	4 ea	60	14	1.6	0	0	0	3	1	12	0.4	7	323	0.07	0.08	0.6	6	87.6
Avocado, Calif, fresh	½ ea	120	212	2.5	21	3.1	0	8	5.9	13	1.4	14	734	0.13	0.15	2.3	9	78.6
Bagel, plain, 3½" diameter	1 ea	68	187	7.1	1	0.1	0	36	1.6	50	2.4	363	0	0.37	0.21	3.1	0	59.84
Banana, fresh, med	1 ea	140	129	1.4	1	0.3	0	33	3.4	8	0.4	1	113	0.06	0.14	0.8	13	26.74
Bar, granola, hard	1 ea	24	113	2.4	5	0.6	0	15	1.3	15	0.7	71	36	0.06	0.03	0.4	0	5.52
Beans, black, mature, ckd w/o salt	1 cup	172	227	15.2	1	0.2	0	41	15	46	3.6	2	10	0.42	0.1	0.9	0	255.9
Beans, chickpea/garbanzo, mature, ckd	1 cup	164	269	14.5	4	0.4	0	45	12.5	80	4.7	11	44	0.19	0.1	0.9	2	282.0
Beans, frijoles/refried, cnd	½ cup	145	136	8	2	0.7	12	23	7.7	51	2.4	434	0	0.04	0.02	0.5	9	15.95
Beans, green, snap/string, ckd	½ cup	65	23	1.2	0	0	0	5	2.1	30	0.8	2	433	0.05	0.06	0.4	6	21.64
Beans, kidney, red, mature, cnd	1 cup	185	157	9.7	1	0.1	0	29	11.8	44	2.3	631	0	0.19	0.16	0.8	2	93.61
Beans, lima, fordhook, immature, ckd f/fzn w/o salt, drained	½ cup	85	85	5.2	0	0.1	0	16	4.9	19	1.2	45	162	0.06	0.05	0.9	11	18.02
Beans, mung, mature, sprouted, raw	½ cup	52	16	1.6	0	0	0	3	0.9	7	0.5	3	11	0.04	0.06	0.4	7	31.62
Beans, pinto, mature, ckd w/o salt	1 cup	171	234	14	1	0.2	0	44	14.7	82	4.5	3	3	0.32	0.16	0.7	4	294.1
Beef, chuck arm pot roast, brsd, choice, ¼" trim	3 oz	85	296	22.9	22	8.6	84	0	0	8	2.6	50	0	0.06	0.2	2.7	0	7.65
Beef, corned, cnd	3 oz	85	212	23	13	5.3	73	0	0	10	1.8	855	0	0.02	0.12	2.1	0	7.65
Beef, ground, hamburger patty, brld, well done, 16% fat	3 oz	85	225	24.3	13	5.3	84	0	0	8	2.4	70	0	0.06	0.27	5	0	9.35
Beef, ground, hamburger patty, brld, well done, 18% fat	3 oz	85	238	24	15	5.9	86	0	0	10	2.1	76	0	0.05	0.2	5.1	0	9.35
Beef, liver, fried	3 oz	85	184	22.7	7	2.3	410	7	0	9	5.3	90	30689	0.18	3.52	12.3	20	187
Beef, T-bone steak, brld, choice, ¼" trim	3 oz	85	263	19.7	20	7.7	57	0	0	7	2.3	54	0	0.08	0.18	3.4	0	5.95
Beef, top sirloin steak, lean, brld, choice, ¼" trim	3 oz	85	172	25.8	7	2.6	76	0	0	9	2.9	56	0	0.11	0.25	3.6	0	8.5
Beer	12 fl-oz	360	148	1.1	0	0	0	13	0.7	18	0.1	18	0	0.02	0.09	1.6	0	21.6
Beer, light	12 fl-oz	354	99	0.7	0	0	0	5	0	18	0.1	11	0	0.03	0.11	1.4	0	14.51
Beets, cnd, drained, diced	½ cup	80	25	0.7	0	0	0	6	1.4	12	1.5	155	9	0.01	0.03	0.1	3	24.16
Biscuits, homemade	1 ea	35	124	2.5	6	1.5	1	16	0.5	82	1	203	29	0.12	0.11	1	0	21.35
Blueberries, fresh, bilberries	½ cup	73	41	0.5	0	0	0	10	2	4	0.1	4	73	0.04	0.04	0.3	9	4.67
Brandy, 86 proof	1 oz	28	70	0	0	0	0	0	0	0	0	0	0	0	0	0	0	0
Bread, banana, prep f/recipe w/veg shortening	1 pce	50	169	2.2	6	1.5	22	28	0.7	9	0.7	99	46	0.09	0.1	0.7	1	5.5
Bread, cracked wheat	1 pce	25	65	2.2	1	0.2	0	12	1.4	11	0.7	134	0	0.09	0.06	0.9	0	15.25
Bread, French	1 pce	35	96	3.1	1	0.2	0	18	1.7	26	0.9	213	0	0.18	0.12	1.7	0	33.25
Bread, mixed grain	1 pce	26	65	2.6	1	0.2	0	12	1.7	24	0.9	127	0	0.11	0.09	1.1	0	20.8
Bread, pita pocket, white	1 ea	60	165	5.5	1	0.1	0	33	1.3	52	1.6	322	0	0.36	0.2	2.8	0	57
Bread, pumpernickel	1 pce	32	80	2.8	1	0.1	0	15	2.1	22	0.9	215	0	0.1	0.1	1	0	25.6
Bread, rye	1 pce	25	65	2.1	1	0.2	0	12	1.5	18	0.7	165	2	0.11	0.08	1	0	21.5
Bread, white, f/recipe w/2% milk	1 pce	25	71	2	1	0.3	1	12	0.5	14	0.7	90	20	0.1	0.1	0.9	0	22.75
Bread, whole wheat	1 pce	25	62	2.4	1	0.1	0	12	1.7	18	0.8	132	0	0.09	0.05	1	0	12.5
Broccoli, med stalk, 8" long, ckd w/o add salt	1 ea	140	39	4.2	0	0.1	0	7	4.1	64	1.2	36	1943	0.08	0.16	0.8	104	70
Broccoli, spear, raw, 5" long	1 ea	114	32	3.4	0	0.1	0	6	3.4	55	1	31	1758	0.07	0.14	0.7	106	80.94
Brownie, chocolate, w/walnuts, prep f/rec	1 ea	20	93	1.2	6	1.5	15	10	0.4	11	0.4	69	153	0.03	0.04	0.2	0	5.8
Brussels Sprouts, ckd, drained	½ cup	78	30	2	0	0.1	0	7	2	28	0.9	16	561	0.08	0.06	0.5	48	46.8
Buns, hamburger	1 ea	40	114	3.4	2	0.5	0	20	1.1	56	1.3	224	0	0.19	0.12	1.6	0	38

Food	Amount	Weight (g)	Calories	Protein (g)	Fat (g)	Sat. Fat (g)	Cholesterol (g)	Carbohydrate (g)	Fiber (g)	Calcium (mg)	Iron (mg)	Sodium (mg)	Vit A (IU)	Thiamin (Vit B_1) (mg)	Riboflavin (Vit B_2) (mg)	Niacin (mg)	Vit C (mg)	Folate (mcg)
Buns, hot dog/frankfurter	1 ea	40	114	3.4	2	0.5	0	20	1.1	56	1.3	224	0	0.19	0.12	1.6	0	38
Burger/Patty, vegetarian, Gardenburger, original	1 ea	71	130	8	3	1	11	18	5	84	0	290	50	0.11	0.15	1.1	0	10.08
Burger/Patty, vegetarian, soy	1 ea	71	142	14.9	6	1	0	6	3.3	21	1.5	390	0	0.64	0.43	7.1	0	55.38
Butter, salted	1 Tbs	5	36	0	4	2.5	11	0	0	1	0.1	41	153	0	0	0	0	0.15
Buttermilk, skim, cultured	1 cup	245	99	8.1	2	1.3	9	12	0	285	0.1	257	81	0.08	0.38	0.1	2	12.25
Cabbage, ckd w/o add salt, drained, shredded	½ cup	85	19	0.9	0	0	0	4	2	26	0.1	7	112	0.05	0.05	0.2	17	17
Cabbage, raw, shredded	½ cup	45	11	0.6	0	0	0	2	1	21	0.3	8	60	0.02	0.02	0.1	14	19.35
Cake, angel food, cmrcl prep	1 pce	60	155	3.5	0	0.1	0	35	0.9	84	0.3	449	0	0.06	0.29	0.5	0	21
Cake, carrot, w/cream cheese icing	1 pce	96	419	4.4	25	4.7	52	45	1.2	24	1.2	236	3310	0.13	0.15	1	1	11.52
Cake, chocolate, w/chocolate icing, 1/8th	1 pce	69	253	2.8	11	3.3	29	38	1.9	30	1.5	230	59	0.02	0.09	0.4	0	11.73
Cake, devils food, marshmallow iced	1 pce	99	408	3.5	21	5.8	52	52	1.2	47	1.3	338	0				0	12.3
Cake, pound, w/butter	1 pce	30	116	1.7	6	3.5	66	15	0.1	10	0.4	119	182	0.04	0.07	0.4	0	2.11
Cake, white, w/chocolate icing	1 pce	71	259	1.8	8	3.7	13	46	0.8	55	0.5	219	166	0.05	0.07	0.3	0	21
Calamari/Squid, fried, mixed species	1 cup	150	262	26.9	11	2.8	390	12	0	58	1.5	459	52	0.08	0.69	3.9	6	
Candy Bar, Almond Joy, fun size	1½ oz	42	196	1.8	11	7.3	2	24	2	26	0.6	61	5	0.01	0.06	0.2	0	9.5
Candy Bar, Mars almond	1 ea	50	234	4.1	12	3.6	8	31	1	84	0.6	85	94	0.02	0.16	0.5	0	6
Candy Bar, Milky Way, 2.1 oz bar	1 ea	60	254	2.7	10	4.7	8	43	1	78	0.5	144	65	0.02	0.13	0.2	1	0.82
Candy Bar, Special Dark sweet chocolate	1 ea	41	226	2	13	8.3	4	25	0.7	11	1	3	14	0.01	0.03	0.1	0	1.4
Candy, caramels, plain/chocolate	1 oz	28	107	1.3	2	1.8	2	22	0.3	39	0	69	9	0	0.05	0.1	0	0
Candy, hard, all flvrs	1 oz	28	110	0	0	0	0	27	0	1	0.1	11	0	0	0	0	0	
Candy, Kisses, milk chocolate	1 oz	28	144	1.9	9	5.2	6	17	1	53	0.4	23	52	0.02	0.08	0.1	0	2.24
Candy, M & M's peanut chocolate	1 oz	28	144	2.7	7	2.9	3	17	1	28	0.3	13	26	0.03	0.05	1	0	9.8
Candy, M & M's plain chocolate	1 oz	28	138	1.2	6	3.7	4	20	0.7	29	0.3	17	57	0.02	0.06	0.1	0	1.68
Candy, milk chocolate, w/almonds	1 oz	28	147	2.5	10	4.8	5	15	1.7	63	0.5	21	21	0.02	0.12	0.4	2	3.36
Carrots, ckd w/o add salt, drained, slices	½ cup	73	33	0.8	0	0	0	8	2.4	23	0.5	48	17924	0.02	0.04	0.4	8	10.15
Carrots, raw, whole, 7½" long	1 ea	81	35	0.8	0	0	0	8	2.4	22	0.4	28	22784	0.08	0.05	0.8	8	11.34
Catsup/Ketchup	1 Tbs	15	16	0.2	0	0	0	4	0.2	3	0.1	178	152	0.01	0.01	0.2	2	2.25
Cauliflower, ckd, drained	½ cup	63	14	1.2	0	0	0	3	1.7	10	0.2	9	11	0.03	0.03	0.3	28	27.72
Celery, raw, med stalk, 8" long	1 ea	40	6	0.3	0	0	0	1	0.7	16	0.2	35	54	0.02	0.02	0.1	3	11.2
Cereal, 100% Bran, rte, dry	½ cup	33	89	4.1	2	0.3	0	24	9.8	23	4.1	229	0	0.79	0.89	10.5	10	23.43
Cereal, All-Bran, rte, dry	¼ cup	21	55	2.6	1	0.1	0	16	6.8	74	3.1	43	525	0.27	0.29	3.5	3	63
Cereal, Alpha-Bits, rte, dry	1 cup	28	110	2.2	1	0.1	0	24	1.2	8	2.7	178	1235	0.36	0.42	4.9	10	98.84
Cereal, bran flakes, rte, dry	¾ cup	30	96	2.8	1	0.1	0	24	5.3	17	8.1	220	750	0.38	0.43	5	12	76.59
Cereal, Cheerios	1 cup	23	84	2.4	1	0.3	0	18	2	42	6.2	218	958	0.29	0.33	3.8	12	93.24
Cereal, Chex, corn, rte, dry	1 cup	28	105	2	0	0.1	0	24	0.5	94	8.4	270	0	0.35	0.02	4.7	6	92
Cereal, Chex, wheat, rte, dry	1 cup	46	159	4.8	1	0.2	0	37	5.1	92	13.8	412	16	0.34	0.06	4.6	6	88.25
Cereal, corn flakes, rte, dry	1 cup	25	91	1.6	0	0.1	0	22	0.7	2	7.8	266	625	0.32	0.35	4.2	12	98.84
Cereal, Corn Pops, rte, dry	1 cup	28	107	1	0	0.1	0	26	0.4	2	1.7	111	700	0.36	0.39	4.7	14	98.84
Cereal, Cream of Wheat, quick, ckd w/water	1 cup	244	132	3.7	0	0.1	0	27	1.2	51	10.5	142	0	0.24	0.29	1.5	0	109.8
Cereal, Crispy Rice, rte, dry	¾ cup	22	87	1.4	0	0	0	19	0.3	4	0.6	161	971	0.41	0.46	5.4	12	108.6
Cereal, Frosted Flakes, rte, dry	1 cup	35	135	1.4	0	0.1	0	32	0.7	20	5.1	226	847	0.42	0.49	5.6	17	105
Cereal, Frosted Mini Wheats, rte, dry	1 cup	55	186	5.2	1	0.2	0	45	5.9	43	15.4	2	0	0.38	0.44	5.4	10	110
Cereal, granola, rte, dry	½ cup	57	257	6	10	1.3	0	38	3.6	19	1.8	92	737	0.18	0.06	0.6	0	8.55
Cereal, Grape Nuts, rte, dry	½ cup	57	205	6.2	1	0.2	0	46	5	14	15.9	348	1323	0.37	0.42	4.9	16	98.04
Cereal, Honey Bran, rte, dry	½ cup	30	102	2.6	1	0.2	0	25	3.3	134	4.8	173	16	0.39	0.45	5.3	6	20.1
Cereal, Life, plain, rte, dry	1 cup	44	167	4.3	2	0.3	0	35	2.8	67	12.3	240	2488	0.55	0.62	7.3	6	146.9
Cereal, Mueslix, five grain muesli, rte, dry	1 cup	82	289	6.2	5	0.7	0	63	5.6	8	8.9	107	0	0.75	0.84	9.8	1	196.8
Cereal, Nutri-Grain, wheat, rte, dry	1 oz	28	101	2.4	0	0.1	0	24	1.8	10	0.8	190	0	0.36	0.42	4.9	15	98.84
Cereal, oatmeal, unsalted, ckd w/water	½ cup	120	74	3.1	1	0.2	0	13	2	10	0.8	1	19	0.13	0.02	0.2	0	4.8

Food	Amount	Weight (g)	Calories	Protein (g)	Fat (g)	Sat. Fat (g)	Cholesterol (g)	Carbohydrate (g)	Fiber (g)	Calcium (mg)	Iron (mg)	Sodium (mg)	Vit A (IU)	Thiamin (Vit B_1) (mg)	Riboflavin (Vit B_2) (mg)	Niacin (mg)	Vit C (mg)	Folate (mcg)
Cereal, raisin bran, rte, dry	1 cup	49	155	3.9	1	0.1	0	38	6.4	22	9	299	623	0.31	0.35	4.2	0	82.81
Cereal, Shredded Wheat, sml biscuits, rte, dry	1 cup	19	68	2.1	0	0.1	0	15	1.9	7	0.8	2	0	0.05	0.05	1	0	9.5
Cereal, Smacks, rte, dry	1 cup	37	141	2.4	1	0.4	0	32	1.3	4	2.5	70	1028	0.52	0.59	6.8	21	136.9
Cereal, Special K, rte, dry	1 cup	21	78	4.3	0	0	0	15	0.7	3	5.9	169	508	0.36	0.4	4.7	10	63
Cereal, Total, wheat, rte, dry	1 cup	33	116	3.3	1	0.2	0	26	2.9	284	19.8	218	1375	1.65	1.87	22.1	66	439.8
Cereal, Wheaties, rte, dry	1 cup	29	106	3.1	1	0.2	0	23	2	53	7.8	215	725	0.36	0.41	4.8	14	96.57
Cheese Puffs/Cheetos	1 oz	28	155	2.1	10	1.8	1	15	0.3	16	0.7	294	74	0.07	0.1	0.9	0	33.6
Cheese Spread, low fat, low sod	1 pce	34	61	8.4	2	1.5	12	1	0	233	0.1	2	92	0.01	0.13	0	0	3.06
Cheese, American, proc, shredded	1 oz	28	105	6.2	9	5.5	26	0	0	172	0.1	401	339	0.01	0.1	0	0	2.18
Cheese, blue	1 oz	28	99	6	8	5.2	21	1	0	148	0.1	391	202	0.01	0.11	0.3	0	10.19
Cheese, cheddar, diced	1 oz	28	113	7	9	5.9	29	0	0	202	0.2	174	297	0.01	0.11	0	0	5.1
Cheese, feta	1 oz	28	74	4	6	4.2	25	1	0	138	0.2	313	125	0.04	0.24	0.3	0	8.96
Cheese, monterey jack, shredded	1 oz	28	105	6.9	8	5.3	25	0	0	209	0.2	150	266	0	0.11	0	0	5.1
Cheese, mozzarella, part skm milk, low moist, shredded	1 oz	28	78	7.7	5	3	15	1	0	205	0.1	148	197	0.01	0.1	0	0	2.77
Cheese, parmesan, grated	1 Tbs	5	23	2.1	2	1	4	0	0	69	0	93	35	0	0.02	0	0	0.4
Cheese, ricotta, part skm	1 oz	28	39	3.2	2	1.4	9	1	0	76	0.1	35	121	0.01	0.05	0	0	3.67
Cheese, Swiss, shredded	1 oz	28	105	8	8	5	26	1	0	269	0	73	237	0.01	0.1	0	0	1.79
Cheesecake	1 pce	85	273	4.7	19	8.4	47	22	0.4	43	0.5	176	465	0.02	0.16	0.2	0	15.3
Cherries, sweet, fresh	10 ea	75	54	0.9	1	0.2	0	12	1.7	11	0.3	0	160	0.04	0.04	0.3	5	3.15
Chicken, broiler/fryer, breast, rstd	1 ea	98	193	29.2	8	2.1	82	0	0	14	1	70	91	0.06	0.12	12.5	0	3.92
Chicken, broiler/fryer, dark meat, w/o skin, rstd	3 oz	85	174	23.3	8	2.3	79	0	0	13	1.1	79	61	0.06	0.19	5.6	0	6.8
Chicken, broiler/fryer, drumstick, rstd	1 ea	52	112	14.1	6	1.6	47	0	0	6	0.7	47	52	0.04	0.11	3.1	0	4.16
Chicken, broiler/fryer, meat only, w/o skin, rstd	3 oz	85	162	24.6	6	1.7	76	0	0	13	1	73	45	0.06	0.15	7.8	0	5.1
Chips, corn	1 oz	28	151	1.8	9	1.3	0	16	1.4	36	0.4	176	26	0.01	0.04	0.3	0	5.6
Chips, tortilla, chili & lime	18 pce	28	110	2	2	0	0	22	2	60	3.6	200	0				0	
Chips, tortilla, plain	1 oz	28	140	2	7	1.4	0	18	1.8	43	0.4	148	55	0.02	0.05	0.4	0	2.8
Cod, batter fried	3½ oz	100	173	17.4	8	1.6	50	7	0.2	29	0.7	91	30	0.07	0.1	2.3	2	8.71
Cod, stmd/poached	3½ oz	100	102	22.4	1	0.1	46	0	0	9	0.3	80	28	0.02	0.05	2.2	3	6.6
Coffee, brewed	¾ cup	180	4	0.2	0	0	0	1	0	9	0.1	4	0	0	0	0.4	0	0.18
Collards, ckd w/o add salt	½ cup	95	25	2	0	0	0	5	2.7	113	0.4	9	2973	0.04	0.1	0.5	17	88.35
Cone, ice cream, wafer/cake type	1 ea	115	480	9.3	8	1.4	0	91	3.4	29	4.1	164	0	0.29	0.41	5.1	0	117.3
Cookie, chocolate chip, prep w/marg f/rec	2 ea	20	98	1.1	6	1.6	6	12	0.6	8	0.5	72	127	0.04	0.04	0.3	0	6.6
Cookie, chocolate sandwich, creme filled	4 ea	40	189	1.9	8	1.5	0	28	1.3	10	1.6	242	1	0.03	0.07	0.8	0	17.2
Cookie, fig bar	4 ea	56	195	2.1	4	0.6	0	40	2.6	36	1.6	196	18	0.09	0.12	1	0	15.12
Cookie, oatmeal raisin, prep f/rec	2 ea	26	113	1.7	4	0.8	9	18	0.8	26	0.7	140	167	0.06	0.04	0.3	0	7.8
Cookie, peanut butter, prep f/rec	2 ea	24	114	2.2	6	1.1	7	14	0.5	9	0.5	124	144	0.05	0.05	0.8	0	13.2
Cookie, shortbread, cmrcl, plain	4 ea	32	161	2	8	2	6	21	0.6	11	0.9	146	28	0.11	0.11	1.1	0	18.88
Cookie, vanilla, wafer type, 12–17% fat	10 ea	40	176	2	6	1.5	20	29	0.8	19	1	125	11	0.11	0.13	1.2	0	20
Coriander, raw	¼ cup	4	1	0.1	0	0	0	0	0.1	4	0.1	1	111	0.03	0.06	0.1		0.41
Corn, yellow, vac pack, cnd	½ cup	83	66	2	0	0.1	0	16	1.7	4	0.3	226	200	0.03	0.06	1	7	40.92
Cornbread, prep f/dry mix	1 ea	60	188	4.3	6	1.6	37	29	1.4	44	1.1	467	123	0.15	0.16	1.2	0	33
Cornmeal, yellow, degermed, enrich, dry	½ cup	120	439	10.2	2	0.3	0	93	8.9	6	5	4	496	0.86	0.49	6	0	224.4
Cottage Cheese, 2% fat	½ cup	113	101	15.5	2	1.4	9	4	0	77	0.2	459	79	0.03	0.21	0.2	0	14.8
Cottage Cheese, creamed, sml curd	½ cup	105	109	13.1	5	3	16	3	0	63	0.1	425	171	0.02	0.17	0.1	0	12.81
Crab, blue, cnd, drained	1 cup	135	134	27.7	2	0.3	120	0	0	136	1.1	450	7	0.11	0.11	1.8	4	57.38
Crackers, cheese	1 ea	10	50	1	3	0.9	1	6	0.2	15	0.5	100	16	0.06	0.04	0.5	0	8
Crackers, graham, plain/honey, 2½ square	2 ea	14	59	1	1	0.2	0	11	0.4	3	0.5	85	3	0.03	0.04	0.6	0	8.4
Crackers, matzoh, plain, svg	1 ea	28	111	2.8	0	0.1	0	23	0.8	4	0.9	1	0	0.11	0.08	1.1	0	32.76

Food	Amount	Weight (g)	Calories	Protein (g)	Fat (g)	Sat. Fat (g)	Cholesterol (g)	Carbohydrate (g)	Fiber (g)	Calcium (mg)	Iron (mg)	Sodium (mg)	Vit A (IU)	Thiamin (Vit B_1) (mg)	Riboflavin (Vit B_2) (mg)	Niacin (mg)	Vit C (mg)	Folate (mcg)
Crackers, rye, wafers	2 ea	14	47	1.3	0	0	0	11	3.2	6	0.8	111	1	0.06	0.04	0.2	0	6.3
Crackers, saltine	1 ea	11	48	1	1	0.3	0	8	0.3	13	0.6	143	0	0.06	0.05	0.6	0	13.64
Crackers, standard, reg, snack type, round	1 ea	3	15	0.2	1	0.1	0	2	0	4	0.1	25	0	0.01	0.01	0.1	0	2.31
Crackers, triscuit	1 ea	5	24	0.5	1	0.2	0	3	0.5	1	0.2	26	0	0.01	0.01	0.1	0	0.36
Crackers, wheat	1 ea	2	9	0.2	0	0.1	0	1	0.1	1	0.1	16	0			0	0	
Cream Cheese	1 oz	28	98	2.1	10	6.2	31	1	0	22	0.3	83	400	0	0.06	0	0	3.7
Cream, light	1 Tbs	15	29	0.4	3	1.8	10	1	0	14	0	6	95	0	0.02	0	0	0.34
Cream, whipping, heavy	1 Tbs	15	52	0.3	6	3.5	21	0	0	10	0	6	221	0	0.02	0	0	0.56
Croissant, butter	1 ea	57	231	4.7	12	6.6	38	26	1.5	21	1.2	424	424	0.22	0.14	1.2	0	35.34
Cucumber, w/o skin, raw, sliced	½ cup	60	7	0.3	0	0	0	2	0.4	8	0.1	1	44	0.01	0.01	0.1	2	8.4
Dates, fresh, whole	10 ea	83	228	1.6	0	0.2	0	61	6.2	27	1	2	42	0.07	0.08	1.8	0	10.46
Dinner, chicken, cacciatore, w/noodles, low cal, fzn	1 ea	308	311	22.5	10	2.4	59	33	3.4	29	3.2	934	732	0.28	0.4	8	26	32.22
Doughnut, cake	1 ea	47	198	2.3	11	1.7	17	23	0.7	21	0.9	257	27	0.1	0.11	0.9	0	22.09
Doughnut, raised, glazed	1 ea	60	242	3.8	14	3.5	4	27	0.7	26	1.2	205	8	0.22	0.13	1.7	0	25.8
Egg Substitute, Egg Beaters, new	¼ cup	61	30	6	0	0	0	0	0	20	1.1	125	300	0	0.85	0	0	32.0
Egg Whites, raw	1 ea	33	16	3.5	0	0	0	0	0	2	0.6	54	0	0	0.15	0	0	0.99
Egg Yolks, raw, lrg	1 ea	17	61	2.8	5	1.6	218	0	0	23	0.6	7	331	0.03	0.11	0	0	24.82
Eggs, hard ckd/bld, lrg	1 ea	50	78	6.3	5	1.6	212	0	0	25	0.6	62	280	0.03	0.26	0	0	22
Eggs, scrambled, plain, lrg	1 ea	64	106	7.1	8	2.4	225	1	0	45	0.8	179	436	0.03	0.28	0.1	0	19.2
Eggs, whole, fried	1 ea	46	92	6.2	7	1.9	211	1	0	25	0.7	162	394	0.03	0.24	0	0	17.48
Entree, lasagna, w/meat, prep f/rec	1 pce	220	352	20.7	14	7.2	52	36	2.5	243	2.8	351	902	0.21	0.3	3.8	13	17.82
Entree, macaroni & cheese, prep f/rec w/margarine	½ cup	100	215	8.4	11	4.4	21	20	0.6	181	0.9	543	430	0.1	0.2	0.9	0	5.15
Entree, meatloaf, beef	1 pce	111	232	20.2	14	5.6	107	5	0.2	37	2.1	185	148	0.06	0.28	3.3	1	14.28
Entree, quiche, lorraine	1 pce	242	724	20.5	56	25.9	304	34	1	318	2.6	303	1323	0.36	0.67	2.8	1	26.48
Entree, spaghetti, w/meatballs, prep f/rec	1 cup	248	332	18.6	12	3.3	74	39	7.7	124	3.7	1009	1587	0.25	0.3	4	22	9.99
Entree, spaghetti, w/tomato sauce & cheese, prep f/rec	1 cup	250	260	8.8	9	2	8	37	2.5	80	2.2	955	1075	0.25	0.17	2.2	12	8
Figs, dried, unckd	1 ea	21	54	0.6	0	0.1	0	14	2.5	30	0.5	2	28	0.01	0.02	0.1	0	1.57
Fish Sticks/Portions, heated t/fzn, 4x1x.5	2 ea	56	152	8.8	7	1.8	63	13	0	11	0.4	326	59	0.07	0.1	1.2	0	10.19
Flour, all purpose, white, bleached, enrich	1 cup	125	455	12.9	1	0.2	0	95	3.4	19	5.8	6	0	0.98	0.62	7.4	0	192.5
Flour, whole wheat	1 cup	120	407	16.4	2	0.4	0	87	14.6	41	4.7	6	0	0.54	0.26	7.6	0	52.8
Frankfurter/Hot Dog, beef & pork, 10 pack	1 ea	57	182	6.4	17	6.1	28	1	0	6	0.7	638	0	0.11	0.07	1.5	0	2.28
Frankfurter/Hot Dog, beef, 8 pack	1 ea	57	180	6.8	16	6.9	35	1	0	11	0.8	585	0	0.03	0.06	1.4	0	2.28
Frankfurter/Hot Dog, turkey	1 ea	45	102	6.4	8	2.7	48	1	0	48	0.8	642	0	0.02	0.08	1.9	0	3.6
Frozen Yogurt, vanilla/strawberry, nonfat, sml scoop	4 oz	113	112	5.6	0	0.1	2	22	0	196	0.1	75	7	0.05	0.23	0.1	1	11.99
Fruit Cocktail, in heavy syrup, cnd	1 cup	245	179	1	0	0	0	46	2.5	15	0.7	15	502	0.04	0.05	0.9	5	6.37
Fruit Cocktail, in juice	1 cup	248	114	1.1	0	0	0	29	2.5	20	0.5	10	756	0.03	0.04	1	7	6.2
Fruit Punch, prep f/pwd	1 cup	240	89	0	0	0	0	23	0	38	0.1	34	0	0	0	0	28	0.24
Fudge, chocolate, prep f/rec	1 oz	28	107	0.5	2	1.4	4	22	0.2	12	0.1	17	53	0	0.02	0	0	0.56
Grapefruit, pink, fresh, 3¾" diameter	½ ea	123	37	0.7	0	0	0	9	1.7	14	0.1	0	319	0.04	0.02	0.2	47	15.01
Grapes, tokay/empress/red flame, fresh	10 ea	50	36	0.3	0	0.1	0	9	0.5	6	0.1	1	36	0.05	0.03	0.2	5	1.95
Haddock, fillet, brd, fried	3 oz	85	184	17.1	9	1.9	65	7	0.2	53	1.5	145	69	0.08	0.09	3.7	0	11.6
Halibut, Greenland, fillet, bkd/brld	3 oz	85	203	15.7	15	2.6	50	0	0	3	0.7	88	51	0.06	0.09	1.6	0	0.85
Honey, strained, extracted	1 Tbs	21	64	0.1	0	0	0	17	0	1	0.1	1	0	0	0.01	0	0	0.42
Hot Cocoa/Choc, prep f/rec w/whole milk	1 cup	250	192	9.8	6	3.6	20	29	2	315	1.1	128	515	0.1	0.44	0.4	2	15
Hummus/Hummos, raw	1 cup	246	421	12.1	21	3.1	0	50	12.5	123	3.9	600	62	0.23	0.13	1	19	146.1
Instant Breakfast, prep f/dry mix w/nonfat milk	1 cup	282	216	15.7	1	0.7	9	36	0.2	407	4.8	268	2343	0.4	0.42	5.5	31	118.2

Food	Amount	Weight (g)	Calories	Protein (g)	Fat (g)	Sat. Fat (g)	Cholesterol (g)	Carbohydrate (g)	Fiber (g)	Calcium (mg)	Iron (mg)	Sodium (mg)	Vit A (IU)	Thiamin (Vit B₁) (mg)	Riboflavin (Vit B₂) (mg)	Niacin (mg)	Vit C (mg)	Folate (mcg)
Instant Breakfast, prep f/dry mix w/whole milk	1 cup	281	280	15.4	9	5.4	38	36	0.2	396	4.9	262	2151	0.41	0.47	5.5	31	117.7
Jam/Preserves, pkt	1 ea	14	39	0.1	0	0	0	10	0.2	3	0.1	4	2	0	0	0	1	4.62
Jelly	1 Tbs	18	51	0	0	0	0	13	0.2	1	0	5	3	0	0	0	1	0.18
Juice, apple, unswtnd, cnd/btld	½ cup	124	58	0.1	0	0	0	14	0.1	9	0.5	4	1	0.03	0.02	0.1	1	0.12
Juice, cranberry cocktail	1 cup	253	144	0.7	0	0	0	36	0.3	8	0.4	5	10	0.02	0.02	0.1	90	0.51
Juice, grape, unswtnd, btld/cnd	½ cup	127	77	0.7	0	0	0	19	0.1	11	0.3	4	10	0.03	0.05	0.3	0	3.3
Juice, grapefruit, unswtnd, cnd	½ cup	124	47	0.6	0	0	0	11	0.1	9	0.2	1	9	0.05	0.02	0.3	36	12.9
Juice, grapefruit, unswtnd, prep f/fzn conc	1 cup	247	101	1.4	0	0	0	24	0.2	20	0.3	2	22	0.1	0.05	0.5	83	8.89
Juice, lemon, fresh	1 Tbs	15	4	0.1	0	0	0	1	0.1	1	0	0	3	0	0	0	7	1.94
Juice, orange, prep f/fzn	½ cup	125	56	0.9	0	0	0	13	0.2	11	0.1	1	98	0.1	0.02	0.3	49	54.75
Juice, prune, w/o pulp	½ cup	88	60	0.7	0	0	0	14	0.5	2	0.9	4	54	0.1	0.1	1	3	
Juice, tomato, w/salt, cnd	1 cup	244	41	1.9	0	0	0	10	1	22	1.4	881	1357	0.11	0.08	1.6	45	48.56
Kale, ckd w/o add salt, drained	½ cup	55	15	1	0	0	0	3	1.1	40	0.5	13	4070	0.03	0.04	0.3	23	7.32
Kiwifruit/Chinese Gooseberries, fresh, med	1 ea	76	46	0.8	0	0	0	11	2.6	20	0.3	4	133	0.02	0.04	0.4	74	28.88
Lamb, leg, whole, lean, rstd, choice, ¼" trim	3 oz	85	162	24.1	7	2.3	76	0	0	7	1.8	58	0	0.09	0.25	5.4	0	19.55
Lamb, loin chop, lean, brld, choice, ¼" trim	3 oz	84	181	25.2	8	2.9	80	0	0	16	1.7	71	0	0.09	0.24	5.8	0	20.16
Lemonade, white, fzn conc	12 oz	340	615	0.1	1	0.1	0	160	1.4	24	2.4	14	323	0.09	0.33	0.3	60	34
Lentils, sprouts, stir fried	1 cup	124	125	10.9	1	0.1	0	26	4.8	17	3.8	12	51	0.27	0.11	1.5	16	83.08
Lentils, unsalted, ckd	1 cup	200	232	18	1	0.1	0	40	15.8	38	6.7	4	16	0.34	0.15	2.1	3	361.6
Lettuce, butterhead, Boston/bibb, leaf, raw	2 pce	15	2	0.2	0	0	0	0	0.2	5	0	1	146	0.01	0.01	0	3	11
Lettuce, romaine, raw, chpd	1 cup	55	8	0.9	0	0	0	1	0.9	20	0.6	4	1430	0.06	0.06	0.3	13	74.64
Lobster, northern, stmd	1 cup	145	142	29.7	1	0.2	104	2	0	88	0.6	551	126	0.01	0.1	1.6	0	16.1
Lunchmeat Spread, liverwurst, cnd	1 oz	28	87	3.6	7	2.5	33	2	0.5	0	2.3	193	3818		0.04	0.7	1	
Lunchmeat, bologna, beef & pork	1 pce	28	88	3.3	8	2.9	15	1	0	3	0.4	285	0	0.05			0	1.4
Lunchmeat, bologna, turkey	2 pce	57	113	7.8	9	2.9	56	1	0	48	0.9	500	0	0.03	0.09	2	0	3.99
Lunchmeat, roast beef, deli style, pouch	3 oz	85	96	17.2	3	1.1	41	1	0	5	1.6	860	0				0	
Lunchmeat, turkey breast, rstd, fat free	1 pce	28	24	4.2	3	0.1	9	1	0	3	0.3	334	0				0	
Mayonnaise, imit, low cal	1 Tbs	15	35	0	3	0.5	4	2	0	0	0	75	14	0	0	0	0	
Mayonnaise, soybean oil, w/salt	1 tsp	5	36	0.1	4	0.6	3	0	0	1	0	28	0	0	0	0	0	0.38
Melon, cantaloupe/musk, med 5" diameter	¼ ea	239	84	2.1	1	0.2	0	20	1.9	26	0.5	22	7705	0.09	0.05	1.4	101	40.63
Melon, honeydew, fresh, wedge, 1/8 melon	1 pce	129	45	0.6	0	0	0	12	0.8	8	0.1	13	52	0.1	0.02	0.8	32	7.74
Milk Shake, chocolate, fast food	10 fl-oz	340	432	11.6	13	7.9	44	70	2.7	384	1.1	330	316	0.2	0.83	0.5	2	11.9
Milk, evaporated, whole, w/add vit A, cnd	½ cup	126	169	8.6	10	5.8	37	13	0	329	0.2	133	500	0.06	0.4	0.2	2	9.95
Milk, low fat, 1%, w/add vit A	1 cup	244	102	8	3	1.6	10	12	0	300	0.1	123	500	0.1	0.41	0.2	2	12.44
Milk, low fat, 2%, chocolate	1 cup	250	179	8	5	3.1	17	26	1.2	284	0.6	150	500	0.09	0.41	0.3	2	12
Milk, low fat, 2%, w/add vit A	1 cup	244	121	8.1	5	2.9	18	12	0	297	0.1	122	500	0.1	0.4	0.2	2	12.44
Milk, nonfat/skim, w/add vit A	1 cup	245	86	8.4	0	0.3	4	12	0	302	0.1	126	500	0.09	0.34	0.2	2	12.74
Milk, whole, 3.3%	1 cup	244	150	8	8	5.1	33	11	0	291	0.1	120	307	0.09	0.4	0.2	2	12.2
Milkshake, strawberry, fast food	10 fl-oz	340	384	11.6	10	5.9	37	64	1.4	384	0.4	282	408	0.15	0.66	0.6	3	10.2
Mixed Vegetables, cnd, drained	1 cup	182	86	4.7	1	0.1	0	17	5.5	49	1.9	271	21198	0.08	0.09	1.1	9	42.95
Muffin, English, plain	1 ea	57	134	4.4	1	0.1	0	26	1.5	99	1.4	264	0	0.25	0.16	2.2	0	46.17
Muffin, English, plain, tstd	1 ea	52	133	4.4	1	0.1	0	26	1.5	98	1.4	262	0	0.2	0.14	2	0	38.48
Muffin, wheat bran, prep f/rec w/whole milk	1 ea	45	130	3.2	6	1.2	16	19	3.2	84	1.9	265	363	0.15	0.2	1.8	4	23.4
Mushrooms, raw, pces/slices	1 cup	35	9	1	0	0	0	1	0.4	2	0.4	1	0	0.03	0.15	1.4	1	4.2
Mustard Greens, ckd w/o add salt, drained	½ cup	70	10	1.6	0	0	0	1	1.4	52	0.5	11	2122	0.03	0.04	0.3	18	51.38
Nuts, almonds, dried, unblanched, whole	¼ cup	36	208	7.7	18	1.4	0	7	4.2	89	1.5	0	0	0.09	0.29	1.4	0	10.44
Nuts, Brazil, dried, shelled, 32 kernels	1 oz	28	184	4	19	4.5	0	4	1.5	49	1	1	4	0.28	0.03	0.5	0	1.12
Nuts, cashews, dry rstd, salted	1 cup	137	786	21	63	12.5	0	45	4.1	62	8.2	877	0	0.27	0.27	1.9	0	94.8
Nuts, coconut, unswtnd, dried	½ cup	65	429	4.5	42	37.2	0	16	10.6	17	2.2	24	0	0.04	0.06	0.4	1	5.85

Food	Amount	Weight (g)	Calories	Protein (g)	Fat (g)	Sat. Fat (g)	Cholesterol (g)	Carbohydrate (g)	Fiber (g)	Calcium (mg)	Iron (mg)	Sodium (mg)	Vit A (IU)	Thiamin (Vit B$_1$) (mg)	Riboflavin (Vit B$_2$) (mg)	Niacin (mg)	Vit C (mg)	Folate (mcg)
Nuts, peanuts, oil rstd, unsalted, chpd	1 oz	28	163	7.4	14	1.9	0	5	1.9	25	0.5	2	0	0.07	0.03	4	0	35.2
Nuts, pecans, dried, halves	1 oz	28	193	2.6	20	1.7	0	4	2.7	20	0.7	0	22	0.18	0.04	0.3	0	6.16
Nuts, walnuts, black, dried, chpd	1 oz	28	170	6.8	16	1	0	3	1.4	16	0.9	0	83	0.06	0.03	0.2	1	18.34
Oil, canola	1 cup	218	1927	0	218	15.5	0	0	0	0	0	0	0	0	0	0	0	0
Oil, corn	1 Tbs	15	133	0	15	1.9	0	0	0	0	0	0	0	0	0	0	0	0
Oil, olive	1 Tbs	15	133	0	15	2	0	0	0	0	0.1	0	0	0	0	0	0	0
Oil, peanut	1 cup	216	1909	0	216	36.5	0	0	0	0	0.1	0	0	0	0	0	0	0
Oil, safflower, greater than 70% linoleic	1 Tbs	15	133	0	15	0.9	0	0	0	0	0	0	0	0	0	0	0	0
Oil, soybean	1 tsp	5	44	0	5	0.7	0	0	0	0	0	0	0	0	0	0	0	0
Okra, bindi, ckd w/o add salt f/raw, drained, pods	8 ea	85	27	1.6	0	0	0	6	2.1	54	0.4	4	489	0.11	0.05	0.7	14	38.85
Olives, w/o pits, ripe, lrg, cnd	10 ea	44	51	0.4	5	0.6	0	3	1.4	39	1.5	384	177	0	0	0	0	0
Olives, w/o pits, ripe, sml, cnd	10 ea	32	37	0.3	3	0.5	0	2	1	28	1.1	279	129	0	0	0	0	0
Onions, yellow, ckd w/o add salt, drained, chpd	½ cup	105	46	1.4	0	0	0	11	1.5	23	0.3	3	0	0.04	0.02	0.2	5	15.75
Oranges, fresh, med	1 ea	180	85	1.7	0	0	0	21	4.3	72	0.2	0	369	0.16	0.07	0.5	96	54.54
Oysters, eastern, brd, fried, med	1 ea	45	89	3.9	6	1.4	36	5	0.1	28	3.1	188	136	0.07	0.09	0.7	2	13.95
Oysters, eastern, raw, wild	½ cup	120	82	8.5	3	0.9	64	5	0	54	8	253	120	0.12	0.11	1.7	4	12
Pancake, buckwheat, prep f/incomplete dry mix, 4"	1 ea	27	56	2.1	2	0.5	18	8	0.6	69	0.5	144	63	0.05	0.07	0.4	0	4.59
Pancake, plain, homemade, 4"	1 ea	73	166	4.7	7	1.5	43	21	1.1	160	1.3	320	143	0.15	0.21	1.1	0	27.74
Papaya, fresh, med	½ ea	227	89	1.4	0	0.1	0	22	4.1	54	0.2	7	645	0.06	0.07	0.8	140	86.26
Pasta, egg noodles, enrich, ckd	½ cup	80	106	3.8	1	0.2	26	20	0.9	10	1.3	6	16	0.15	0.07	1.2	0	51.2
Pasta, macaroni noodles, enrich, ckd	½ cup	70	99	3.3	0	0.1	0	20	0.9	5	1	1	0	0.14	0.07	1.2	0	49
Pasta, spaghetti noodles, enrich, salted, ckd	1 cup	140	197	6.7	1	0.1	0	40	2.4	10	2	140	0	0.29	0.14	2.3	0	98
Pasta, spaghetti noodles, whole wheat, ckd	1 cup	125	155	6.7	1	0.1	0	33	5.6	19	1.3	4	0	0.14	0.06	0.9	0	6.25
Pastry, cinnamon danish	1 ea	110	443	7.7	25	6.2	23	49	1.4	78	2.2	408	13	0.33	0.29	3.2	0	68.2
Peaches, fresh, sliced	½ cup	85	37	0.6	0	0	0	9	1.7	4	0.1	0	455	0.01	0.03	0.8	6	2.89
Peaches, in heavy syrup, cnd	½ tsp	96	71	0.4	0	0	0	19	1.2	3	0.3	6	319	0.01	0.02	0.6	3	3.07
Peaches, in juice, cnd, whole	½ tsp	77	34	0.5	0	0	0	9	0.9	5	0.2	3	293	0.01	0.01	0.4	3	2.62
Peanut Butter, smooth, salted	1 Tbs	32	190	8.1	16	3.3	0	6	1.9	12	0.6	149	0	0.03	0.03	4.3	0	23.68
Pears, bartlett, fresh, med	1 ea	180	106	0.7	1	0	0	27	4.3	20	0.4	0	36	0.04	0.07	0.2	7	13.14
Pears, in heavy syrup, cnd, halves	½ ea	103	76	0.2	0	0	0	20	1.6	5	0.2	5	0	0.01	0.02	0.2	1	1.24
Pears, in juice, cnd, halves	½ ea	77	38	0.3	0	0	0	10	1.2	7	0.2	3	5	0.01	0.01	0.2	1	0.92
Peas, cnd, drained	½ cup	85	59	3.8	0	0.1	0	11	3.5	17	0.8	214	653	0.1	0.07	0.6	8	37.65
Peas, green, ckd f/fzn w/o add salt, drained	½ cup	80	62	4.1	0	0.1	0	11	4.4	19	1.3	70	534	0.23	0.08	1.2	8	46.88
Peppers, bell, green, sweet, raw, med	1 ea	200	54	1.8	0	0.1	0	13	3.6	18	0.9	4	1264	0.13	0.06	1	179	44
Peppers, bell, red, sweet, sml	1 ea	74	20	0.7	0	0	0	5	1.5	7	0.3	1	4218	0.05	0.02	0.4	141	16.28
Peppers, bell, yellow, sweet, raw, lrg	1 ea	186	50	1.9	0	0.1	0	12	1.7	20	0.9	4	443	0.05	0.05	1.7	341	48.36
Pickles, dill	1 ea	135	24	0.8	0	0.1	0	6	1.6	12	0.7	1731	444	0.02	0.04	0.1	3	1.35
Pickles, sweet, med	1 ea	35	41	0.1	0	0	0	11	0.4	1	0.2	329	44	0	0.01	0.1	0	0.35
Pie, apple, bkd f/fzn, 1/6th of 8"	1 pce	118	280	2.2	13	4.5	0	40	1.9	13	0.5	314	146	0.03	0.03	0.3	4	25.96
Pie, bluberry, prep f/rec, 1/8th of 9"	1 pce	158	387	4.3	19	4.6	0	53	2.2	11	1.9	292	66	0.24	0.21	1.9	1	36.34
Pie, cherry, prep f/rec, 1/8th of 9"	1 pce	118	319	3.3	14	3.5	0	45	1.8	12	2.2	225	483	0.17	0.15	1.5	1	31.86
Pie, chocolate cream, rts, 1/6th of 8"	1 pce	175	532	4.5	34	8.7	9	59	3.5	63	1.9	238	9	0.06	0.19	1.2	0	22.75
Pie, lemon meringue, rts, 1/6th of 8"	1 pce	140	375	2.1	12	2.5	63	56	1.7	78	0.9	204	245	0.09	0.29	0.9	4	18.2
Pie, pecan, rts, 1/6th of 8"	1 pce	138	552	5.5	26	4.9	44	79	4.8	23	1.4	585	242	0.13	0.17	0.3	2	37.26
Pie, pumpkin, rts, 1/6th of 8"	1 pce	114	239	4.4	11	2	23	31	3.1	68	0.9	321	3915	0.06	0.17	0.2	1	22.8
Pineapple, chunks, fresh	½ cup	78	38	0.3	0	0	0	10	0.9	5	0.3	1	18	0.07	0.03	0.3	12	8.27
Pineapple, in heavy syrup, cnd, tidbits	½ cup	128	100	0.4	0	0	0	26	1	18	0.5	1	18	0.12	0.03	0.4	9	5.89
Pineapple, in juice, cnd	½ cup	125	75	0.5	0	0	0	20	1	18	0.3	1	48	0.12	0.02	0.4	12	6
Popcorn, air popped, plain	1 cup	6	23	0.7	0	0	0	5	0.9	1	0.2	0	12	0.01	0.02	0.1	0	1.38

Food	Amount	Weight (g)	Calories	Protein (g)	Fat (g)	Sat. Fat (g)	Cholesterol (g)	Carbohydrate (g)	Fiber (g)	Calcium (mg)	Iron (mg)	Sodium (mg)	Vit A (IU)	Thiamin (Vit B₁) (mg)	Riboflavin (Vit B₂) (mg)	Niacin (mg)	Vit C (mg)	Folate (mcg)
Popcorn, ckd in oil, salted	1 cup	11	55	1	3	0.5	0	6	1.1	1	0.3	97	17	0.01	0.01	0.2	0	1.87
Pork, bacon/cracklings, brld/pan fried/rstd	2 pce	15	86	4.6	7	2.6	13	0	0	2	0.2	239	0	0.1	0.04	1.1	0	0.75
Pork, cured, ham, reg, 11% fat, rstd	3 oz	85	151	19.2	8	2.7	50	0	0	7	1.1	1275	0	0.62	0.28	5.2	0	2.55
Pork, ham, whole, rstd	3 oz	85	232	22.8	15	5.5	80	0	0	12	0.9	51	0	0.54	0.27	3.9	0	8.5
Pork, ribs, spareribs, brsd	3 oz	85	337	24.7	26	9.5	103	0	0	40	1.6	79	8	0.35	0.32	4.7	0	3.4
Potato Chips, plain, salted	10 pce	20	107	1.4	7	2.2	0	11	0.9	5	0.3	119	0	0.03	0.04	0.8	6	9
Potatoes, au gratin, prep w/milk & butter f/dry mix	1 cup	245	228	5.6	10	6.3	37	31	2.2	203	0.8	1076	522	0.05	0.2	2.3	8	16.17
Potatoes, baked, w/flesh & skin, long	1 ea	202	220	4.6	0	0.1	0	51	4.8	20	2.7	16	0	0.22	0.07	3.3	26	22.22
Potatoes, hash browns, prep f/fzn	½ cup	78	170	2.5	9	3.5	0	22	1.6	12	1.2	27	0	0.09	0.02	1.9	5	5.07
Potatoes, mashed, w/whole milk	½ cup	105	81	2	1	0.3	2	18	2.1	27	0.3	318	20	0.09	0.04	1.2	7	8.61
Potatoes, sweet, flesh, bkd in skin, med, peeled	1 ea	146	150	2.5	0	0	0	35	4.4	41	0.7	15	31860	0.11	0.19	0.9	36	33
Pretzels, hard, salted, twisted	1 oz	28	107	2.5	1	0.2	0	22	0.9	10	1.2	480	0	0.13	0.17	1.5	0	47.88
Prunes, dried	5 ea	61	146	1.6	0	0	0	38	4.3	31	1.5	2	1212	0.05	0.1	1.2	2	2.26
Pudding, choc, rte, 5oz can	5 oz	142	189	3.8	6	1	4	32	1.4	128	0.7	183	51	0.04	0.22	0.5	3	4.26
Pudding, tapioca, 5oz can	5 oz	142	169	2.8	5	0.9	1	28	0.1	119	0.3	226	0	0.03	0.14	0.4	1	4.26
Pudding, vanilla, 5oz can	5 oz	142	185	3.3	5	0.8	10	31	0.1	125	0.2	192	30	0.03	0.2	0.4	0	0
Raisins, seedless, unpacked	1 oz	28	84	0.9	0	0	0	22	1.1	14	0.6	3	2	0.04	0.02	0.2	1	0.92
Raspberries, fresh	1 cup	123	60	1.1	1	0	0	14	8.3	27	0.7	3	160	0.04	0.11	1.1	31	31.98
Raspberries, swtnd, fzn	1 cup	250	400	10	1	0	0	62	5.5	368	3.1	245	400	0.09	0.53	0.8	1	27.5
Rice, brown, ckd	½ cup	96	107	2.5	1	0.2	0	22	1.7	10	0.4	5	0	0.09	0.02	1.5	0	3.84
Rice, white, reg, ckd	½ cup	103	134	2.8	0	0.1	0	29	0.4	10	1.2	0	0	0.17	0.01	1.5	0	59.74
Rice, wild, ckd	½ cup	100	101	4	0	0	0	21	1.8	3	0.6	3	0	0.05	0.09	1.3	0	26
Rolls, hard, white	1 ea	50	146	4.9	2	0.3	0	26	1.1	48	1.6	272	0	0.24	0.17	2.1	0	47.5
Salad Dressing, blue cheese/roquefort	1 Tbs	15	76	0.7	8	1.5	3	1	0	12	0	164	32	0	0.02	0	0	1.21
Salad Dressing, french	1 Tbs	16	69	0.1	7	1.5	0	3	0	2	0.1	219	208	0	0	0	0	0.67
Salad Dressing, French, low cal	1 Tbs	15	20	0	1	0.1	0	3	0	2	0.1	118	195	0	0	0	0	0
Salad Dressing, Italian	1 Tbs	15	70	0.1	7	1.1	0	2	0	2	0	118	12	0	0	0	0	0.73
Salad Dressing, Italian, diet, 2cal/tsp, cmrcl	1 Tbs	15	16	0	1	0.2	1	1	0	0	0	118	0	0	0	0	0	0
Salad Dressing, ranch	1 Tbs	15	80	0	8	1.2	5	0	0	0	0	105	0	0	0	0	0	
Salad Dressing, thousand island	1 Tbs	15	57	0.1	5	0.9	4	2	0	2	0.1	105	48	0	0	0	0	0.94
Salad Dressing, thousand island, low cal	1 Tbs	15	24	0.1	2	0.2	2	2	0	2	0.1	150	48	0	0	0	0	0.84
Salad, chicken, w/celery	½ cup	78	268	10.6	25	3.1	48	1	0.2	16	0.6	201	155	0.03	0.07	3.3	1	8.46
Salad, pasta, garden primavera, prep f/dry	¾ cup	142	280	8	12	2.5	0	34	0.2	80	1.8	730	200	0.15	0.17	2	0	
Salad, potato	½ cup	125	179	3.4	10	1.8	85	14	1.6	24	0.8	661	261	0.1	0.07	1.1	12	8.38
Salad, tuna	1 cup	205	383	32.9	19	3.2	27	19	0	35	2	824	199	0.06	0.14	13.7	5	16.4
Salami, beef & pork, dry	1 oz	28	117	6.4	10	3.4	22	1	0	2	0.4	521	0	0.17	0.08	1.4	0	0.56
Salmon, pink, w/bone, cnd, not drained	3 oz	85	118	16.8	5	1.3	47	0	0	181	0.7	471	47	0.02	0.16	5.6	0	13.09
Salmon, sockeye, fillet, bkd/brld	3 oz	85	184	23.2	9	1.6	74	0	0	6	0.5	56	178	0.18	0.15	5.7	0	4.25
Salsa, homemade, Mexican sauce	1 Tbs	15	3	0.1	0	0	0	1	0.2	1	0	1	57	0.01	0	0.1	2	1.74
Sandwich, bacon, lettuce & tomato, on soft white	1 ea	130	323	10.8	18	4.7	22	30	1.7	54	2.1	619	271	0.36	0.2	3.4	12	35.5
Sandwich, egg salad, on soft white	1 ea	111	361	9.1	24	4.2	149	29	1.2	67	2.1	499	239	0.25	0.3	1.9	0	35.39
Sandwich, peanut butter & jam, on soft white, unsalted	1 ea	100	348	11.5	15	3.1	2	46	3	60	2.2	290	2	0.27	0.17	5.3	0	40.04
Sandwich, reuben, grilled	1 ea	237	458	27.6	29	9.8	80	25	2.2	286	4.2	1933	453	0.21	0.34	2.8	13	37.79
Sardines, Atlantic, w/bones, cnd in oil, drained	1 oz	28	58	6.9	3	0.4	40	0	0	107	0.8	141	63	0.02	0.06	1.5	0	3.3
Sauce, soy, made f/soy & wheat	1 Tbs	16	9	1.3	0	0	0	1	0.1	3	0.3	871	0	0.01	0.03	0.4	0	2.56
Sauce, teriyaki, rts	1 Tbs	18	15	1.1	0	0	0	3	0	4	0.3	690	47	0.01	0.01	0.2	0	3.6
Sauerkraut, w/liquid, cnd	½ cup	118	22	1.1	0	0	0	5	2.9	35	1.7	780	21	0.02	0.03	0.2	17	27.97

Food	Amount	Weight (g)	Calories	Protein (g)	Fat (g)	Sat. Fat (g)	Cholesterol (g)	Carbohydrate (g)	Fiber (g)	Calcium (mg)	Iron (mg)	Sodium (mg)	Vit A (IU)	Thiamin (Vit B₁) (mg)	Riboflavin (Vit B₂) (mg)	Niacin (mg)	Vit C (mg)	Folate (mcg)
Sausage, pork, smkd, link	1 ea	68	265	15.1	22	7.7	46	1	0	20	0.8	1020	0	0.48	0.17	3.1	1	3.4
Scallops, brd, fried, mixed species, lrg	2 ea	31	67	5.6	3	0.8	19	3	0	13	0.3	144	23	0.01	0.03	0.5	1	11.47
Seaweed, spirulina, dried	1 cup	119	345	68.4	9	3.2	0	28	4.3	143	33.9	1247	678	2.83	4.37	15.3	12	111.8
Shrimp/Prawns, brd, fried, lrg	7 ea	85	206	18.2	10	1.8	150	10	0.3	57	1.1	292	161	0.11	0.12	2.6	1	6.89
Shrimp/Prawns, ckd, lrg	3 oz	85	84	17.8	1	0.2	166	0	0	33	2.6	190	186	0.03	0.03	2.2	2	2.98
Soda, cola	12 fl-oz	369	151	0	0	0	0	38	0	11	0.1	15	0	0	0	0	0	0
Soda, cola/Coke, diet, w/sacc, low sod	12 fl-oz	340	0	0	0	0	0	0	0	14	0.1	54	0	0	0	0	0	0
Soda, ginger ale	12 fl-oz	366	124	0	0	0	0	32	0	11	0.7	26	0	0	0	0.1	0	0
Soda, lemon lime	12 fl-oz	340	136	0	0	0	0	35	0	7	0.2	37	0	0	0	0	0	0
Soda, root beer	12 fl-oz	340	139	0	0	0	0	36	0	17	0.2	44	0	0	0	0	0	0
Sole/Flounder, fillet, bkd/brld	3 oz	85	99	20.5	1	0.3	58	0	0	15	0.3	89	32	0.07	0.1	1.9	0	7.82
Soup, beef bouillon/broth, cnd, prep w/water	1 cup	240	17	2.7	1	0.3	0	0	0	14	0.4	782	0	0	0.05	1.9	0	4.8
Soup, chicken noodle, prep w/water	1 cup	241	75	4	2	0.7	7	9	0.7	17	0.8	1106	711	0.05	0.06	1.4	0	21.69
Soup, clam chowder, Manhattan, prep f/cnd	1 cup	244	112	12.3	2	0	10	11	3.1	41	1.8	725	2297				4	
Soup, clam chowder, New England, prep w/milk	1 cup	248	164	9.5	7	3	22	17	1.5	186	1.5	992	164	0.07	0.24	1	3	9.67
Soup, cream of chicken, prep w/milk	1 cup	248	191	7.5	11	4.6	27	15	0.2	181	0.7	1047	714	0.07	0.26	0.9	1	7.69
Soup, cream of mushroom, prep w/milk	1 cup	245	201	6	13	5.1	20	15	0.5	176	0.6	906	152	0.08	0.28	0.9	2	9.8
Soup, minestrone, prep w/water	1 cup	241	82	4.3	3	0.6	2	11	1	34	0.9	911	2338	0.05	0.04	0.9	1	36.15
Soup, pea, split, w/ham, prep w/water	1 cup	245	184	10	4	1.7	7	27	2.2	22	2.2	975	431	0.14	0.07	1.4	1	2.45
Soup, tomato, prep w/milk	1 cup	248	161	6.1	6	2.9	17	22	2.7	159	1.8	744	848	0.13	0.25	1.5	68	20.83
Soup, tomato, prep w/water	1 cup	245	86	2.1	2	0.4	0	17	0.5	12	1.8	698	691	0.09	0.05	1.4	67	14.7
Soup, vegetable beef, prep w/water	1 cup	245	78	5.6	2	0.9	5	10	0.5	17	1.1	794	1899	0.04	0.05	1	2	10.54
Soup, vegetable, vegetarian, prep w/water	1 cup	250	75	2.2	2	0.3	0	12	0.5	22	1.1	852	3118	0.05	0.05	0.9	2	11
Sour Cream, cultured	1 Tbs	14	30	0.4	3	1.8	6	1	0	16	0	7	111	0	0.02	0	0	1.51
Spinach, ckd w/o add salt, drained	½ cup	103	24	3.1	0	0	0	4	2.5	140	3.7	72	8436	0.1	0.24	0.5	10	150.1
Spinach, raw, chpd	1 cup	55	12	1.6	0	0	0	2	1.5	54	1.5	43	3693	0.04	0.1	0.4	15	106.9
Spinach, w/o add salt, cnd, drained	½ cup	103	24	2.9	1	0.1	0	4	2.5	131	2.4	28	9039	0.02	0.14	0.4	15	100.7
Squash, acorn, ckd	1 cup	245	83	1.6	0	0	0	22	6.4	64	1.4	632	7	0.25	0.02	1.3	16	27.69
Squash, summer, ckd w/o add salt, drained	½ cup	90	18	0.8	0	0.1	0	4	1.3	24	0.3	7	258	0.04	0.04	0.5	5	18.09
Squash, winter, avg, bkd, mashed	½ cup	103	40	0.9	1	0.1	0	9	2.9	14	0.3	1	3664	0.09	0.02	0.7	10	28.84
Strawberries, fresh, whole	1 cup	149	45	0.9	1	0	0	10	3.4	21	0.6	1	40	0.03	0.1	0.3	84	26.37
Strawberries, slices, swtnd, fzn	1 cup	250	240	1.3	0	0	0	65	4.8	28	1.5	8	60	0.04	0.13	1	104	37.25
Stuffing, bread, prep f/dry mix	½ cup	70	125	2.2	6	1.2	0	15	2	22	0.8	380	219	0.1	0.07	1	0	70.7
Sugar, beet/cane, brown, packed	1 tsp	5	19	0	0	0	0	5	0	4	0.1	2	0	0	0	0	0	0.05
Sugar, white, granulated	1 tsp	4	15	0	0	0	0	4	0	0	0	0	0	0	0	0	0	0
Syrup, maple	1 Tbs	20	52	0	0	0	0	13	0	13	0.2	2	0	0	0	0	0	0
Taco Shells	1 ea	10	47	0.7	2	0.3	0	7	0.7	20	0.2	67	33	0.05	0.04	0.2	0	9.44
Tangerines/Mandarin oranges, fresh, med	1 ea	116	51	0.7	0	0	0	13	2.7	16	0.1	1	1067	0.12	0.03	0.2	36	23.66
Tea, brewed	1 cup	180	2	0	0	0	0	1	0	5	0	5	0	0	0.03	0	0	9.36
Tempeh	1 cup	166	320	30.8	18	3.7	0	16	9	184	4.5	15	0	0.13	0.59	4.4	0	39.67
Tofu, firm, silken	½ cup	126	78	8.7	3	0.5	0	3	0.1	40	1.3	45	0	0.13	0.05	0.3	0	15
Tomatoes, red, ripe, raw, med, whole	1 ea	100	21	0.9	0	0	0	5	1.1	5	0.4	9	623	0.06	0.05	0.6	19	5.95
Tomatoes, red, ripe, w/o add salt, cnd, in liquid	½ cup	121	23	1.1	0	0	0	5	1.2	36	0.7	179	720	0.05	0.04	0.9	17	9.44
Tortilla/Taco/Tostada Shell, corn	1 ea	148	693	10.7	33	5	0	92	11.1	237	3.7	543	518	0.34	0.08	2	0	8.88
Trout, rainbow, fillet, bkd/brld, wild	3 oz	85	128	19.5	5	1.4	59	0	0	73	0.3	48	42	0.13	0.1	4.9	2	16.15
Tuna, light, cnd in oil, drained	3 oz	85	168	24.8	7	1.3	15	0	0	11	1.2	301	66	0.03	0.1	10.5	0	4.51
Tuna, light, cnd in water, drained	3½ oz	99	115	25.3	1	0.2	30	0	0	11	1.5	335	55	0.03	0.07	13.1	0	3.96
Turkey, average, w/o skin, rstd	3 oz	85	144	24.9	4	1.4	65	0	0	21	1.5	60	0	0.05	0.15	4.6	0	5.95

Food	Amount	Weight (g)	Calories	Protein (g)	Fat (g)	Sat. Fat (g)	Cholesterol (g)	Carbohydrate (g)	Fiber (g)	Calcium (mg)	Iron (mg)	Sodium (mg)	Vit A (IU)	Thiamin (Vit B$_1$) (mg)	Riboflavin (Vit B$_2$) (mg)	Niacin (mg)	Vit C (mg)	Folate (mcg)
Turnip Greens, ckd f/fzn, drained	½ cup	73	22	2.4	0	0.1	0	4	2.5	111	1.4	11	5822	0.04	0.05	0.3	16	28.76
Turnips, ckd w/add salt, raw, cubes	½ cup	78	16	0.6	0	0	0	4	1.6	17	0.2	39	0	0.02	0.02	0.2	9	7.18
Veal, loin, brsd	3 oz	85	241	25.7	15	5.7	100	0	0	24	0.9	68	0	0.03	0.26	7.7	0	11.9
Veal, loin, lean, brsd	3 oz	85	192	28.5	8	2.2	106	0	0	27	0.9	71	0	0.04	0.29	8.5	0	12.75
Vinegar, balsamic, 60 grain	1 Tbs	15	21	0	0	0	0	5	0	2	0.1	3	0	0.08	0.08	0.1	0	
Watermelon, fresh, diced	1 cup	160	51	1	1	0.1	0	11	0.8	13	0.3	3	586	0.13	0.03	0.3	15	3.52
Wheat, bulgur, ckd	1 cup	135	112	4.2	0	0.1	0	25	6.1	14	1.3	7	0	0.08	0.04	1.4	0	24.3
Wheat, flakes, rolled, dry	1 cup	30	97	3.5	0	0	0	21	4.4	18	1	0	0	0.13	0.03	1.4	0	
Wheat, germ, tstd	1 Tbs	6	23	1.7	1	0.1	0	3	0.8	3	0.5	0	0	0.1	0.05	0.3	0	21.12
Whiskey, 90 proof	2 fl-oz	42	110	0	0	0	0	0	0	0	0	0	0	0	0	0	0	0
Wine, cooler	4 oz	113	56	0.1	0	0	0	7	0	6	0.3	9	1	0.01	0.01	0.1	2	1.34
Wine, red	⅙ cup	30	22	0.1	0	0	0	1	0	2	0.1	2	0	0	0.01	0	0	0.6
Wine, Rose	2 fl-oz	59	42	0.1	0	0	0	1	0	5	0.2	3	0	0	0.01	0	0	0.65
Wine, white, med	2 fl-oz	59	40	0.1	0	0	0	0	0	5	0.2	3	0	0	0	0	0	0.12
Yogurt, fruit, low fat, 10g prot/8 oz	1 cup	227	231	9.9	2	1.6	10	43	0	345	0.2	133	104	0.08	0.4	0.2	1	21.11
Yogurt, plain, low fat, 12g prot/8 oz	8 oz	226	143	11.9	4	2.3	14	16	0	413	0.2	159	149	0.1	0.48	0.3	2	25.31
FAST FOOD RESTAURANTS																		
General																		
Burrito, bean	1 ea	166	342	10.8	10	5.3	3	55	6.3	86	3.5	754	254	0.48	0.46	3.1	1	66.4
Chili, con carne	1 cup	255	258	24.8	8	3.5	135	22	4	69	5.2	1015	1675	0.13	1.15	2.5	2	45.9
Cole Slaw, fast food	1 cup	120	178	1.8	13	1.9	6	15	2	41	0.9	324	409	0.05	0.04	0.1	10	46.8
English Muffin, w/butter	1 ea	63	189	4.9	6	2.4	13	30	1.9	103	1.6	386	136	0.25	0.31	2.6	1	56.7
Entree, enchilada, cheese	1 ea	230	451	13.6	27	14.9	62	40		458	1.9	1106	1638	0.12	0.6	2.7	0	92
Hot Dog, plain	1 ea	98	242	10.4	15	5.1	44	18		24	2.3	670	0	0.24	0.27	3.6	0	48.02
Pancake, w/butter & syrup	2 ea	232	520	8.3	14	5.9	58	91	1.2	128	2.6	1104	281	0.39	0.56	3.4	3	51.04
Sandwich, chicken, fillet, plain	1 ea	157	444	20.8	25	7.4	52	33	1.1	52	4	826	86	0.28	0.2	5.9	8	86.35
Sundae, hot fudge, fast food	1 ea	164	295	5.9	9	5.2	21	49		215	0.6	189	230	0.07	0.31	1.1	2	9.84
Arby's																		
Salad, chef	1 ea	273	136	12.3	6	2.6	84	9		113	3.3	529	3321	0.26	0.25	4.6	35	
Sandwich, beef, Arby Q	1 ea	190	389	17.6	15	5.4	29	48		70	9.2	1268		0.27	0.39	9.2		
Sandwich, beef, French dip & swiss cheese	1 ea	154	369	24.7	16	7.5	58	31	0.9	232	3.6	1237	0	0.18	0.47	7.4	0	16.35
Sandwich, beef 'n cheddar	1 ea	194	508	24.6	26	7.7	52	43		150	6.1	1166	0	0.42	0.63	9.8	1	
Sandwich, chicken, grilled, deluxe	1 ea	195	365	20	17	3	37	35		59	2.1	764	339	0.27	0.25	11.5	7	
Sandwich, roast beef, regular	1 ea	155	383	22	18	6.9	43	35	1.1	60	4.9	936	0	0.28	0.48	11	1	14
Sauce, Arby's	½ oz	14	15	0.1	0	0	0	3			0.4	113						
Sauce, horsey	½ oz	14	110	0.1	5	1.2	0	3		20		105						
Burger King Corporation																		
Cheeseburger, Whopper	1 ea	294	730	33	46	16	115	46	3	250	4.5	1350	750	0.34	0.48	7	9	
Croissant, w/egg, sausage & cheese	1 ea	110	375	13.8	29	10	162	16	0.6	94	2.2	712	250				9	
Hamburger, Whopper	1 ea	270	640	27	39	11	90	45	3	80	4.5	870	500	0.33	0.41	7	9	
Onion Rings, reg svg	3 ea	30	75	1	3	0.5	0	10	1.5	24	0.3	196	0				0	
Potatoes, french fries, salted, med svg	1 ea	116	370	5	20	5	0	43	3	0	1.1	240	0				4	
Sandwich, chicken, broiler	1 ea	168	373	20.3	20	4.1	54	28	1.4	41	3.7	325	203				4	
Sandwich, fish, big	1 ea	255	700	26	41	6	90	56	3	60	2.7	980	100				1	
Dunkin Donuts, Inc.																		
Croissant, plain	1 ea	18	81	1.2	5	1.2	2	8	0	6	0.5	78	0				0	
Hidden Valley																		
Salad Dressing, ranch, reduced fat & cal	2 Tbs	28	58	0.5	5	0.9	10	2	0	11	0.1	237	15				0	
International Dairy Queen Inc.																		
Frozen Yogurt Cone, med	4 oz	113	148	5.1	1	0.3	3	32	0	143	1	91	0	0.05	0.2	1	1	
Frozen Yogurt, nonfat	4 oz	113	133	4	0	0		28	0	133	1	93	0				0	

Food	Amount	Weight (g)	Calories	Protein (g)	Fat (g)	Sat. Fat (g)	Cholesterol (g)	Carbohydrate (g)	Fiber (g)	Calcium (mg)	Iron (mg)	Sodium (mg)	Vit A (IU)	Thiamin (Vit B₁) (mg)	Riboflavin (Vit B₂) (mg)	Niacin (mg)	Vit C (mg)	Folate (mcg)
Hamburger, homestyle	1 ea	138	290	17	12	5	45	29	2	60	2.7	630	200	0.29	0.25	3.9	4	
Ice Cream Cone, vanilla, med	1 ea	142	237	5.7	6	4.3	22	38	0	179	1.3	115	538	0.06	0.26	0.1	2	
Milk Shake, vanilla, med	1 ea	397	520	12	14	8	45	88	0.3	400	1.4	230	400	0.12	0.6	0.8	0	
Onion Rings, svg	3 oz	85	241	3.8	12	3	0	29	2.3	15	1.1	135	0	0.09	0.05	0.4	0	
Sandwich, fish, fillet	1 ea	182	396	17.1	17	3.7	48	42	2.1	43	1.9	674	0	0.32	0.24	3.2	0	
Sundae, chocolate, med	1 ea	184	315	6.3	8	4.7	24	56	0	197	1.1	165	590	0.06	0.27	0.3	0	
Jack In the Box																		
Bowl, chicken, teriyaki	1 ea	502	670	26	4	1	15	128	3	100	4.5	1730	6500				24	
Cheeseburger, Jumbo Jack	1 ea	296	640	31	38	15	105	44	2	250	4.5	1340	750	0.44	0.54	2	9	
Hamburger	1 ea	104	250	12	9	3.5	30	30	2	100	3.6	610	0	0.16	0.28	2.1	0	
Hamburger, sourdough, jack	1 ea	233	690	34	45	15	105	37	2	200	4.5	1180	750	0.68	0.5	8.4	9	
Sandwich, chicken, supreme	1 ea	305	830	33	49	7	65	66	3	200	3.6	2140	500	0.49	0.4	13.7	9	
Kentucky Fried Chicken Corporation																		
Chicken, leg, original recipe	1 ea	54	124	11.5	8	1.8	66	4	0	18	0.6	374	89				1	
Chicken, wing, hot & spicy	1 ea	55	210	10	15	4	55	9	1	20	0.7	350	100				1	
Chicken, wing, original recipe	1 ea	45	134	8.6	10	2.4	53	5	0	19	0.3	396	96				1	
Long John Silver's																		
Dinner, fish & fries, batter fried, 2pce	1 ea	261	610	27	37	7.9	60	52		40	1.8	1480		0.38	0.34	8	9	
McDonald's Nutrition Information Center																		
Biscuit, sausage & egg	1 ea	175	541	17.7	36	9.8	241	34	1	98	2.7	1140	295	0.53	0.57	4.1	0	27.73
Cheeseburger	1 ea	115	304	14.3	12	5.7	38	33	1.9	190	2.6	779	285	0.31	0.29	3.6	2	22.37
Cheeseburger, Quarter Pounder	1 ea	186	493	26	28	12.1	88	35	1.9	279	4.2	1200	465	0.37	0.4	6.3	2	31.06
Chicken, nuggets, McNuggets, 4 pce, svg	1 ea	71	190	12	11	2.5	40	10	0	9	0.7	340	0	0.08	0.11	5	0	
Danish, apple	1 ea	115	394	5.5	18	5.5	44	56	1.1	88	1.2	318	548	0.33	0.19	2.2	1	5.03
Frozen Yogurt Cone, vanilla, low fat	3 oz	85	142	3.8	4	2.8	19	22	0	94	0.3	71	283				1	33.16
Hamburger, Big Mac	1 ea	204	529	24.6	29	9.4	80	42	2.8	236	4.2	1011	283	0.46	0.42	5.7	3	46.53
Hamburger, Quarter Pounder	1 ea	160	391	21.4	20	7.4	65	34	1.9	140	4.2	763	93	0.37	0.3	6.3	2	25.63
McMuffin, egg	1 ea	138	294	17.2	12	4.6	238	27	1	203	2.7	802	507	0.5	0.45	3.3	1	33.47
McMuffin, sausage	1 ea	135	434	15.7	28	9.6	54	31	1.2	241	2.2	892	241	0.68	0.33	4.5	0	18.95
Milk Shake, vanilla, sml	1 ea	289	355	10.8	9	5.9	39	58	0	345	0.4	246	296	0.12	0.5	0.3	1	
Muffin, apple bran, fat free	1 ea	75	197	3.9	2	0.3	0	40	4	66	0.9	250	0	0.14	0.14	1.3	1	5.03
Pie, apple	1 ea	307	1037	12	52	14	0	136	2	80	4.3	797		0.71	0.43	5.6	96	33.16
Potatoes, french fries, sml svg	1 ea	68	210	3	10	1.5	0	26	2	9	0.4	135	0	0.05	0	1.9	9	25.57
Potatoes, hash browns	1 ea	55	135	1	8	1.6	0	15	1	7	0.4	342	0	0.08	0.02	0.9	2	8.64
Salad, garden, shaker	1 ea	149	100	7	6	3	75	4	2	150	1.1	120	1500				15	
Sandwich, Filet O Fish	1 ea	131	378	13.4	21	3.8	42	35	1.7	126	1.5	731	168	0.29	0.21	2.3	0	26.73
Sauce, sweet & sour, pkt 1	1½ oz	32	57	0	0	0	0	13	0	2	0.2	160	343		0.01	0.1	0	
Pizza Hut, Inc.																		
Pizza, cheese, pan, med, 12"	2 pce	205	495	22.8	21	9.5	47	53	3.8	273	2.8	951	1000	0.57	0.61	5.2	7	
Pizza, cheese, thin n' crispy, med, 12"	2 pce	148	350	18.8	14	6.8	43	36	3.4	247	1.8	911	922	0.39	0.39	4.8	5	
Pizza, pepperoni, pan, med, 12"	2 pce	211	539	22.4	24	8.1	49	57	4.1	209	3.3	1157	966	0.63	0.49	5.4	8	0
Pizza, pepperoni, personal pan	1 ea	255	637	27	28	10	55	69	5	250	4	1339	1164	0.56	0.66	8.2	10	
Pizza, supreme, pan, med, 12"	2 pce	255	581	28	28	11.2	56	52	5.6	219	4.3	1428	912	0.8	0.79	6	10	
Subway International																		
Sandwich, chicken breast, rstd, on white, 6"	1 ea	246	332	26	6	1	48	41	3	35	3	967	617				15	
Sandwich, Italian bmt, on white, 6"	1 ea	246	445	21	21	8	56	39	3	44	4	1652	753				15	
Sandwich, meatball, on white, 6"	1 ea	260	404	18	16	6	33	44	3	32	4	1035	712				16	
Sandwich, roast beef, deli style	1 ea	180	245	13	4	1	13	38	2	23	3	638	565				14	
Sandwich, tuna, w/lt mayonnaise, on wheat, 6"	1 ea	253	391	19	15	2	32	46	3	38	3	940	729				15	
Sandwich, turkey, on white, 6"	1 ea	232	273	17	4	1	19	40	3	30	4	1391	601				15	

Food	Amount	Weight (g)	Calories	Protein (g)	Fat (g)	Sat. Fat (g)	Cholesterol (g)	Carbohydrate (g)	Fiber (g)	Calcium (mg)	Iron (mg)	Sodium (mg)	Vit A (IU)	Thiamin (Vit B₁) (mg)	Riboflavin (Vit B₂) (mg)	Niacin (mg)	Vit C (mg)	Folate (mcg)
Taco Bell Inc.																		
Burrito, beef, big supreme	1 ea	298	520	24	23	10	55	54	11	150	2.7	1520	3000	0.4			5	
Burrito, seven layer	1 ea	234	438	13.2	19	5.8	21	55	10.7	165	3	1058	1240				5	
Burrito, supreme	1 ea	255	440	17	19	8	35	51	10	150	9	1230	2500		2.1	2.9	5	
Taco	1 ea	83	192	9.6	11	4.3	27	13	3.2	85	1.1	351	532	0.05	0.15	1.3	0	
Taco, soft	1 ea	92	225	9.2	10	4.1	26	12	3.1	82	1.1	337	511	0.39	0.22	2.7	0	
Wendy's Foods International																		
Cheeseburger, w/bacon, jr	1 ea	170	393	20.5	19	7.5	58	35	1.9	171	3.6	895	390	0.31	0.32	6.6	9	28.85
Chicken, nuggets	6 pce	94	292	13.9	20	3.6	37	14	0	24	0.5	589	0	0.15	0.14	9	1	
Frosty, dairy dessert, med	1 ea	298	440	11	11	7	50	73	0	410	1.4	260	1000	0.14	0.62	0.4	0	22.9
Hamburger, bacon classic, big	1 ea	251	517	30.1	26	10.7	88	41	2.4	206	4.5	1298	622	0.4	1.36	5.3	13	
Salad, caesar, w/o dressing, side	1 ea	130	151	12.4	8	3.4	25	9	2	190	1.6	538	2501				22	
Salad, chicken, grilled, w/o dressing	1 ea	338	195	22.1	8	1.7	46	10	4	188	2.1	676	5872				35	
Salad, garden, deluxe, w/o dressing	1 ea	271	110	6.7	6	1	1	10	3.9	189	1.5	319	5883				35	
Salad, taco, w/o chips	1 ea	510	411	28.7	20	10.5	69	31	8.7	403	4.5	1132	2582	0.29	0.5	3.2	28	88.27
Sandwich, chicken, brd	1 ea	208	433	27.4	16	3.1	54	47	1.8	93	2.7	754	217	0.43	0.32	13.3	13	
Sandwich, chicken, club	1 ea	220	483	30.6	20	4.4	64	48	1.9	95	2.9	957	222				14	
Sandwich, chicken, grilled	1 ea	177	283	22.6	7	1.5	61	34	1.8	84	2.7	698	201				9	
CONVENIENCE FOODS & MEALS																		
El Charrito																		
Entree, enchilada, beef, family size, 6 pack	1 ea	200	353	11.8	17	6.5	33	39	5.2	196	2.4	837	1961				3	
Healthy Choice																		
Dinner, fish, herb baked, fzn	1 ea	273	300	14.1	6	1.3	31	48	4.4	35	0.6	424	2650				0	
Dinner, meatloaf, traditional, fzn	1 ea	340	316	15.3	5	2.5	37	52	6.1	48	2.2	459	745				55	
Entree, burrito, chicken, con queso, fzn	1 ea	216	253	10.1	4	1.8	25	43	4.3	29	1.3	426	1084				4	
Entree, lasagna, roma, fzn	1 ea	284	311	19.3	7	2.2	26	44	4.4	111	2.7	430	371	0.22	0.19	1.5	4	
Entree, spaghetti, bolognese, fzn	1 ea	284	280	14	6	2	30	43	5	40	3.6	470	500				15	
Lean Cuisine																		
Entree, chow mein, chicken, w/rice	1 ea	241	198	12.3	5	0.9	33	26	1.9	19	0.3	482	95	0.14	0.16	4.7	6	
Entree, lasagna, w/meat sauce	1 ea	291	270	19	6	2.5	25	34	5	150	1.8	560	500	0.15	0.25	3	12	
Entree, ravioli, cheese	1 ea	241	250	12	8	3	55	32	4	200	1.1	500	750	0.06	0.25	1.2	6	48
Entree, spaghetti, w/meatballs, fzn	1 ea	290	322	19.4	8	2.2	6	43	4.9	102	2.6	502	0					
The Budget Gourmet																		
Dinner, chicken, teriyaki, 3 dish	1 ea	340	360	20	12		55	44		80	1.4	610	1500	0.15	0.34	6	12	
Dinner, veal, parmigiana, 3 dish	1 ea	340	440	26	20		165	39		30	4.5	1160	5000	0.45	0.6	6	6	
Entree, beef, sirloin tips, w/country gravy	1 ea	334	365	18.8	21		47	25		71	0.4	670	882	0.18	0.2	4.7	3	
Entree, linguini, w/shrimp	1 ea	284	330	15	15		75	33		10	3.6	1250	5000	0.3	0.17	3	2	
The Budget Gourmet-Slim Select																		
Entree, stroganoff, beef	1 ea	238	269	17.3	10		58	28		58	2.6	537	288	0.25	0.33	3.8	9	
Weight Watchers																		
Entree, chow mein, chicken	1 ea	255	200	12	2	0.5	25	34	3	40	0.7	430	1499				36	

This food composition table has been prepared for West-Wadsworth Publishing Company and is copyrighted by ESHA Research in Salem, Oregon—the developer and publisher of the Food Processor®, Genesis® R&D, and the Computer Chef® nutrition software systems. The major sources for the data are from the USDA, supplemented by more than 1200 additional sources of information. Because the list of references is so extensive, it is not provided here, but is available from the publisher.

Answer Key

CHAPTER 1

1. a   2. b   3. d   4. c   5. e   6. e   7. e   8. b   9. e   10. c

CHAPTER 2

1. d   2. b   3. c   4. c   5. e   6. a

CHAPTER 3

1. b   2. a   3. e   4. d   5. e   6. e

CHAPTER 4

1. a   2. a   3. e   4. d   5. e   6. e

CHAPTER 5

1. c   2. e   3. e   4. c   5. b   6. a   7. a

CHAPTER 6

1. a   2. e   3. b   4. c   5. a   6. e   7. c   8. b   9. b   10. a

CHAPTER 7

1. d   2. c   3. d   4. c   5. a   6. d   7. a   8. a   9. e   10. e

CHAPTER 8

1. c   2. d   3. c   4. b   5. d   6. e   7. d

CHAPTER 9

1. e   2. b   3. d   4. a   5. b   6. e   7. b   8. b   9. e   10. e

CHAPTER 10

1. c   2. d   3. e   4. a   5. b   6. c   7. a   8. c   9. d   10. e

CHAPTER 11

1. b   2. a   3. e   4. e   5. e   6. c   7. e   8. e   9. e   10. e

CHAPTER 12
1. b   2. e   3. e   4. a   5. e   6. b   7. d   8. a   9. b   10. e

CHAPTER 13
1. b   2. b   3. e   4. e   5. b   6. d   7. d   8. e

CHAPTER 14
1. d   2. e   3. a   4. b   5. d   6. a   7. c   8. a

Photo Credits

Cover Image
© John Terrence Turner/Getty Images

p. xi © George Doyle/Stockbyte Platinum/Getty Images; **p. xii** © Ken Reid/Taxi/Getty Images; **p. xiii** © Eric Glenn/DK Stock/Getty Images; **p. xiv** © Lori Adamski Peek/Stone/Getty Images; **p. xv** © Kate Power/Taxi/Getty Images; **p. xvi** © Digital Vision/Getty Images

Chapter 1
p. 1 © George Doyle/Stockbyte Platinum/Getty Images; **p. 2** © Fitness & Wellness, Inc.; **p. 3** John Crawley; **p. 6** © Fitness & Wellness, Inc.; **p. 7** John Crawley; **p. 8** © Fitness & Wellness, Inc.; **p. 9** John Crawley; **p. 10** (left) © 2000 PhotoDisc, Inc.; **p. 10** (right) © 2001 PhotoDisc, Inc.; **p. 11** © Fitness & Wellness, Inc.; **p. 12** © Fitness & Wellness, Inc.; **p. 13** © Fitness & Wellness, Inc.; **p. 16** © 2001 Photo Disc, Inc.

Chapter 2
p. 25 © Skip Brown/National Geographic/Getty Images; **p. 28** © Chuck Scheer, Boise State University; **p. 32** © Fitness & Wellness, Inc.; **p. 33** © 2001 PhotoDisc, Inc.; **p. 35** (left) © Steve Raymer/CORBIS; **p. 35** (right) © Fitness & Wellness, Inc.; **p. 36** © Fitness & Wellness, Inc.; **p. 38** Chuck Scheer, Boise State University

Chapter 3
p. 47 © Dianne Collins/Photonica/Getty Images; **p. 48** © 2001 Photo Disc, Inc.; **p. 50** © Fitness & Wellness, Inc.; **p. 54** (left) © Fitness & Wellness, Inc.; **p. 54** (right) Jerry Hawkins; **p. 56** © Fitness & Wellness, Inc.; **p. 57** © Fitness & Wellness, Inc.

Chapter 4
p. 73 © A. J. James/Digital Vision/Getty Images; **p. 74** © Fitness & Wellness, Inc.; **p. 75** (left) © Fitness & Wellness, Inc.; **p. 75** (right) © 2001 PhotoDisc, Inc.; **p. 76** © Fitness & Wellness, Inc.; **p. 78** © Fitness & Wellness, Inc.; **p. 79** © © 2001 PhotoDisc, Inc.; **p. 81** © Fitness & Wellness, Inc.

Chapter 5
p. 87 © Jed Share/Photographer's Choice/Getty Images; **p. 89** © 2001 PhotoDisc, Inc.; **p. 90** © 2001 PhotoDisc, Inc.; **p. 91** © 2001 PhotoDisc, Inc.; **p. 92** © Fitness & Wellness, Inc.; **p. 94** © Fitness & Wellness, Inc.; **p. 140** © Fitness & Wellness, Inc.; **p. 141** © Fitness & Wellness, Inc.; **p. 146** © Fitness & Wellness, Inc.

Chapter 6
p. 105 © Ken Reid/Taxi/Getty Images; **p. 106** © Fitness & Wellness, Inc.; **p. 107** © Fitness & Wellness, Inc.; **p. 109** (left) © David Madison Sports Images; **p. 109** (right) © Fitness & Wellness, Inc.; **p. 111** Chuck Scheer, Boise State University; **p. 114** © Fitness & Wellness, Inc.; **p. 115** © Fitness & Wellness, Inc.; **p. 116** © Fitness & Wellness, Inc.; **p. 117** © Fitness & Wellness, Inc.; **p. 118** © Fitness & Wellness, Inc.

Chapter 7
p. 127 © Dennis O'Claire/Photographer's Choice/Getty Images; **p. 129** © Fitness & Wellness, Inc.; **p. 130** © Fitness & Wellness, Inc.; **p. 131** © Fitness & Wellness, Inc.; **p. 133** © Aero-belt Aerobics; **p. 136** © Nautilus Sports/Medical Industries, Inc.; **p. 137** Eric Risberg; **p. 138** © Fitness & Wellness, Inc.; **p. 141** © Doug Olmstead. Courtesy of United Spirit Association, Sunnyvale, CA; **p. 142** © Fitness & Wellness, Inc.; **p. 146** © Fitness & Wellness, Inc.; **p. 154** © Fitness & Wellness, Inc.; **p. 155** © Fitness & Wellness, Inc.; **p. 156** © Fitness & Wellness, Inc.; **p. 157** (top) © Fitness & Wellness, Inc.; **p. 157** (middle three) © Fitness & Wellness, Inc.; **p. 157** (bottom two) © Universal Gym Equipment, Inc.; **p. 158** (top) © Nautilus Sports/Medical Industries, Inc; **p. 158** (all others) © Universal Gym Equipment, Inc.; **p. 159** (top four) © Universal Gym Equipment, Inc.; (bottom two) © Nautilus Sports/Medical Industries, Inc.; **p. 160** (top two) © Universal Gym Equipment, Inc.; **p. 157** (all others) © Fitness & Wellness, Inc.; **p. 161** © Fitness & Wellness, Inc.; **p. 162** © Fitness & Wellness, Inc.; **p. 163** © Fitness & Wellness, Inc.; **p. 164** © Fitness & Wellness, Inc.

Chapter 8
p. 173 © Eric Glenn/DK Stock/Getty Images; **p. 174** (left) © Tony Freeman/PhotoEdit, (middle, right) © Matthew Farruggio; **p. 175** © 2001 PhotoDisc, Inc.; **p. 178** © Fitness & Wellness, Inc.; **p. 180** © Polara Studios, Inc.; **p. 181** © Thomas Harm and Tom Peterson/Quest Photographic, Inc.; **p. 185** © 2001 PhotoDisc, Inc.; **p. 194** (left) © 2001 PhotoDisc, Inc.; **p. 194** (right) © 2001 PhotoDisc, Inc.

Chapter 9
p. 209 © Andy Whale/Photonica/Getty Images; **p. 211** © Fitness & Wellness, Inc.; **p. 212** (left) © Fitness & Wellness, Inc.; **p. 212** (right) © Life Management, Inc.; **p. 213** © Fitness & Wellness, Inc.; **p. 220** © Fitness & Wellness, Inc.

Chapter 10
p. 229 © Lori Adamski Peek/Stone/Getty Images; **p. 231** © Fitness & Wellness, Inc.; **p. 232** © Fitness & Wellness, Inc.; **p. 236** © Topham/The Image Works; **p. 243** © Fitness & Wellness, Inc.; **p. 245** © Fitness & Wellness, Inc.; **p. 251** (center bottom) Eric Risberg; **p. 251** (all others) © Fitness & Wellness, Inc.

Chapter 11
p. 265 © Lori Adamski Peek/Stone/Getty Images; **p. 268** © Fitness & Wellness, Inc.; **p. 269** © Fitness & Wellness, Inc.; **p. 274** © Fitness & Wellness, Inc.; **p. 277** (top left) Chuck Scheer, Boise State University; (all others) © Fitness & Wellness, Inc.; **p. 278** © Fitness & Wellness, Inc.; **p. 280** © Fitness & Wellness, Inc.

Chapter 12
p. 287 © Kate Powers/Taxi/Getty Images; **p. 290** © Fitness & Wellness, Inc.; **p. 291** © Fitness & Wellness, Inc.; **p. 293** University of Colorado Health Sciences Center; **p. 297** University of Colorado Health Sciences Center; **p. 301** © Fitness & Wellness, Inc.; **p. 302** © Fitness & Wellness, Inc.

Chapter 13

p. 311 © David Trood/The Image Bank/Getty Images; p. 316 The American Cancer Society; p. 319 U.S. Department of Justice, Drug Enforcement Administration; p. 320 U.S. Department of Justice, Drug Enforcement Administration; p. 327 © 2001 PhotoDisc, Inc.

Chapter 14

p. 339 © Digital Vision/Getty Images; p. 343 © State of Colorado, Department of Health; p. 344 © 2001 PhotoDisc, Inc.; p. 345 State of Colorado, Department of Health

Appendixes

p. 357 © Bryan Peterson/Taxi/Getty Images

Glossary

A

Acquired immunodeficiency syndrome (AIDS) The final stage of HIV infection, characterized by opportunistic infections that are rare or harmless in people with normal immune function.

Adaptation energy stores Reserves of physical, mental, and emotional energy that give us the ability to cope with stress.

Addiction An abnormal or disordered relationship with an object, event, or behavior.

Adequate Intakes (AI) The average amount of a nutrient that appears to be sufficient to maintain a specific criteria; used as a guide for nutrient intake when an RDA cannot be determined.

Aerobic Refers to an activity that requires oxygen to produce the necessary energy (ATP) to carry out the activity.

Affirmations Positive statements that reinforce the positive aspects of personality and experience.

Air displacement Technique to assess body composition by calculating the body volume from the air displaced by an individual sitting inside a small chamber.

Alarm stage The first phase of the general adaptation syndrome, characterized by the release of stress hormones.

Altruism The act of giving of oneself out of a genuine concern for other people; unselfish devotion to the interests and welfare of others.

Amino acids Building blocks of protein ("amino" means "containing nitrogen").

Anaerobic Activity that does not require oxygen to produce the necessary energy (ATP) to carry out the activity.

Android obesity Obesity pattern in individuals who tend to store fat in the trunk or abdominal area.

Anger A feeling of extreme hostility, indignation, or exasperation; rage.

Anorexia nervosa An eating disorder characterized by self-imposed starvation to lose and maintain very low body weight.

Anthropometric measurement techniques Measurement of body girths at different sites.

Antibodies Substances produced by the white blood cells in response to an invading agent.

Antioxidants Compounds that protect other compounds from oxidation by being oxidized itself and damaging cells and body fluids.

Anxiety A state of intense worry that is not grounded in reality.

Aquaphobic Having a fear of water.

Atrophy Decrease in size of a cell, often stemming from non-use.

Autogenics A relaxation technique in which the person is trained, with the aid of specialized equipment, to relax all major muscle groups through a form of self-hypnosis, followed by imagery.

Autoimmune disorder A condition in which the immune system attacks the body.

Autoinoculation Spreading an infection to other parts of one's own body.

B

Ballistic stretching Exercises performed using jerky, rapid, and bouncy movements.

Basal metabolic rate (BMR) The lowest level of oxygen consumption necessary to sustain life.

Behavior modification A process to permanently change destructive or negative behaviors and replace them with positive behaviors.

Behavioral health The effects of lifestyle behaviors on health.

Benign Noncancerous.

Beta-carotene A vitamin A precursor made by plants; an orange pigment with antioxidant activity.

Binge drinking Imbibing at least five alcoholic beverages in one sitting for men, and four for women.

Binge-eating disorder An eating disorder characterized by uncontrollable episodes of eating excessive amounts of food within a relatively short time.

Bioelectrical impedance Technique to assess body composition by running a weak electrical current through the body.

Biofeedback A relaxation technique that involves measuring and controlling physiological functions.

Blood pressure A measure of the force exerted against the walls of blood vessels by the blood flowing through them.

Bod Pod Commercial name of the equipment used for assessing body composition through the air displacement technique.

Body composition The fat and non-fat components of the human body; important in assessing recommended body weight.

Body mass index (BMI) A technique to determine thinness and excessive fatness that incorporates height and weight to estimate critical fat values at which the risk for disease increases.

Bone integrity A component of physiologic fitness used to determine risk for osteoporosis based on bone mineral density.

Bulimia nervosa An eating disorder characterized by a pattern of binge eating and purging in an attempt to lose weight and maintain low body weight.

Burnout A state of physical and mental exhaustion in which few resources remain.

C

Calories Units used to measure energy; determined from the heat food releases when burned; calories reflect the extent to which a food's energy can be stored in body fat.

Cancer A group of more than a hundred diseases in which cells grow at an uncontrolled rate, mature in an abnormal way, and invade nearby tissues.

Cancer-prone personality Also called the Type C personality, an emotionally unexpressive person who demonstrates ambivalence and is at increased risk for cancer; sometimes called Type C personality.

Carbohydrates Nutrients composed of carbon, oxygen, and hydrogen atoms; carbohydrates provide about half of all energy needed by muscles and other tissues and is the preferred fuel for the brain and nervous system.

Carcinogens Cancer-causing substances.

Cardiac arrhythmias Irregular heart rhythms.

Cardiac output Amount of blood ejected by the heart in one minute.

Cardiorespiratory endurance The ability of the lungs, heart, and blood vessels to deliver adequate amounts of oxygen to the cells to meet the demands of prolonged physical activity.

Cardiovascular diseases The array of conditions that affect the heart and the blood vessels.

Cellulite A term frequently used in reference to fat deposits that bulge out; these deposits are nothing but enlarged fat cells from excessive accumulation of body fat.

Chancre A painless, red-rimmed sore that develops at the site where syphilis bacteria enter the body.

Chlamydia An STI caused by bacteria that infects the mucous membranes that line the genitals, rectum, anus, mouth, and eyes.

Cholesterol A waxy substance, technically a steroid alcohol, found only in animal fats and oil; used in making cell membranes, as a building block for some hormones, in the fatty sheath around nerve fibers, and in other necessary substances; necessary for synthesis of sex hormones, adrenal hormones, and vitamin D.

Chronic diseases Illnesses that linger over time and may get progressively worse.

Chylomicrons Triglyceride-transporting molecules in the blood.

Complete proteins Dietary proteins that contain all nine essential amino acids in the same relative amounts that humans require.

Complex carbohydrates Polysaccharides composed of straight or branched chains of monosaccharides.

Conflict The stress that results from two opposing and incompatible goals, demands, or needs.

Coronary heart disease (CHD) Condition in which the arteries that supply the heart muscle with oxygen and nutrients are narrowed by fatty deposits, such as cholesterol and triglycerides.

Coronary-prone personality A hard-driving, competitive person who is also hostile, angry, suspicious, and at increased risk for heart attack; also known as Type A personality.

Crack A particularly dangerous and addictive form of cocaine.

C-reactive protein (CRP) A protein whose blood levels increase with inflammation, at times hidden deep in the body; elevation of this protein is an indicator of potential cardiovascular events.

D

Daily Values (DV) Reference values of daily requirements developed by the Food and Drug Administration (FDA) specifically for use on food labels.

Diabetes mellitus A disease in which the body doesn't produce or utilize insulin properly.

Diastolic blood pressure Pressure exerted by the blood against the walls of the arteries during the relaxation phase (diastole) of the heart.

Dietary fiber Food substance that is not digested in the small intestine and provides the bulk needed to keep the digestive system running smoothly; found in vegetables, fruits, grains, and legumes.

Dietary Reference Intakes (DRI) A set of nutrient values for the dietary nutrient intakes of healthy people; includes Estimated Average Requirements, Recommended Dietary Allowances, Adequate Intakes, and Tolerable Upper Intake Levels.

Denial Refusal or inability to acknowledge that a problem exists.

Distress Negative stress, usually consisting of too much stress in a short time, chronic stress over a prolonged time, or a combination of stressors.

Dual energy X-ray absorptiometry (DEXA) Method to assess body composition that uses very low-dose beams of X-ray energy to measure total body fat mass, fat distribution pattern, and bone density.

Duration of exercise How long a person exercises.

Dynamic Strength-training method that uses muscle contractions with movement.

E

Emotional wellness The ability to understand your own feelings, accept your limitations, and achieve emotional stability.

Empty calories A food or beverage that provides calories but little or no nutrients.

Energy The capacity to do work or produce heat.

Energy-balancing equation A principle holding that as long as caloric input equals caloric output, the person will not gain or lose weight. If caloric intake exceeds output, the person gains weight; when output exceeds input, the person loses weight.

Environmental wellness The capability to live in a clean and safe environment that is not detrimental to health.

Essential amino acids Amino acids that the body cannot produce at all or produces in amounts insufficient to meet its needs; they must be provided by the diet.

Essential fat Minimal amount of body fat needed for normal physiological functions; constitutes about 3 percent of total weight in men and 12 percent in women.

Essential hypertension Persistent high blood pressure that has no known cause.

Estimated Average Requirement (EAR) The amount of a nutrient that will maintain a specific biochemical or physiological function in half of the population.

Estimated energy requirement (EER) The average dietary energy (caloric) intake that is predicted to maintain energy balance in a healthy adult of defined age, gender, weight, height, and level of physical activity, consistent with good health.

Eustress Positive, desirable stress.

Exercise Physical activity that requires planned, structured, and repetitive bodily movement done to improve or maintain one or more components of physical fitness.

Exercise ECG An exercise test during which workload is increased gradually (until the person reaches maximal fatigue) with blood pressure and 12-lead electrocardiographic monitoring throughout the test.

Exhaustion The final stage in the general adaptation syndrome, characterized by depletion of the body's resources and loss of adaptive abilities.

Explanatory style The way people perceive the events in their lives, from an optimistic or a pessimistic perspective.

External locus of control One's prevailing belief that the things that happen are unrelated to one's own behavior and are determined by outside forces.

F

Faith Belief and trust in God or something that can't be proved.

Family A unique cluster of people who enjoy a special relationship by reason of love, marriage, procreation, and mutual dependence.

Fat Lipids in food or in the body that provide the body with a continuous fuel supply, protect it from mechanical shock, and carry fat-soluble vitamins.

Fear A state of escalated worry and apprehension that causes distinct physical and emotional reactions.

Fetal alcohol syndrome A set of mental and physical characteristics in a newborn caused by moderate-to-heavy alcohol drinking during pregnancy.

Fighting spirit Determination; the open expression of emotions, whether negative or positive.

Fight-or-flight response A series of rapid-fire physical reactions to stress that provides maximum physical readiness to face threats in the environment.

Flexibility The achievable range of motion at a joint or group of joints without causing injury.

Forgiveness The ability to release from the mind all past hurts and failures, all sense of guilt and loss.

Free fatty acids (FFA) Fats formed by glycerol and three fatty acids. Also known as triglycerides.

Freebasing Smoking cocaine that has been separated from its hydrochloric salt by mixing it with a volatile chemical.

Frequency of exercise How often a person engages in an exercise session.

G

Gateway drugs Drugs (such as tobacco and alcohol) that were followed by use of other, more dangerous drugs.

General adaptation syndrome A three-stage attempt of the body to react and adapt to stressors that disrupt its normal balance.

Genital warts An STI caused by the human papilloma virus (HPV) and characterized by warts around the genitals or mouth.

Girth measurements Technique to assess body composition by measuring circumferences at specific body sites.

Glucose intolerance A condition characterized by slightly elevated blood glucose levels.

Glycemic index An index that is used to rate the plasma glucose response of carbohydrate-containing foods with the response produced by the same amount of carbohydrate from a standard source, usually glucose or white bread.

Glycogen A storage form of carbohydrate in the liver and muscle.

Gonorrhea An STI caused by bacteria that infects the cervix, rectum, urethra, or mouth.

Gynoid obesity Obesity pattern in people who store fat primarily around the hips and thighs.

H

Hardiness A set of personality traits marked by commitment, control, and challenge.

Hassles Seemingly minor, irritating, everyday annoyances that increase the level of stress.

HDL cholesterol Cholesterol-transporting molecules in the blood ("good cholesterol").

Health A state of complete well-being and not just the absence of disease or infirmity.

Health locus of control The extent to which people believe their behavior affects their health status.

Health-related fitness Fitness programs prescribed to improve the overall health of the individual.

Healthy life expectancy (HLE) Number of years a person is expected to live in good health; this number is obtained by subtracting ill-health years from overall life expectancy.

Hepatitis B A form of hepatitis spread through exposure to the contaminated blood or body fluids of an infected person; can cause long-term liver damage.

Herpes genitalis An infection caused by the herpes simplex-2 virus and characterized by blistering sores on the genitals.

Homeostasis A stable sense of physiological balance wherein all of the body's systems are functioning normally.

Homocysteine An amino acid that, when allowed to accumulate in the blood, may lead to plaque formation and blockage of arteries.

Hope Positive anticipation and expectation, characterized by optimism.

Hopelessness A mental state marked by negative expectations about the future; despairing.

Hostility An ongoing accumulation of anger and irritation; a permanent, deep-seated type of anger that hovers quietly until some trivial incident causes it to erupt.

Human immunodeficiency virus (HIV) The virus that weakens and destroys the immune system and gradually leads to AIDS.

Human papilloma virus (HPV) The virus that causes genital warts; some strains of the virus also have been linked to cervical cancer.

Hydrogenation A chemical process by which hydrogens are added to monounsaturated or polyunsaturated fats to reduce the number of double bonds and make the product more saturated (solid) and more resistant to spoilage.

Hydrostatic weighing Underwater technique to assess body composition; considered the most accurate of the body composition assessment techniques.

Hypertension Chronically elevated blood pressure.

Hypertrophy An increase in the size of the cell (for example, muscle hypertrophy).

Hypokinetic diseases Illnesses caused by lack of physical activity.

I

Imagery Vivid mental visualization.

Immunity The function that guards the body from invaders, both internal and external.

Incomplete proteins Dietary proteins that do not contain all the essential amino acids in sufficient quantities for human protein synthesis.

Insulin Hormone secreted by the pancreas; essential for proper metabolism of blood glucose (sugar) and maintenance of blood glucose level.

Insulin resistance Inability of the cells to respond appropriately to insulin.

Intensity of exercise In cardiorespiratory exercise, how hard a person has to exercise to improve or maintain fitness.

Internal locus of control One's prevailing belief that events are a consequence of one's own actions and, thus, potentially can be controlled.

Irradiation Sterilizing a food by exposure to energy waves; kills microorganisms and insects.

Isokinetic Strength-training method in which the speed of the muscle contraction is kept constant because the equipment (machine) provides an accommodating resistance to match the user's force through the range of motion.

Isometric Strength-training method that uses muscle contractions that produce little or no movement, such as pushing or pulling against immovable objects.

J

Jaundice Liver condition in which the skin and whites of the eyes appear yellow.

L

LDL cholesterol Cholesterol-transporting molecules in the blood ("bad cholesterol").

Lean body mass Body weight without body fat.

Life expectancy Number of years a person is expected to live based on the person's birth year.

Lifetime sports Activities that a person can do throughout the lifespan.

Loneliness A state of mind that occurs when a person's network of social relationships is significantly deficient in either quality or quantity.

Lymphocytes Specialized immune system cells.

M

Major minerals Essential mineral nutrients found in the human body in amounts larger than 5 grams; also called "macrominerals."

Malignant Cancerous.

Maximal exercise test Any test that requires the participant's all-out or nearly all-out effort.

Maximal heart rate (MHR) Highest heart rate for a person, primarily related to age.

Maximal oxygen uptake (VO$_{2max}$) The maximum amount of oxygen the body is able to utilize per minute of physical activity, commonly expressed in ml/kg/min; the best indicator of cardiorespiratory or aerobic fitness.

Meditation To sit quietly while focusing on breathing; a mental exercise to help gain control over thoughts.

Mental wellness A state in which your mind is engaged in lively interaction with the world around you.

Metabolic fitness A component of physiologic fitness that denotes reduction in the risk for diabetes and cardiovascular disease through a moderate-intensity exercise program in spite of little or no improvement in cardiorespiratory fitness.

Metabolic syndrome An array of metabolic abnormalities that contribute to development of atherosclerosis triggered by insulin resistance; these conditions include low HDL-cholesterol, high triglycerides, high blood pressure, and an increased blood clotting mechanism.

Metabolism All energy and material transformations that occur within living cells; necessary to sustain life.

Metastasis The process that occurs when cancer cells from one growth break off, enter the bloodstream or lymph system, and are carried to a distant part of the body, where they cause another cancerous growth to begin.

Minerals Inorganic elements that the body needs to provide specific body functions.

Mode of exercise Form of exercise.

Moderate-intensity physical activity Physical activity that uses 150 calories of energy per day or 1,000 calories per week.

Monounsaturated fats Fatty acids that lack two hydrogen atoms and have one double bond between carbons; found in olive oil, canola oil, and peanut oil.

Morphologic fitness A component of physiologic fitness used in reference to body composition (fat) factors such as percent body fat, body fat distribution, and body circumference.

Motivation The desire and will to do something.

Muscular endurance The ability of a muscle to exert submaximal force repeatedly over a period of time.

Muscular strength The ability to exert maximum force against resistance.

N

Nicotine A poisonous, addictive component of tobacco, inhaled by smokers or absorbed through the lining of the mouth by people who use smokeless tobacco.

Nonresponders Individuals who exhibit small or no improvements in fitness as compared to others who undergo the same training program.

Nutrients Substances obtained from food and used in the body to promote growth, maintenance, and repair. The essential nutrients are those the body cannot make for itself in sufficient quantity to meet physiological needs and, therefore, must be obtained from food.

Nutrition The science of foods, the nutrients and other substances they contain, and their actions within the body.

O

Obesity An excessive accumulation of body fat, usually at least 30 percent above recommended body weight; a body mass index (BMI) of 30 or higher.

Occupational wellness The ability to perform your job skillfully and effectively under conditions that provide personal and team satisfaction and adequately reward each individual.

Oncogenes Pieces of genetic material that serve as markers to predict later mutation and development of certain cancers, probably by encouraging mutation of related cells.

One repetition maximum (1 RM) The maximal amount of resistance (weight) that an individual is able to lift in a single effort.

Open-circuit indirect calorimetry (direct gas analysis) The most precise way to determine VO$_{2max}$, using a metabolic cart to measure the amount of oxygen consumed by the body.

Optimism A tendency to expect the best possible outcome.

Overweight An excess amount of weight against a given standard, such as recommended percent body fat; a body mass index (BMI) greater than 25 but less than 30.

Oxygen free radicals Substances formed during metabolism that attack and damage proteins and lipids, in particular the cell membrane and DNA, leading to conditions such as heart disease, cancer, and emphysema.

P

Pedometer An electronic device that senses body motion and counts footsteps; some pedometers also record distance, calories burned, speeds, "aerobic steps," and time spent being physically active.

Pelvic inflammatory disease (PID) A severe infection of the lining of the abdominal cavity in women, usually caused by bacterial STIs.

Percent body fat Proportional amount of fat in the body based on the person's total weight; includes both essential fat and storage fat; also termed fat mass.

Perfectionism The compulsive pursuit of unrealistically high standards.

Personality The whole of a person's behavioral characteristics.

Pessimism A tendency to view life situations with negativity and gloom.

Physical activity Bodily movement produced by skeletal muscles that requires energy expenditure and produces progressive health benefits.

Physical fitness The ability to meet the ordinary as well as the unusual demands of daily life safely and effectively without being overly fatigued and still have energy left for leisure and recreational activities.

Physical wellness Flexibility, endurance, strength, and optimism about your ability to take care of health problems.

Physiologic fitness A form of skill-related fitness used with reference to biological systems that are affected by physical activity and the role of activity in preventing disease.

Physiological addiction A change in the body's biochemistry so that the substance is required for functioning.

Polyunsaturated fats Fatty acids that lack four hydrogen atoms and have two or more double bonds between carbons; found in safflower, sunflower, corn, soybean, and cottonseed oils.

Precancerous Describes any of the conditions in which a benign (noncancerous) condition has the potential to become cancerous.

Principle of individuality Training concept stating that genetics plays a major role in individual responses to exercise training and that these differences must be considered when designing exercise programs for different people.

Prodrome The stage of infection when early symptoms erupt; in the case of herpes, a sensation in which the skin starts to itch or tingle; precedes onset of the blisters and sores.

Progressive overload principle Training concept stating that the demands placed on a system (for example, cardiorespiratory or muscular) must be increased systematically and progressively over time to cause physiological adaptation (development or improvement).

Progressive relaxation A method of reducing stress that consists of tensing, then relaxing, small muscle groups.

Progressive resistance training A gradual increase in resistance lifted over a period of time when training with weights.

Proprioceptive neuromuscular facilitation (PNF) Stretching technique in which muscles are stretched out progressively with intermittent isometric contractions.

Protein A nutrient composed of amino acids necessary for growth or tissue repair; protein also functions as enzymes, hormones, regulators of fluid and electrolyte balance, acid-base regulators, transporters, and antibodies.

Psychological addiction A strong craving for a substance or behavior.

Psychoneuroimmunology (PNI) The scientific investigation of how the brain affects the body's immune cells and how the immune system can be affected by behavior.

Pubic lice Commonly called "crabs," tiny parasites that feed on the small blood vessels of the skin beneath the pubic hair.

R

Random acts of kindness To engage in behavior that helps another person.

Rate of perceived exertion (RPE) A perception scale to monitor or interpret the intensity of aerobic exercise.

Recommended body weight Body weight at which there seems to be no harm to human health; healthy weight.

Recommended Dietary Allowances (RDA) The average daily amount of a nutrient considered adequate to meet the known nutrient needs of most healthy people—a goal for dietary intakes by individuals.

Recovery stage The return to homeostasis after a stressful event.

Reframing Changing the way you look at things.

Relapse To slip or fall back into unhealthy behavior(s) or fail to maintain healthy behaviors.

Relaxation response The body's ability to enter a scientifically defined state of relaxation.

Religion The system of how to know God, accompanied by rituals and places of worship.

Resistance Amount of weight lifted in strength training.

Resistance stage The second phase of the general adaptation syndrome, characterized by meeting the perceived challenge.

Responders Individuals who exhibit improvements in fitness as a result of exercise training.

Resting heart rate Heart rate after a person has been sitting quietly for 15–20 minutes.

Resting metabolic rate (RMR) The energy requirement to maintain the body's vital processes in the resting state.

Resting metabolism The amount of energy (expressed in milliliters of oxygen per minute or in total calories per day) an individual requires during resting conditions to sustain proper body function.

Retroviruses Viruses that invade a cell's genetic structure and are passed on to each succeeding generation of cells as the cells divide.

Reverse cholesterol transport A process in which HDL molecules attract cholesterol and carry it to the liver, where it is changed to bile and eventually excreted in the stool.

S

Saturated fats Fats carrying the maximum possible numbers of hydrogen atoms; usually found in animal products such as butter and lard.

Scabies Tiny mites that burrow under the skin; may be spread by sexual or nonsexual contact.

Secondhand smoke A mixture of smoke exhaled by smokers and smoke from the burning portion of a cigarette, pipe, or cigar.

Self-esteem A sense of positive self-regard and self-respect.

Set Number of repetitions in strength training (e.g., one set of 12 repetitions).

Setpoint Weight control theory holding that the body has an established weight and strongly attempts to maintain that weight.

Sexually transmitted disease (STD) A disease that is passed from one person to another through sexual contact.

Sexually transmitted infection (STI) An infection that is passed from one person to another through sexual contact.

Simple carbohydrates Sugars in the form of fruits and milk or honey, sucrose, corn syrup, and fructose.

Skill-related fitness Fitness components important for success in skillful activities and athletic events.

Skinfold thickness Technique to assess body composition by measuring a double thickness of skin at specific body sites.

Slow-sustained stretching Technique whereby the muscles are lengthened gradually through a joint's complete range of motion and the final position is held for a few seconds.

Social network The size, density, durability, intensity, and frequency of social contacts.

Social support The human resources that people provide to each other.

Social wellness The ability to relate well to others, both within and outside the family unit.

Specificity of training Targeting the specific body system or area the person is attempting to improve (aerobic endurance, anaerobic capacity, strength, flexibility).

Sphygmomanometer An inflatable bladder contained within a cuff and a mercury gravity manometer (or an aneroid manometer) from which the blood pressure is read.

Spiritual health Dimension of health related to a person's moral or religious nature; a relationship with a Higher Being.

Spiritual wellness The sense that life is meaningful, that life has purpose, and that some power brings all humanity together; the ethics, values, and morals that guide us and give meaning and direction to life.

Spirituality A belief in and a person's relationship with a Higher Being.

Spontaneous remission Inexplicable recovery from incurable illness.

Spot reducing Fallacious theory holding that exercising a specific body part will result in significant fat reduction in that area.

Storage fat Body fat in excess of essential fat; stored in adipose tissue.

Stress An automatic biological response to stressors, or demands made on an individual; the result of any event or condition that requires adaptation.

Stressor Any situation or demand that requires adaptation.

Subcutaneous fat Fat deposits directly under the skin.

Subluxation Partial dislocation of a joint.

Suppressor genes Pieces of genetic material that are part of a cell's normal protective mechanism against development of cancer.

Synergistic effect A phenomenon in which the effects of using more than one drug simultaneously are different and greater than using any of the drugs alone.

Syphilis An STI caused by bacteria, occurring in four stages; untreated, it is fatal.

Systolic blood pressure Pressure exerted by the blood against the walls of the arteries during the forceful contraction (systole) of the heart.

T

THC (delta-9-tetrahydrocannabinol) The psychoactive ingredient in marijuana.

Tolerable Upper Intake Level (TUIL) The maximum amount of a nutrient that seems to be safe for most healthy people and beyond which there is an increased risk of adverse effects.

Toxic core Type A personality traits most detrimental to health: anger, cynicism, suspiciousness, and excessive self-involvement.

Trace minerals Essential mineral nutrients found in the human body in amounts less than 5 grams; also called "microminerals."

Transtheoretical model Behavioral modification model proposing that change is accomplished through a series of progressive stages in keeping with a person's readiness to change.

Triglycerides Fats formed by glycerol and three fatty acids. Also known as "free fatty acids."

Type 1 diabetes Insulin-dependent diabetes mellitus (IDDM), a condition in which the pancreas produces little or no insulin; also known as juvenile diabetes because it is seen primarily in young people.

Type 2 diabetes Non-insulin-dependent diabetes mellitus (NIDDM), a condition in which insulin is not processed properly; also known as adult-onset diabetes.

Type A personality Sometimes referred to as "hurry sickness," a person who is hard-driving and competitive and also hostile, angry, and suspicious; also known as coronary-prone behavior.

Type B personality Known as the relaxed personality, a person who is easy-going and generally free of hostility, anger, and suspicion.

Type C personality Also called the cancer-prone personality, an emotionally unexpressive person who demonstrates ambivalence and is at increased risk for cancer.

Type D personality A distressed personality characterized by negative emotions, social inhibition, and isolation.

U

Underweight Extremely low body weight.

USDA Food Guide A food group plan that assigns foods to major food groups; developed by U.S. Department of Agriculture.

V

Vegetarians People who omit meat, fish, and poultry from their diet.

Very low-calorie diet A diet that allows an energy intake (consumption) of 800 calories or less per day.

Vigorous activity Any activity that requires a MET level equal to or greater than 6 METs (21 ml/kg/min).

Vitamins Organic, essential nutrients required in small amounts to perform specific functions that promote growth, maintenance, or repair.

W

Waist circumference (WC) A waist girth measurement to assess potential risk for disease based on intra-abdominal fat content.

Warm-up Starting a workout slowly.

Weight-regulating mechanism (WRM) A feature of the hypothalamus of the brain that controls how much the body should weigh.

Wellness Full integration of physical, mental, emotional, social, environmental, occupational, and spiritual well-being into a quality life.

Worry A state in which we dwell on something so much that we become apprehensive.

Y

Yoga An exercise technique involving stretching, used to relieve stress and induce calm.

Yo-yo dieting Constantly losing and gaining weight.

Index